Forthcoming Monographs

THE RADIOLOGY OF VERTEBRAL TRAUMA

John A. Gehweiler, Jr., M.D., Raymond L. Osborne, Jr., M.D., and R. Frederick Becker, Ph.D.

ARTHROGRAPHY: PRINCIPLES AND TECHNIQUES

Tom W. Staple, M.D.

CLINICAL PEDIATRIC AND ADOLESCENT UROGRAPHY

Alfred L. Weber, M.D., and Richard C. Pfister, M.D.

RADIOLOGY OF THE GALLBLADDER AND BILE DUCTS

Robert N. Berk, M.D., and Arthur R. Clemett, M.D.

RADIOLOGY OF THE LIVER

James McNulty, M.B., F.F.R.

PEDIATRIC ORTHOPAEDIC RADIOLOGY

M. B. Ozonoff, M.D.

XEROMAMMOGRAPHIC PATHOLOGY

Michael D. Lagios, M.D., H. Joachim Burhenne, M.D., and F. Margolin, M.D.

E. JAMES POTCHEN, M.D., *Consulting Editor*
Professor and Chairman
Department of Radiology
Michigan State University
East Lansing, Michigan

Published

GASTROINTESTINAL ANGIOGRAPHY
Stewart R. Reuter, M.D., and Helen C. Redman, M.D.

THE RADIOLOGY OF JOINT DISEASE
D. M. Forrester, M.D., and John W. Nesson, M.D.

THE HAND IN RADIOLOGIC DIAGNOSIS
Andrew K. Poznanski, M.D.

RADIOLOGY OF THE ILEOCECAL AREA
Robert N. Berk, M.D., and Elliott C. Lasser, M.D.

FUNDAMENTALS OF ABDOMINAL AND PELVIC ULTRASONOGRAPHY
George R. Leopold, M.D., and W. Michael Asher, M.D. & Cdr., MC USN.

RADIOLOGY OF THE ORBIT
G. A. S. Lloyd, B.M., B.Ch. Oxf., F.F.R., D.M.R.D.

SPECIAL PROCEDURES IN CHEST RADIOLOGY
Stuart S. Sagel, M.D.

RADIOLOGY OF RENAL FAILURE
Harry J. Griffiths, M.D.

RADIOLOGY OF THE ALIMENTARY TRACT IN INFANTS AND CHILDREN
Edward B. Singleton, M.D., Milton L. Wagner, M.D., and Robert V. Dutton, M.D.

RADIOLOGIC DIAGNOSIS OF RENAL PARENCHYMAL DISEASE
Alan J. Davidson, M.D.

Volume 3 in the Series
SAUNDERS MONOGRAPHS IN CLINICAL RADIOLOGY

RADIOLOGY OF THE PANCREAS AND DUODENUM

S. BOYD EATON, JR., M.D.

Clinical Assistant Professor of Radiology,
Emory University School of Medicine;
Radiologist, West Paces Ferry Hospital and St. Joseph's Infirmary,
Atlanta, Georgia

JOSEPH T. FERRUCCI, JR., M.D.

Associate Radiologist,
Massachusetts General Hospital;
Assistant Professor of Radiology,
Harvard Medical School,
Boston, Massachusetts

Anatomical drawings by Paul G. Andriesse

W. B. SAUNDERS COMPANY • Philadelphia • London • Toronto

W. B. Saunders Company: West Washington Square
Philadelphia, PA 19105

1 St. Anne's Road
Eastbourne, East Sussex BN21 3UN, England

1 Goldthorne Avenue
Toronto, Ontario M8Z 5T9, Canada

Radiology of the Pancreas and Duodenum ISBN 0-7216-3310-2

Print No.: 9 8 7 6 5 4 3

To
Daphne and Brenda

CONTRIBUTORS

CRISTOS ATHANASOULIS, M.D. Assistant Professor of Radiology, Harvard Medical School; Assistant Radiologist, Massachusetts General Hospital, Boston, Massachusetts

STANLEY BAUM, M.D. Radiologist, Massachusetts General Hospital; Professor of Radiology, Harvard Medical School, Boston, Massachusetts

S. BOYD EATON, JR., M.D. Clinical Assistant Professor of Radiology, Emory University School of Medicine; Radiologist, West Paces Ferry Hospital and St. Joseph's Infirmary, Atlanta, Georgia

JOSEPH T. FERRUCCI, JR., M.D. Assistant Professor of Radiology, Harvard Medical School; Associate Radiologist, Massachusetts General Hospital, Boston, Massachusetts

PAUL C. KAHN, M.D. Director of Nuclear Medicine and Ultrasound, New England Center Hospital, Boston, Massachusetts; Professor of Radiology, Tufts University School of Medicine, Boston, Massachusetts

MAJIC S. POTSAID, M.D. Associate Professor of Radiology, Harvard Medical School; Associate Radiologist, Massachusetts General Hospital, Boston, Massachusetts

WELLAND F. SHORT, M.D. Associate Professor of Clinical Radiology, University of Pittsburgh, Pittsburgh, Pennsylvania

EDITOR'S FOREWORD

This third volume in Saunders Monographs in Clinical Radiology is designed to clarify the clinical utility, opportunities, and frustrations in the various radiologic evaluations of the pancreas and duodenum. As Dr. Margulis states in his Introduction, well-organized, honest, and up-to-date appreciation of the role of diagnostic radiology in this difficult diagnostic area may well serve not only to teach the current status but also to stimulate and clarify future research efforts.

While still a Harvard medical student, Dr. Eaton demonstrated outstanding capabilities in diagnostic radiology. In residency at the Massachusetts General Hospital, he and his colleague Dr. Ferrucci were attracted by the more difficult and complex arenas of gastrointestinal diagnosis. Dr. Ferrucci has remained at the Massachusetts General Hospital, where he continues his work in the Gastrointestinal Section. Dr. Eaton has moved on to Atlanta, Georgia and Emory University. Both men have helped to broaden the application of radiologic tools to the assessment of duodenal and pancreatic pathology.

The quality of this book is consistent with the aura of excellence established by the first two volumes of Saunders Monographs in Clinical Radiology. By providing a useful and stimulating learning experience, it fulfills the major goal of the series.

E. JAMES POTCHEN, M.D.

PREFACE

For decades the pancreas has been considered a hidden organ. Internists, surgeons and radiologists have so often been frustrated by the difficulties of diagnosis in this region that the gland has taken on an aura of almost mysterious fascination. During the past few years, however, major advances in pancreatic radiology have produced a significant change: the theme of this monograph is that nearly all pancreatic disease can now be demonstrated radiologically by the time that clinical manifestations become apparent. True "early diagnosis" (that is, identification of disease before the development of related symptoms) remains a rarity, but the chief problems related to this organ must now be considered those of improving treatment rather than diagnosis—a change of emphasis about which radiologists can be justifiably proud. It is timely that radiologic diagnosis of pancreatic disease has achieved respectable accuracy. The rapidly increasing frequency of pancreatic carcinoma has been the subject of numerous recent articles and editorials. This malignancy is currently the fourth commonest cause of cancer death in men, and its incidence now exceeds that of gastric cancer.

One of the roentgen methods developed chiefly for detection of pancreatic disease—hypotonic duodenography—has had the important side effect of greatly improving radiographic demonstration of primary duodenal disease. This technique has advanced the accuracy of duodenal roentgenology far beyond its traditional limits.

This monograph attempts to present the entire scope of current radiologic knowledge pertinent to diagnosis of pancreatic and duodenal disease. In order to even approach this goal, the publishers have allowed us to employ a dual-level organizational format. Most chapters are primarily concerned with the radiologic findings which can be produced by pancreatic disease. The emphasis of such chapters is on the techniques necessary for demonstrating these signs, the mechanisms responsible for their development, the radiologic criteria for establishing their presence, and the differential considerations important for their diagnostic application. Other chapters are more clinically oriented. They stress the clinical features with which radiologic findings must be correlated and develop a strategy for appropriate employment of radiologic techniques in specific clinical circumstances.

Organization of a book along these lines necessitates a certain degree of "planned redundancy." Material covered in one section is frequently presented again, in a different context, in another chapter. This approach fits well with our belief that almost no one reads a reference text from cover to cover as he might a novel. Rather, such monographs are consulted for specific problems as they arise. This book is designed to provide reasonably complete answers within any given chapter without need for searching back and forth throughout the book to locate essential information. An extensive bibliography is provided at the end of each chapter for those readers who wish to explore individual points more exhaustively. The dual-level format also accommodates our observation that radiologists tend to encounter two main types of professional problems. A perplexing roentgen finding may be noted on a given examination. In these circumstances, further information concerning the significance, reliability and necessary differential related to this particular observation may be desirable. Alternatively, the specific clinical details of an individual patient's case may be presented by a clinician requesting radiologic consultation about the most appropriate examination to be ordered and its likelihood of success. The dual-level organization we have employed has been chosen so that readers can approach the book from either of these "radiologic" or "clinical" points of view and obtain reasonably complete information within a single section or chapter.

S. BOYD EATON, JR., M.D.
JOSEPH T. FERRUCCI, JR., M.D.

ACKNOWLEDGMENTS

It has been possible to create this monograph only because a very large number of radiologists and other physicians have generously allowed us to reproduce roentgenograms, scintigraphic images and echograms which are particularly appropriate for demonstrating important principles of pancreatic and duodenal radiology. The following list of these benefactors fails utterly to convey our sense of gratitude and indebtedness; without the material given us by these colleagues, we would have been unable to assemble anything like the collection of illustrations which highlights this text.

Herbert L. Abrams, M.D.
John R. Amberg, M.D.
Karl T. Benedict, M.D.
Walter Berdon, M.D.
Marcia K. Bilbao, M.D.
Stanley Bohrer, M.D.
Joseph J. Bookstein, M.D.
John Bryan, M.D.
H. Joachim Burhenne, M.D.
James L. Clements, M.D.
R. Dale Cooper, M.D.
Jack R. Dreyfuss, M.D.
James J. DuBois, M.D.
Alice Ettinger, M.D.
Donald J. Fleischli, M.D.
Atis K. Freimanis, M.D.
Morton G. Glickman, M.D.
Henry I. Goldberg, M.D.
Joseph Hanelin, M.D.
E. Ralph Heinz, M.D.
Malcolm C. Hill, M.D.
James Hoffman, M.D.
John M. Howard, M.D.
W. Breck Howard, M.D.
A. Everette James, M.D.
Roberto B. Jimenez, M.D.
Norman Joffe, M.D.
Mansho T. Khilnani, M.D.
Myo M. Kyaw, M.D.
Ted F. Leigh, M.D.
George R. Leopold, M.D.
Ann Lewicki, M.D.
Lincoln Lum, M.D.
Robert C. McEligot, M.D.
William C. McGarity, M.D.
Joseph A. Marasco, M.D.
Alexander R. Margulis, M.D.
Luis F. Mattoso, M.D.
Robert D. Milledge, M.D.
Hideyo Minagi, M.D.
James G. Moore, M.D.
George L. Nardi, M.D.
Robert A. Nebesar, M.D.
Harry Newman, M.D.
Robert E. Paul, M.D.
Kent D. Pearson, M.D.
James Petersen, M.D.
James J. Pollard, M.D.
Maurice M. Reeder, M.D.
Stewart R. Reuter, M.D.
Laurence L. Robbins, M.D.
Josef Rosch, M.D.
Robert C. Seidler, M.D.
Thomas E. Shea, M.D.
Douglas J. Sheft, M.D.
Parry D. Soder, M.D.
Peter Sones, M.D.
Arch W. Templeton, M.D.
H. Stephen Weens, M.D.
A. Justin Williams, M.D.
Justin L. Williams, M.D.
Jack Wittenberg, M.D.
Stanley M. Wyman, M.D.

A listing of this sort almost certainly has to be incomplete; to any individuals who have been inadvertently omitted, we tender our apologies and our sincere thanks.

Paul Andriesse and Stan Bennett of the medical art and medical photography departments at the Massachusetts General Hospital have our admiration for their professional skills and our lasting gratitude for coming to our aid when such help often meant major additions to their already overburdened workloads.

Jack Hanley, Daphne Moo-Young and Herb Powell of the W. B. Saunders Company have given us invaluable technical advice and assistance. They have become our friends during the course of this project.

Our secretaries: Diane McMahon, Linda Vinceguerra, Roselynn Wall and Lillyan Spark have worked ably and indefatigably. Anyone who has written a book knows that such individuals are indispensable and that they cannot be adequately thanked.

Finally, we would like to thank our children who have often been neglected due to the demands of this project, our parents who have meant more to us than is currently fashionable to acknowledge, and our wives, Daphne and Brenda, who have unceasingly given us encouragement, support, patience and inspiration.

S.B.E.
J.T.F.

CONTENTS

INTRODUCTION

The pancreas, the diagnostically silent area, has excited radiologists almost since the beginning of diagnostic radiology. Diagnostic signs have been indirect for many many years and frustrations multiplied with every new approach. Even the terminology became confused. Radiologists have been publishing papers describing early signs of pancreatic disease, in which the emphasis was on minimal signs but not necessarily on reliable signs of early disease. As a matter of fact, the disease usually must be in its advanced stage for minimal signs to be present. This led to repeated disappointments, as sober and critical evaluation followed the enthusiastic claims which introduced each new procedure. This course of events was true for upper gastrointestinal examinations with cineradiography, hypotonic duodenography, arteriography (selective and superselective with multiple vessel injections), percutaneous transhepatic cholangiography, pancreatography, selenium methionine scanning, ultrasonography, and so forth.

This book by Dr. Eaton and Dr. Ferrucci is a well-organized, honest and up-to-date rendition of total radiologic knowledge of the pancreas and duodenum. It describes the current approaches in a critical, erudite manner, as well as the reasons for their success and the causes of their failures.

Especially valuable is the way in which the book deals with disease and diagnostic problems as a starting point for developing a radiologic strategy—a strategy for selecting those radiologic procedures that have the greatest likelihood of giving a diagnostic answer for a particular patient. I found, in this respect, that Chapter 5, "The Radiology of Jaundice," and Chapter 12, "Tailored Radiologic Evaluation of Suspected Pancreaticoduodenal Disease," were highly commendable. It is refreshing to have such a scholarly book with so much condensed experience and information written by two young gastrointestinal radiologists. One can only hope that they will continue to produce such admirable work.

ALEXANDER R. MARGULIS, M.D.

Chapter 1

ANATOMIC CONSIDERATIONS

Over the years, radiology of the pancreas has really meant radiology of the abdominal viscera adjacent to the pancreas. Until recently, it has been impossible to demonstrate directly the pancreas itself by radiographic study and, accordingly, secondary effects, produced by pathologic involvement of contiguous structures, have constituted the evidence used for radiologic diagnosis. Because of this, the anatomic relationships of the pancreas have assumed great significance for radiologists. They have been carefully studied, and a considerable body of experience, bearing on radiologically demonstrable pathologic interactions between the pancreas and its neighbors, has been amassed.

The duodenum occupies a central position within the abdomen and serves as a readily accessible indicator of a pathologic condition involving adjacent portions of many abdominal viscera. Because of the duodenum's intimate relation to the pancreas, radiologic study of it has been particularly valuable for identification of pancreatic disease, but abnormalities of many other organs can also produce duodenal manifestations.

It is the purpose of this chapter to describe the anatomic relations of the pancreas and duodenum and to discuss the significance of these relationships in the production of radiologic signs important for diagnosis of disease involving this region.

GROSS ANATOMIC INTERRELATIONSHIPS

Pancreaticoduodenal Interrelationships

The value of barium duodenal examination as a diagnostic procedure for pancreatic disease depends entirely upon the intimate anatomic relationship between the duodenum and the pancreas. Radiologic abnormalities in any portion of the duodenum may reflect the effects of an underlying pathologic condition involving the pancreas (Fig. 1–1).

The duodenal bulb lies above and anterior to the upper portion of the head of the pancreas. The descending duodenum lies lateral and slightly posterior

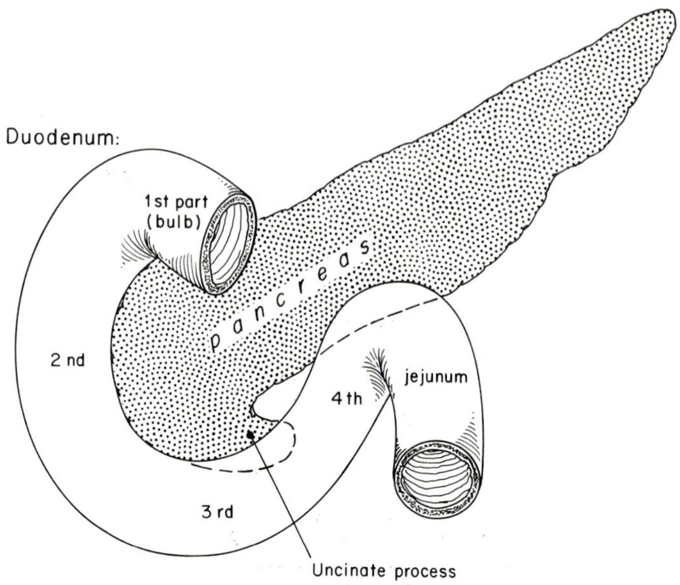

Figure 1–1. Gross relationships between the pancreas and the duodenum.

to the right margin of the head of the pancreas, while the third (horizontal) portion of the duodenum passes below and slightly posterior to the inferior margin of the head of the pancreas. The ascending (fourth) portion of the duodenum lies to the left and somewhat anterior to the uncinate process, and the duodenojejunal flexure (at the ligament of Treitz) lies below the body of the pancreas.

Whether or not a pathologic process arising in the pancreas will produce an effect upon the duodenum depends chiefly upon whether the process comes in contact with the pancreaticoduodenal interface. Distention of the duodenum (as during hypotonic duodenography) tends to increase the area of the pancreaticoduodenal interface and improve chances for radiologic demonstration of pancreatic disease. Acute pancreatitis, which generally involves the whole organ, produces at least some radiologically identifiable duodenal abnormality in 92 per cent of the patients studied by barium examination (Bergkvist, 1959). Chronic pancreatitis has been reported to produce duodenal changes in 80 per cent—an almost equally high percentage (Rubinstein, 1971).

In contrast with inflammatory processes, pancreatic malignancies usually involve only a portion of the pancreas, and whether or not the duodenal loop is affected depends more on the location of the lesion than on its size alone (Russell, 1965). For example, ampullary neoplasms produce abnormalities demonstrable by hypotonic duodenography in 92 per cent of the patients in whom they occur (Jacquemet, 1965). Since the head of the pancreas is most closely related to the duodenal loop, lesions in this region have a somewhat better chance of producing abnormalities than do those in the body or tail. In 82 to 84 per cent of the patients, tumors arising in the head of the pancreas can be detected by hypotonic duodenography (Eaton, 1968; Bilbao, 1968). The body and tail of the pancreas are less intimately associated with the duodenum than is the head, but this consideration is somewhat offset by the fact that malignancies arising in this area are usually further advanced than are head lesions by the time the patient reports symptoms. Accordingly, the incidence of duodenal abnormalities is only slightly less. Mani (1966) found distal duodenal roentgen manifestations in 61 per cent of his 46 patients with tumors arising in the body or tail.

Extrahepatic Biliary Tree

The posteroinferior surface of the body of the *gallbladder* usually lies against the anterolateral aspect of the upper descending duodenum (Fig. 1–2). The posteroinferior aspect of the neck of the gallbladder is adjacent to the anterosuperior surface of the apex of the duodenal bulb. The *cystic duct* is quite variable in course and configuration; it passes over the superior surface of the duodenal bulb and may or may not come in contact with that structure. Where the cystic duct joins the common hepatic duct, the *common bile duct* is formed. The common bile duct passes inferiorly in the free border of the hepatoduodenal ligament in company with the portal vein and hepatic artery. It then runs behind the duodenal bulb (usually the apical portion) before becoming embedded in a somewhat vertical groove or channel on the dorsal surface of the head of the pancreas. Its course is directed obliquely toward the posteromedial wall of the second portion of the duodenum. In its lower extent (Fig. 1–3), it often becomes intimately related to the wall of the duodenum, running directly alongside it without intervening pancreatic tissue for 1 or 2 cm. before actually piercing it (Kune, 1964). The external diameter of the common bile duct is fairly constant, averaging 8 or 9 mm in width. The internal diameter is also fairly constant, averaging 7 or 8 mm in width, down to a point just before the duct pierces the duodenal wall. At this level, the internal caliber ordinarily narrows to an average value of about 4 mm.

The site of the *duodenal papilla* is variable. In about 75 per cent of the patients, it is located on the posteromedial aspect of the descending duodenum usually in its mid or lower portion; in about 18 per cent, it is located near the inferior duodenal flexure and, in most of the remaining patients, it is situated on the superior aspect of the third (horizontal) portion of the duodenum (Schwartz, 1962). The papilla rarely may be in the proximal duodenum or even in the gastric antrum (Hess, 1965).

On specimen radiographs, Poppel (1953) demonstrated that the normal duodenal papilla may be as large as 3 cm. in greatest diameter. More recently, however, evidence has been presented that, on routine barium studies in living

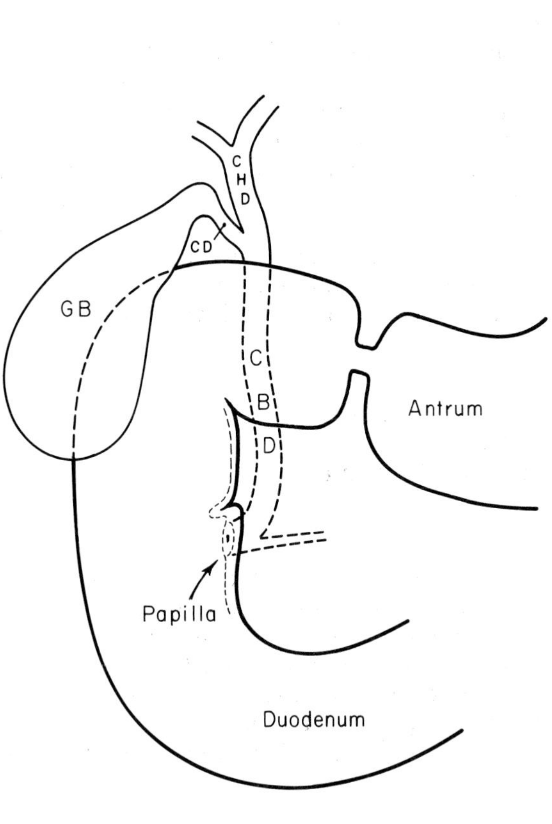

Figure 1–2. Gross relationships between the biliary tree and the duodenum.

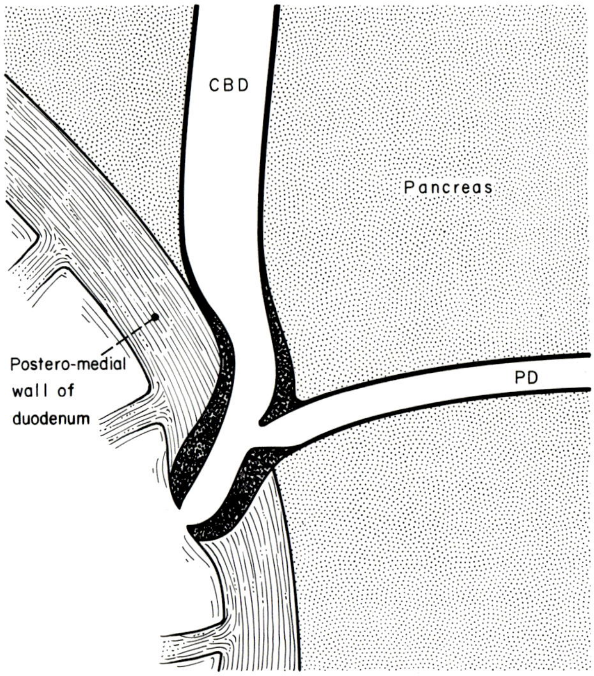

Figure 1–3. Gross relationships between the distal common bile duct and the duodenal wall. (Modified from Kune, G. A.: Surgical anatomy of the common bile duct. Arch. Surg., 89:995–1004, 1964.)

patients, only about 1 per cent of the papillae exceed 1.5 cm. in greatest dimension (Eaton, 1972).

Pathologic abnormalities of the extrahepatic biliary tree can be demonstrated by a number of radiologic techniques. Oral, intravenous, and percutaneous cholangiography are most direct, but angiography, barium studies, and ultrasonography are also occasionally applicable to the investigation of these structures. A detailed review of extrahepatic biliary tract radiology is found in Chapter 5.

Relations of the Pancreas and Duodenum to Other Abdominal Viscera

Veins

The pancreas is situated immediately adjacent to a number of important portal and systemic venous channels (Fig. 1–4). Both neoplastic and inflammatory pathologic conditions arising in the pancreas frequently produce distortion and/or obstruction of these veins. Such changes can be demonstrated directly by angiography (see Chapter 7), and various sequelae (e.g., collateral varices, splenomegaly, and so forth) arising from such involvement can be shown by other radiologic techniques. In general, when any of these venous structures is shown unequivocally to be involved by pancreatic malignancy, total surgical extirpation of the tumor will be impossible and, therefore, any surgery contemplated should be for palliation (Sato, 1967).

As it ascends, the *inferior vena cava* passes behind the third portion of the duodenum and the head of the pancreas. Since it lies in direct contiguity to the posterior surface of the head of the pancreas, tumors arising within it and growing dorsally may distort it; most commonly, the anterior and left caval walls are affected (Filler, 1962). The *left renal vein* runs behind the head, uncinate process, and body of the pancreas while the *right renal vein,* shorter than the left, passes behind the upper descending duodenum and the upper right portion of the head of the pancreas. Tumors arising in practically any portion of the pan-

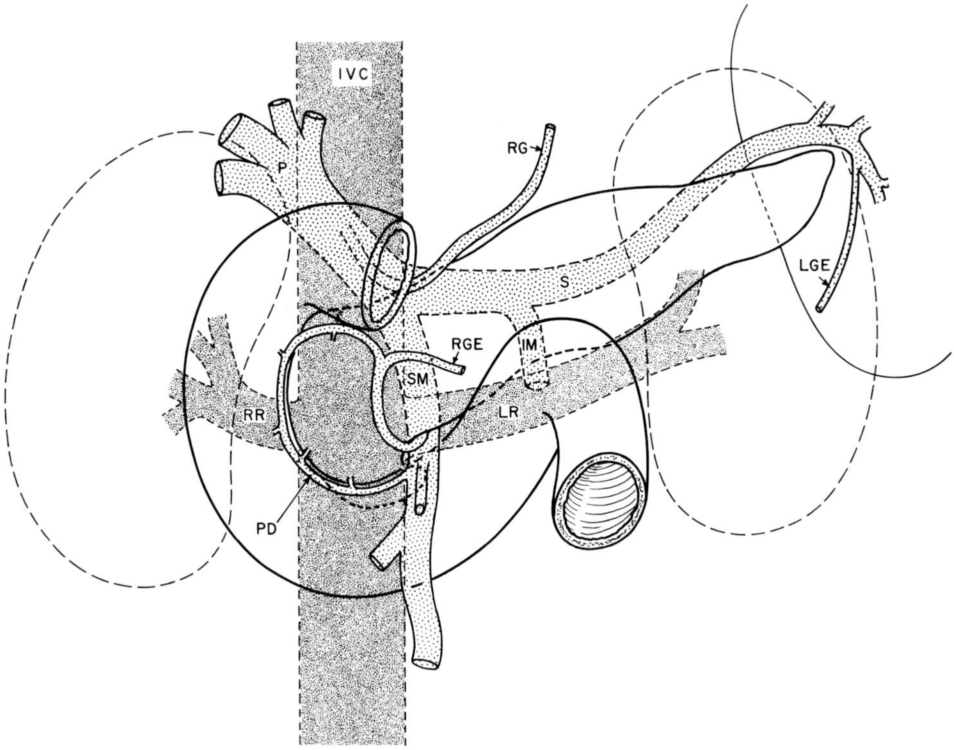

Figure 1–4. Venous anatomy of the pancreaticoduodenal region.
Portal venous system: P, portal vein; SM, superior mesenteric vein; S, splenic vein; IM, inferior mesenteric vein; RG, right gastric vein; RGE, right gastroepiploic; PD, pancreaticoduodenal; LGE, left gastroepiploic.
Systemic venous system: IVC, inferior vena cava; RR, right renal vein; LR, left renal vein.

creas, except the most distal segment of the tail may encroach upon the renal veins. In practice, this is most common with tumors of the body. Cope (1969) demonstrated left renal vein compression or invasion in 8 of 14 patients (57 per cent) with pancreatic carcinoma. There were some instances of right renal venous involvement, but this was less common and occurred only when changes in the left renal vein were also present.

The *splenic vein* runs transversely in a groove-like indentation along the posterosuperior aspect of the tail or the body of the pancreas. The *inferior mesenteric vein* ascends behind the body of the pancreas to drain into the splenic vein. As the *superior mesenteric* vein ascends, it passes anterior to the junction of the third and fourth portions of the duodenum and to the uncinate process of the pancreas. It then dips behind the neck of the pancreas where it unites with the splenic vein to form the portal vein. The *portal vein* ascends obliquely behind the upper part of the head of the pancreas, then passes posterior to the apical portion of the duodenal bulb before it reaches the porta hepatis. All these components of the portal venous system lie in direct contact with the pancreas. Changes occurring as a result of a pancreatic pathologic condition can be demonstrated by splenoportography (Rosch, 1964) and by arteriography (when filming is continued into the venous phase of the examination) (Nebesar, 1967). While both pancreatitis and pseudocysts can affect the portal venous system, pancreatic cancers are especially prone to producing such changes. Buranasiri (1972) found involvement of at least one vein in 46 of 47 patients (98 per cent) with pancreatic carcinoma.

The superior mesenteric vein was affected in most patients with carcinoma of the head of the pancreas, and the splenic vein, in most patients with carcinoma of the body and tail (see Chapter 7).

Arteries

Like the peripancreatic veins, the arteries adjacent to the pancreas are frequently affected by a pathologic condition arising within it. Cancer and, less commonly, pancreatitis may produce localized distortion and even occlusion, while pseudocysts frequently displace the nearby arteries in an arcuate fashion around their margins. While arteries in this area may thus "reflect" the effects of adjacent visceral disease, they may also "produce" dysfunction. The aorta and superior mesenteric artery enclose the third portion of the duodenum like the jaws of a nutcracker. This arrangement may, in special circumstances, produce significant functional duodenal obstruction, a topic discussed at length in Chapter 10. Any discussion of arterial anatomy in this area is hindered by the frequency with which anatomic variations occur. Coverage of all these possible ramifications is beyond the scope of this work, and readers interested in further analysis of this subject are referred to the monograph by Nebesar and his associates (1969).

The *aorta* passes behind the proximal body of the pancreas and more inferiorly behind the third (horizontal) portion of the duodenum (Fig. 1–5). The *celiac axis* arises from the anterior aspect of the aorta at the superior border of the body of the pancreas. Many variations of celiac anatomy occur, but it generally gives off a left gastric branch, then bifurcates into the common hepatic and splenic arteries. The *common hepatic artery* usually originates from the celiac axis at the superior border of the body of the pancreas and runs to the right along the upper margin of the head of the pancreas. It then passes upward behind the duodenal bulb in consort with the portal vein and common bile duct. In this region, it gives off the *gastroduodenal* artery. This vessel descends behind the duodenal bulb, gives rise to the anterior and posterior superior pancreaticoduodenal arcades, and continues on as the right gastroepiploic artery. The *superior pancreaticoduodenal arcades* provide blood to the entire duodenum and pancreatic head. They anastomose with branches of the inferior pancreaticoduodenal branch of the superior mesenteric artery and can thus provide collateral pathways in cases of mesenteric occlusive disease (Baum, 1965).

The *splenic artery* usually arises from the celiac axis at the superior margin of the body of the pancreas and runs to the left along the upper border of the body of the pancreas where it commonly creates a groove-like indentation. The vessel is frequently quite tortuous but is seldom very far from the pancreas. Near the tail of the pancreas, the splenic artery usually comes to lie anterior to pancreatic tissue just before passing to the hilum of the spleen. The splenic artery commonly sends out branches to provide blood for the body and tail of the pancreas. While it may arise from the celiac, common hepatic, or even the superior mesenteric artery, the *dorsal pancreatic artery* usually arises from the proximal portion of the splenic artery. When it does, it passes inferiorly and often ends by forming the *transverse pancreatic artery*. This vessel runs along the posteroinferior aspect of the pancreas and frequently anastomoses with branches from the pancreaticoduodenal arcades and/or with the *pancreatic magna* branch of the splenic artery. The latter vessel commonly arises from the splenic artery and runs inferiorly behind the junction of the pancreatic body and tail.

The *superior mesenteric artery* arises from the anterior surface of the aorta about 1½ cm. below the origin of the celiac axis. At its origin, the superior mesenteric artery lies behind the neck of the pancreas. It then passes inferiorly and forward, anterior to the uncinate process of the pancreas, and then anterior to the third portion of the duodenum. The *inferior pancreaticoduodenal artery* is usually the first branch of the superior

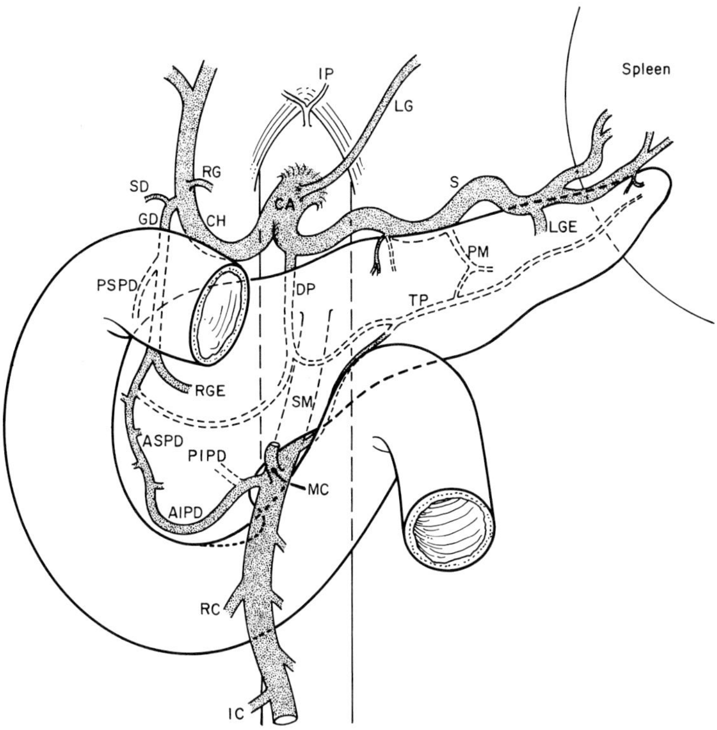

Figure 1–5. Arterial anatomy of the pancreaticoduodenal region. CA, celiac axis; LG, left gastric artery; S, splenic artery; LGE, left gastroepiploic artery; PM, pancreatica magna artery; DP, dorsal pancreatic artery; TP, transverse pancreatic artery; CH, common hepatic artery; RG, right gastric artery; SD, superior duodenal artery (retroduodenal artery); GD, gastroduodenal artery; PSPD, posterior superior pancreaticoduodenal artery; RGE, right gastroepiploic artery; ASPD, anterior superior pancreaticoduodenal artery; SM, superior mesenteric artery; PIPD, posterior inferior pancreaticoduodenal artery; AIPD, anterior inferior pancreaticoduodenal artery; MC, middle colic artery; IC, ileocolic artery; RC, right colic artery; IP, inferior phrenic artery.

mesenteric artery. It arises at the point where the latter crosses the third portion of the duodenum and passes to the right. Its branches anastomose with the superior pancreaticoduodenal arcades of the gastroduodenal artery.

In 10 to 20 per cent of all individuals, an *aberrant* (or replaced) *right hepatic artery* arises from the proximal portion of the superior mesenteric artery (Fig. 1–6). When present, this vessel passes obliquely upward behind the head of the pancreas and the duodenal bulb before reaching the hepatoduodenal ligament through which it travels, together with the common bile duct and portal vein, to reach the porta hepatis. Prior knowledge of the presence of such a vessel is important if pancreaticoduodenotomy is to be attempted, since it can be injured easily if the surgeon is unaware of its presence (Hess, 1965).

The tendency of pancreatic malignancy to produce arterial abnormalities has formed the basis for arteriographic diagnosis of this condition. The incidence of such changes varies widely with the reported series, but recent studies have shown that they can be demonstrated in over 70 per cent of the patients with such a disease (Bookstein, 1969; Fredens, 1969). Encasement (an abnormal arterial narrowing) is the most common single abnormality, but occlusion, tumor vascularity, and occasionally arterial displacement can also occur. Chronic pancreatitis can also produce hypervascularity and encasement (Moskowitz, 1968), while arterial displacement is common in pancreatic pseudocysts (Fu, 1969). Kadell (1967) has emphasized that pseudocysts can also produce serious gastrointestinal hemorrhage by erosion of major adjacent arteries.

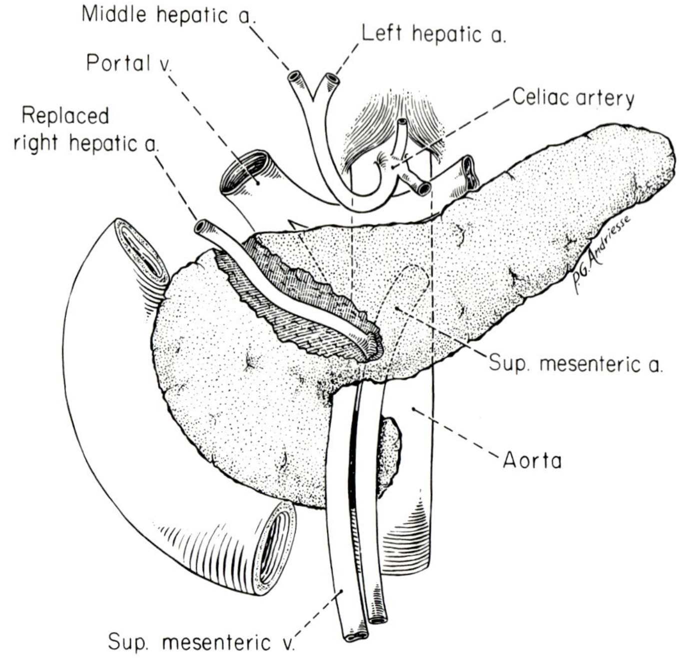

Figure 1–6. Replaced (aberrant) right hepatic artery. (From Nebesar, R. A., et al.: Celiac and superior mesenteric arteries. Boston, Little, Brown & Co., 1969.)

Lesions centered in the head of the pancreas tend to produce arterial changes in the gastroduodenal artery or pancreaticoduodenal arcades. Lesions in the body involve the celiac axis, common hepatic and proximal splenic arteries, as well as the smaller, intrapancreatic arteries (the dorsal and transverse pancreatic arteries and the pancreatica magna). Lesions in the uncinate process may distort the superior mesenteric artery or the inferior pancreaticoduodenal artery. A pathologic condition arising in the tail of the pancreas generally affects the distal splenic artery and, in some cases, the pancreatica magna and/or the transverse pancreatic artery.

Kidneys

The relationship between the duodenum and the *right kidney* is somewhat variable. Generally, the posterolateral aspect of the upper descending duodenum passes in front of the anterior aspect of the right renal hilum (Fig. 1–7). In certain individuals, however, the descending duodenum may lie anterior to a portion of the anteromedial surface of the kidney itself (usually the lower pole). In occasional patients, the right margin of the head of the pancreas may overlap the medial aspect of the anterior surface of the right kidney (Dietz, 1969), but this is the exception rather than the rule. Mass lesions arising in the right kidney can produce extrinsic indentation defects on the posterior and/or lateral aspect of the descending duodenum, can directly invade the descending duo-

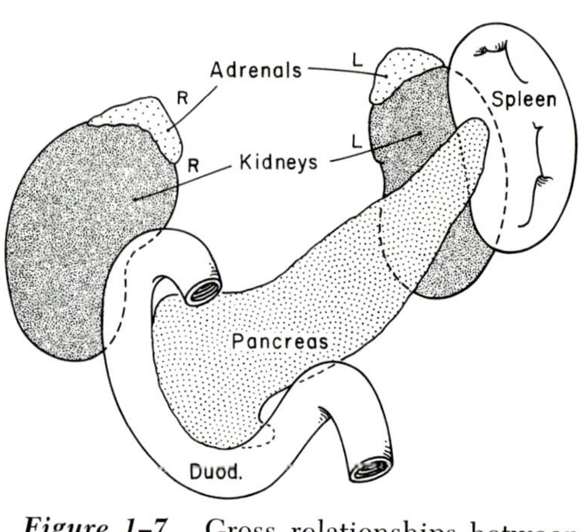

Figure 1–7. Gross relationships between the retroperitoneal upper abdominal viscera.

denum, or can produce a generalized displacement of the descending duodenum to the left or anteriorly. Bluth (1961) has presented six cases of various right renal mass lesions to illustrate these points. Disease arising in the duodenum can also involve the right kidney; both benign and malignant duodenorenal fistulae have been reported (King, 1950). Involvement of the right kidney by pancreatic cysts or tumors is rare but occasionally has occurred (Guerrier, 1970).

The posterior aspect of the body of the pancreas is in direct contact with the anterior surface of the middle and/or upper part of the *left kidney*. Many instances of left renal involvement by pseudocysts or cancers arising in the body or tail of the pancreas have been encountered (Gorder, 1969; Marshall, 1965). The most common type is inferior and lateral displacement of the upper pole of the left kidney but, in some cases, a pancreatic pathologic condition may mimic almost exactly the roentgen features of an intrarenal cyst or tumor. Although the left kidney does not ordinarily come in contact with the duodenum, large masses arising in it may create an extrinsic indentation on the left aspect of the duodenojejunal junction, sometimes producing displacement of this anatomic landmark to the right.

Right Adrenal Gland

The anteroinferior aspect of the *right adrenal gland* is occasionally in contact with the posterior surface of the superior duodenal flexure or upper descending duodenum. In some instances, enlargement of the right adrenal has produced anterior displacement of the upper descending duodenum (Ganem, 1956; Messenger, 1955).

Spleen

"The head of the pancreas lies nestled in the arms of the duodenum while the spleen gets all the tail," an aphorism concerning anatomy, has probably been in vogue for at least as long as there have been medical students. In fact, the posterior aspect and left extremity of the tail of the pancreas are in contact with the inferior anteromedial aspect of the visceral surface of the spleen, just below the splenic hilum (Fig. 1–7). This close relationship underlies the diagnostic problems which may be presented by mass lesions arising in this region. Pancreatic malignancies or pseudocysts may be mistaken for splenic tumors, cysts, or hematoma, and vice versa. Furthermore, pancreatic pseudocysts may actually grow into the splenic pulp itself, producing intrasplenic masses actually of pancreatic origin (Warshaw, 1972). A pathologic condition arising in the body or tail of the pancreas fairly commonly produces splenic vein occlusion (see Chapters 3 and 7). In such circumstances, splenomegaly usually results. Mani (1966) found ten instances of splenic enlargement in 46 patients with carcinoma of the body or tail of the pancreas.

Stomach

A large part of the anterior aspect of the pancreas is closely related to the posterior wall of the stomach, being separated only by the potential space of the lesser peritoneal sac (Fig. 1–8). The pylorus and gastric antrum lie in

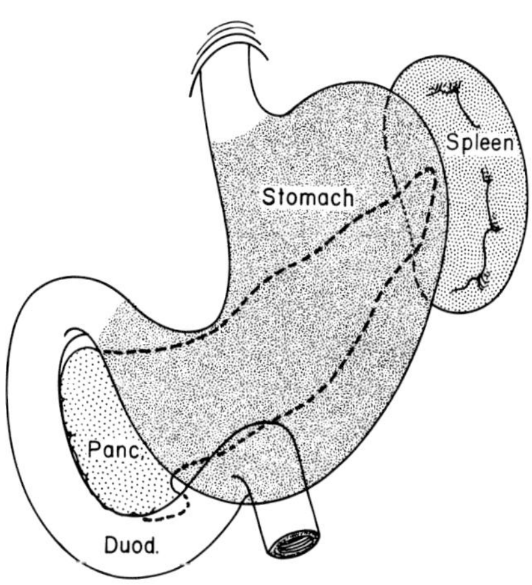

Figure 1–8. Gross relationships between the stomach and the pancreas.

front of the upper anterior surface of the head and neck of the pancreas, while the body and lesser curvature of the stomach are usually anterior to the body of the pancreas. The tail of the pancreas lies behind the junction of the gastric body and fundus.

Roentgen abnormalities of the stomach are common in patients with pancreatic disease and depend upon the close proximity of the two organs. The portion of the stomach involved depends upon the site of the pancreatic pathologic condition. Thus in the series reported by Eyler (1962), the "pad sign" (upward and anterior displacement of the gastric antrum) was most commonly associated with a mass in the head of the pancreas, while Mani (1966) observed that masses arising in the body of the pancreas usually indented or invaded the gastric body. In both series, lesions involving the tail of the pancreas commonly produced abnormalities of the fundus of the stomach. Pseudocysts also cause radiographically demonstrable gastric abnormalities. These occur in 60 to 70 per cent of the patients studied by barium meal examination (Shockman, 1967; Thomford, 1969), and again their specific nature depends upon the location of the underlying cyst. In some cases, pancreatic neoplasms (and even pseudocysts) produce such extensive gastric involvement that the roentgen findings suggest primary gastric malignancy (Chait, 1960). Even on pathologic examination at autopsy, the primary site may not be identified with certainty in some of these patients (Castleman, 1972).

Colon

The right colic (hepatic) flexure is adjacent to the lateral aspect of the descending duodenum (Fig. 1–9). In certain individuals, this relationship is sufficiently close to produce a variable degree of mutual indentation (Poppel, 1960). The posterior surface of the transverse colon crosses the anterior aspect of the middle third of the descending duodenum. Thereafter, it is related posteriorly to the anterior surface of the greater part of the right half of the head of the pancreas. The posterosuperior aspect of the left colic (splenic) flexure is contiguous to the left extremity of the inferior margin of the body of the pancreas and to the anteroinferior surface of the tail of the pancreas.

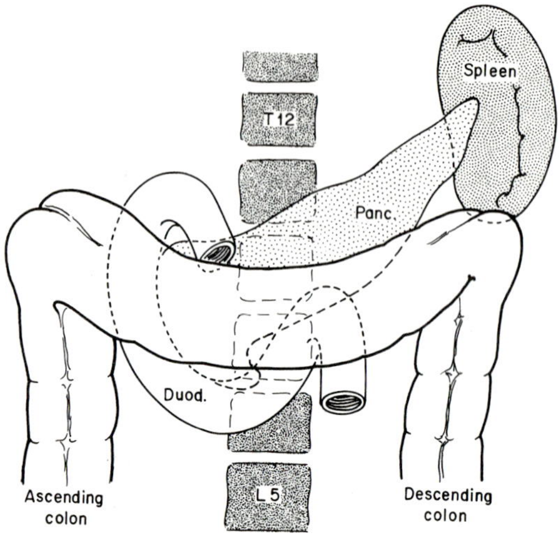

Figure 1–9. Gross relationships between the colon and the pancreas.

The proximity of the hepatic flexure and right transverse colon to the descending duodenum explains the occasional production of duodenal deformity by carcinoma arising in this portion of the colon. Treitel (1970) has reported three instances of this (see also Chapter 4). The colon is often secondarily involved by pancreatic disease. This is due to the close anatomic relationship between these two viscera and to the peritoneal reflections (i.e., the transverse mesocolon and phrenicocolic ligament) connecting them. Pancreatitis (Brascho, 1962; Mohiuddin, 1971), pancreatic pseudocysts (Shockman, 1967), and pancreatic cancer (Mani, 1966) all can produce radiographic abnormalities. These range from a localized ileus, through displacement, to mass indentation and actual stricture (see Chapter 3). The splenic flexure is most commonly involved.

Liver

The anterosuperior aspect of the apical portion of the duodenal bulb is ordinarily in contact with the most medial portion of the visceral surface of the *right lobe* of the liver and with the inferior aspect of the *quadrate lobe.* Posteriorly, the duodenal bulb and superior duodenal flexure are close to, if not actually contiguous with, the anterior portion of the inferior surface of the *caudate lobe.* The *porta hepatis* is not normally in contact with the duodenum, but is situated just superior to the apical portion of the duodenal bulb.

None of these portions of the liver ordinarily produce any extrinsic indentation on the barium-filled duodenum but, when a mass lesion arises in any of these areas, an appropriately located duodenal indentation may result (Meyers, 1958; Whalen, 1972) (see Chapter 4).

Lymph Nodes

A number of important lymph node groups and chains are present in the pancreaticoduodenal area (Fig. 1–10). The pancreaticolienal chain of lymph nodes, located along the posterosuperior surface of the body and tail of the pancreas adjacent to the splenic artery and vein, receives drainage from the body and tail of the pancreas. Lymph from the head of the pancreas chiefly flows to the subpyloric and pancreaticoduodenal nodes. The former group is more prominent and lies below the superior duodenal flexure; the latter lies in the groove between the pancreas and duodenum, both anteriorly and posteriorly. To a lesser extent, drainage from portions of the head, neck, and proximal body of the pancreas may be directed upward toward the hepatic nodes, along the hepatic artery, and in the porta hepatis or, inferiorly, toward the superior mesenteric, mesocolic and paraaortic nodal groups. These are generally related to the inner margin of the fourth (ascending) portion of the duodenum and to the duodenojejunal junction.

From the standpoint of roentgen diagnosis, peripancreatic lymphatic structures have triple significance. First,

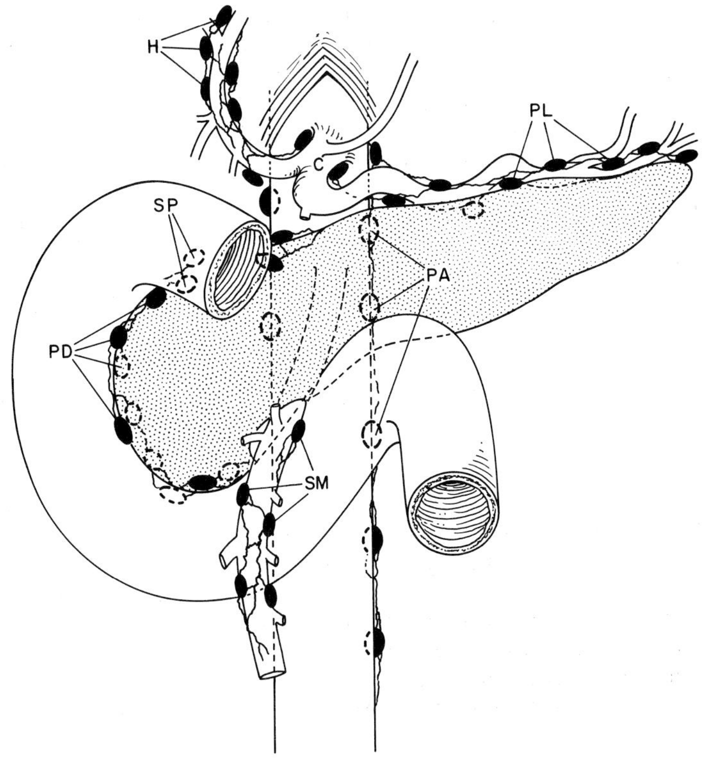

Figure 1–10. Lymphatic drainage of the pancreas and duodenum. C, celiac nodes; H, hepatic nodes; PL, pancreaticolienal nodes; PA, paraaortic nodes; SP, subpyloric nodes; PD, pancreaticoduodenal nodes; SM, superior mesenteric nodes.

nodal metastases may produce or augment compression of adjacent veins (e.g., the left renal vein) (Cope, 1969). Secondly, metastatic or infectious lymphadenopathy may produce duodenal deformity readily demonstrable on barium examination (Renert, 1971; McCort, 1953). There is widespread intermingling of pancreatic lymphatics with those of adjacent abdominal viscera. In addition, pancreatic lymphatics communicate freely with those of the retroperitoneal space and the posterior abdominal wall. As a result, lymphnodal metastases from cancers arising far from the pancreaticoduodenal area can produce striking abnormalities of the duodenum. Von Capeller (1957) reported such findings in a patient with ovarian cancer, and the authors of this monograph have encountered several cases of this abnormality due to metastases from the breast or lung (see Chapter 4). In the third place, paraaortic nodal involvement occasionally can be demonstrated by lymphangiography. Pancreatitis may produce large nodes with normal architecture, whereas metastatic tumor produces discrete filling defects of varying size. Furthermore, the abdominal portion of the thoracic duct is closely related to the posterior surface of the neck of the pancreas. Inflammation or malignancy arising in the pancreas may thus produce displacement and even obstruction of the thoracic duct (Dodd, 1970). This phenomenon may contribute to the chylous ascites which occasionally complicates pancreatic disease.

Peritoneal Reflections

Lesser Omentum

This structure extends between the liver and the lesser curvature of the stomach and the first portion of the duodenum (Fig. 1–11, *C*). The right portion of the lesser omentum (between the liver and duodenum) is termed the hepatoduodenal ligament (Fig. 1–11, *A* and *C*). The right border of this structure is a free margin in which run the hepatic artery, the perihepatic lymphatics, the common bile duct, and the portal vein. This free margin constitutes the anterior boundary of the epiploic foramen—the entry into the lesser peritoneal sac. The hepatoduodenal ligament can be identified radiographically by demonstrating the structures which run within it.

Cystogastrocolic Ligament

This is an anomalous peritoneal band which extends from the gallbladder across the anterior aspect of the duodenal bulb and the superior duodenal flexure to the greater omentum or transverse colon (Fig. 1–11, *B*). It is present in approximately 22 per cent of all patients (Kellogg, 1927). Unlike the hepatoduodenal ligament, the cystogastrocolic ligament is a structure of little or no pathologic or surgical significance. However, it occasionally produces abnormalities on barium meal examination. Samuel (1952) has described roentgen findings which can simulate bulbar or pyloric deformity similar to that observed in patients with acid-peptic ulcer disease. In some instances, the appearance produced by the band may simulate common bile duct impression on the bulb.

Mesenteric Root

The mesentery proper is a fan-shaped fold of peritoneum which attaches the jejunum and ileum to the posterior wall of the abdomen. Its root (Fig. 1–11, *C*), a narrow strip beginning at the duodenojejunal junction, is directed inferiorly and obliquely across the anteromedial aspect of the ascending (fourth) portion of the duodenum, the anterior surface of the uncinate process of the pancreas, and the anterior aspect of the third portion of the duodenum. Inflammatory processes involving the mesenteric small bowel or arising in the pancreas can produce marked thickening of the mesenteric root. Simon (1962) has described this occurrence in acute pancreatitis, small-bowel infarction, and acute re-

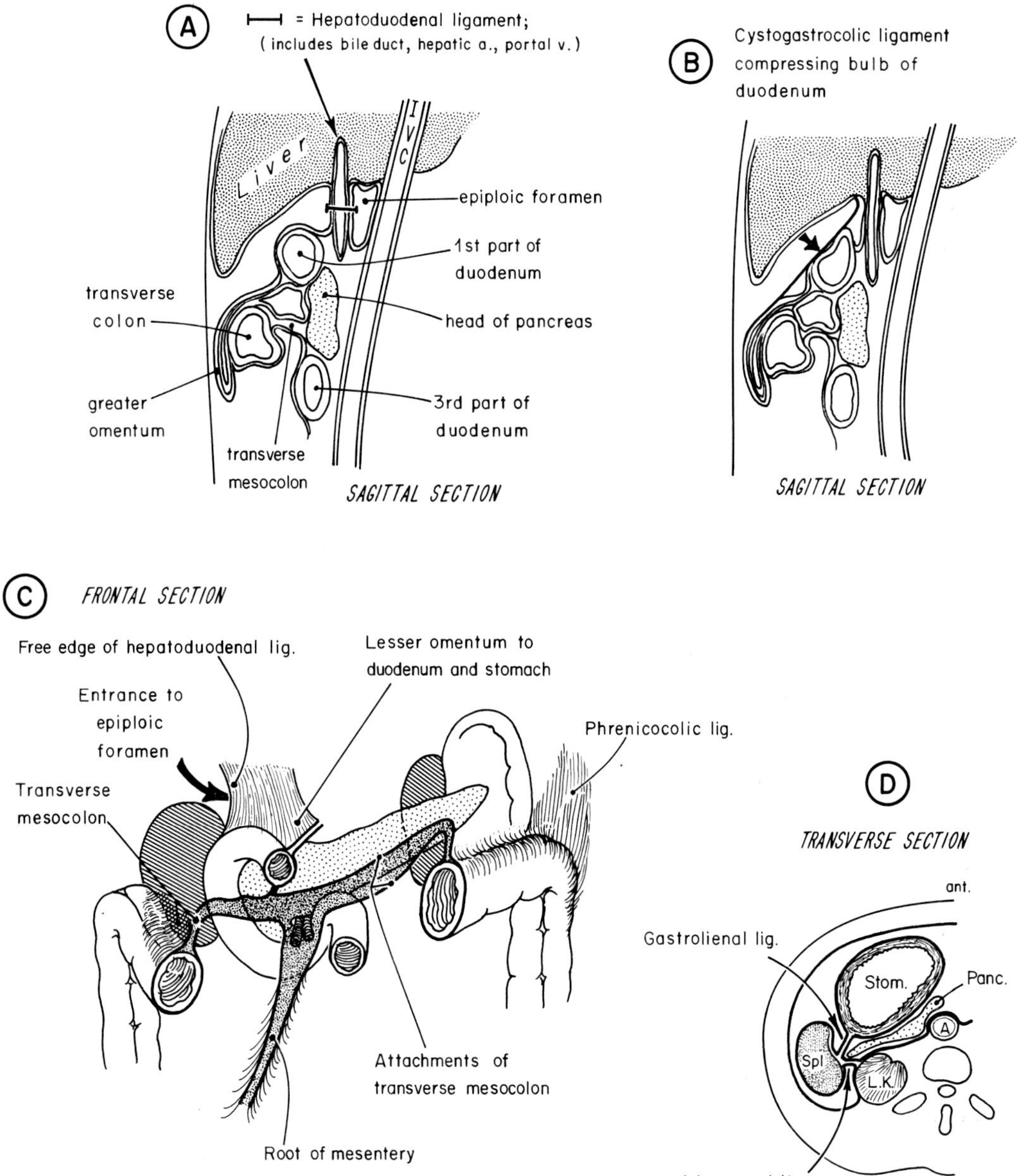

Figure 1–11. Peritoneal reflections important in pancreaticoduodenal radiology.

gional enteritis. In each case, the edematous mesenteric root produced compression and partial obstruction of the third portion of the duodenum. The radiographic appearance differed from that of the superior mesenteric artery syndrome in that the obstruction was unrelieved by changes in the patient's position.

Phrenicocolic Ligament

This is a peritoneal fold which extends from the anatomic splenic flexure of the colon to the parietal peritoneum overlying the posterolateral aspect of the diaphragm (Fig. 1–11, *C*). At the level of the phrenicocolic ligament, the intraperitoneal transverse colon becomes the retroperitoneal descending colon. The phrenicocolic ligament is medially continuous with the transverse mesocolon (Fig. 1–11, *C*) and with the gastrolienal and lienorenal ligaments (Fig. 1–11, *D*) (Meyers, 1970). Since the tail of the pancreas is situated within the leaves of the lienorenal ligament, enzymes released during episodes of acute pancreatitis have direct access to the splenic flexure. Both the "colon cut-off" sign (Brascho, 1962), which can accompany acute pancreatitis, and other splenic flexure abnormalities (e.g., extrinsic indentation, spasm, stricture, and so forth), which can be seen in either acute or chronic pancreatitis (Schwartz, 1957), are probably the result of transmission of pancreatic inflammatory products to the splenic flexure by means of the phrenicocolic ligament.

Transverse Mesocolon

This peritoneal reflection anchors the posterosuperior aspect of the transverse colon to the retroperitoneal abdominal structures. Its parietal attachment (Fig. 1–11, *C*) crosses the anterior aspect of the mid-descending duodenum and the mid portion of the anterior surface of the pancreas. It passes just superior to the duodenojejunal junction, then runs along the anteroinferior margin of the body and tail of the pancreas (Whalen, 1972). The importance of this structure in radiologic diagnosis is analogous to that of the phrenicocolic ligament: inflammatory and malignant processes arising in the pancreas have ready access to the transverse colon by passing between the leaves of the transverse mesocolon (Stuart, 1956; Brascho, 1962). The colon cut-off sign is the typical roentgen manifestation of this process (see Chapter 2).

Spine

The third portion of the duodenum usually crosses the spine somewhere between the upper border of the third lumbar vertebral body and the mid portion of the fourth lumbar vertebral body (Fig. 1–9). The head of the pancreas most often lies anterior to the second and third lumbar vertebrae, while the body of the gland is directed transversely upward to the left and lies in the region of the first lumbar segment. Although neither the pancreas nor the duodenum is in direct contact with the spine, their relatively close proximity has a certain degree of radiologic significance. Forceful compression of the duodenum against the spine by blunt abdominal trauma can result in duodenal rupture or hematoma formation. Either of these forms of injury can be demonstrated radiologically (see Chapter 10). Arteriomesenteric duodenal compression depends, in all cases, on the presence of the spine and aorta posterior to the third portion of the duodenum, and can be induced in previously asymptomatic patients by orthopedic correction of spinal curvature (Evarts, 1971). The influence of the spine on the pancreas is less significant than that on the duodenum, but there is a definite flattening of the neck of the pancreas from front to back as it crosses the spine. The diminution in pancreatic mass produced by this flattening has resulted in numerous false-positive diagnoses when relatively "cold" areas have been depicted in the neck of the pancreas by ^{75}Se selenomethionine imaging (Riccobono, 1968).

INTRINSIC DUODENAL ANATOMY

General Features

The duodenum ordinarily is 25 to 30 cm. in length. The first portion is essentially intraperitoneal and freely movable. Beyond the superior duodenal flexure (i.e., where the descending duodenum commences), the duodenum is retroperitoneal and fixed in its position. The first portion is usually short but, occasionally, the postbulbar segment is elongated, and considerable redundancy may be present in this area (see Chapter 4). At the superior and inferior duodenal flexures (the latter marks the junction of the second and third portions), there may be considerable infolding of the inner wall, producing a pseudotumoral effect (Goldstein, 1969; Nelson, 1971) (see Chapter 4). The duodenojejunal junction usually can be identified on barium studies, but the position of this landmark varies widely: it can be found at any level from the eleventh thoracic to the fourth lumbar vertebra, and from 4 cm. above to 5 cm. below the level of the superior duodenal flexure (Eaton, 1972).

Internal Anatomy

When the duodenal bulb is well distended, its mucosal surface is relatively flat and featureless although a few longitudinal folds are occasionally present. Even when maximally distended by hypotonic duodenography, however, the circular mucosal folds of Kerckring are normally visible in the duodenum beyond the superior duodenal flexure. These folds (or plicae) generally are oriented transversely, perpendicular to the long axis of the duodenum, though some branching interconnections are occasionally present.

The major duodenal papilla is visible as a rounded indentation on the inner duodenal margin in 20 to 30 per cent of barium duodenal studies (Ferrucci, 1970; Eaton, 1972). This papilla's greatest dimension exceeds 1.5 cm. in only about 1 per cent of all such examinations, except when peri-Vaterian disease is present. The minor duodenal papilla, anatomically present in nearly all patients, is almost never visible on radiologic examination, except when a pathologic condition exists (Stiennon, 1957). It usually is located about 2.5 cm. above the major papilla.

Although the major papilla can be identified in only a minority of barium upper gastrointestinal examinations, the site of the papilla can be localized in over 60 per cent of such studies when certain accessory anatomic features are sought (Ferrucci, 1970) (Fig. 1–12; see also Fig. 4–23). These include the *promontory*, a shoulder-like luminal projection of the inner duodenal margin. A notch-like indentation of the inner duodenal margin often marks the superior

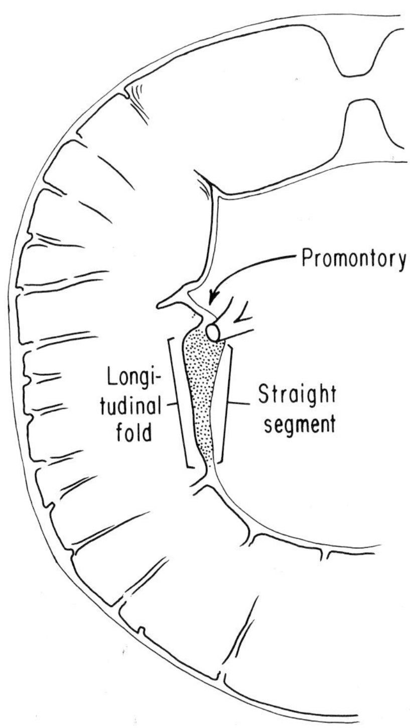

Figure 1–12. Schematic representation of the descending duodenum showing the typical arrangement of the promontory, straight segment, longitudinal fold and papilla.

aspect of the promontory. The common bile duct enters the duodenum at the promontory in all instances in which the latter exists as an identifiable feature. When a promontory is visible, the duodenal wall below usually is relatively flat for several centimeters. This *straight segment* is normal and must be distinguished from the pathologic flattening and fold effacement along the inner duodenal border which may be seen in chronic or resolving acute pancreatitis. Since the normal straight segment is found only in the lower descending duodenum, flattening involving the upper descending duodenum is usually a reliable sign of disease. The *longitudinal fold* is a well-recognized anatomic structure which surrounds and extends inferiorly from the major duodenal papilla. On duodenal radiographs, it appears as a linear structure parallel to the straight segment, producing a double contour which should not be mistaken for a pathologic mass indentation defect (see Chapter 4).

One or more of this triad of radiographic features (the promontory, straight segment, and longitudinal fold) are present in over 60 per cent of barium duodenal examinations. When these features can be identified, the location of the duodenal papilla can be determined accurately even though the papilla itself is not visible (see Chapter 4).

INTRINSIC PANCREATIC ANATOMY

Embryologic Development

The pancreas develops from separate dorsal and ventral anlagen. The former arises from that portion of the foregut which later becomes the duodenum. It grows upward and posteriorly and forms, in the adult, a portion of the pancreatic head, the uncinate process, and the body and tail of the pancreas. The ventral pancreas arises from the primitive bile duct and, during the course of embryologic growth, together with the developing common bile duct, rotates backward behind the duodenum. The ventral pancreas comes to lie behind that portion of the dorsal pancreas closest to the duodenum and, in the adult, forms most of the pancreatic head. Shortly after meeting, the two components fuse, establishing a communication between their two ductal systems. Eventually, that of the ventral pancreas forms the main pancreatic duct (of Wirsung) while that of the dorsal pancreas persists as the accessory pancreatic duct (of Santorini).

Anatomic Features

The ducts of Santorini and Wirsung intercommunicate in 75 per cent of adults. The accessory pancreatic duct enters the duodenum at the minor papilla which is located about 2.5 cm. above the major papilla in most patients. In about 5 per cent of adults, the minor papilla actually receives most of the pancreatic exocrine drainage. The main pancreatic duct and the common bile duct enter into the duodenum via a common channel in about 80 per cent of the cases (Hand, 1963) (see Chapter 8).

In adults, the pancreas is generally about 12 to 15 cm. in length and weighs between 85 and 90 gm. It is divided into head, body, and tail. A somewhat constricted portion, the neck, can be identified between the head and body in some patients.

Functional Considerations

Exocrine Activity

Each day the normal pancreas secretes 1500 to 2000 ml. of alkaline juice into the duodenal lumen. This secretion helps to neutralize the acidity of gastric contents reaching the duodenum, and contains an immense amount of digestive enzyme protein. Trypsinogen, chymotrypsinogen (inactive precursors of trypsin and chymotrypsin), amylase, lipase, and carboxypeptidase are among the chief pancreatic enzymes; these play an important role in the digestion of all the major foodstuffs. Such digestive enzyme proteins are synthesized by the pancreatic acinar cells which have been shown to incorporate amino acids into proteins more rapidly than do the cells of any other tissue (Hansson, 1959; Awwad, 1967). This activity permits imaging of the pancreas after intravenous administration of ^{75}Se selenomethionine —a radiopharmaceutical which serves as an effective amino acid analogue. When the main pancreatic duct is blocked (e.g., by tumor) or when a substantial portion of the gland has been destroyed (e.g., by recurrent pancreatitis), pancreatic digestive enzyme synthesis is markedly diminished and pancreatic steatorrhea may be the clinical consequence (see Chapter 6).

The physiologic control of pancreatic exocrine secretion is complex. When the acidic gastric contents come in contact with the duodenal mucosa, *secretin* is released from the duodenal mucosa into the blood stream. This agent, the first hormone ever described, causes the pancreas to secrete a large volume of watery fluid, rich in bicarbonate and poor in enzymes. Centrilobular cells within the pancreatic acini seem responsible for the elaboration of bicarbonate in pancreatic juice. Various other food materials in the duodenal lumen cause the release of *pancreozymin,* another duodenal hormone. This agent promotes the release of pancreatic enzymes from the acinar cells into the pancreatic ductules, but has little influence on the total amount or bicarbonate content of pancreatic juice secretion. *Vagal stimulation* has effects similar to those of pancreozymin.

Endocrine Activity

Scattered throughout the pancreatic parenchyma are the islets of Langerhans. These small independent functional units contain three types of cells. Beta cells, the most numerous, are concerned with the production and release of insulin. Alpha and delta cells appear to represent the sites of glucogen and gastrin synthesis.

In view of these different cellular constituents, it follows that islet cell tumors can produce quite different clinical manifestations. "Insulinomas," the most common form of islet cell neoplasm, are derived from beta-cells and produce hyperinsulinism. The incidence of malignancy in these lesions is relatively low. On the other hand, "gastrinomas" are usually malignant (an incidence of 60 per cent). Tumors of this sort, associated with the Zollinger-Ellison syndrome, are derived from non-beta cells. There are often multiple pancreatic tumors in patients with hypergastrinism and, in about 25 per cent of all such patients, there are other endocrine tumors as well (e.g., parathyroid, pituitary, and so forth).

REFERENCES

Awwad, H. K., Adelstein, S. J., Potchen, E. J., et al: The interconversion and reutilization of injected 75-Se-selenomethionine in the rat. J. Biol. Chem., *242*:492–500, 1967.

Baum, S., Stein, G. N., and Baue, A.: Extrinsic pressure defects on the duodenal loop in mesenteric occlusive disease. Radiology, *85*:866–874, 1965.

Bergkvist, A., and Seldinger, S. I.: Contrast roentgenography in differential diagnosis between perforated ulcer and acute pancreatitis. Acta Chir. Scand., *118*:137–145, 1959.

Bilbao, M. K., Rösch, J., Frische, L. H., and Dotter, C. T.: Hypotonic duodenography in the diagnosis of pancreatic disease. Seminars Roentgen., *3*:280–287, 1968.

Bluth, I., and Vitale, P.: Right renal enlargements causing alterations in the descending duodenum. Radiology, *76*:777–784, 1961.

Bookstein, J. J., Reuter, S. R., and Martel, W.: Angiographic evaluation of pancreatic carcinoma. Radiology, *93*:757–764, 1969.

Brascho, D. J., Reynolds, T. N., and Zanca, P.: The radiographic "colon cut-off sign" in acute pancreatitis. Radiology, *79*:763–769, 1962.

Buranasiri, S., and Baum, S.: The significance of the venous phase of celiac and superior mesenteric arteriography in evaluating pancreatic carcinoma. Radiology, *102*:11–20, 1972.

Castleman, B.: Personal communication, 1972.

Chait, H., and Faegenburg, D. H.: Illusory neoplasms of the stomach and duodenum as a manifestation of carcinoma of the pancreas. Radiology, *74*:771–777, 1960.

Cope, C., and Isard, H. J.: Left renal vein entrapment. A new diagnostic finding in retroperitoneal disease. Radiology, *92*:867–872, 1969.

Dietz, W.: Infrapancreatic right kidney. Amer. J. Roentgen., *107*:69–70, 1969.

Dodd, G. D.: Lymphography in diseases of the liver and pancreas. Radiol. Clin. N. Amer., *8*:69–84, 1970.

Eaton, S. B., Fleischli, D. J., Pollard, J. J., et al: Comparison of current radiologic approaches to diagnosis of pancreatic diseases. New Eng. J. Med., *279*:389–396, 1968.

Eaton, S. B., Ferrucci, J. T., Margulis, A. R., and Weens, H. S.: Unfamiliar roentgen findings in pancreatic disease. Amer. J. Roentgen., *116*:396–405, 1972.

Evarts, C. M., Winter, R. B., and Hall, J. E.: Vascular compression of duodenum associated with treatment of scoliosis. J. Bone Joint Surg. [Amer.], *53A*:431–444, 1971.

Eyler, W. R., Clark, M. D., and Rian, R. L.: An evaluation of roentgen signs of pancreatic enlargement. J.A.M.A., *181*:967–971, 1962.

Ferrucci, J. T., Benedict, K. T., Page, D. L., et al: Radiographic features of the normal hypotonic duodenogram. Radiology, *96*:401–408, 1970.

Filler, R. M., Harris, S. H., and Edwards, E. A.: Characteristics of the inferior-cava venogram in retroperitoneal cancer. New Eng. J. Med., *266*:1194–1197, 1962.

Fredens, M., Egeblad, M., and Holst-Nielsen, F.: The value of selective angiography in the diagnosis of tumors of the pancreas and liver. Radiology, *93*:765–769, 1969.

Fu, W. R., and Stanton, L. W.: Angiographic study of pseudocysts of the pancreas. J. Canad. Ass. Radiol., *20*:176–179, 1969.

Ganem, E. J., Wallwork, D. W., and West, G. V.: Anterior displacement of the descending duodenum as an aid in the diagnosis of retroperitoneal tumor: roentgenologic sign of possible significance in some cases of enlargement of the right adrenal gland. New Eng. J. Med., *254*:552–555, 1956.

Goldstein, H. M., and Zboralske, F. F.: Tubeless hypotonic duodenography. J.A.M.A., *210*: 2086–2088, 1969.

Gorder, J. L., and Stargardter, F. L.: Pancreatic pseudocysts simulating intrarenal masses. Amer. J. Roentgen., *107*:65–68, 1969.

Guerrier, K., and Persky, L.: Pancreatic disease simulating renal abnormality. Amer. J. Surg., *120*:46–49, 1970.

Hand, B. H.: An anatomical study of the choledochoduodenal area. Brit. J. Surg., *50*:486–494, 1963.

Hansson, E.: The formation of pancreatic juice proteins studied with labeled amino acids. Acta Physiol. Scand., *46*: Suppl. 161, 1959.

Hess, W.: *Surgery of the Biliary Passages and the Pancreas.* Princeton, N.J., D. Van Nostrand Company, Inc. 1965, p. 21.

Jacquemet, P., Liotta, D., and Mallet-Guy, P.: Early Radiologic Diagnosis of Diseases of the Pancreas and Ampulla of Vater: Elective Exploration of the Ampulla of Vater and Head of the Pancreas by Hypotonic Duodenography. Springfield, Ill., Charles C Thomas, Publisher, 1965.

Kadell, B. M., and Riley, J. M.: Major arterial involvement by pancreatic pseudocysts. Amer. J. Roentgen., *99*:632–636, 1967.

Kellogg, E. L., and Kellogg, W. A.: Chronic duodenal stasis. Radiology, *9*:23–38, 1927.

King, J. D.: Spontaneous renoduodenal fistulas. Radiology, *54*:82–86, 1950.

Kune, G. A.: Surgical anatomy of common bile duct. Arch. Surg., *89*:995–1004, 1964.

Mani, J. R., Zboralske, F. F., and Margulis, A. R.: Carcinoma of the body and tail of the pancreas. Amer. J. Roentgen., *96*:429–446, 1966.

Marshall, S., Lapp, M., and Schulte, J. W.: Lesions of the pancreas mimicking renal disease. J. Urol., *93*:41–45, 1965.

McCort, J. J.: Roentgenographic appearance of metastases to the central lymph nodes of the superior mesenteric artery in carcinoma of the right colon. Radiology, *60*:641–646, 1953.

Messenger, H. M., and Monroe, L.: An unusual cause of duodenal deformity in Addison's disease. Gastroenterology, *29*:313–317, 1955.

Meyers, H. I., and Jacobson, G.: Displacements of stomach and duodenum by anomalous lobes of the liver. Amer. J. Roentgen., *79*:789–792, 1958.

Meyers, M. A.: Roentgen significance of the phrenicocolic ligament. Radiology, *95*:539–545, 1970.

Mohiuddin, S., Sakiyalak, P., Gullick, H. D., et al: Stenosing lesions of the colon secondary to pancreatitis. Arch. Surg., *102*:229–231, 1971.

Moskowitz, H., Chait, A., and Mellius, H. Z.: "Tumor encasement" of the celiac axis due to chronic pancreatitis. Amer. J. Roentgen., *104*:641–645, 1968.

Nebesar, R. A., Kornblith, P. L., Pollard, J. J., and Michels, N. A.: Celiac and Superior Mesenteric Arteries. Boston, Little, Brown, and Company, 1969.

Nebesar, R. A., and Pollard, J. J.: A critical evaluation of selective celiac and superior mesenteric angiography in the diagnosis of pancreatic diseases, particularly malignant tumor: facts and "artifacts." Radiology, *89*:1017–1027, 1967.

Nelson, J. A., and Sheft, D. J.: A duodenal pseudopolyp. Presented at the 57th Scientific Assembly and Annual Meeting of the Radiological Society of North America, Chicago, 1971.

Poppel, M. H.: Duodenocolic apposition. Amer. J. Roentgen., *83*:851–856, 1960.

Poppel, M. H., Jacobson, H. G., and Smith, R. W.: The Roentgen Aspects of the Papilla and Ampulla of Vater. Springfield, Ill., Charles C Thomas, Publisher, 1953.

Renert, W. A., and Hecht, H. L.: Lymphangiographic demonstration of impression upon the duodenum by retroperitoneal lymph nodes. Brit. J. Radiol., *44*:189–194, 1971.

Riccobono, K. J.: Pancreatic scanning. Seminars Roentgen., *3*:310–317, 1968.

Rosch, J., and Herfort, K.: Splenoportographic diagnosis of pancreatic disease. Geriatrics, *19*:725–734, 1964.

Rubinstein, Z. J., Bank, S., Marks, I. N., et al: Hypotonic duodenography in chronic pancreatitis. Brit. J. Radiol., *44*:142–149, 1971.

Russell, W. M., and Margulis, A. R.: Impression on the duodenal loop resulting from tumor of the pancreas: a roentgenographic evaluation. Amer. J. Roentgen., *94*:449–452, 1965.

Samuel, E.: The cystogastrocolic band: radiological considerations. Brit. J. Radiol., *25*:19–21, 1952.

Sato, T., Kakizaki, G., Saito, Y., et al: A combined method for diagnosis in malignant jaundice. Arch. Surg., *95*:207–216, 1967.

Schwartz, A., and Birnbaum, D.: Roentgenologic study of the topography of the choledochoduodenal junction. Amer. J. Roentgen., *87*:772–776, 1962.

Schwartz, S., and Nadelhaft, J.: Simulation of colonic obstruction at the splenic flexure by pancreatitis: roentgen features. Amer. J. Roentgen., *78*:607–616, 1957.

Shockman, A. T., and Marasco, J. A.: Pseudocysts of the pancreas. Amer. J. Roentgen., *101*:628–638, 1967.

Simon, M., and Lerner, M. A.: Duodenal compression by the mesenteric root in acute pancreatitis and inflammatory conditions of the bowel. Radiology, *79*:75–81, 1962.

Stiennon, O. A.: The anatomical basis for the epsilon sign of Frostberg. Amer. J. Roentgen., *75*:282–290, 1956.

Stuart, C.: Acute pancreatitis: new radiodiagnostic sign. J. Fac. Radiol., *8*:50–58, 1956.

Thomford, N. R., and Jesseph, J. E.: Pseudocyst of the pancreas. A review of fifty cases. Amer. J. Surg., *118*:86–94, 1969.

Treitel, H., Meyers, M. A., and Maza, V.: Changes in the duodenal loop secondary to carcinoma of the colon. Brit. J. Radiol., *43*:209–213, 1970.

Von Capeller, D., and Cummins, A. J.: Solitary duodenal metastasis eight years after radiation of carcinoma of the cervix. Gastroenterology, *33*:655–658, 1957.

Warshaw, A. L., Chesney, T. McC., Evans, G. W., and McCarthy, H. F.: Intrasplenic dissection by pancreatic pseudocysts. New Eng. J. Med., *287*:72–75, 1972.

Whalen, J. P., Evans, J. A., and Meyers, M. A.: Vector principle in the differential diagnosis of abdominal masses, right upper quadrant. Amer. J. Roentgen., *115*:318–333, 1972.

Chapter 2

PLAIN FILM FEATURES OF PANCREATIC DISEASE

Plain films of the abdomen, chest, and extremities often yield useful and, on occasion, diagnostic information pertinent to the detection of pancreatic disease. Although such findings usually arise in association with inflammatory processes and are most commonly encountered during episodes of acute illness, certain features can be detected during relatively quiescent stages of chronic pancreatitis, and other manifestations occur in patients with neoplastic conditions. In most instances, abnormalities demonstrated by plain films are only of suggestive value and serve as indications for further, more specific, radiologic studies. In some patients, however, the clinical situation is so grave that more elaborate examinations are considered hazardous. In these cases, accurate interpretation of the plain film findings assumes special significance.

OSSEOUS ABNORMALITIES

Intramedullary Fat Necrosis

Several reports of osseous abnormality, apparently associated with pancreatitis, have appeared during the past decade (Immelman, 1964; Gerle, 1965; and Bank, 1966). Three distinct types of changes have been described. The first consists of multiple, small, irregular osteolytic areas often associated with periosteal new bone formation (Fig. 2–1). This sort of abnormality is seen most commonly in the radius, ulna, phalanges, and metacarpals. These changes, thought to represent bone resorption associated with active intramedullary fat necrosis, become apparent during or shortly after attacks of acute pancreatitis. Both of the other kinds of bony changes associated with pancreatitis occur in patients with chronic disease. The *metadiaphyseal type* consists of relatively well-circumscribed areas of dense calcification occurring in the medullary cavities of long bones—most often, the distal femur or proximal tibia. This calcification may appear as a group of punctate densities or as a conglomeration of linear streaks (Fig. 2–2). The *epiphyseal type* resembles aseptic necrosis and occurs in the ends of long bones—especially the femoral and humeral heads. In early stages, a fine radiolucent band develops in the immediate subcortical area. Later, a well-defined area of increased density appears as the trabecular pattern becomes smudged and indistinct (Fig. 2–3). Still later, there is cystic change, fragmentation, and collapse. Ultimately, the findings of degenerative arthritis develop.

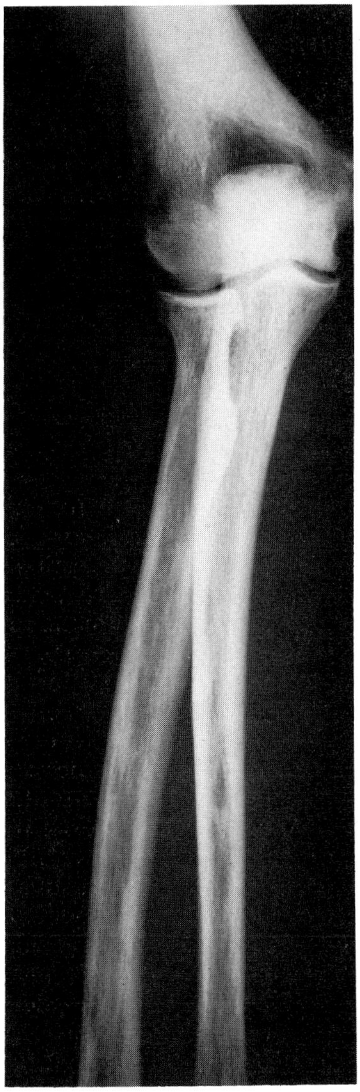

Figure 2–1. Intramedullary fat necrosis (early phase). Multiple areas of poorly defined osteolysis in distal radial and ulnar shafts in a patient with acute pancreatitis.

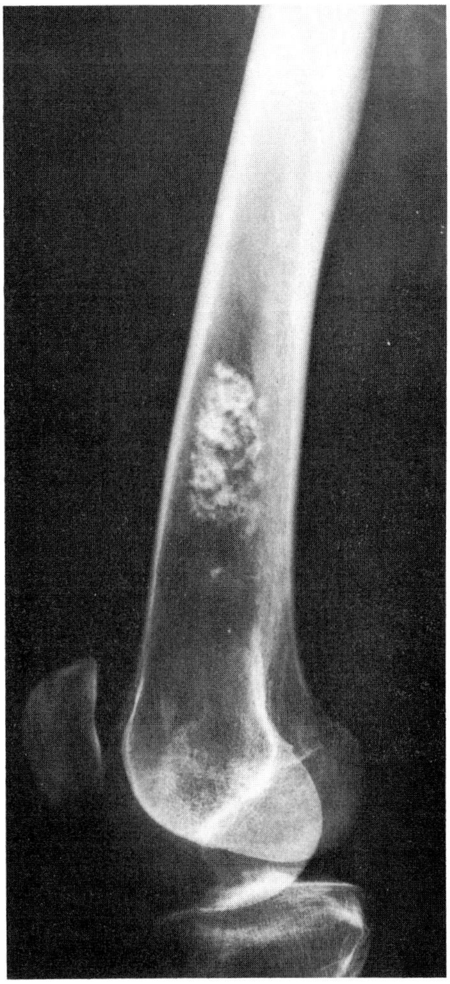

Figure 2–2. Bone infarction (metadiaphyseal fat necrosis) in a patient with chronic pancreatitis.

The pathophysiology of bony changes in pancreatitis is only speculative, but a logical, if unproven, hypothesis has been advanced to explain them. High

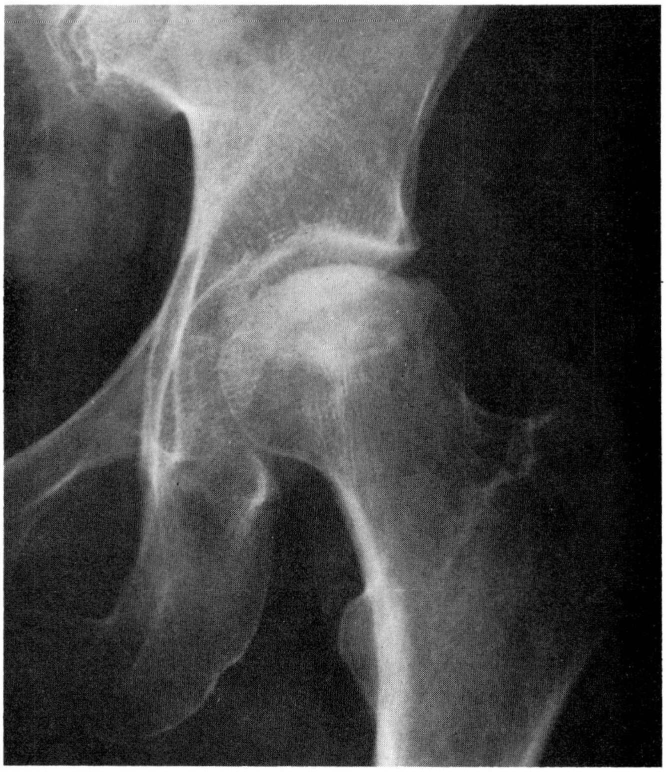

Figure 2–3. Aseptic necrosis (epiphyseal fat necrosis) in a patient with chronic pancreatitis. Note flattening and increased density of femoral head.

levels of circulating serum lipase, released by pancreatic inflammation, result in "metastatic" medullary fat necrosis. Such fat necrosis has been produced experimentally both by inducing severe pancreatitis and by injecting lipase intravenously in animals (Scarpelli, 1956). The associated inflammatory reaction produces compression of the small intramedullary arteries and arterioles; inflammatory vascular injury and thrombosis also develop, and the over-all effect is osseous ischemia and bone infarction. The resulting bone resorption can be identified as radiologically evident osteolysis. Considerably later, dystrophic calcification occurs in metaphyseal areas, and changes of aseptic necrosis develop in the femoral or humeral heads.

Intramedullary fat necrosis can be associated with mild localized bone pain, skin lesions similar to erythema nodosum, and small subcutaneous nodules. [The latter two findings probably represent the effects of concomitant subcutaneous fat necrosis. In rare cases, such fat necrosis results in soft-tissue calcification which has been identified in some patients with pancreatitis (Gerle, 1965).] Most patients with pancreatitis are not subjected to systematic roentgen study of the skeletal system. Accordingly, the true incidence of osseous changes is unknown. Scarpelli (1956) found intramedullary fat necrosis in seven of 67 patients (10.4 per cent) examined at autopsy as a result of hemorrhagic pancreatitis. In the series reported by Gerle (1965) and Bank (1966), six of 100 patients with pancreatitis (6 per cent) had radiologically evident bony changes. Of interest is the fact that in at least two patients with pancreatic carcinoma, radiographic evidence of medullary fat necrosis has been present (Jackson, 1952).

Although, in most instances, understanding of the relationship between pancreatic inflammation, intramedullary fat necrosis, and bone infarction is of little practical value, it may occasionally help to explain an otherwise confusing clinical picture (e.g., the coexistence of limb pains and acute abdominal discomfort). In other patients, it may be valuable to obtain a skeletal survey when a diagnosis of chronic pancreatitis is suspected but not readily documented. Demonstration of typical osseous abnormalities can provide useful supportive evidence of the disease in such circumstances.

Osseous Metastasis

Pancreatic carcinoma fairly commonly metastasizes to the skeleton. The spine, ribs, sternum, and mandible have all been reported as sites of such involvement (Frantz, 1959). In one series (Turner, 1940), 6.3 per cent of the pancreatic tumors exhibited bony metastases, the great majority of which were osteolytic. In rare instances, however, metastases from the pancreas may stimulate an osteoblastic response (Geyman, 1947; Gillison, 1970) (Fig. 2–4). One additional form of bony involvement by pancreatic malignancy has been described. The bodies of the twelfth thoracic and the three upper lumbar vertebrae are in close relation to the head and body of the pancreas. Malignancies arising in this portion of the pancreas and growing posteriorly can involve any of these vertebrae by direct extension (Borak, 1943). Such involvement may be destructive (Mani, 1966) or osteoblastic (Gillison, 1970).

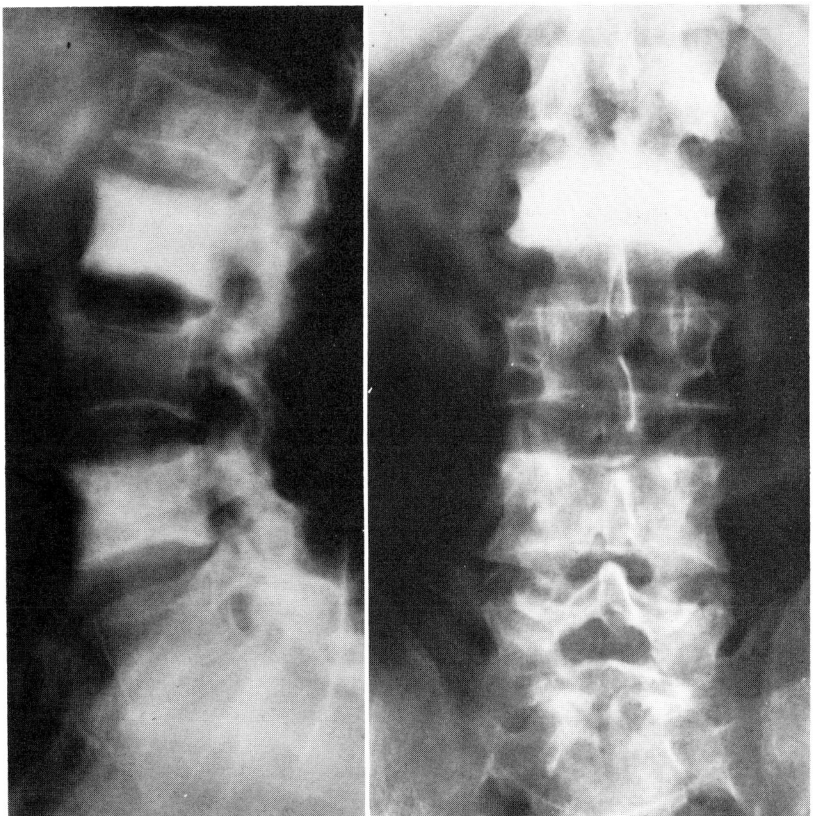

Figure 2–4. Osteoblastic metastasis to the lumbar spine from carcinoma of the pancreas. Histologically proven at autopsy. (Courtesy of Dr. Norman Joffe.)

INTRATHORACIC ABNORMALITIES

Pleuropulmonary Manifestations of Acute Pancreatitis

Acute episodes of pancreatitis are commonly associated with pleuropulmonary abnormalities. Although these are largely nonspecific, it is important to know that they can occur since, in occasional instances, clinical and radiographic evidence of chest disease is so prominent that the underlying pancreatic inflammation may not be suspected (Roseman, 1960). In other cases, appropriate weighing of chest findings may clarify readily apparent, but confusing or nonspecific, intraabdominal roentgen manifestations of the disease.

The incidence of pleuropulmonary abnormalities in patients with acute pancreatitis has ranged from 14 per cent (Fishbein, 1962) to 71 per cent (Lipp, 1950). Such manifestations are almost always observed at the lung bases, and the most frequently noted abnormalities are hemidiaphragmatic elevation, platelike subsegmental atelectasis, consolidation (either pneumonia or segmental atelectasis), and pleural effusion. Except for the last, these findings occur with almost exactly equal frequency at both lung bases and are commonly bilateral (Fig. 2–5).

Pleural effusion is considerably more common on the left side than on the right (Table 2–1). Identification of pleural effusion in a patient who could have acute pancreatitis is of major diagnostic significance, not because of any radiologic specificity, but because it allows for simultaneous determination of amylase activity in the serum and pleural fluid. Hammarsten (1959) and his associates were among the first to emphasize the importance of this procedure. They analyzed pleural fluid aspirated from four patients with acute pancreatitis, and found it to have an amylase content higher than that of serum in all instances. When serial determinations were made, pleural fluid amylase returned to normal more slowly than did the serum amylase activity. They also analyzed pleural fluid amylase in 12 patients with diseases other than pancreatitis; in 11, pleural fluid amylase levels were lower than simultaneously drawn serum levels. Subsequent reports (Roseman, 1960; Fishbein, 1962; and Goldman, 1962) have also described pleural fluid amylase activity to be greater than that of serum in patients with acute pancreatitis. Fraser and Paré (1970) have accepted an elevated level of pleural fluid amylase as a criterion for positive diagnosis of pancreatitis in patients with pleural effusions.

Pulmonary abnormalities similar to those found in acute pancreatitis also accompany pancreatic pseudocyst. In two recent reports (Caravati, 1966; Thomford, 1969), about 35 per cent of the patients had chest roentgenographic findings. Pleural effusions, usually on the left side, occurred in 17 and 20 per cent of the two series, respectively. Pleural fluid amylase activity, when determined, was higher than that of serum.

Basilar pleuropulmonary abnormalities occur in a variety of upper abdominal inflammatory conditions other than pancreatic inflammatory disease. Subdiaphragmatic abscess, gastric or intestinal perforation, acute cholecystitis, and even acute appendicitis may all produce chest findings similar to those seen in acute pancreatitis. Pancreatitis does seem to cause such changes more often than do the other conditions. Fishbein (1962) analyzed the chest roentgenograms of 100 patients with acute cholecystitis and found pleuropulmonary abnormalities in only 6 per cent of them. Freimanis and Nelson (1964) feel that, under appropriate clinical circumstances, a left pleural effusion is a likely indicator of pancreatitis. The authors of this monograph feel that whenever a pleural effusion (especially one on the left) is demonstrated in a patient who could have acute pancreatitis, serum and pleural fluid amylase activities should be simultaneously determined. This diagnostic maneuver is quick, simple, inexpensive, and of conclusive diagnostic value.

The mechanism of pleuropulmonary changes in acute pancreatitis is not fully understood. Direct spread of inflammation (via chemical and enzymatic irrita-

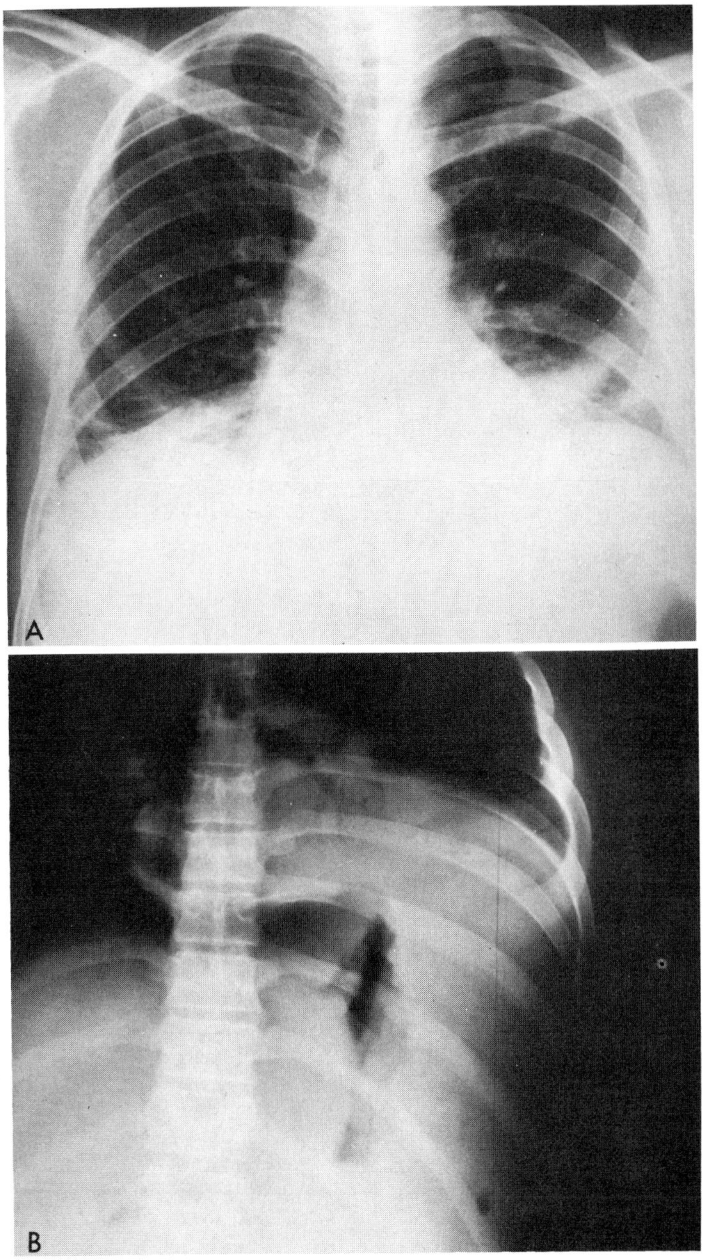

Figure 2–5. Pleuropulmonary changes in acute pancreatitis.

A, Bibasilar subsegmental atelectasis and diaphragmatic elevation.

B, Consolidation of left lower lobe (air bronchogram) with left pleural effusion. Note the gastric deformity produced by adjacent pancreatic edema. *A* and *B* are in different patients.

TABLE 2–1. Pleural Effusion in Acute Pancreatitis

	NO. OF EFFUSIONS	RIGHT	BILATERAL	LEFT
Fishbein (1962)	6	1	1	4
Schieppati (1946)	5	1		4
Coffey (1952)	6			6
Hammarsten (1959)				
Literature review	31	3	7	21
Personal series	4	1		3
Stein (1959)	1			1
TOTALS	53	6 (11%)	8 (15%)	39 (74%)

tion) through the diaphragm itself (with which the tail of the pancreas is ordinarily in direct anatomic contiguity), through hiatal orifices between the chest and the abdomen, and through the retroperitoneal tissues seems the likeliest possibility. There are rich transdiaphragmatic lymphatic connections which may play a role in the spread of inflammation.

Mediastinal Pseudocyst

On occasion, thoracic abnormalities other than those already described can accompany acute pancreatitis; pericardial effusion, pancreatobronchopleural fistula, and hemothorax are among these. Still another condition recently has attracted considerable attention. This is the development of pseudocysts in the mediastinum. At least ten such cases have now been reported (Table 2–2). As Poppel (1959) has pointed out, inflammatory collections arising in the pancreas tend to migrate in the direction offering least resistance. Extension into any adjacent potential space along tissue planes or through any opening contiguous with the cyst is possible. Pancreatic pseudocysts reach the mediastinum via the esopha-

TABLE 2–2. Roentgen Characteristics of Mediastinal Pseudocysts

	LOCATION OF MASS IN MEDIASTINUM (ALL ON LEFT)	DISPLACEMENT OF ESOPHAGUS	EFFUSION
Edlin (1951)	Posteroinferior	?	Left
Clauss (1958)	Posteroinferior	Posteriorly and to left	None
Poppel (1959)	Inferior	To left	Left*
	Posteroinferior	Anteriorly	?
Roseman (1960)	Posteroinferior	Anteriorly	Left
McClintock (1965)	Posteroinferior	Anteriorly and to left	Bilateral*
Galligan (1966)	Posteroinferior	Anteriorly and to left	None
Laird (1966)	Inferior	?	Left
Gee (1969)	Posteroinferior	?	Left*
Weidmann (1969)	Posteroinferior	Posteriorly and to left	Bilateral

*Elevated pleural fluid amylase concentration.

geal hiatus or through the aortic diaphragmatic opening. These pseudocysts present radiographically as posteroinferior mediastinal masses. On frontal chest roentgenograms, they are usually situated in a left retrocardiac position, and a left or bilateral pleural effusion is usually present (Fig. 2–6). (In at least three instances, elevated pleural fluid amylase has been detected.) Esophagography reveals compression and displacement of the lower esophagus which is usually deviated to the left anteriorly or posteriorly. On occasion, the mediastinal extension may represent an actual abscess rather than a pseudocyst (Roseman, 1960).

Mediastinal pseudocysts have occurred

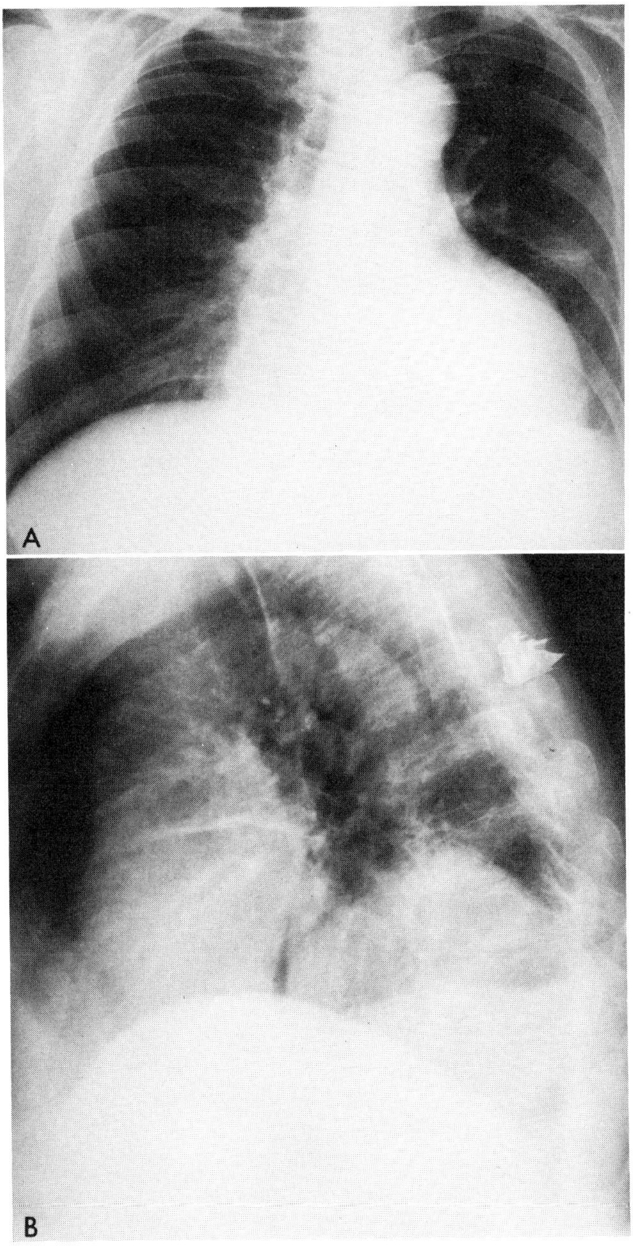

Figure 2–6. Mediastinal pseudocyst. Location in the posteromedial mediastinum is typical as is the associated left pleural effusion.

in both children and adults, usually in patients who have previously had pancreatitis. Nearly all patients have had abdominal pain, and chest discomfort, dyspnea, and dysphagia are frequently present. This diagnosis should be suspected in any patient with a posteroinferior mediastinal mass, a pleural effusion, and a history suggesting past or present pancreatitis.

Pulmonary Metastases

Pancreatic carcinomas commonly metastasize to the lungs (Frantz, 1959), and such metastases are occasionally symptom-producing. Gullick (1959) has noted the relative frequency with which pulmonary metastases can give rise to the presenting clinical complaint, especially in patients with primary lesions in the body or tail of the pancreas. The most common such presentation is that of bronchogenic carcinoma. Bronchoscopic biopsy or bronchial cytology may support misdiagnosis in these cases. Pulmonary metastasis rarely may present clinically as acute bronchopneumonia (Grant, 1954).

At autopsy, pancreatic tumors originating in the head of the organ are found to have produced pulmonary metastases in 11 to 25 per cent of the cases. Those arising in the body or tail spread to the lungs more often (in 27 to 50 per cent). Mediastinal lymph node involvement is somewhat less common, occurring in 1 to 20 per cent, and pleural metastasis occurs in 2 to 8 per cent (Leach, 1950; Bell, 1957; and Gullick, 1959).

Roentgenographically, two patterns of pulmonary metastasis can be observed. Extension of tumor into the lung from pre-existing mediastinal lymph node involvement gives rise to large masses of tumor in the hilus of the lungs, whereas hematogenous dissemination results in multiple nodules in the lung periphery (Fig. 2–7). In a series of 13 patients (Leach, 1950), peripheral lung metastases were seen in six in the absence of mediastinal lymph node involvement and, in seven, masses of secondary tumor were located in the hilus of the lung in association with large cancerous lymph nodes. This latter appearance led to an erroneous diagnosis of bronchogenic carcinoma in three instances.

INTRAABDOMINAL MANIFESTATIONS

Abnormalities of the Bowel Gas Pattern

Of all the secondary manifestations of acute pancreatitis, abnormalities of the bowel gas pattern are probably the most common. A number of different appearances have been described as occurring in pancreatitis. Though all are nonspecific, they may be the only radiologic evidence available for interpretation, so an appreciation of their nature and of differential diagnostic alternatives requiring consideration is important.

Tumors of the tail of the pancreas may indent the gastric air bubble as seen on upright chest radiographs (Fig. 2–8). Observations of this sort, though interesting, require barium upper gastrointestinal study for confirmation.

Felson (1968) has popularized the term *gasless abdomen.* This gasless appearance can be normal, but has been observed in numerous patients with acute pancreatitis (Fig. 2–9). A gasless abdomen can also be produced by high intestinal obstruction and can, uncommonly, be seen in mesenteric infarction (Tomchik, 1970). The reverse pattern—generalized adynamic ileus involving both colon and small bowel—can also be seen. Cantwell (1959) observed this phenomenon in six of 51 patients. A *sentinel loop,* a localized segment of gas-filled, dilated small bowel, has long been considered to suggest the presence of adjacent inflammation (Fig. 2–10). Although this finding is nonspecific, it does occur commonly in acute pancreatitis. Stein and his associates (1959) observed a sentinel loop in fully 55 per cent of the patients in their series. Other reports have noted this finding less often

(*Text continued on page 32*)

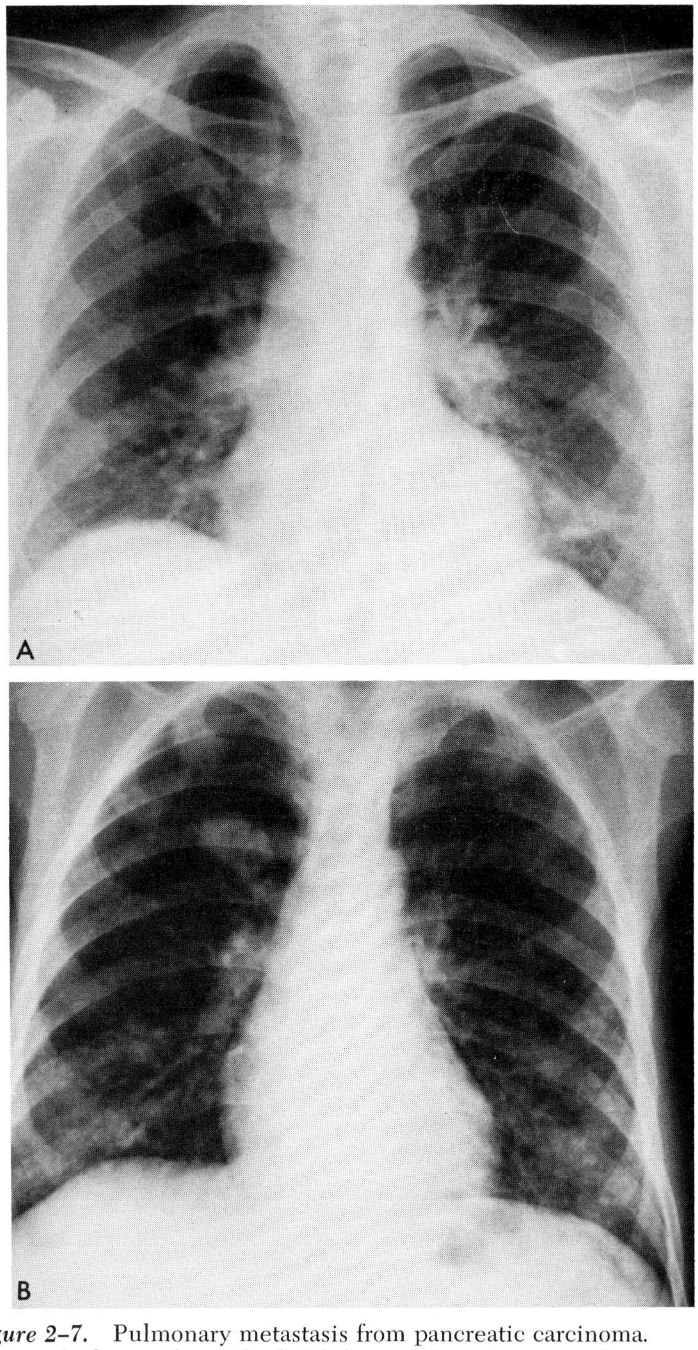

Figure 2–7. Pulmonary metastasis from pancreatic carcinoma. *A*, Lymphadenopathy at the left hilum; *B*, hematogenous dissemination.

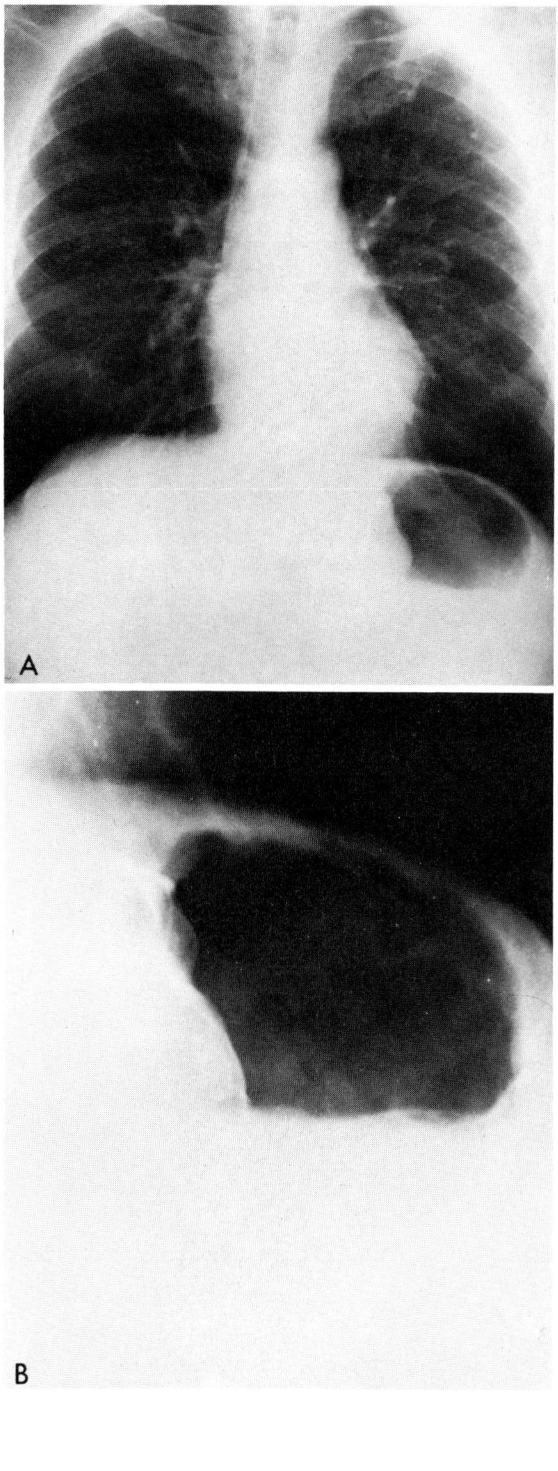

Figure 2–8. Carcinoma of the tail of the pancreas.

A, Note the indentation on the medial aspect of the gastric cardia seen on chest examination.

B, Barium gastrointestinal examination confirms the presence of extrinsic indentation.

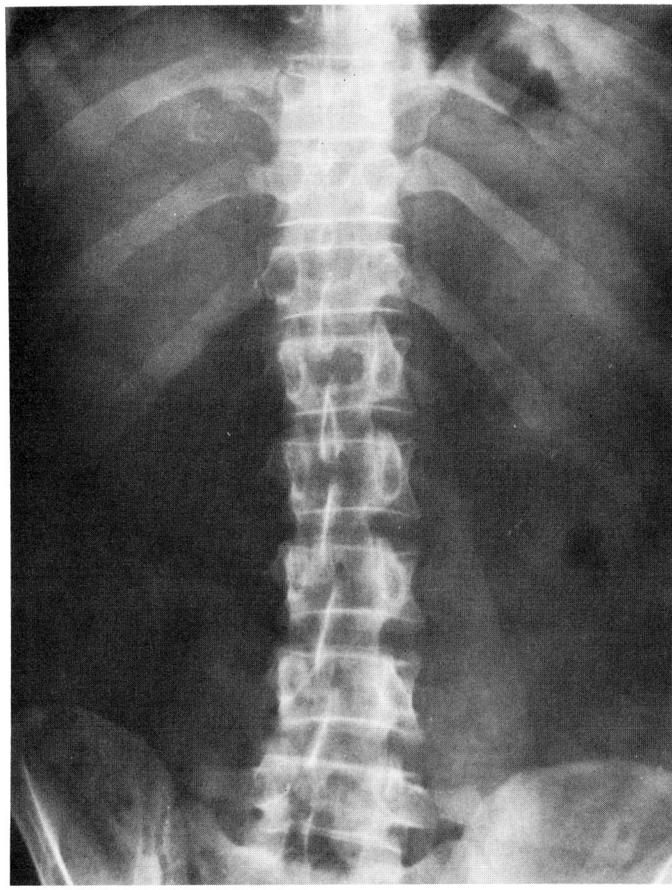

Figure 2–9. "Gasless abdomen" in acute pancreatitis. Some gas is present, but the over-all amount is markedly diminished.

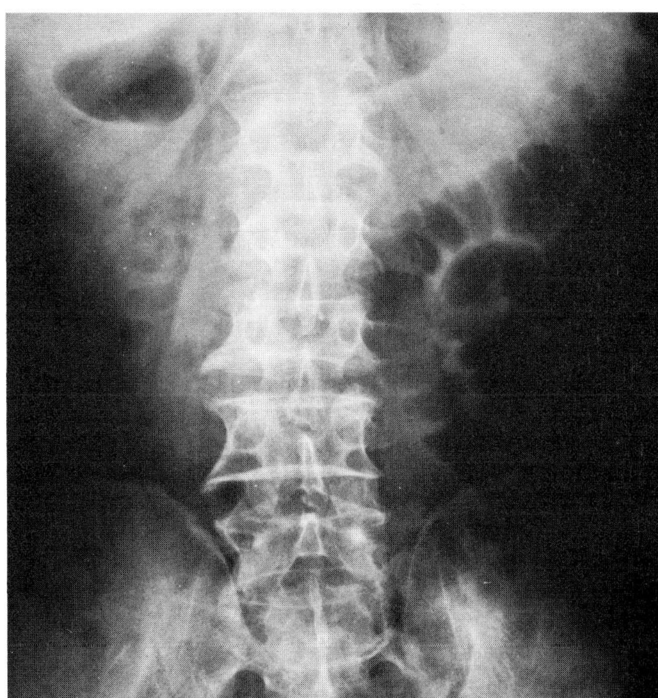

Figure 2–10. "Sentinel loop" in acute pancreatitis.

(Brascho, 1962: 33 per cent; Weens, 1964: 10 per cent) and, in Weens's material, the sign was seen as often in acute cholecystitis as in acute pancreatitis. Almost all radiologists with extensive emergency-room experience have seen sentinel loops in a variety of different acute abdominal conditions.

One type of sentinel loop phenomenon which has greater diagnostic significance than most is localized *duodenal ileus* (Fig. 2–11). Some degree of duodenal air-filling was present in fully 42 per cent of the patients with acute pancreatitis in one series (Weens, 1964), and marked gaseous dilatation of the duodenum was present in 24 per cent. Even this finding is nonspecific since it can occur in both acute pancreatitis and acute cholecystitis. Weens and Walker (1964) observed adynamic duodenal ileus with approximately the same frequency in both conditions, but the authors of this monograph have seen it much more commonly in acute pancreatitis.

The *colon cut-off sign* originally was described (Price, 1956) as an "isolated gaseous distention of the ascending colon and hepatic flexure, with sharp delimitation of the gas shadow just to the left of the hepatic flexure." Other early descriptions (e.g., Stuart, 1956) also emphasized the absence of gas in the mid-transverse colon. Brascho and his coauthors (1962), however, stressed that gaseous distention of the right and transverse colon, with abrupt cut-off of the air column at the splenic flexure, was actually a much more common manifestation of acute pancreatitis (Fig. 2–12). They observed a colon cut-off sign in 30 of 54 patients with acute pancreatitis (56 per cent). In 28 of the 30 patients with positive signs (93 per cent), the cut-off was at or just beyond the splenic flexure. Other authors have encountered

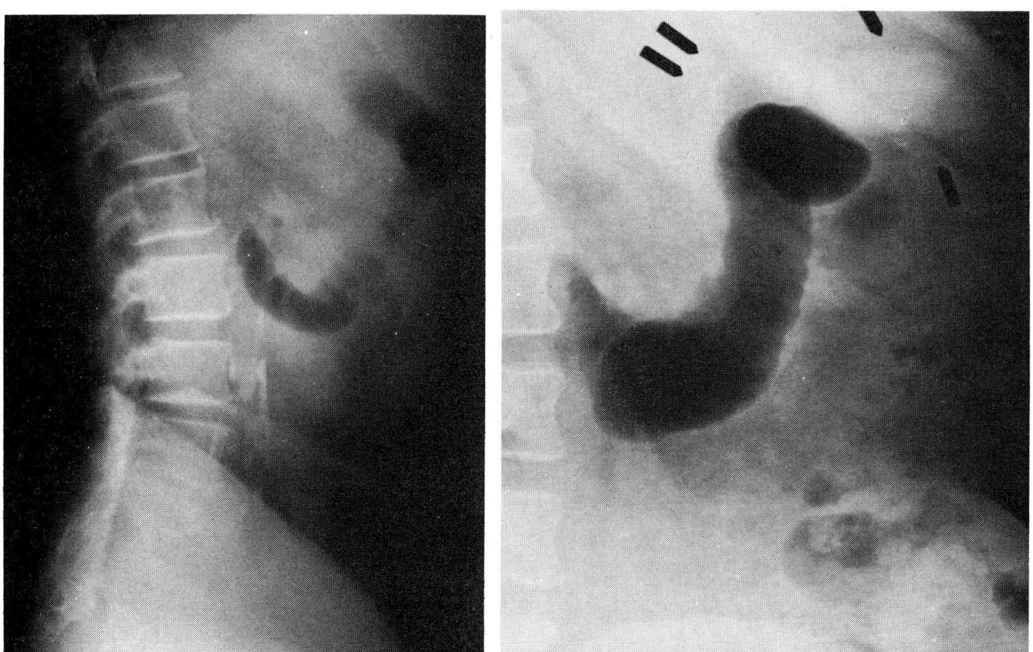

Figure 2–11. Duodenal ileus in acute pancreatitis: two examples. Note edema of folds in descending duodenum (*A*) and edema of duodenal papilla (*B*). Arrows in (*B*) delineate opacified gallbladder and common bile duct. (*B*, From Wees, H. S., and Walker, L. A.: The radiologic diagnosis of acute cholecystitis and pancreatitis. Radiol. Clin. N. Amer., 2:89–106, 1964.)

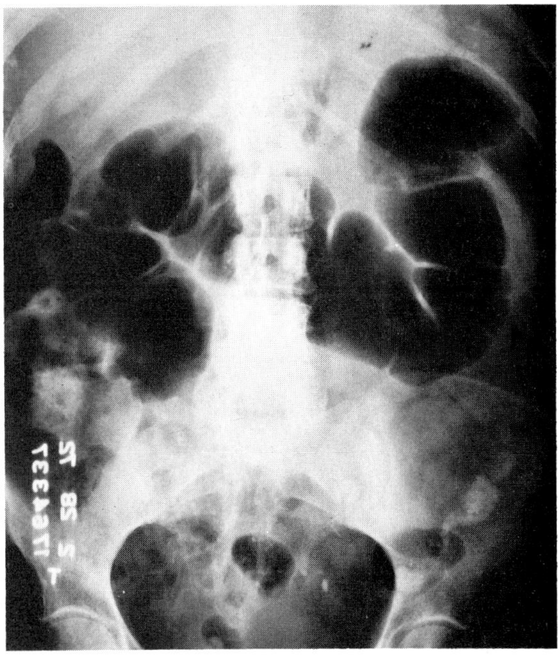

Figure 2–12. Colon cut-off sign (commonly accepted pattern). Gas distends the transverse colon in a patient with acute pancreatitis.

the colon cut-off sign much less often. Cantwell (1959) observed the original (i.e., collapsed transverse colon) sign in only one of 51 patients. Weens (1964) could find only four examples of either variety in his series of 50 unselected patients with acute pancreatitis. The personal experience of the authors of this monograph leads us to agree with Brascho, that cut-off occurs most often at the splenic flexure and with Weens, that the sign is infrequently encountered.

The pathophysiologic mechanism for the colon cut-off phenomenon is interesting. The transverse mesocolon connects the transverse colon with the anterior surface of the pancreas. Because of this relationship, the inflammatory exudate produced by acute pancreatitis can easily spread via the mesocolon to involve the transverse colon secondarily. The type of colonic response probably depends on the degree of inflammatory irritation produced. When there is only a low-grade influence, hypercontractility forces gas out of the transverse colon, giving rise to the originally described type of hepatic-flexure colon cut-off. More severe colonic involvement results in paralysis of the transverse colon, with secondary passive distention of the cecum and ascending colon—i.e., the more commonly encountered splenic-flexure colon cut-off (Poppel, 1968; Rosch, 1967). The colon thus responds to adjacent pancreatic inflammation in much the same way as the duodenum does (Bergkvist, 1959).

While a clear-cut (sic) colon cut-off sign should prompt a radiologic suggestion of acute pancreatitis, there are diagnostic alternatives. Colonic obstruction at the splenic flexure can mimic the radiographic appearance exactly, but clinical manifestations are usually quite dissimilar. On the other hand, mesenteric vascular thrombosis and even nonocclusive ischemic colitis can simulate both the radiographic and clinical appearance of acute pancreatitis. Tomchik and his associates (1970) observed a splenic-flexure cut-off pattern in 12 of 67 patients (18 per cent) with bowel infarctions.

Intraabdominal Fat Necrosis

One of the most characteristic histologic features of acute pancreatitis is focal necrosis of pancreatic and peripancreatic fat (Spjut, 1968). This finding is often grossly visible at surgery or at autopsy and has occasionally been demonstrated on plain abdominal roentgenograms (Baylin, 1944; Merner, 1958; Weens, 1964; and Berenson, 1971). The condition is almost pathognomonic of acute pancreatitis [one instance associated with enzyme-producing pancreatic cancer has been reported (Jackson, 1952)] and is the result of the action of pancreatic lipase. During acute episodes of pancreatitis, activated enzymes (including lipase) are present within the pancreatic parenchyma and reach adjacent intraabdominal tissues by direct inflammatory extension. Hydrolysis of involved fatty tissue results; ordinarily, the degree of such change is variable, producing foci of rather extensive fatty breakdown interspersed with relatively unaffected areas. The free fatty acids released by hydrolysis become saponified, and the calcium salts thus deposited in heavily involved sites produce the white, opaque, plaque-like areas which are so often observed on the pancreas, mesentery, omentum, and peritoneum at surgery.

Radiographically, intraabdominal fat necrosis is recognized as an indistinct mottling which may be localized in the area of the pancreas or may spread throughout the abdomen. Irregular, rounded areas of water density are intermingled with relatively radiolucent patches of normal fat density (Fig. 2–13). It is important to note that the abnormally dense areas which, when contrasted with adjacent tissue of normal fat density, produce the mottled pattern are not of calcium density. Because calcium does become deposited in areas of fat necrosis, it may seem logical to assume that the associated foci of increased density reflect an increased calcium content in the tissue. Although this may contribute to the roentgen findings, the major factor is hydrolysis in affected areas; this process alone probably accounts for most of the radiographically demonstrable findings (Baylin, 1944; Berenson, 1971).

Pancreatic Gas Abscess

An uncommon but very significant feature of acute pancreatic inflammation

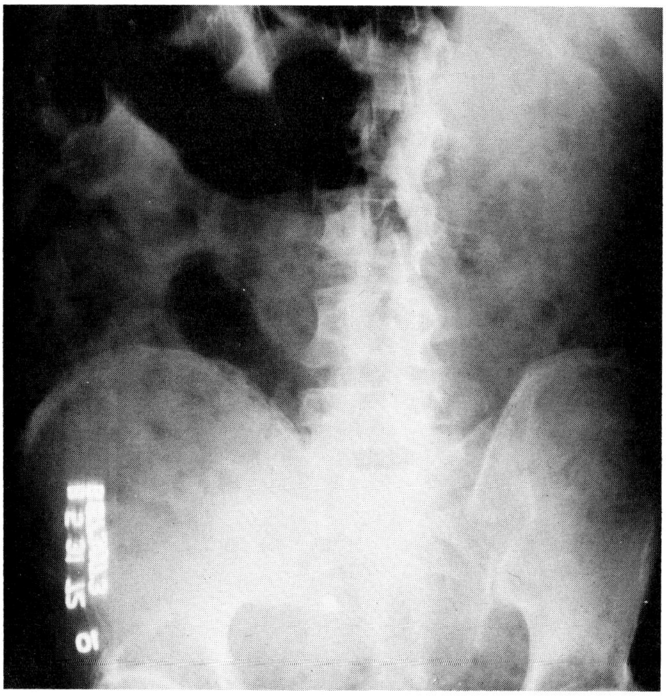

Figure 2–13. Intraabdominal fat necrosis. Note indistinctly mottled radiolucencies throughout the abdomen. The presence of fat necrosis was confirmed at surgery.

is the development of gas within the pancreas. In approximately 3 to 4 per cent of the patients with acute pancreatitis, inflammation progresses to the point of abscess formation. This development is of major clinical concern since mortality from pancreatic abscess is high (29 to 57 per cent) (Table 2–3). In discussing the management of this condition, surgeons invariably stress the importance of early diagnosis, because prompt surgical drainage offers practically the only chance for cure (Altemeier, 1963; Evans, 1969). In this regard, identification of gas within the pancreas can be of great importance.

Although several prior reports described the presence of gas within pancreatic abscesses, Felson (1957) was the first to emphasize the importance of this roentgen finding. The most common appearance is that of multiple small gas bubbles distributed within the region of the pancreas and lesser sac (Fig. 2–14, *A*, *C*). The margins of the process are ill-defined and the collection is constant in location. When contrast material is given orally, the retrogastric location of the process can be confirmed (Fig. 2–14, *B*, *D*), but this is often possible on lateral abdominal roentgenograms made without contrast material. A less common type of intrapancreatic gas collection is a single large pocket of gas or a single long air-fluid level (Fig. 2–15). This finding has even more dire prognostic significance than do multiple gas bubbles.

A collection of small vesicles of air within the upper abdomen has to be distinguished from a lesser sac abscess unrelated to pancreatic disease (e.g., after penetration of gastric or duodenal ulcer); this is uncommon since most processes of this kind produce pancreatitis secondarily and become, in essence, pancreatic abscesses. Other forms of disease which at least must be considered would include emphysematous gastritis, subphrenic abscess, and pneumatosis cystoides intestinalis. A more common differential problem is the exclusion of mixed air and fluid within the stomach, or of mixed air and feces within the transverse colon. If such differentiation cannot be made on the basis of appropriately positioned plain films, contrast studies will usually resolve the problem.

Pancreatic Calcification

Alcoholic pancreatitis is the commonest cause of pancreatic lithiasis. There are, however, a number of less frequent but interesting and important etiologic possibilities which should be considered when such calcification is demonstrated radiologically (Ring, 1973).

Alcoholic Pancreatitis

In the United States, pancreatitis occurs most commonly in patients who also

TABLE 2–3. Intrapancreatic Gas in Patients with Pancreatic Abscess

	NO. OF PATIENTS	NO. OF PATIENTS WITH INTRAPANCREATIC GAS	NO. OF DEATHS
Farringer (1967)	7	2	2
Bolooki (1968)	74	5	42
Evans (1969)	17	4	10
Altemeier (1963)	32	2	14
Felson (1957)	6	6	4
TOTALS	136	19 (14%)	72 (54%)

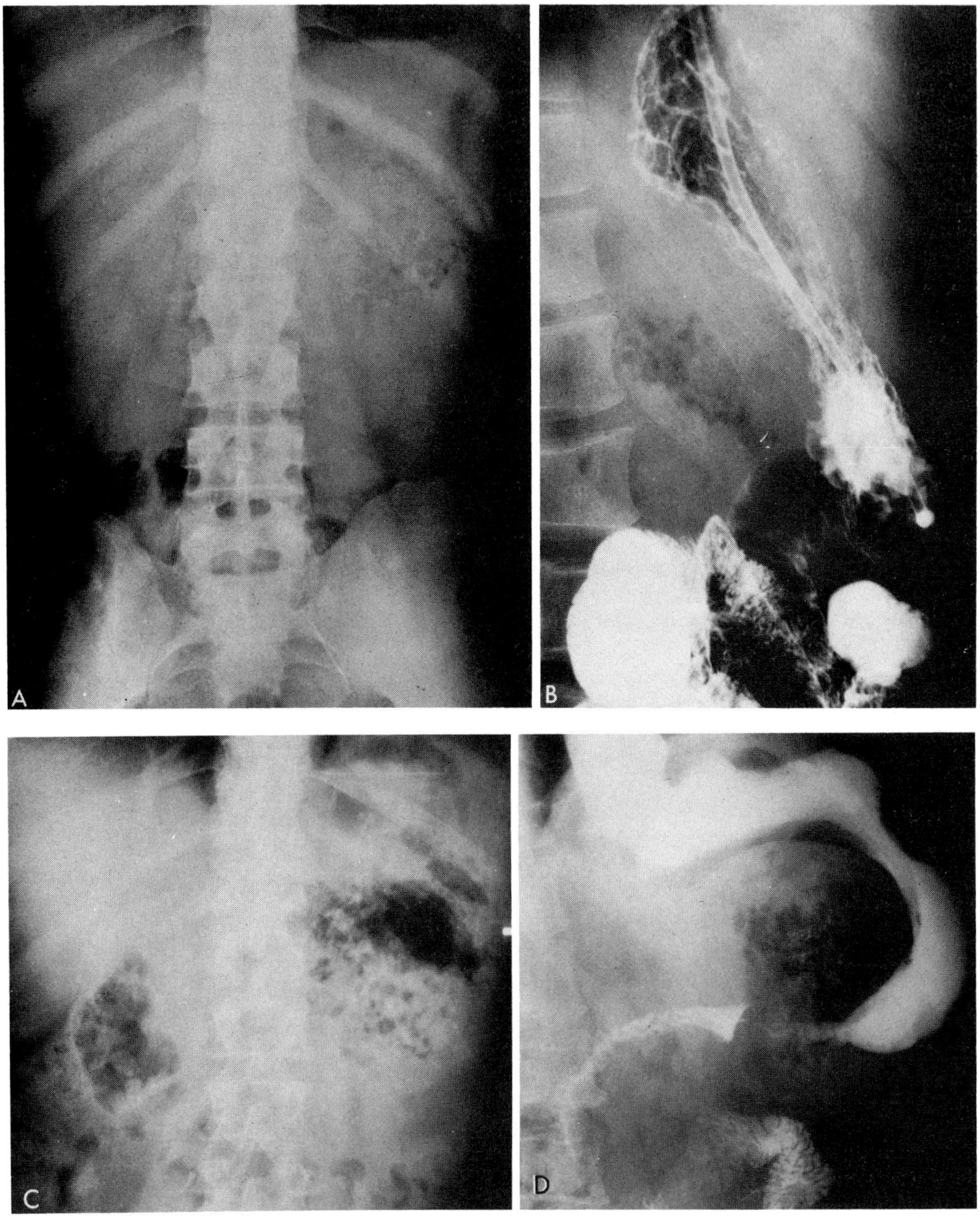

Figure 2–14. Pancreatic gas abscess: two cases. *A* and *C* show multiple small bubbles of gas in upper left midabdomen. *B* and *D* are upper gastrointestinal barium examinations which demonstrate the retrogastric location of the respective abscesses.

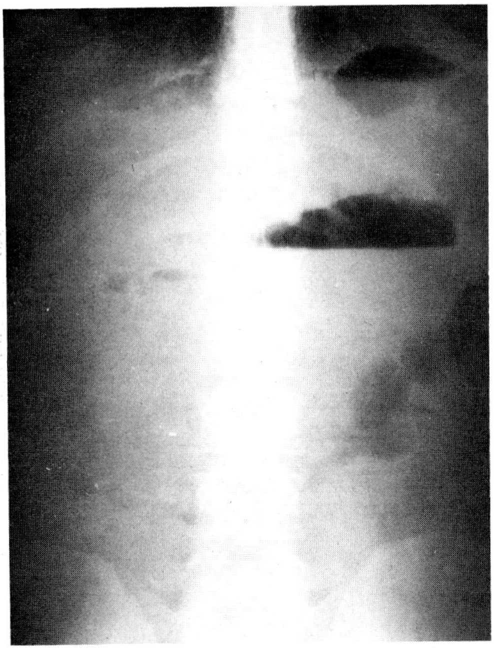

Figure 2–15. Pancreatic abscess. Large air and fluid collection in the region of the pancreas, with a prominent air-fluid level on this upright roentgenogram.

have biliary tract disease or who suffer from alcoholism; the former, however, seldom produces pancreatic calcification. The incidence of pancreatic lithiasis in patients with "gallstone pancreatitis" is only 2 per cent or less (Howard, 1960). On the other hand, 20 to 40 per cent of all patients with chronic alcoholic pancreatitis develop intrapancreatic calcific deposits (Sarles, 1965; Owens, 1958). Conversely, in most series of patients with pancreatic calcification, about 85 to 90 per cent of them are alcoholics (Howard, 1960).

Calcification encountered in chronic alcoholic pancreatitis usually develops only after 5 to 10 years of episodic abdominal pain (Howard, 1960), and consists almost exclusively of intraductal calculi (McGeorge, 1957). These calcifications appear radiographically as numerous irregular, small concretions deposited throughout the gland (Fig. 2–16). Calcifications are limited to the head or tail of the pancreas in about a quarter of all cases, but solitary pancreatic calculi are rare. True calcification of pancreatic parenchyma can occur after trauma or infarction where there has been intraparenchymal hemorrhage. Pancreatic calcification can be observed in 12 to 20 per cent of all patients who develop pseudocysts as a complication of pancreatitis. Usually the pattern of calcification is similar to that seen in patients with uncomplicated chronic pancreatitis but, occasionally, a rim of

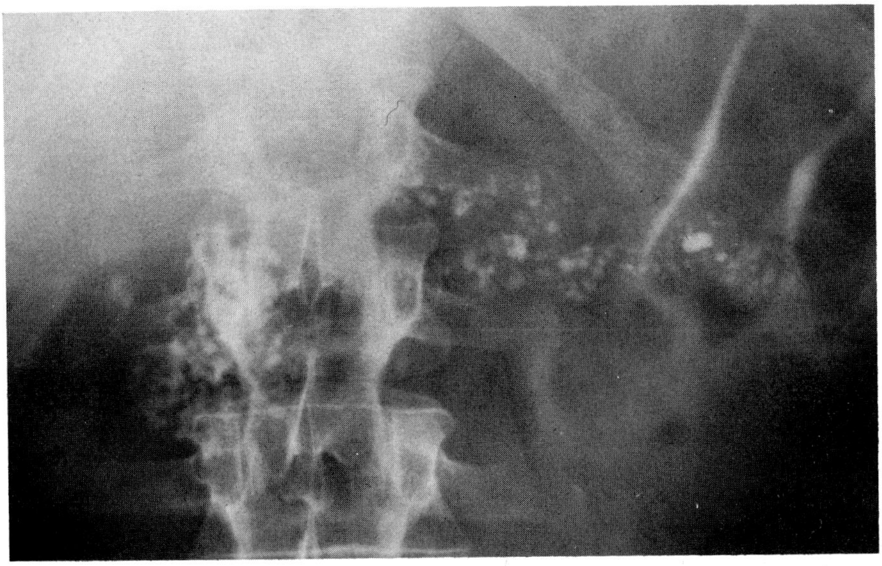

Figure 2–16. Alcoholic pancreatitis. Calculi, distributed throughout the pancreas, vary in size but are generally small.

calcification outlines the pseudocyst (Fig. 2–17).

Hereditary Pancreatitis

Hereditary pancreatitis is an autosomal dominant disorder characterized by recurrent episodes of abdominal pain usually beginning in childhood and continuing despite all efforts at therapy. More than 100 patients, members of over 20 kindreds, have now been reported (Kattwinkel, 1973). In some of these families, aminoaciduria has been an associated feature (Gross, 1962). No consistent anatomic abnormality of the pancreas, ducts, or ampulla has been found in the more than 40 patients who have undergone surgical exploration.

Many patients with hereditary pancreatitis ultimately develop pancreatic cancer; fully 21 per cent of all deaths in patients with this disorder have been the result of pancreatic malignancy. An even higher proportion of these individuals develop pancreatic lithiasis. Thirteen of the 22 patients (59 per cent) studied by Kattwinkel (1973) had radiographically visible calcifications. The calcifications are typically rounded and are often larger than those found in other pancreatic diseases (Fig. 2–18). This appearance may allow a radiologic diagnosis, especially in relatively young, nonalcoholic patients.

Hyperparathyroidism

It is now accepted that pancreatitis may develop in patients with hyperparathyroidism. This association has been estimated to occur in 6.5 to 18.9 per cent of all patients with hyperparathyroidism (Schmidt, 1970; Ludwig, 1966). Though the exact mechanism remains open to question, most authors agree that the former disorder occurs as a result of the latter, a relationship substantiated by numerous instances in which parathyroidectomy was followed by remission of pancreatitis (Mixter, 1962; Herskovic, 1967).

About half of the patients whose hyperparathyroidism is complicated by pancreatitis develop chronic disease and, in these individuals, pancreatic calcification is frequently detected. This finding was noted in 45 per cent of the

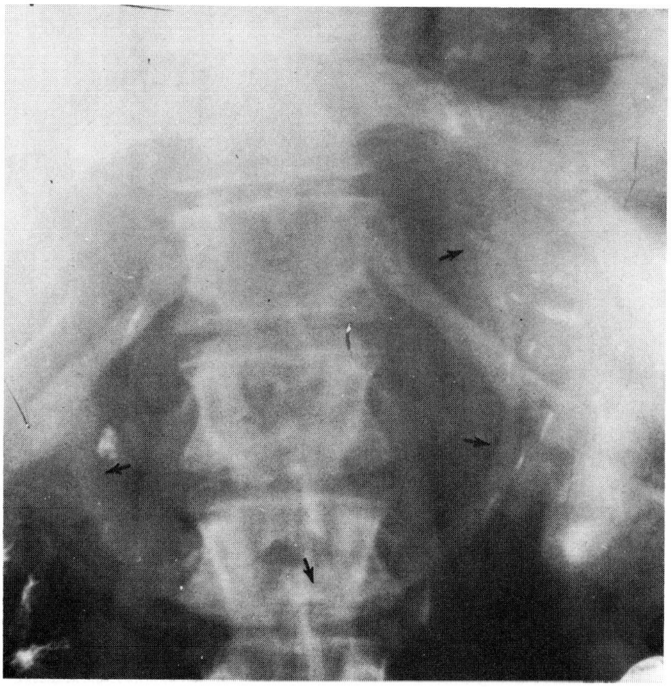

Figure 2–17. Pancreatic pseudocyst. A faint rim of calcification *(arrows)* outlines the cyst.

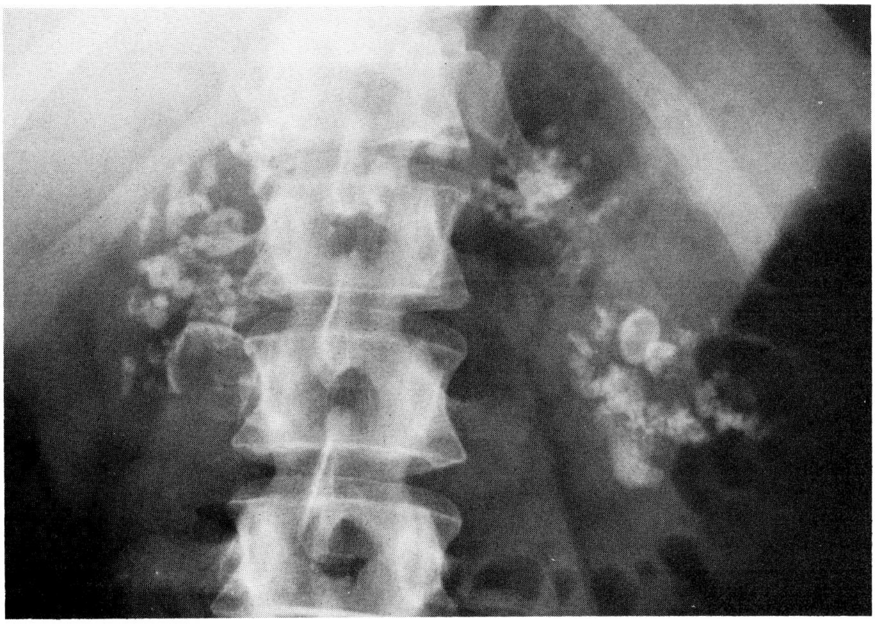

Figure 2–18. Hereditary pancreatitis. Note the large calculi present, a feature typical of hereditary pancreatitis.

62 American patients studied by Mixter (1962) and in 25 per cent of the 24 European patients analyzed by Schmidt (1970). Based on published reports, there is nothing unique about the pancreatic lithiasis present in hyperparathyroidism, but there is a very high incidence of associated nephrocalcinosis and nephrolithiasis in such cases (Fig. 2–19). Renal calcification was present in 70 per cent of the patients reported by Ludwig (1966), regardless of whether or not pancreatic calcification was present. Six patients with hyperparathyroidism and pancreatic calcification studied by Stobbe (1970) all had a significant

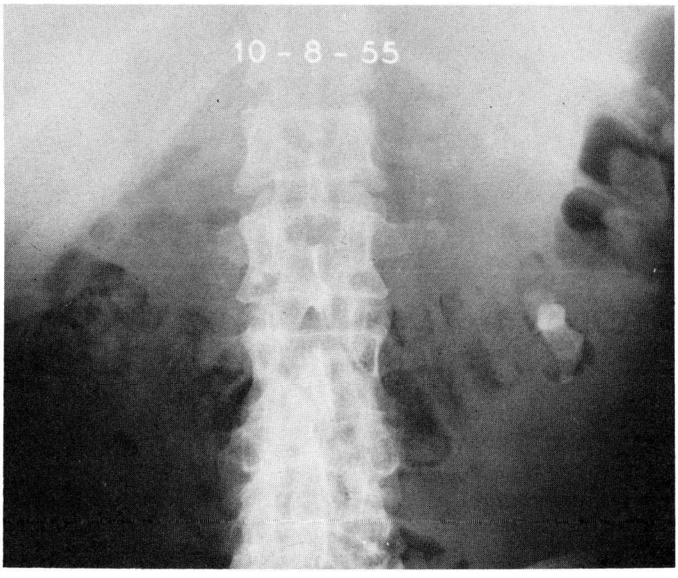

Figure 2–19. Hyperparathyroidism. Note staghorn calculus in the left renal pelvis, together with diffuse pancreatic calcification. (From Gross, J. B.: Some recent developments pertaining to pancreatitis. Ann. Intern. Med. *49*:796–819, 1958.)

degree of nephrocalcinosis. Since pancreatitis may develop before there is any overt evidence of hyperparathyroidism (Cope, 1957; Warshaw, 1968), it is incumbent upon radiologists to suggest the possibility of parathyroid disease whenever renal and pancreatic calcifications are found together.

Kwashiorkor (Protein Malnutrition)

In the emerging nations of the world, pancreatic calcification is frequently associated with protein malnutrition. The patients involved may develop histologic abnormalities of the pancreatic acinar cells in early childhood (Blackburn, 1969), and often manifest pancreatic lithiasis before reaching adulthood (Zuidema, 1959; Olurin, 1969). Abdominal pain is a less prominent feature in these patients than in Western patients, but complications such as diabetes and steatorrhea are more common and tend to develop at an earlier age. In most African and Asian patients, there has been no history of alcoholism, but in Uganda many patients with pancreatic calcification have had a history of heavy drinking in addition to low protein nutrition (Shaper, 1964).

The calcification present in such patients is radiographically similar to that seen in Western patients with chronic alcoholism (Fig. 2–20), but the historic and geographic factors involved should allow prompt diagnosis.

Cystic Fibrosis

Pancreatic calcification is found at autopsy in many patients with cystic fibrosis (Anderson, 1938) and, occasionally, such calcification may be apparent on abdominal radiographs (Singleton, 1968). Reeves (1948) reported such calcification in a patient who was only 4 years old. Patients with roentgenographically visible pancreatic calcification usually have fairly advanced pancreatic fibrosis associated with diabetes mellitus (Rosan, 1962; Grossman, 1966). Typically, the calcification is finely granular in appearance (Fig. 2–21); individual calculi are almost invariably smaller than the fairly large deposits which characterize hereditary pancreati-

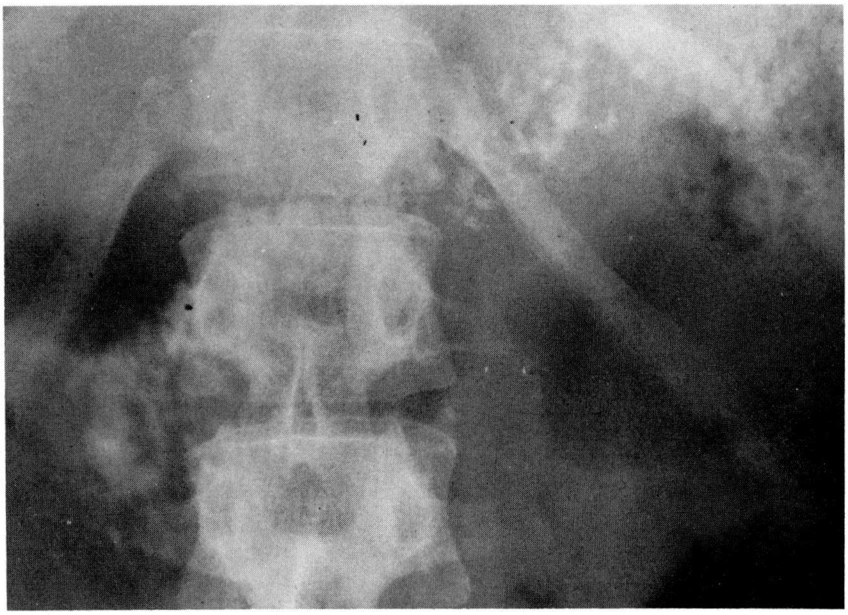

Figure 2–20. Kwashiorkor. Calculi are distributed throughout the pancreas. By radiographic criteria alone, they are indistinguishable from those found in alcoholic pancreatitis. (Courtesy of Dr. Stanley Borher.)

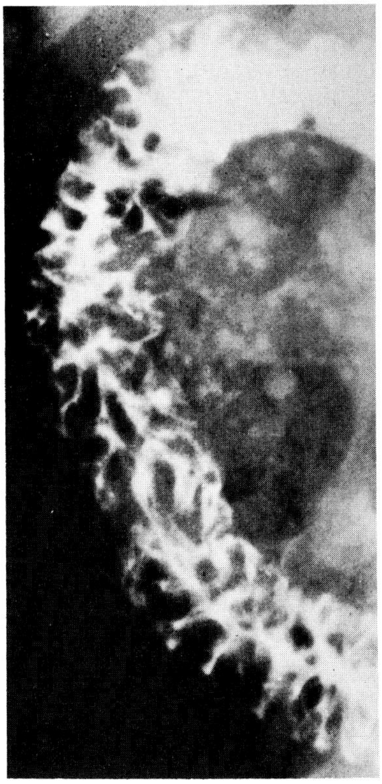

Figure 2–21. Cystic fibrosis. Numerous small calculi are present in the head of the pancreas. (Courtesy of Dr. Walter Berdon.)

tis. These two conditions account for the great majority of pediatric pancreatic lithiasis encountered in this country, so it is of some interest that the patterns of calcification are often radiographically distinct. In most instances, however, the diagnosis of cystic fibrosis will have been made before pancreatic calcification is manifested. Rarely, alcoholism can produce chronic pancreatitis and pancreatic lithiasis in the pediatric age group (Schmidt, 1964).

Idiopathic Pancreatic Calcification

Most series of patients with radiographically demonstrable pancreatic calcification include at least a few individuals in whom there have been no clinical manifestations of pancreatic disease (McGeorge, 1957; Kelley, 1957). The causes for calcification in these patients are not fully understood. Some cases may represent the effects of "painless pancreatitis" (Goulston, 1962), but this does not appear to explain all the cases without clinical signs. Stobbe (1970) recently studied histologic material from 22 patients with symptomless pancreatic lithiasis (only one was an alcoholic). In each case, the calculi were found "upstream" from an area of nonspecific pancreatic ductal obstruction. Pathologically, these patients had ductal dilatation, periductal fibrosis, parenchymal atrophy, and fatty replacement in the involved portions of the pancreas. These findings were felt to represent the effects of obstructive atrophy rather than chronic inflammation.

Pancreatic Calcification and Pancreatic Cancer

There is an increased incidence of pancreatic cancer in patients with chronic pancreatitis (Paulino-Netto, 1960; Ansari, 1968). This relationship is true for alcoholic pancreatitis, and even more so for hereditary pancreatitis; one-fifth of all the deaths which have occurred in patients studied for the latter disorder have been due to pancreatic cancer (Kattwinkel, 1973). The incidence of pancreatic cancer has been reported to be particularly high in patients with pancreatic calcification. Paulino-Netto (1960) suggested that 20 per cent of all patients with pancreatic lithiasis might have concurrent pancreatic carcinoma. Subsequently, Johnson (1963) reviewed 677 cases and found only 24 (3.7 per cent) with coexisting carcinoma. In Guien's (1972) series of French patients with pancreatic calcification, only 2 per cent had carcinoma. Conversely, in two recent studies of patients with pancreatic cancer, only three of 183 (1.6 per cent) had pancreatic lithiasis (Ansari, 1968; Rastogi, 1967). A consideration of these statistics reveals that benign disease will be present in over 95 per cent of all the patients with radiologically demonstrable pancreatic lithiasis. Thus, while the incidence of pancreatic cancer in patients with pancreatic calcification is very significantly higher than that for the general population, this roentgen finding should still be considered an indicator of benign rather than malignant pancreatic disease.

In those uncommon instances in which pancreatic cancer and pancreatic lithiasis coexist, the calcium usually represents the effect of pre-existing pancreatitis and is diffusely present throughout the gland. In occasional instances, however, malignant pancreatic ductal obstruction has produced lithiasis which is restricted to that portion of the organ upstream from the obstruction (Stobbe, 1970).

In one widely publicized instance, pancreatic calculi secondary to chronic pancreatitis were observed to disappear in a patient who later developed pancreatic carcinoma (Tucker, 1963). The same phenomenon (i.e., disappearing calcification) has been noted in patients with chronic pancreatitis alone (Baltaxe, 1967; Stein, 1965). Along the same lines, displacement of pre-existing calcification may define the growth of pseudocysts (Alexander, 1952) (Fig. 2–22).

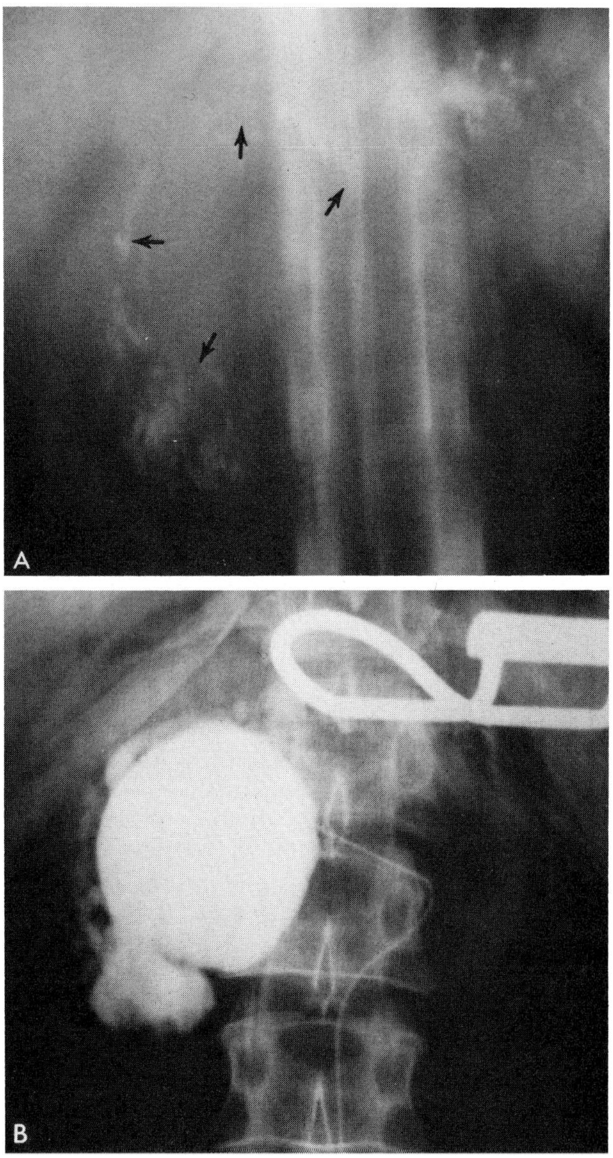

Figure 2–22. Pancreatic pseudocyst.

A, An anteroposterior laminogram reveals displacement of pre-existing pancreatic calcification by a rounded mass within the head and proximal body of the pancreas.

B, Intraoperative cystogram. Note how closely the cyst contour corresponds to the area defined by displacement of calcification as shown in *A*.

Tumor Calcification

For all practical purposes, adenocarcinoma of the pancreas is not associated with tumor calcification. Actual tumor calcification does occur, however, in approximately 10 per cent of the patients with cystadenoma or cystadenocarcinoma of the pancreas (Piper, 1962; Becker, 1965). In many instances, the calcification found in such tumors is nonspecific in its radiographic appearance but, occasionally, a radiating "sunburst" pattern is present (Haukohl, 1950). This configuration correlates with gross pathologic findings in which cystic spaces are seen to separate spoke-like stromal elements which radiate from a central nidus. When such calcification is observed, a specific plain-film diagnosis can be made (Fig. 2–23).

One other rare pancreatic tumor, the cavernous lymphangioma, calcifies and again the pattern of calcification may allow plain-film diagnosis (Fig. 2–24). In such cases, a collection of phleboliths in and adjacent to the pancreas is the characteristic feature (Dodds, 1969).

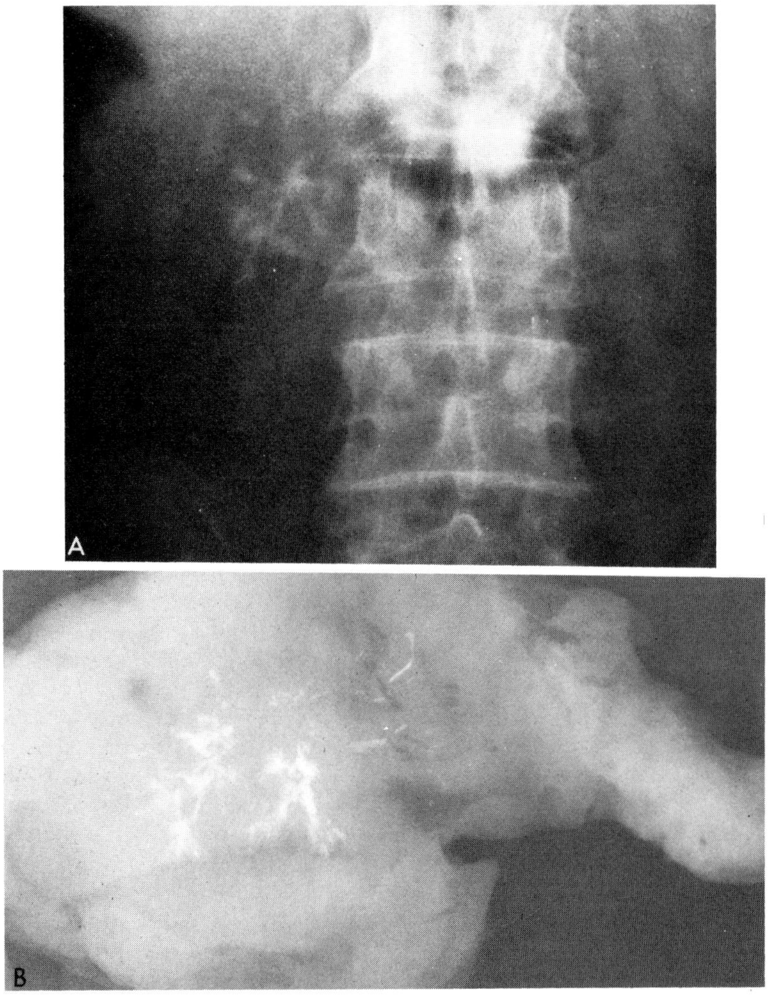

Figure 2–23. Pancreatic cystadenocarcinoma.
A, Supine abdominal roentgenogram reveals a "sunburst" pattern of calcification.
B, Postmortem roentgenogram better demonstrates the nature of calcification.

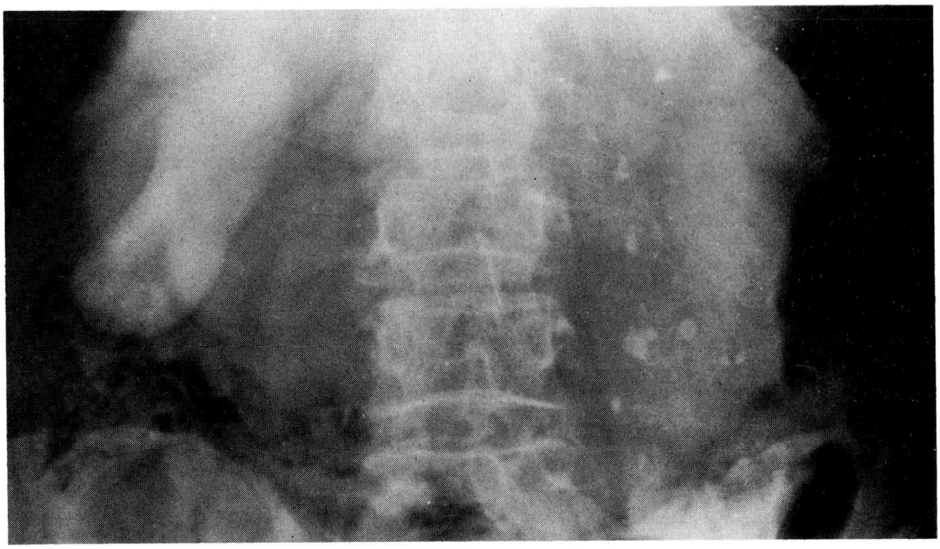

Figure 2–24. Cavernous lymphangioma of the pancreas. Multiple phleboliths are located in and adjacent to the tail of the pancreas. (From Dodds, W. J., Margolin, F. R., and Goldberg, H. I.: Cavernous lymphangioma of the pancreas. Radiol. Clin. Biol., *38*:267–270, 1969.)

Miscellaneous Intraabdominal Abnormalities

Splenomegaly

Enlargement of the spleen in a patient clinically suspected of having pancreatic disease should direct attention to the possibility of splenic and/or portal venous involvement, thereby adding some support to the provisional clinical diagnosis (Longstreth, 1971). In one series, the spleen was enlarged (presumably due to splenic vein obstruction) in ten of 46 patients (22 per cent) with carcinoma arising in the body or tail of the pancreas (Mani, 1966). This experience is similar to that reported in the older literature (Duff, 1939: 25 per cent). Neoplasms occurring in the head of the pancreas produce secondary splenomegaly less often, but can do so via portal venous obstruction. Pancreatitis (Rosch, 1962) and pseudocysts (Varriale, 1963) can also block the splenic or portal veins, resulting in splenomegaly (Fig. 2–25). Detection of splenomegaly on plain abdominal roentgenograms should be followed up by a careful search for esophageal and/or gastric varices on barium upper gastrointestinal examination (see Chapter 3).

Gallbladder Enlargement

A dilated gallbladder can occasionally be identified on plain abdominal roentgenograms (Fig. 2–26) when its margins indent adjacent gas-containing alimentary structures (usually the hepatic flexure of the colon). In a patient with jaundice, such a finding represents good evidence of the Courvoisier phenomenon. Courvoisier pointed out that a palpable (i.e., enlarged) gallbladder was commonly present in patients whose jaundice was the result of pancreaticoduodenal malignancy. In contrast, patients whose jaundice was due to choledocholithiasis usually had chronic cholecystitis as well. In these patients, the gallbladder was rarely palpable. Experience has shown that absence of Courvoisier's sign has little significance but, when an enlarged gallbladder can be demonstrated, malignant obstruction of the distal common bile duct is very likely. Hess (1965) has found gallbladder dilatation at surgery in 87 per cent of his patients with carcinoma of the head of the pancreas. Criteria for gallbladder enlargement are not well established, but a transverse diameter greater than 5 cm. probably is abnormal (Redman, 1970).

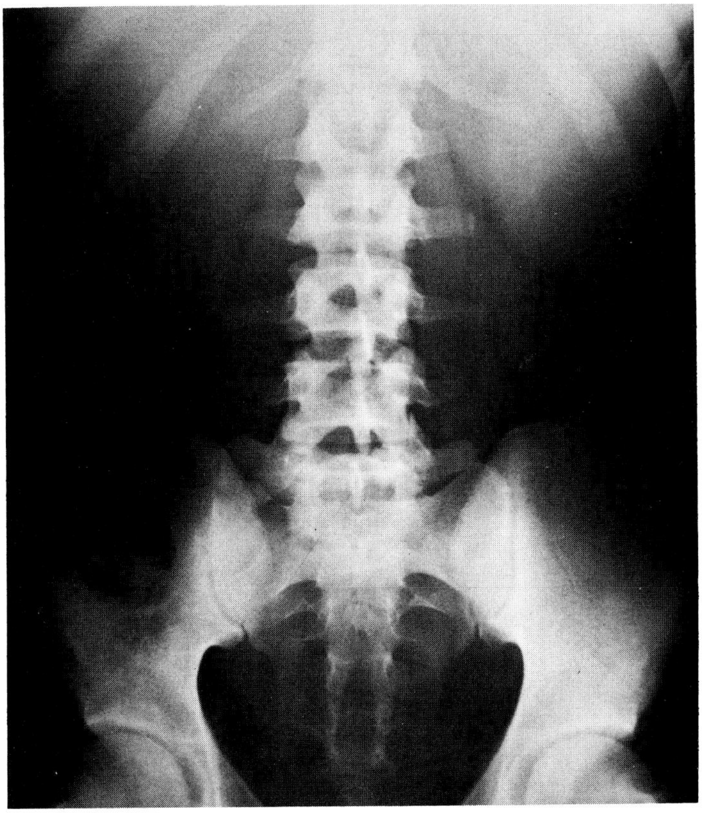

Figure 2–25. Splenomegaly due to splenic vein thrombosis in pancreatitis.

Pancreatic Mass Effect

In rare instances, a soft-tissue mass located in or near the pancreas may give plain-film evidence of pancreatic disease. In some cases, this may take the form of increased separation between the gastric and transverse colonic gas shadows. This occurs most often in acute pancreatitis. In other instances, there may be a poorly defined upper abdominal mass effect which correlates with a clinically palpable mass. This appearance is found most often in patients with large pseudocysts (Fig. 2–27).

Ascites

Although seldom considered a manifestation of pancreatic disease, ascites can result from disorders of the pancreas. Mikal (1950) found ascites in 57 per cent of the patients with cancer of the head of the pancreas, and in 68 per cent of the patients with cancer of the body or tail. In most instances of this kind, ascites indicates the presence of peritoneal metastases. Hess (1965) encountered ascites in 40 per cent of his patients with carcinoma of the body or tail of the pancreas; in every instance, the fluid contained malignant cells, and the underlying tumors were found to be inoperable. Ascites also occurs ocasionally in acute (Poppel, 1968; Rosch, 1967) and chronic (Cameron, 1967) pancreatitis. When pancreatic ascites persists over a long period of time, the possibility of a pancreatic pseudocyst with leakage of cyst contents into the peritoneal cavity should be considered (Schindler, 1970). Rarely, chylous ascites occurs in patients with pancreatic disease. Lymphatic obstruction is usually considered the pathologic mechanism for this phenomenon which can develop either in benign (Gambill, 1960) or in malignant disease (Dodd, 1970) (Fig. 2–28).

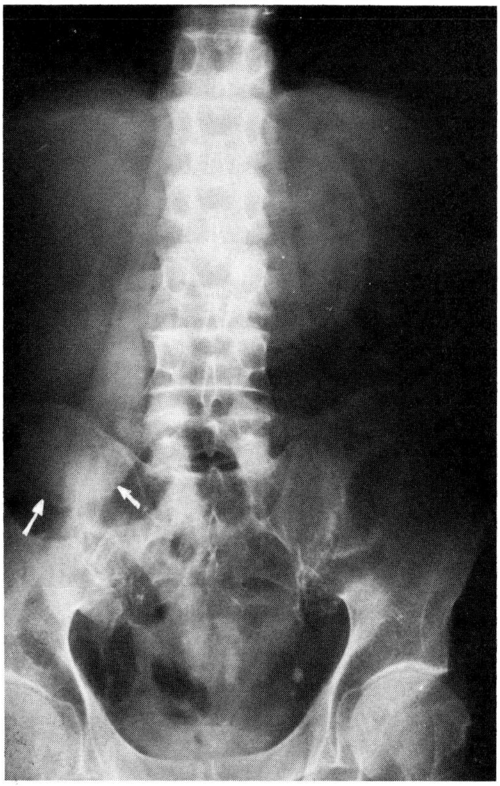

Figure 2–26. Courvoisier gallbladder. The arrows outline the distended gallbladder; the lower pole of the right kidney is visible just above the right iliac crest.

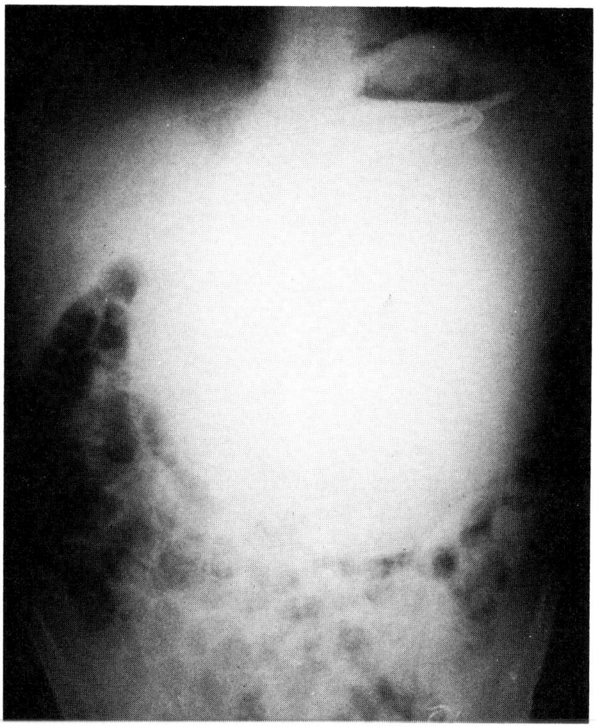

Figure 2–27. Pancreatic pseudocyst. There is a poorly defined mass effect in the left upper abdominal quadrant. This was found at surgery to result from a pancreatic pseudocyst arising from the body and tail of the organ.

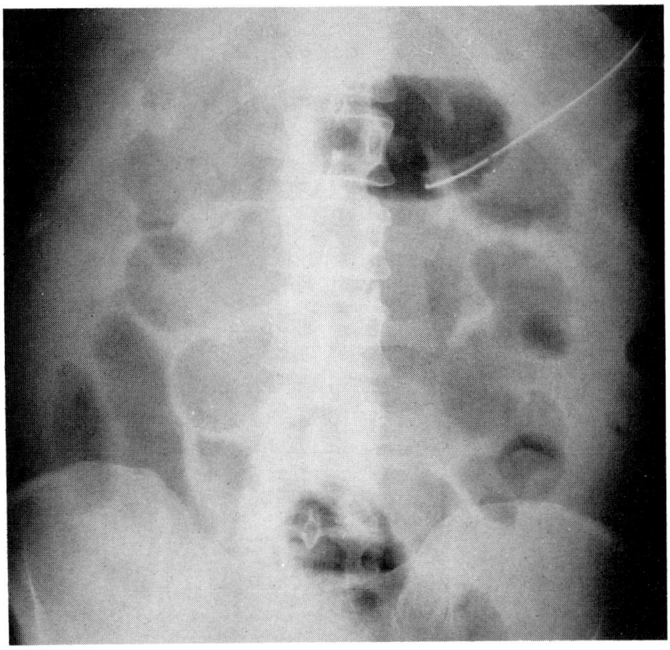

Figure 2–28. Chylous ascites in pancreatic carcinoma. Over 3 liters of milk-white ascitic fluid were removed from the patient's abdomen after this roentgenogram was obtained.

REFERENCES

Alexander, G. H., and Lowder, R. J.: Definition of pancreatic cysts within pancreatic calcification: report of two cases. Gastroenterology, *21*:439–443, 1952.

Altemeier, W. A., and Alexander, J. W.: Pancreatic abscess. A study of 32 cases. Arch. Surg., *87*: 80–89, 1963.

Andersen, D. H.: Cystic fibrosis of the pancreas and its relation to celiac disease: a clinical and pathologic study. Amer. J. Dis. Child., *56*: 344–399, 1938.

Ansari, A., and Burch, G. E.: A correlative study of proven carcinoma of the pancreas in 83 patients. Amer. J. Gastroent., *50*:456–475, 1968.

Baltaxe, H. A., and Leslie, E. V.: Vanishing pancreatic calcifications. Amer. J. Roentgen., 99:642–644, 1967.

Bank, S., Marks, I. N., Farman, J., and Immelman, E. J.: Further observations of calcified medullary bone lesions in chronic pancreatitis. Gastroenterology, *51*:224–230, 1966.

Baylin, G. J., and Weeks, K. D.: Some roentgen aspects of pancreatic necrosis. Radiology, *42*:466–470, 1944.

Becker, W. F., Welsh, R. A., and Pratt, H. S.: Cystadenoma and cystadenocarcinoma of the pancreas. Ann. Surg., *161*:845–863, 1965.

Bell, E. T.: Carcinoma of the pancreas. I. A clinical and pathologic study of 609 necropsied cases. II. The relation of carcinoma of the pancreas to diabetes mellitus. Amer. J. Path., *33*:499–523, 1957.

Berenson, J. E., Spitz, H. B., and Felson, B.: The abdominal fat necrosis sign. Radiology, *100*: 567–571, 1971.

Bergkvist, A., and Seldinger, S. I.: Contrast roentgenography in differential diagnosis between perforated ulcer and acute pancreatitis. Acta Chir. Scand., *118*:137–145, 1959.

Blackburn, W. R., and Vinijchaikul, K.: The pancreas in kwashiorkor. Lab. Invest., *20*:305–318, 1969.

Bolooki, H., Jaffe, B., and Biliedman, M. L.: Pancreatic abscesses and lesser omental sac collections. Surg. Gynec. Obstet., *126*:1301–1308, 1968.

Borak, J.: Roentgen examination of pancreatic tumors. Radiology, *41*:170–180, 1943.

Brascho, D. J., Reynolds, R. N., and Zanca, P.: The radiographic "colon cut-off sign" in acute pancreatitis. Radiology, 79:763–768, 1962.

Caffey, J.: The pancreas. *In* Pediatric X-ray Diagnosis. Chicago, Ill., Year Book Medical Publishers Inc., 1967, pp. 455–457.

Cameron, J. L., Anderson, R. P., and Zuidema, G. D.: Pancreatic ascites. Surg. Gynec. Obstet., *125*:328–332, 1967.

Cantwell, D. E., and Pollock, A. V.: Radiology of acute pancreatitis. J. Fac. Radiol., *10*:95–99, 1959.

Caravati, C. M., Ashworth, J. S., and Frederick, P.: Pancreatic pseudocysts: a medical evaluation. J.A.M.A., *197*:572–576, 1966.

Clauss, R. H., and Wilson, D. W.: Pancreatic pseudocyst of the mediastinum. J. Thorac. Surg., *35*:795–801, 1958.

Coffey, R. J.: Unusual features of acute pancreatic disease. Ann. Surg., *135*:715–720, 1952.
Cope, O., Culver, P. J., Mixter, C. G., and Nardi, G. L.: Pancreatitis: diagnostic clue to hyperparathyroidism. Ann. Surg., *145*:857–863, 1957.
Dodd, G. D.: Lymphography in diseases of the liver and pancreas. Radiol. Clin. N. Amer., *8*:69–84, 1970.
Dodds, W. J., Margolin, F. R., and Goldberg, H. I.: Cavernous lymphangioma of the pancreas. Radiol. Clin. Biol., *38*:267–270, 1969.
Duff, G. L.: Clinical and pathological features of carcinoma of body and tail of pancreas. Bull. Johns Hopkins Hosp., *65*:69–100, 1939.
Edlin, P.: Mediastinal pseudocyst of the pancreas. Gastroenterology, *17*:96–102, 1951.
Evans, F. C.: Pancreatic abscess. Amer. J. Surg., *117*:537–540, 1969.
Farringer, J. L., Robbins, L. B., and Pickens, D. R.: Abscess of the pancreas: diagnosis and treatment. Amer. Surg., *33*:139–142, 1967.
Felson, B.: Gas abscess of pancreas. J.A.M.A., *163*:637–641, 1957.
Felson, B.: Letter from the editor. Seminars Roentgen., *3*:215–216, 1968.
Fishbein, R., Murphy, G. P., and Wilder, R. J.: The pleuropulmonary manifestations of pancreatitis. Dis. Chest, *41*:392–397, 1962.
Frantz, V. K.: Tumors of the pancreas. *In* Atlas of Tumor Pathology, Section VII, Fascicles 27 and 28, Armed Forces Institute of Pathology, Washington, D.C., 1959.
Fraser, R. G., and Paré, J. A. P.: Diagnosis of Diseases of the Chest. Philadelphia, W. B. Saunders Company, 1970, pp. 520–521.
Freimanis, A. K., and Nelson, S. W.: The chest roentgenogram in the diagnosis of acute abdominal disease. Radiol. Clin. N. Amer., *2*: 3–20, 1964.
Galligan, J. J., and Williams, H. J.: Pancreatic pseudocysts in childhood. Amer. J. Dis. Child., *112*:479–482, 1966.
Gambill, E. E., Baggenstoss, A. H., and Priestley, J. T.: Chronic relapsing pancreatitis: fate of fifty-six patients first encountered in the years 1939 to 1943, inclusive. Gastroenterology, *39*:404–413, 1960.
Gambill, E. E., Walters, W., and Scanlon, P. W.: Chronic relapsing pancreatitis with extensive subacute peritonitis and chronic, recurrent massive "chylous ascites." Amer. J. Med. *28*: 668–670, 1960.
Gee, W., Foster, E. D., and Doohen, D. J.: Mediastinal pancreatic pseudocyst. Ann. Surg., *169*:420–424, 1969.
Gerle, R. D., Walker, L. A., Achord, J. L., and Weens, H. S.: Osseous changes in chronic pancreatitis. Radiology, *85*:330–337, 1965.
Geyman, M. J., and Present, A. J.: Carcinoma of the pancreas with generalized bone metastases. Amer. J. Roentgen., *57*:220–223, 1947.
Gillison, E. W., Grainger, R. G., and Fernandez, D.: Osteoblastic metastases in carcinoma of pancreas. Brit. J. Radiol., *43*:818–820, 1970.
Goldman, M., Goldman, G., and Fleischner, F. G.: Pleural-fluid amylase in acute pancreatitis. New Eng. J. Med., *266*:715–716, 1962.
Goulston, S. J. M., and Gallagher, N. D.: Chronic painless pancreatitis. Gut, *25*:252–254, 1962.
Grant, G. H., and Perceral, P. E.: Carcinoma of the pancreas in a girl of 16, presenting as carcinomatosis of the lungs. Brit. Med. J. *1*: 857, 1954.
Gross, J. B., Ulrich, J. A., and Maber, E. T.: Further observations on the hereditary form of pancreatitis. *In* The Exocrine Pancreas, Ciba Foundation Symposium. Edited by A. V. S. DeReuck and M. P. Cameron. Boston, Little, Brown and Company, 1962, pp. 278–305.
Grossman, H., Berdon, W. E., and Baker, D. H.: Gastrointestinal findings in cystic fibrosis. Amer. J. Roentgen., *97*:227–238, 1966.
Guien, C.: General radiology of the pancreas. Clinics Gastroent., *1*:61–83, 1972.
Gullick, H. D.: Carcinoma of the pancreas. A review and critical study of 100 cases. Medicine, *38*:47–84, 1959.
Hammarsten, J. E., Honska, W. L., and Limes, J. L.: Pleural fluid amylase in pancreatitis and other diseases. Amer. Rev. Tuberc. Pulmon. Dis., *79*:606–611, 1959.
Herskovic, T., Keating, F. R., and Gross, J. B.: Coexistent pancreatitis and hyperparathyroidism: observations on 15 cases. Gastroenterology, *52*:1093, 1967.
Hess, W.: Surgery of the Biliary Passages and the Pancreas. Princeton, N. J., D. Van Nostrand Company, Inc., 1965, p. 125.
Haukohl, R. S., and Melamed, A.: Cystadenoma of the pancreas. A report of two cases showing calcification. Amer. J. Roentgen., *63*:234–245, 1950.
Holt, J. F.: Roentgen diagnosis of pancreatic cyst. Radiology, *46*:329–333, 1946.
Howard, J. M.: Pancreatic calcification. *In* Surgical Diseases of the Pancreas. Edited by J. M. Howard and G. L. Jordan. Philadelphia, J. B. Lippincott Company, 1960, p. 203.
Immelman, E. J., Bank, S., Krige, H., and Marks, I. N.: Roentgenologic and clinical features of intramedullary fat necrosis in bones in acute and chronic pancreatitis. Amer. J. Med., *36*: 97–105, 1964.
Jackson, S. H., Savidge, R. S., Stein, L., and Varley, H.: Carcinoma of the pancreas associated with fat-necrosis. Lancet, *263*:962–967, 1952.
Johnson, J. R., and Zintel, H. A.: Pancreatic calcification and cancer of the pancreas. Surg. Gynec. Obstet., *117*:585–588, 1963.
Kattwinkel, J., Lapey, A., diSant 'Agnese, P. A., and Edwards, W. A.: Hereditary pancreatitis: three new kindreds and a critical review of the literature. Pediatrics, *51*:55–69, 1973.
Kelley, M. L., Squire, L. F., Boynton, L. C., and Logan, V. W.: The significance of pancreatic calcifications. New York J. Med., *57*:721–730, 1957.
Laird, C. A., and Clagett, O. T.: Mediastinal pseudocyst of the pancreas in a child: a report of a case. Surgery, *60*:465–469, 1966.
Leach, W. B.: Carcinoma of the pancreas: a clinical and pathological analysis of thirty-nine autopsied cases. Amer. J. Path., *26*:333–347, 1950.

Lipp, W. E., and Aaron, A. H.: Acute pancreatitis: further observations of value in its recognition. New York J. Med., *50*:2043–2047, 1950.

Longstreth, G. F., Newcomer, A. D., and Green, P. A.: Extrahepatic portal hypertension caused by chronic pancreatitis. Ann. Intern. Med., *75*: 903–908, 1971.

Ludwig, G. D., and Chaykin, L. B.: Pancreatitis associated with primary hyperparathyroidism. Med. Clin. N. Amer., *50*:1403–1418, 1966.

Mani, J. R., Zboralske, F. F., and Margulis, A. R.: Carcinoma of the body and tail of the pancreas. Amer. J. Roentgen., *96*:429–446, 1966.

McClintock, J. T., McFee, J. L., and Quimby, R. L.: Pancreatic pseudocyst presenting as a mediastinal tumor. J.A.M.A., *192*:229–230, 1965.

McGeorge, C. K., Wildmann, B. P., Ostrum, H., and Miller, R. F.: Diffuse calcification of the pancreas. Amer. J. Roentgen., *78*:599–606, 1957.

Merner, T. B.: Acute pancreatitis with peritoneal fat necrosis. Amer. J. Roentgen., *80*:67–72, 1958.

Mikal, S., and Campbell, A. J. A.: Carcinoma of the pancreas: diagnostic and operative criteria based on 100 consecutive autopsies. Surgery, *28*:963–969, 1950.

Mixter, C. G., Keynes, W., Chir, M., and Cope, O.: Further experiences with pancreatitis as a diagnostic clue to hyperparathyroidism. New Eng. J. Med., *266*:265–272, 1962.

Olurin, R. O., and Olurin, O.: Pancreatic calcification: a report of 45 cases. Brit. Med. J., *4*:534–539, 1969.

Owens, J. L., and Howard, J. M.: Pancreatic calcification: a late sequel in the natural history of chronic alcoholism and alcoholic pancreatitis. Ann. Surg., *147*:326–338, 1958.

Paulino-Netto, A., Dreiling, D. A., Baronofsky, I. D.: The relationship between pancreatic calcification and cancer of the pancreas. Ann. Surg., *151*:530–537, 1960.

Piper, C. E., ReMine, W. H., and Priestley, J. R.: Pancreatic cystadenomata: report of 20 cases. J. A. M. A., *180*:648–652, 1962.

Poppel, M. H.: Some migratory aspects of inflammatory collections of pancreatic origin. Radiology, *72*:323–329, 1959.

Poppel, M. H.: The roentgen manifestations of pancreatitis. Seminars Roentgen., *3*:227–241, 1968.

Price, C. W. R.: The colon cut-off sign of acute pancreatitis. Med. J. Aust., *1*:313–314, 1956.

Rastogi, H., and Brown, C. H.: Carcinoma of the pancreas. A review of one hundred cases. Cleveland Clinic Quart., *34*:243–263, 1967.

Redman, H. C., and Reuter, S. R.: The angiographic evaluation of gallbladder dilatation. Radiology, *97*:367–370, 1970.

Reeves, R. J., and Moran, F. T.: Diffuse pancreatic calcification. An analysis of six cases. Radiology, *51*:219–224, 1948.

Ring, E. J., Eaton, S. B., Ferrucci, J. T., and Short, W. F.: The differential diagnosis of pancreatic calcification. Amer. J. Roentgen, *117*:446–452, 1973.

Rosan, R. C., Schwachman, H., and Kulczvcki, L. L.: Diabetes mellitus and cystic fibrosis of the pancreas. Laboratory and clinical observations. Amer. J. Dis. Child., *104*:625–634, 1962.

Rosch, J.: Roentgenologic diagnosis of pancreatic disease. Amer. J. Roentgen., *100*:664–672, 1967.

Rosch, J., and Herfort, K.: Contribution of splenoportography to the diagnosis of diseases of the pancreas. Acta Med. Scand., *171*:251–272, 1962.

Roseman, D. M., Kowlessar, O. D., and Sleisenger, M. H.: Pulmonary manifestations of pancreatitis. New Eng. J. Med., *263*:294–296, 1960.

Sarles, H., Sarles, J. C., Camatte, R., et al: Observations on 205 confirmed cases of acute pancreatitis, recurring pancreatitis, and chronic pancreatitis. Gut, *6*:545–559, 1965.

Scarpelli, D. G.: Fat necrosis of bone marrow in acute pancreatitis. Amer. J. Path., *32*:1077–1087, 1956.

Schieppatti, E.: Pleural effusion in acute pancreatitis. Bol. Trab. Acad. Argent. Cir., *30*:1115–1134, 1946.

Schindler, S. C., Schaefer, J. W., Hull, D., et al: Chronic pancreatic ascites. Gastroenterology, *59*:453–459, 1970.

Schmidt, B. J., Barros Barreto, H. P., Barbante, P. J., et al: Pancreatic lithiasis due to malnutrition and alcoholism in a child. J. Pediat., *65*:613–615, 1964.

Schmidt, H., and Creutzfeldt, W.: Calciphylactic pancreatitis and pancreatitis in hyperparathyroidism. Clin. Orthop., *69*:135–145, 1970.

Shaper, A. G.: Aetiology of chronic pancreatic fibrosis with calcification seen in Uganda. Brit. Med. J., *1*:1607–1609, 1964.

Singleton, E. G., and Gray, P. M.: Radiologic evaluation of pancreatic diseases in children. Seminars Roentgen., *3*:267–279, 1968.

Spjut, H. G., and Anderson, M. S.: Pathology of the pancreas. Seminars Roentgen., *3*:217–226, 1968.

Stein, G. N., Kalser, M. H., Sarian, N. N., and Finkelstein, A.: An evaluation of the roentgen changes in acute pancreatitis: correlation with clinical findings. Gastroenterology, *36*:354–361, 1959.

Stein, G. N.: X-ray investigation of the pancreas. *In* Gastroenterology, Vol. 3., 2nd ed. Edited by H. L. Bockus. Philadelphia, W. B. Saunders Company, 1965, pp. 998–1017.

Stobbe, K. C., ReMine, W. H., and Bagganstoss, A. H.: Pancreatic lithiasis. Surg. Gynec. Obstet., *131*:1090–1099, 1970.

Stuart, C.: Acute pancreatitis: new Radiodiagnostic sign. J. Fac. Radiol., *8*:50–58, 1956.

Thomford, N. R., and Jesseph, J. E.: Pseudocyst of the pancreas. A review of fifty cases. Amer. J. Surg., *118*:86–94, 1969.

Tomchik, F. S., Wittenberg, J., and Ottinger, L. W.: Roentgenographic spectrum of bowel infarction. Radiology, *96*:249–260, 1970.

Tucker, D. H., and Moore, I. B.: Vanishing pancreatic calcification in chronic pancreatitis. New Eng. J. Med., *268*:31–33, 1963.

Turner, J. W., and Jaffee, H. L.: Metastatic neoplasm. Amer. J. Roentgen., *43*:479–492, 1940.

Varriale, P., Bonanno, C. A., and Grace, W. J.:

Portal hypertension secondary to pancreatic pseudocysts. Arch. Intern. Med., *112*:191–198, 1963.

Weidmann, P., Rutishauser, W., Siegenthaler, W., et al: Mediastinal pseudocyst of the pancreas. Amer. J. Med., *46*:454–459, 1969.

Weens, H. S., and Walker, L. A.: The radiologic diagnosis of acute cholecystitis and pancreatitis. Radiol. Clin. N. Amer., *2*:89–106, 1964.

Warshaw, A. L., Heizer, W. D., and Laster, L.: Pancreatic insufficiency as the presenting feature of hyperparathyroidism. Ann. Intern. Med., *68*:161–167, 1968.

Zuidema, P. J.: Cirrhosis and dissemininated calcification of the pancreas in patients with malnutrition. Trop. Geograph. Med., *11*:70–74, 1959.

Chapter 3

CONVENTIONAL CONTRAST EXAMINATIONS IN PANCREATIC DISEASE: Extraduodenal Manifestations

Pancreatic disease may produce abnormalities of the distal esophagus, stomach, mesenteric small bowel, or colon. These manifestations are all demonstrable by conventional barium examination, and an understanding of their nature is essential because such findings may be the only radiologic sign of pancreatic disease. Furthermore, awareness of these manifestations may explain apparent diagnostic contradictions when clinical parameters suggest pancreatic disease, but roentgen study reveals only abnormalities of viscera (e.g., the esophagus or colon) not ordinarily considered to reflect pancreatic disease. In occasional instances, abnormal findings demonstrated by excretory urography and intravenous cholangiography may also represent the effects of pancreatic disease. Misdiagnosis is understandably common when such changes occur.

It is the aim of this chapter to illustrate and comment on extraduodenal manifestations of pancreatic disease demonstrable by upper gastrointestinal examination, barium enema, excretory urography, and intravenous cholangiography.

ESOPHAGUS

Varices

When chronic pancreatitis, pancreatic pseudocyst, or pancreatic carcinoma involves the body or tail of the pancreas, stenosis or occlusion of the splenic vein commonly results (Sutton, 1970). Both splenoportography and splenic arteriography have been utilized to demonstrate this phenomenon which is particularly common in carcinoma where over 90 per cent of the patients have been observed to have such changes (Rosch, 1964; Buranasiri, 1972). Not surprisingly, esophageal varices frequently develop when the splenic vein is completely obstructed (Yale, 1971) (Fig. 3–1). Therefore, demonstration of varices by barium study can be considered indirect evidence of pancreatic disease when clinical findings also support the diagnosis. The value of esophageal varices as a sign of pancreatic disease is further increased if primary liver disease (e.g., cirrhosis) is considered unlikely on the basis of clinical and chemical data. One additional qualification concerns those patients in whom prehepatic (or subhepatic) portal hypertension has been present since early childhood. In these cases, primary portal vein thrombosis is nearly always the underlying condition. Such thrombosis may have developed in association with omphalitis or dehydration, but seldom represents a response to pancreatic disease. On the other hand, when prehepatic portal hypertension develops during adult life, pancreatic disease is the most likely etiologic factor (Child, 1964).

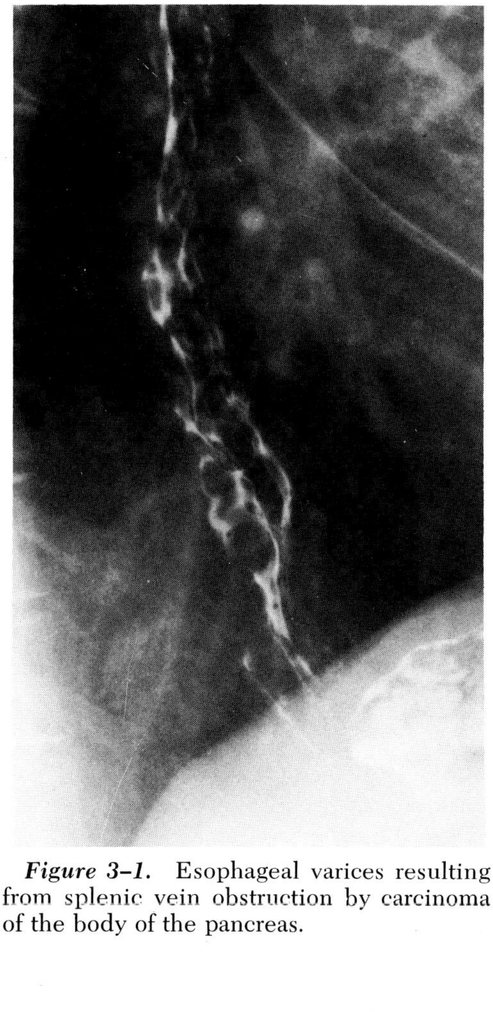

Figure 3–1. Esophageal varices resulting from splenic vein obstruction by carcinoma of the body of the pancreas.

Displacement and/or Stenosis

Changes in the position or configuration of the distal esophagus can be the result of both pseudocysts and malignant tumors of the tail of the pancreas. At least ten cases of *pancreatic pseudocyst* extending through the esophageal and/or aortic diaphragmatic hiatus into the lower middle or posterior mediastinum have now been reported. The cardinal roentgen characteristic of most of these cases has been a posteroinferior mediastinal mass visible on chest radiographs but, in several instances, anterior displacement of the distal esophagus, together with a long, smoothly tapered narrowing of the involved esophageal segment, has also been present (Fig. 3–2). Pleural effusion, pancreatic calcification and evidence of retrogastric mass are other fairly common features (see Table 2–2, Chapter 2). When the supradiaphragmatic components alone are present, a correct diagnosis can only be suspected on the basis of historic features such as alcoholism, previous episodes of pancreatitis, or abdominal trauma. However, when a retrogastric mass is also present and in continuity with the lower mediastinal lesions, pancreatic pseudocyst should be suggested by the roentgen findings alone. Differential considerations would include neurogenic tumor, aortic aneurysm, collateral varicose channels, lymphadenopathy (especially lymphoma), and alimentary tract duplication.

Even when they remain confined to the abdomen, *mass lesions arising from the tail of the pancreas* occasionally de-

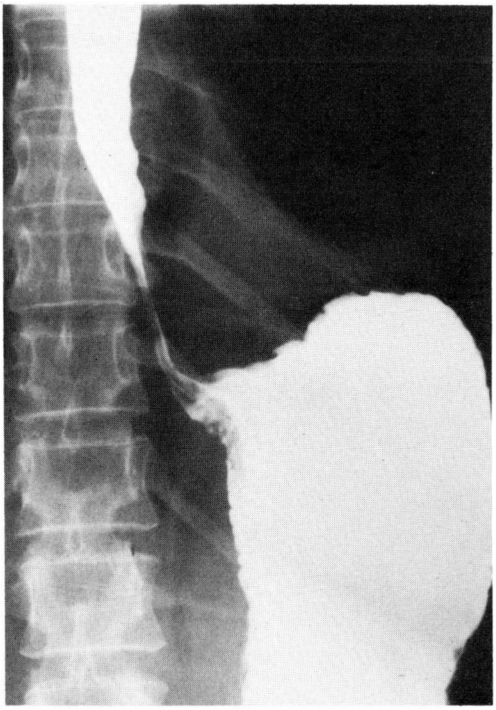

Figure 3–2. Distal esophageal narrowing produced by a mediastinal pseudocyst. The narrowed segment was constant in two separate examinations.

form the distal esophagus (Strang, 1953). Most commonly, tumors in this location produce an upward displacement of the subdiaphragmatic portion of the esophagus, giving it an exaggerated horizontal orientation as it enters the gastric cardia. A mass indentation effect involving the inferior aspect of the subdiaphragmatic esophagus and adjacent stomach is commonly present as well (Fig. 3–3). Actual invasion of the distal esophagus can also occur. A stenotic segment suggestive of primary esophageal or gastric carcinoma is thus produced (Fig. 3–4) and, in such cases, the patient may actually present with dysphagia.

STOMACH

In contrast to the rarity of esophageal changes arising as a result of pancreatic disease, roentgen abnormalities of the stomach are common. Retrospective studies have suggested that over 50 per cent of the patients with cancer arising in any part of the pancreas have gastric findings

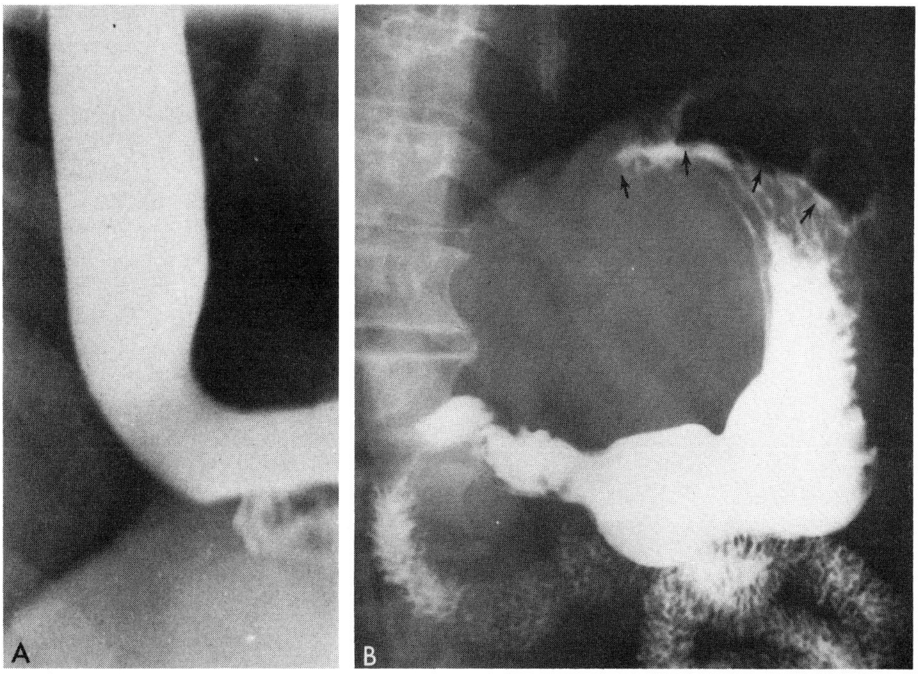

Figure 3–3. Upward displacement of the subdiaphragmatic portion of the esophagus, producing an abnormally horizontal course. Note the extrinsic indentation effect on both the esophagus (*A*) and the adjacent portion of the gastric fundus (*B*). Changes were produced by carcinoma of the tail of the pancreas.

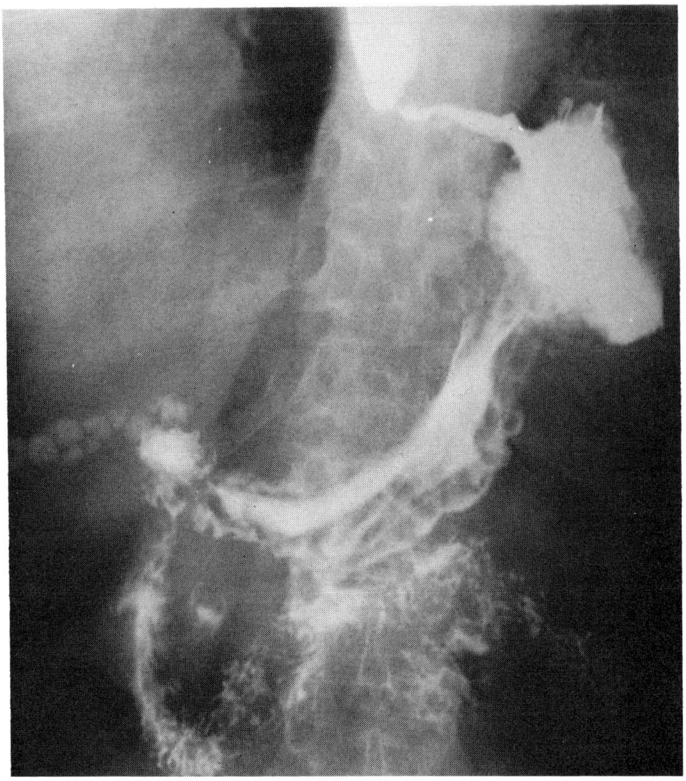

Figure 3–4. Distal esophageal stricture due to invasion by carcinoma of the tail of the pancreas.

(Broadbent, 1951; Eyler, 1962). Lesions of the body and/or tail produce gastric abnormalities more often than do those confined to the head. In one series of 46 tumors confined to the body and/or tail of the organ, the incidence of gastric abnormalities visible in retrospect was 83 per cent (Mani, 1966). Pancreatic pseudocysts produce gastric findings with at least equal frequency. The incidence of such changes has ranged from 70 to 82 per cent in different reviews (Shockman, 1967; Tomford, 1969; and Caravati, 1966). Gastric abnormalities demonstrable by barium study during acute pancreatitis have been less frequently described than have those due to neoplasm or pseudocyst but, in carefully analyzed series, they appear to be present in over 50 per cent of the patients examined (Schultz, 1963).

Several different types of gastric abnormalities have been described in patients with pancreatic disease. Some of these are widely accepted while others are controversial; some are common and others are infrequently encountered; none are absolutely specific and some are frankly misleading.

Widened Retrogastric Space

One of the most commonly cited roentgen findings attributed to pancreatic mass lesions is an increase in the distance between the posterior wall of the stomach and the spine, as determined from lateral roentgenograms made during barium upper gastrointestinal examination. This sign is also one of the most controversial: since the concept was initially introduced (Brown, 1928; Rigler, 1933; and Engel, 1934), there has been widespread disagreement about its theoretical validity, about the best technique for obtaining the measurement, and about the effects of variables such as body habitus, abdominal muscular tone, stomach configuration, ascites, scoliosis, obesity, and so forth.

Early reports concerning this subject contended that the width of retrogastric space should be no greater than the anteroposterior diameter of the adjacent vertebral body (Engel, 1934; Poppel, 1949). Meschan (1953), however, noted a wide range of normal variation, and several authors (Lobsenz, 1949; Beranbaum, 1966) have contended that a retrogastric mass can be identified with confidence only if a constant extrinsic pressure indentation on the posterior gastric wall is demonstrated.

Two recent contributions to the literature of this topic are of particular interest. The first is that of Herbert and Margulis, (1965). These authors studied 200 normal subjects and 72 patients with tumor by means of erect anteroposterior and lateral roentgenograms of the barium-filled stomach. Several different measurements and various other observations (height, weight, age, degree of gastric filling, and so forth) were made and subjected to computer analysis. It was concluded that no single measurement or group of measurements was a valid indicator of retrogastric disease and that only an extrinsic tumor impression has statistical significance for the diagnosis of a retroperitoneal mass.

An opposing view has, however, been posited recently by Poole (1970). This author has used an abdominal compression device to insure that the posterior gastric wall be in actual contact with the retroperitoneal structures during lateral radiography. A nomogram was used to correct for patient weight. The measurements obtained in 33 patients with retrogastric disease were compared with those obtained in 141 normal subjects. In 31 of the former, the antrum-to-spine measurement exceeded the 95 per cent confidence limit of the normal subjects.

This technique appears to have merit, but seems best adapted to lesions situated immediately anterior to the spine. Its validity for lesions arising to the left of the spine in the body or tail of the pancreas may be questioned and, in any case, its value in prospective clinical situations remains to be established.

It is our personal opinion that measurements, at least those obtained from any standard lateral roentgenograms, are by themselves useless for identifying retrogastric disease. Lateral roentgenography is of great value, but the chief sign to be sought is that of extrinsic indentation on the posterior gastric wall, and not that of a widened retrogastric space (Fig. 3–5).

We ordinarily obtain a lateral recumbent roentgenogram, with the patient's right side dependent if a lesion in the pancreatic head is suspected (on the basis of clinical or fluoroscopic findings), and with the left side dependent if a lesion in the body or tail seems more likely.

Extrinsic Indentations

The most common type of gastric abnormality produced by pancreatic disease processes is an impression defect. Mass lesions arising from any part of the pancreas tend to indent or displace the adjacent portion of the gastric wall, thereby creating a concave defect in the expected gastric contour. Although such impressions can be seen occasionally on plain abdominal and chest roentgenograms (see Chapter 2), they usually are identified only on barium upper gastrointestinal examination. The position of the indentation is determined by the location of the pancreatic tumor. Lesions arising in the head of the pancreas tend to indent the greater curvature aspect of the antrum (Fig. 3–6). The posterior wall of the antrum is also commonly indented by such lesions and, infrequently, the lesser curvature of the antrum can be involved. Masses arising in the body of the pancreas usually indent the posterior wall of the body of the stomach. Either the lesser or the greater curve also may be involved (Fig. 3–7). Lesions arising in the tail of the pancreas most commonly indent the gastric fundus along its posterior or lesser curvature aspect (Fig. 3–8).

Masses arising in the head alone or in the head and body of the pancreas may give rise to the *pad sign*. This finding was originally described by Hershenson (1937) and popularized by Case (1940). The pad sign originally referred to the splaying of rugal folds in the antrum,

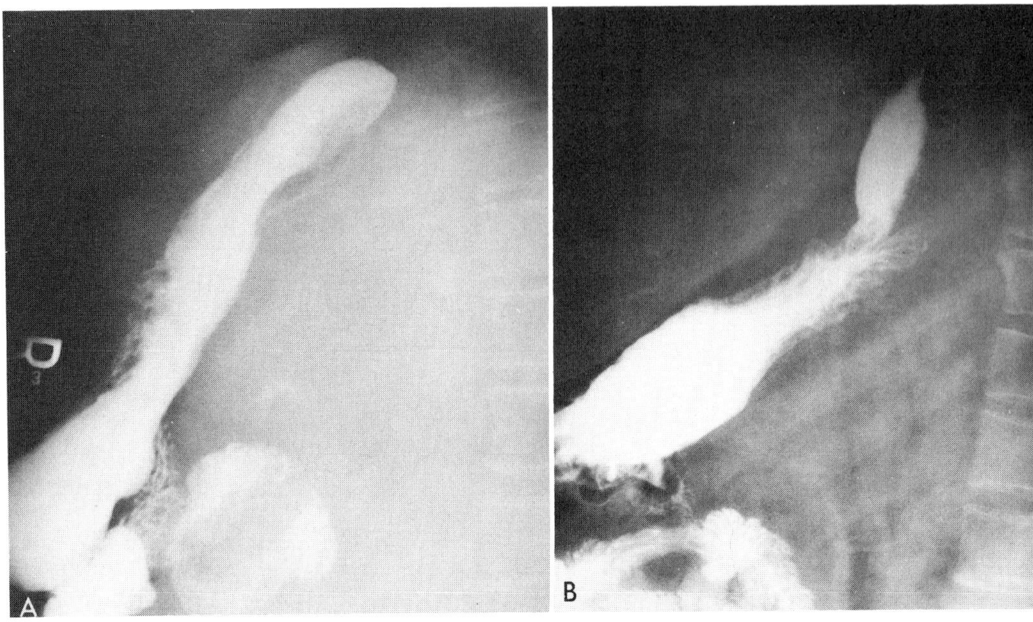

Figure 3–5. "Widened" retrogastric space in patients with acute pancreatitis (*A*) and without pancreatic abnormality (*B*). The latter patient had cirrhosis. These similar roentgenograms demonstrate the difficulty in predicting a pathologic condition in the pancreas, based on anterior gastric displacement alone (i.e., without an associated indentation defect).

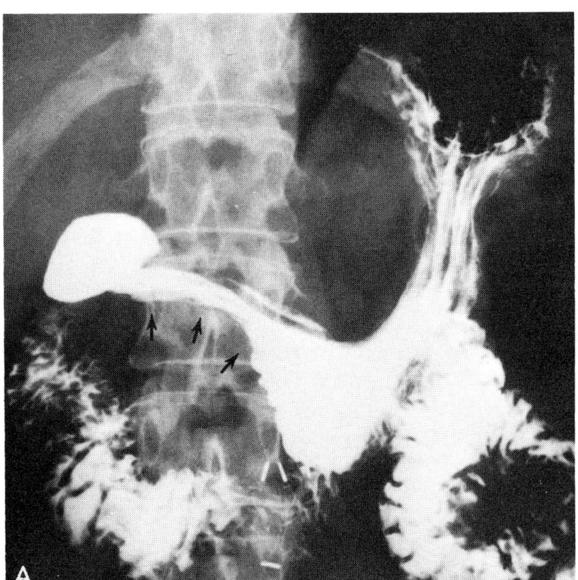

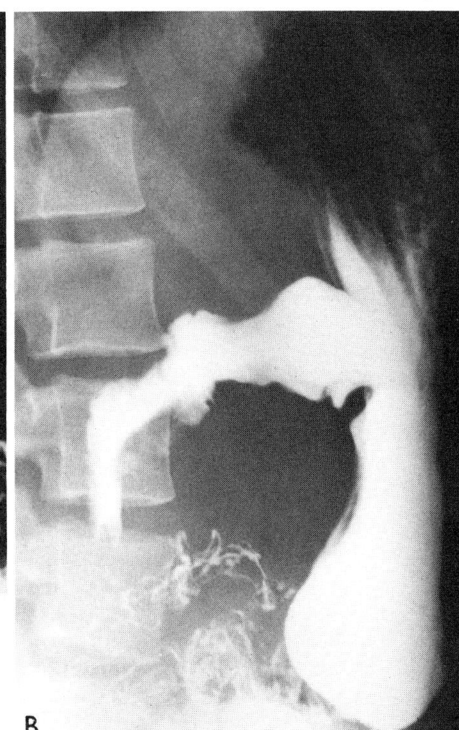

Figure 3–6. Extrinsic indentation of the inferior (*A*) and posterior (*B*) aspect of the gastric antrum. The former patient had reticulum cell sarcoma involving the head of the pancreas, and the latter had carcinoma of the head of the pancreas.

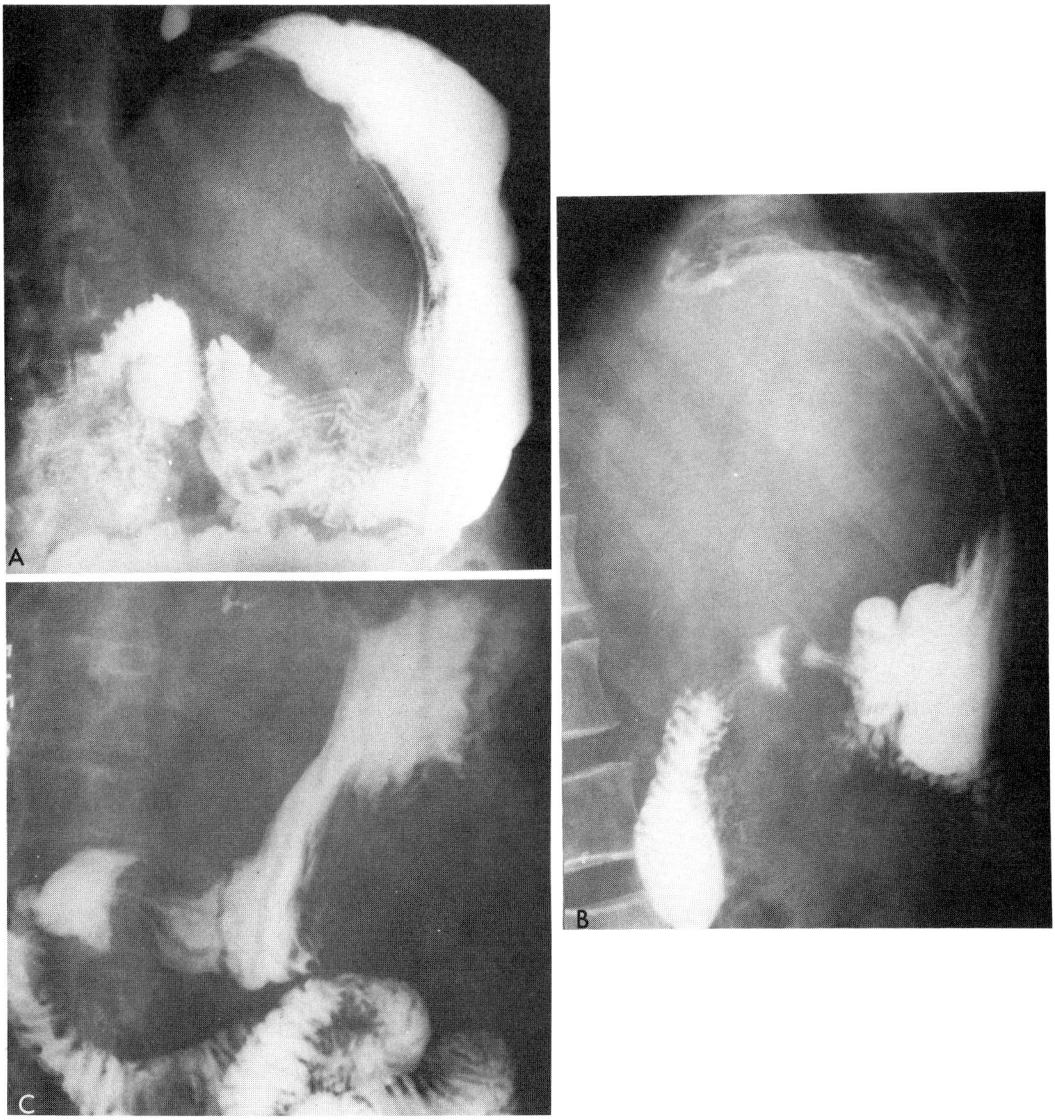

Figure 3–7. Mass lesions arising from the body of the pancreas and indenting the body of the stomach.

A, Pancreatic cancer indenting the lesser curve.

B, Pancreatic pseudocyst indenting the posterior wall.

C, Pancreatic pseudocyst indenting the greater curve.

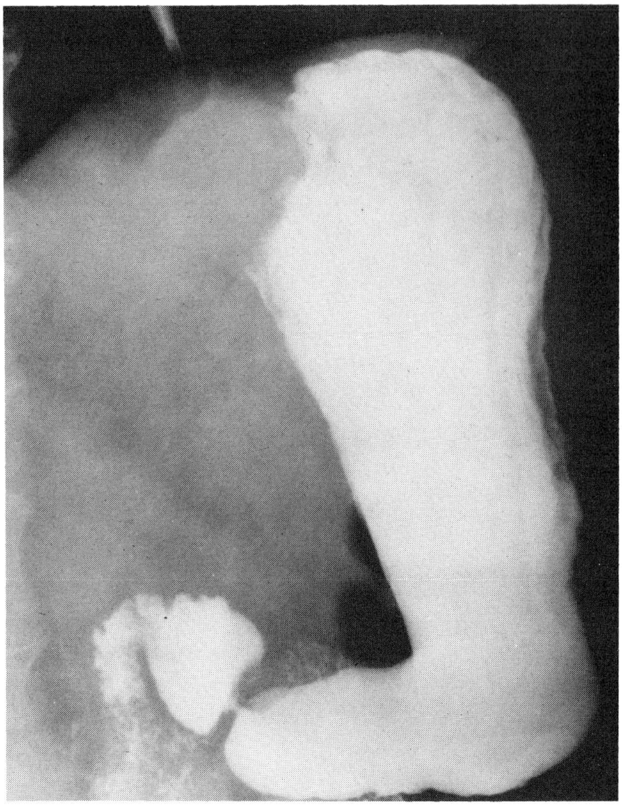

Figure 3–8. Carcinoma of the tail of the pancreas indenting and invading the fundus of the stomach near the cardia.

caused by a mass directly posterior to this portion of the stomach. Over the years, however, the term has taken on a somewhat different meaning. An extrinsic indentation on the posteroinferior aspect of the antrum, with associated draping of rugae over the mass, is now considered characteristic (Fig. 3–9). Splaying of gastric rugae in general is, of course, merely an *en face* manifestation of an extrinsic mass indentation which, if radiographed tangentially, would produce a typical retrogastric contour defect (Fig. 3–10). In one well-analyzed series, contour indentations were observed five times as commonly as was splaying of rugal folds (Mani, 1966).

Demonstration of an extrinsic mass adjacent to the stomach cannot, by itself, distinguish between various types of pancreatic disease. Solid tumors, cysts, and even acute pancreatitis can all give rise to radiologic changes of this nature. Furthermore, mass lesions arising in other organs near the stomach can produce essentially identical gastric findings on barium upper gastrointestinal examination (Table 3–1). Accurate interpretation of an extrinsic mass lesion producing gastric indentation therefore requires careful attention to ancillary roentgen findings present on the barium study, to the results of additional radio-

TABLE 3–1. Abdominal Mass Lesions Capable of Producing Extrinsic Gastric Indentation

Adrenal masses
Aortic aneurysm
Choledochal cyst
Hepatic mass lesions and hepatomegaly
Intramural gastric tumors (e.g., leiomyosarcoma)
Lymphoma
Mesenteric cyst
Pancreatic masses
Renal masses
Retractile mesenteritis
Retroperitoneal sarcoma
Splenic mass lesions and splenomegaly

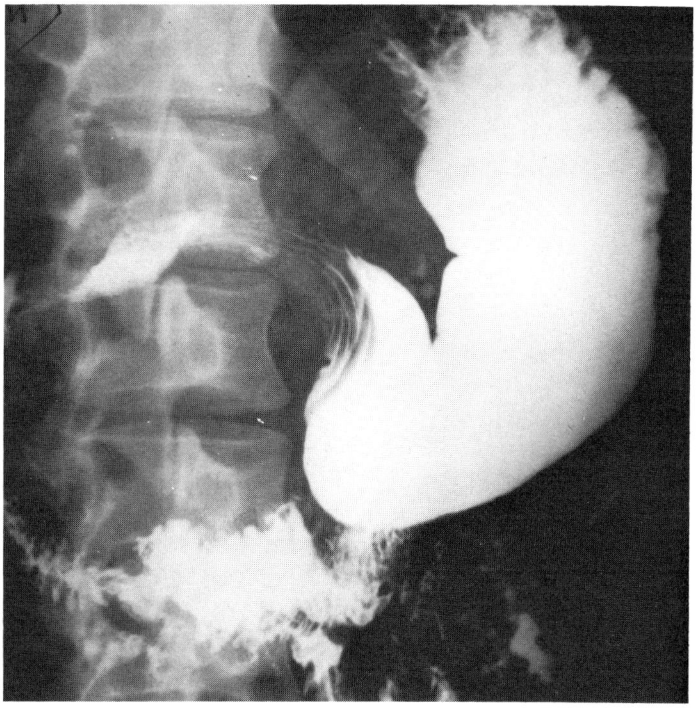

Figure 3–9. Pancreatic pseudocyst (note calcification) producing "antral pad sign" as currently understood. The inferior aspect of the antrum is indented, and rugae are stretched around the mass which arises from the head and body of the pancreas.

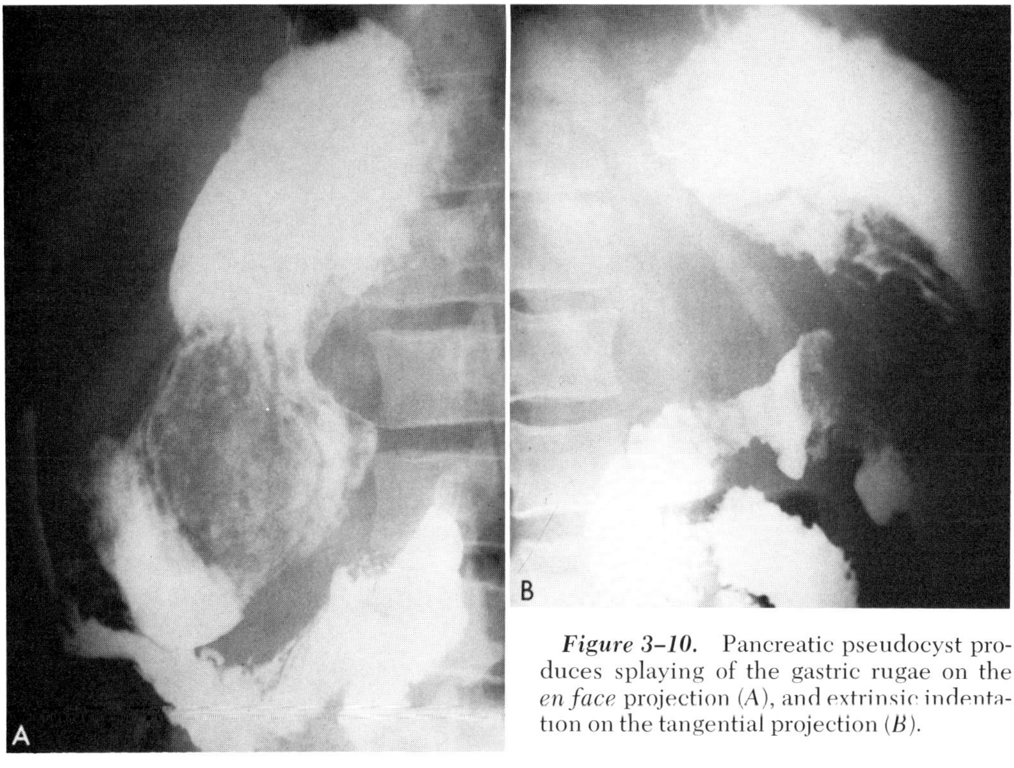

Figure 3–10. Pancreatic pseudocyst produces splaying of the gastric rugae on the *en face* projection (*A*), and extrinsic indentation on the tangential projection (*B*).

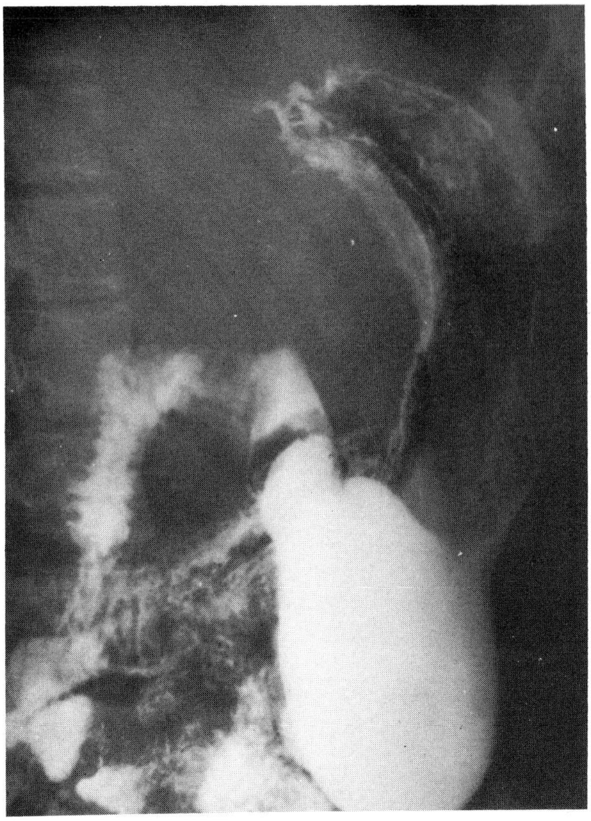

Figure 3–11. Pancreatic pseudocyst produces a smooth extrinsic indentation on the upper posterior wall of the stomach.

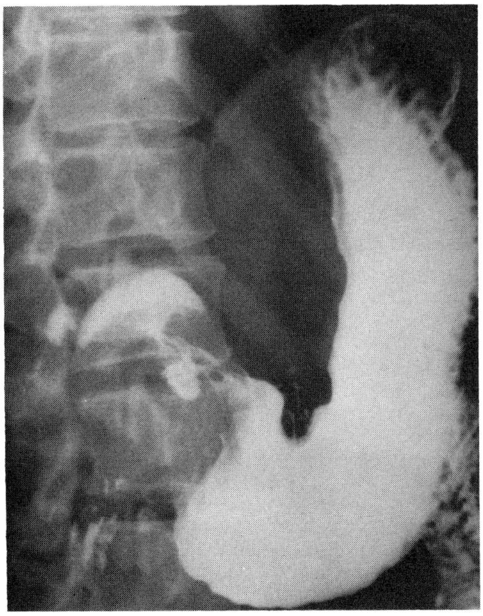

Figure 3–12. Carcinoma arising in the head of the pancreas and invading the gastric antrum, resulting in gastric ulceration.

logic examinations and, most important, to intelligent correlation with the pertinent clinical and laboratory features of the case.

Mural Irregularity

When a pancreatic mass produces a smooth indentation of the gastric wall, the process is usually, though not invariably, noninvasive (at least with respect to the stomach) (Fig. 3–11). In contrast, when the surface of an indentation defect is irregular or frankly ulcerated, inflammatory erosion or malignant invasion is usually present. Gastric ulceration produced by pancreatic disease (Fig. 3–12) nearly always indicates a malignant process, but nonulcerative mural irregularity can be the result of both pancreatic cancers and pseudocysts

(Fig. 3–13). As a rule, irregular indentation of this sort indicates invasion of the gastric wall, but this can be the result of infiltration by malignant tissue or of enzymatic and inflammatory activity present in the walls of pancreatic pseudocysts (Shockman, 1967). Conversely, a smooth indentation suggests an adjacent mass which has not actually invaded the stomach, but again, fails to distinguish be-

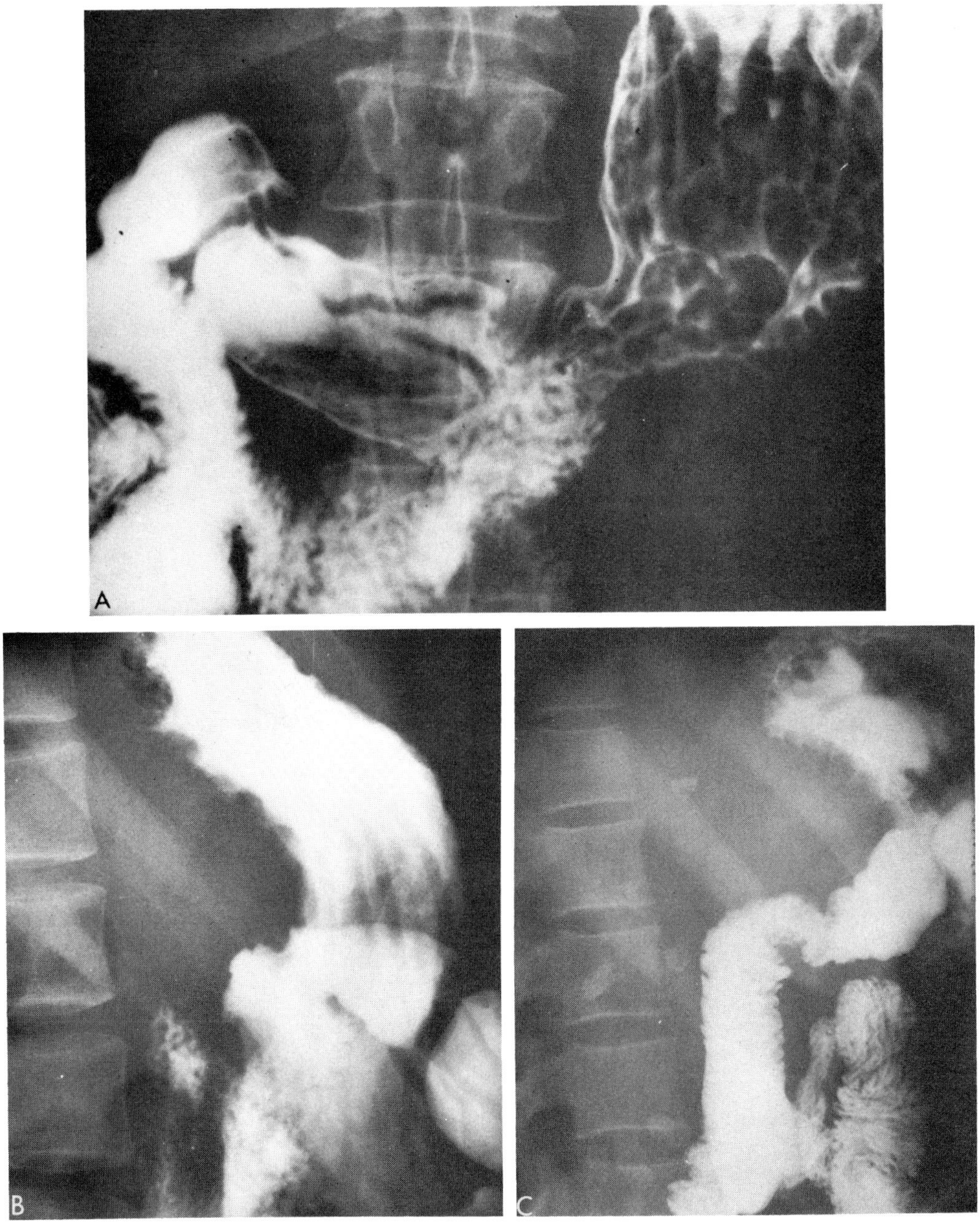

Figure 3–13. Irregular extrinsic indentation of the stomach involving the greater curve (*A*) and the posterior wall (*B* and *C*) in three separate patients. Changes in *A* and *B* resulted from pancreatic carcinoma while those in *C* were due to a pseudocyst.

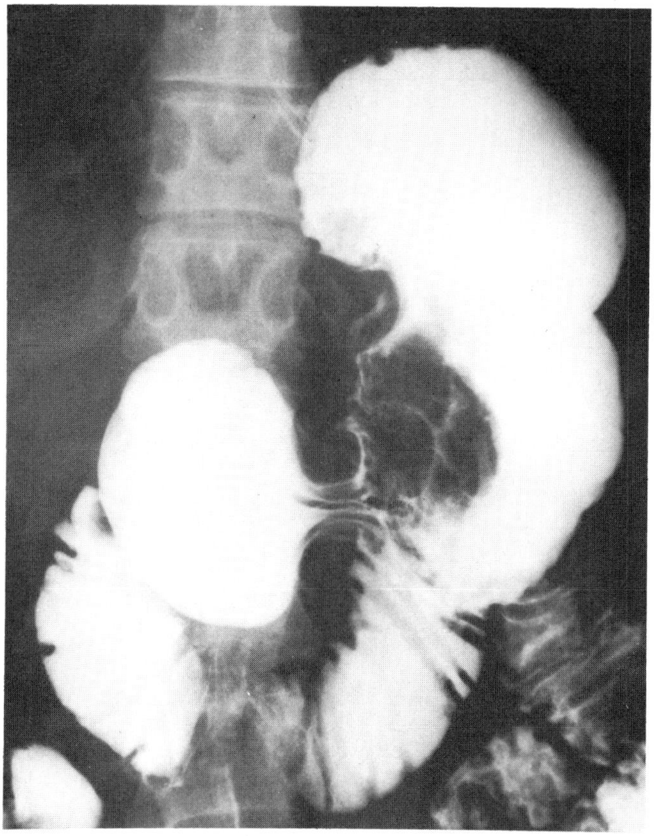

Figure 3–14. Pancreatic pseudocyst simulating fungating primary gastric carcinoma.

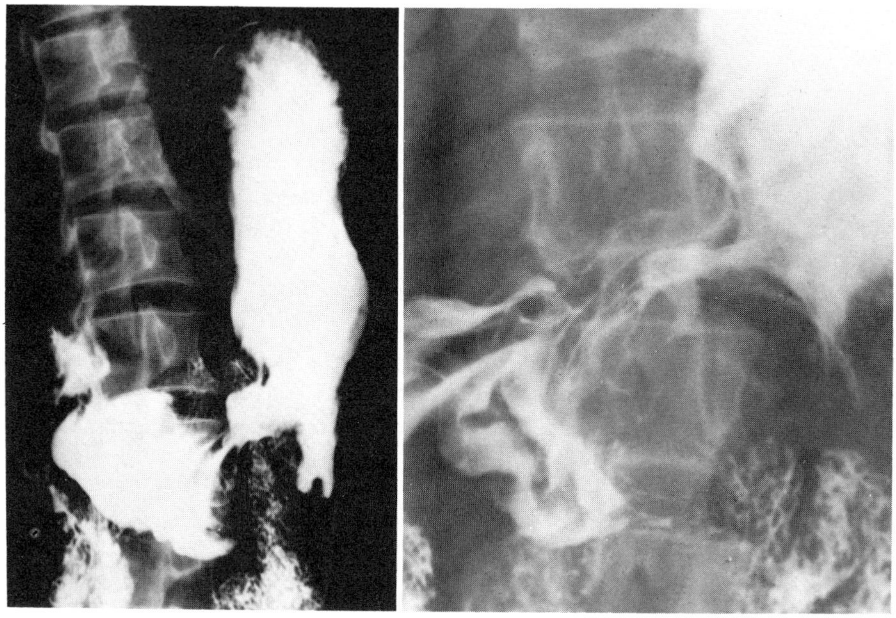

Figure 3–15. Carcinoma arising in the body of the pancreas produces extrinsic indentation and ulceration of the body of the stomach.

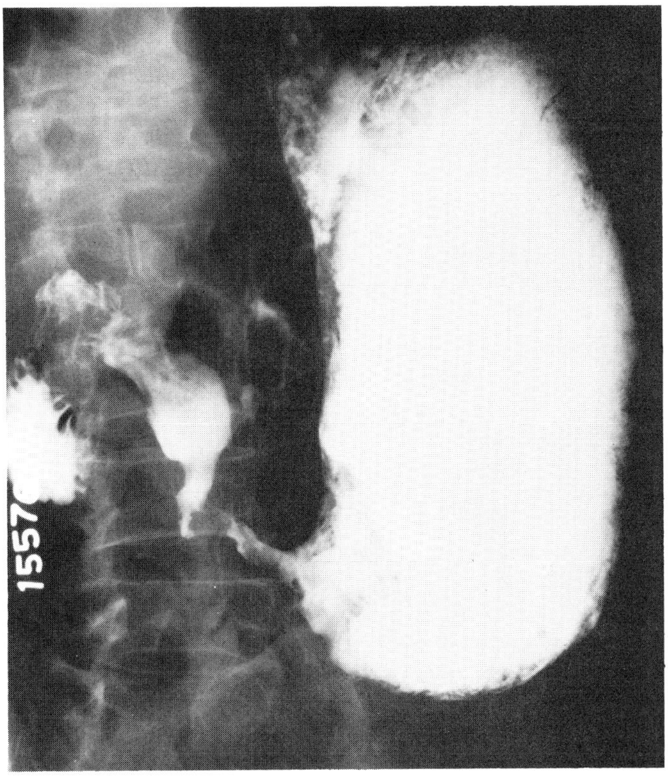

Figure 3–16. Pancreatic carcinoma producing gastric outlet obstruction. The antral stricture resulted from direct invasion by the pancreatic tumor.

tween benign and malignant processes (compare Figs. 3–6, *B* and 3–11; Figs. 3–7, *A* and 3–7, *B*).

In some instances, a pathologic condition arising in the pancreas can produce such significant gastric involvement that upper gastrointestinal barium examination demonstrates findings typical of primary gastric malignancy. Chait (1960) reported ten cases (in a series of 161 patients with pancreatic carcinoma) which were indistinguishable radiologically from primary neoplasms of the stomach. Such cases are almost always the result of extensive invasion of the gastric wall by pancreatic cancer although, rarely, pseudocysts can produce similar diagnostic difficulty (Fig. 3–14). Chait (1960) observed that gastric mucosal tumefaction, malignant-appearing ulceration (Fig. 3–15), and stricture (with and without obstruction) (Fig. 3–16) can all be simulated by pancreatic cancer. In these circumstances, exact radiologic diagnosis by barium meal examination is impossible, and even pathologic assessment at autopsy is frequently inconclusive as to the origin of the neoplasm.

Gastric Sequela of Pancreatic Inflammation

Edematous pancreatic enlargement during acute pancreatitis may, as previously described, produce an extrinsic mass indentation on the gastric contour, but two other types of gastric abnormality are also common. These are disordered gastric motor activity and rugal edema (Rosch, 1967).

Generalized hyperperistalsis or localized spasm (usually in the antrum) is encountered occasionally in patients with acute pancreatitis, especially when the disease is relatively mild. Much more often, however, the stomach is atonic and distended, particularly when the inflammation is severe (Fig. 3–17). Disorders of gastric motility in this condition thus parallel those of the duodenum in which acute pancreatitis produces localized atony or paralytic ileus considerably more often than it does spasm (Bergkvist, 1959).

Edematous rugal folds due to pancreatic inflammation usually occur on the posterior gastric wall or along the greater curvature aspect of the antrum (Fig. 3–18). They can resemble those occurring in lymphoma, gastritis, and Menetrier's disease, but clinical findings usually allow prompt differentiation. Similar rugal enlargement can also be seen in patients with pancreatic cancer (McGlone, 1956; Beranbaum, 1966). Presumably this phenomenon reflects the reactive inflammatory process which surrounds many pancreatic carcinomas (Bowden, 1958). Such an inflammatory response represents a localized focus of pancreatitis perfectly capable of stimulating an edematous reaction in that portion of the gastric wall adjacent to it.

Gastric Varices

As previously described, the body and tail of the pancreas are in intimate anatomic proximity to the splenic vein which runs along their posterior superior surface. Pseudocysts, chronic pancreatitis, and especially carcinomas involving this region therefore frequently produce obstruction of the splenic vein. Gastric varices, with or without associated esophageal varices, may develop (Marks, 1952; Rosch, 1964). While these often have a fairly characteristic appearance (Fig. 3–19), they may be difficult to distinguish from a primary gastric tumor or from gastric invasion by the underlying pancreatic neoplasm. On occasion, a tumor of the body or tail of the pancreas may produce splenic vein obstruction and resultant gastric (and/or esophageal) varices before any other gastrointestinal abnormality develops. This occurred in the case reported by Marks (1952) in which gastric varices and splenomegaly were the only radiologic findings.

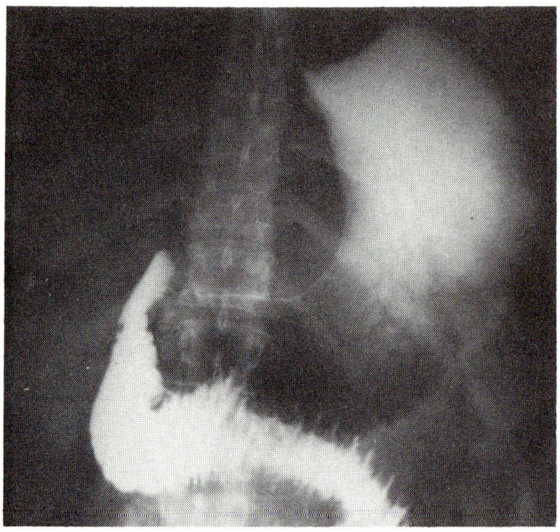

Figure 3–17. Gastric atony in acute pancreatitis. Note the spiculation and fold thickening in the horizontal portion of the duodenum. (Courtesy of Dr. David Morse.)

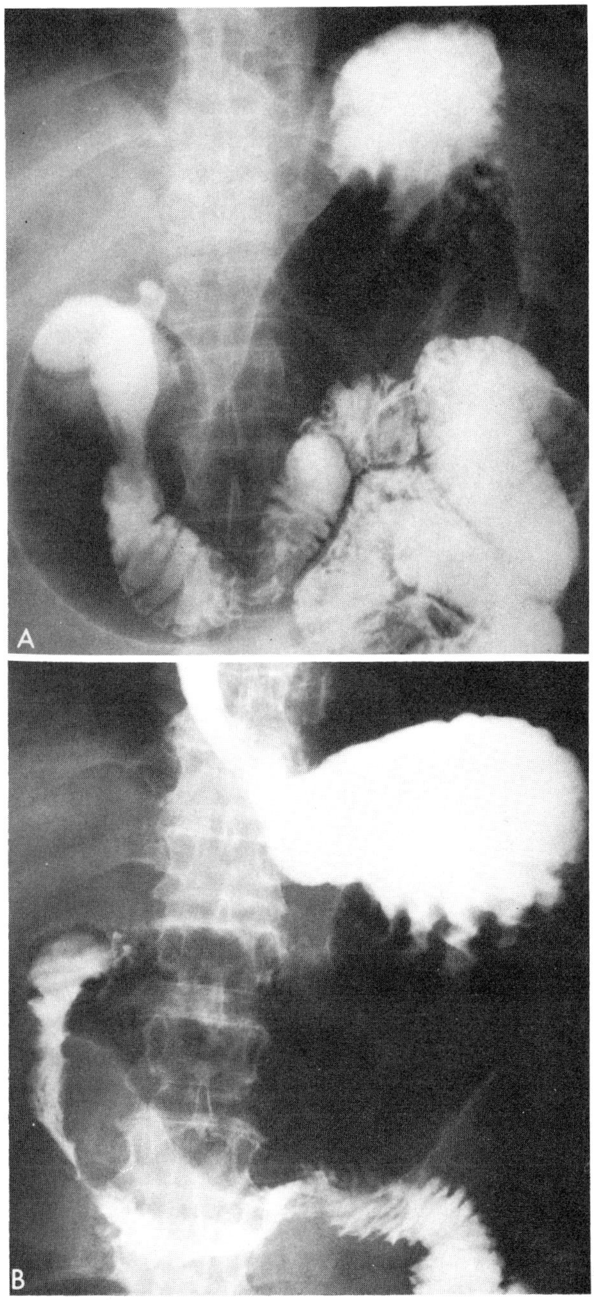

Figure 3–17 (*Continued*). Gastric atony in acute pancreatitis in two additional patients.

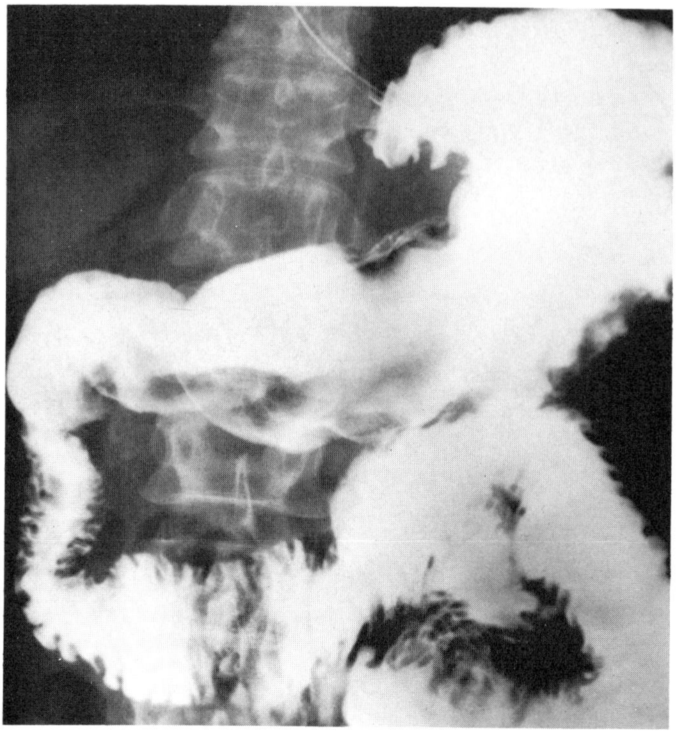

Figure 3–18. Edema of the gastric rugae resulting from acute pancreatitis.

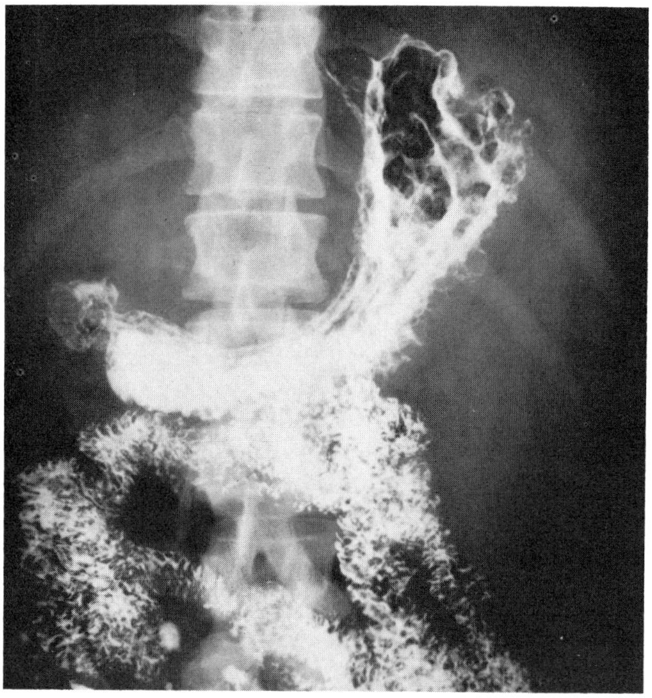

Figure 3–19. Gastric varices resulting from splenic vein obstruction in chronic pancreatitis. Note associated splenomegaly.

MESENTERIC SMALL INTESTINE

Pancreatic disease affects the jejunum and ileum less often than it does the stomach or duodenum, but small-bowel abnormalities are by no means rare. The changes demonstrated radiographically may be the result of direct anatomic contiguity between the pancreas and the involved small-bowel segment (e.g., displacement, atony, localized mucosal distortion) or may reflect an indirect effect of pancreatic disease (e.g., malabsorption, the Zollinger-Ellison syndrome). Both inflammatory and neoplastic pancreatic disease may alter the appearance of the mesenteric small intestine.

Local Mass Phenomena

When a mass arising in the body or tail of the pancreas becomes large enough, any adjacent jejunal loops will be displaced to a position which outlines the periphery of the mass (Fig. 3–20). Often, such lesions also indent the greater curvature of the stomach, thus allowing further delineation of their circumference. In most cases, masses of this sort are subject to the same differential diagnostic considerations as those which indent the stomach alone (Table 3–1); however, in rare instances, the presence of extraluminal gas, usually in the form of numerous small bubbles localized in the region of the pancreas, allows definitive diagnosis of pancreatic abscess.

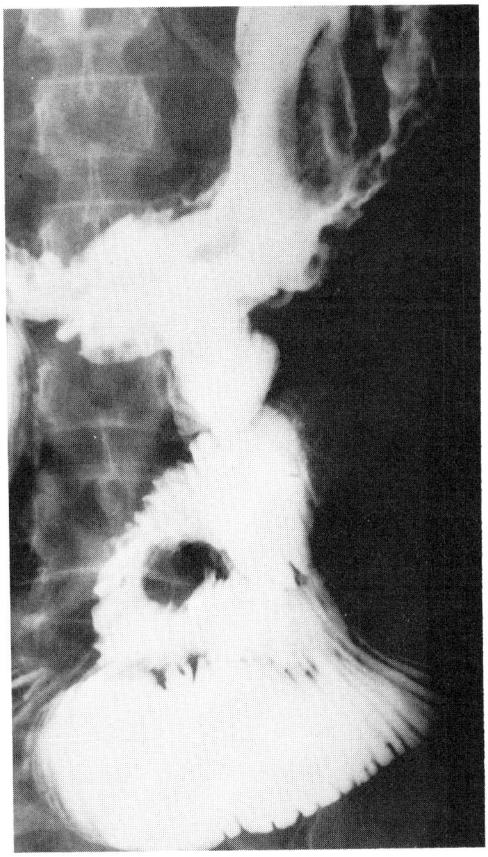

Figure 3–20. Pancreatic abscess producing displacement and an extrinsic indentation effect on the adjacent loops of the jejunum.

Nonspecific Inflammatory Changes

Duodenal ileus is the most common single roentgen feature of acute pancreatitis (Bergkvist, 1959), and reduced motility with abnormal distention is frequently present in the proximal jejunum as well (Fig. 3–21). In other instances, fold edema and spiculation, similar in nature to those more commonly noted in the duodenum, occur in the proximal jejunum in patients with pancreatic inflammatory disease (Fig. 3–22). In the authors' experience, such findings most frequently have been encountered in acute pancreatitis, but Steedman (1967) and Bolooki (1968) have described similar findings in patients with pancreatic abscesses, and Margulis (1967) notes that they can occur secondary to cancer of the body or tail of the pancreas.

Exocrine Pancreatic Insufficiency

There is general agreement that a small-bowel "malabsorption pattern" can often be demonstrated by barium examination in patients with cystic fibrosis (Tucker, 1963; Clemett, 1967). There is, however, some dispute about the occurrence of small-bowel abnormalities in adults with exocrine pan-

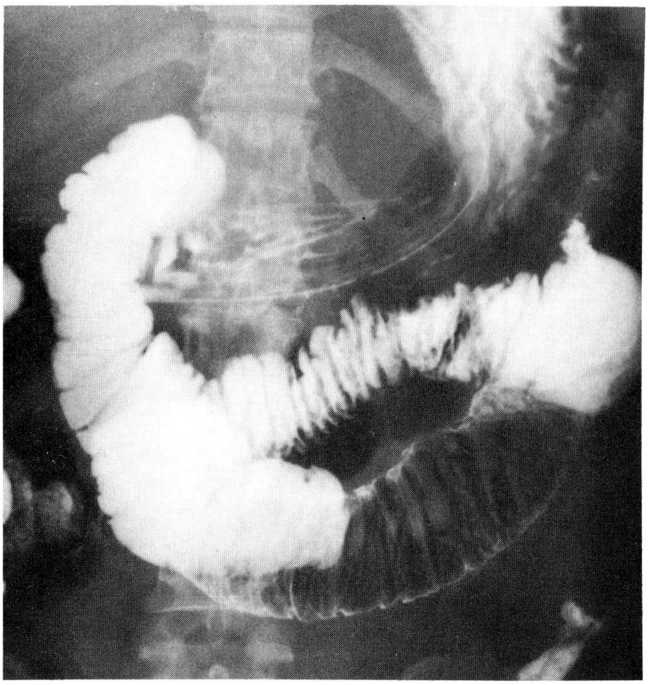

Figure 3–21. Jejunal atony in acute pancreatitis. Note the mucosal abnormalities (spiculation) at the duodenojejunal junction. Conventional examination was performed without use of Pro-Banthine.

creatic insufficiency either due to chronic pancreatitis or to pancreatic cancer. In contrast with most patients suffering from malabsorption, individuals with pancreatic disease have insufficient digestive enzymes (and, in some cases, bile salts) rather than a primary structural abnormality of the small-bowel wall.

Numerous authors have described "disordered motor function" or an "abnormal motility pattern" in patients with malabsorption associated with chronic pancreatitis, carcinoma of the head of the pancreas, or after pancreatic resection. Poppel (1951) summarized the early reports of such phenomena. He felt that roentgen abnormalities did occur, but were nonspecific and insufficient to allow the distinction between an intrinsic small-bowel pathologic condition and pancreatic disease. Abnormal segmentation and "obliteration" of the mucosal-fold pattern were the most common abnormalities noted in these early reports. Rosch (1967) believes that the small intestine often has an abnormal appearance in chronic pancreatitis, especially in advanced stages when secretory function is significantly disturbed. In Marshak's (1966) experience, however, small-bowel examination in patients with pancreatic insufficiency usually reveals no abnormalities. He thinks that a normal roentgen study in patients with documented steatorrhea should actually suggest the diagnosis of underlying chronic pancreatitis.

Isbell and his associates (Isbell, 1969) describe roentgen findings in eight patients with exocrine pancreatic insufficiency (three with pancreatic cancer and five with chronic pancreatitis). Seven had documented steatorrhea and, of these, five had one or more of the small-bowel abnormalities ordinarily considered indicative of malabsorption. Segmentation (i.e., separation of the barium column into clumps of varying size within the small-bowel lumen) was present in all five patients, while thickened folds, dilatation, moulage, and prolonged transit time were less commonly noted. Micropulverized barium was used in these examinations. We have personally studied only a few patients with pancreatic insufficiency and documented malabsorption. In most of these, the small bowel appeared radiographically normal (Fig.

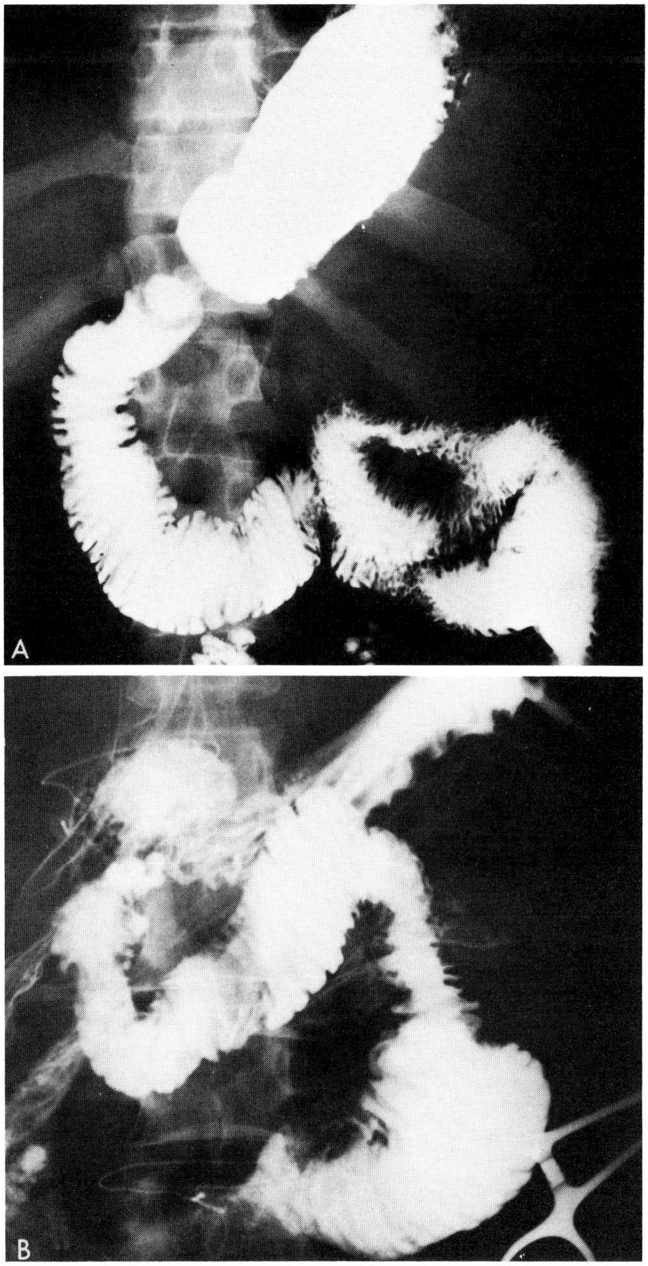

Figure 3–22. Mucosal abnormalities in two separate patients with acute pancreatitis. *A*, Spiculation; *B*, edema.

3–23) but, in occasional instances, nonspecific generalized small-bowel abnormality was present (Fig. 3–24).

Zollinger-Ellison Syndrome

The appearance of the mesenteric small intestine is frequently abnormal in patients with Zollinger-Ellison syndrome (Zboralske, 1968; Nelson, 1968). Prominent findings often occur concomitantly and, together, may allow a specific radiologic diagnosis. One of the most common abnormalities is edema of the jejunal valvulae conniventes; the folds are thickened and the barium-filled interfold grooves may appear spike-like. The jejunum is usually dilated and somewhat hypomotile (although occasionally there is marked hypermotility) (Fig. 3–25). Increased intraluminal fluid content causes

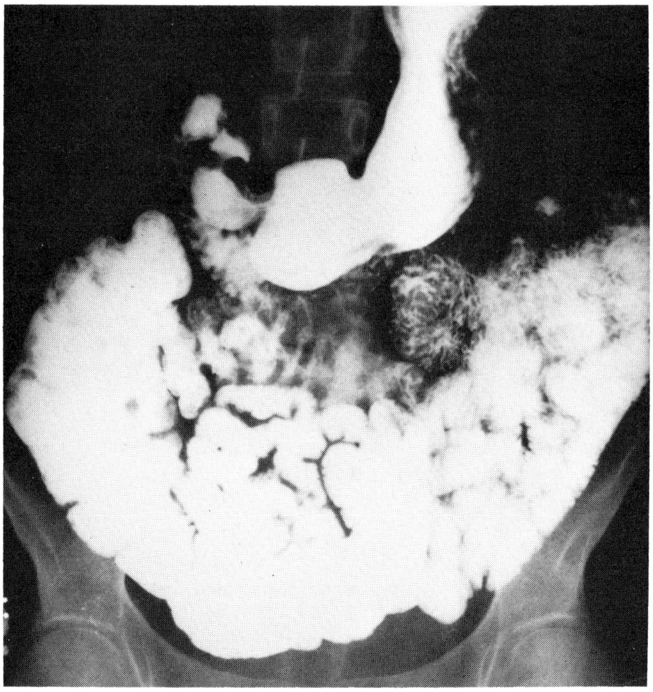

Figure 3–23. Normal small-bowel barium examination in a patient with chronic pancreatitis and malabsorption.

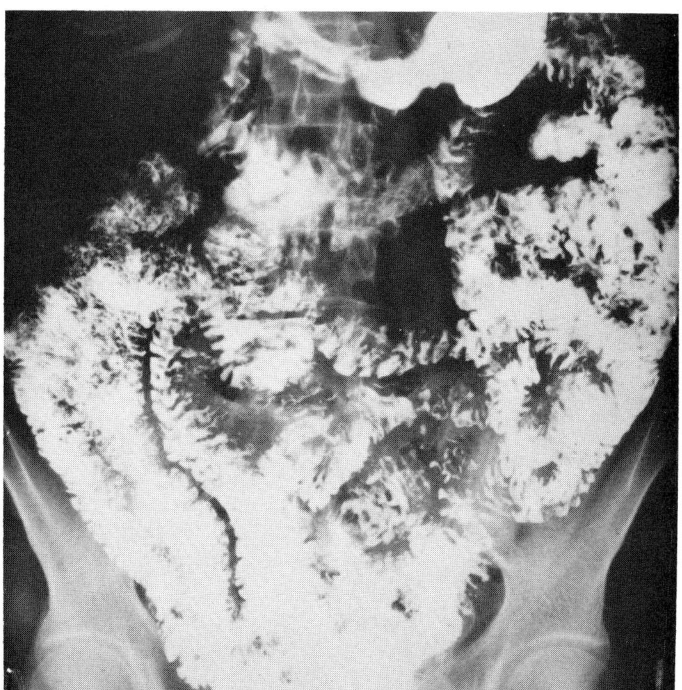

Figure 3–24. Abnormal small-bowel barium examination in a patient with chronic pancreatitis and malabsorption. Note the thickened mucosal folds and modest dilatation.

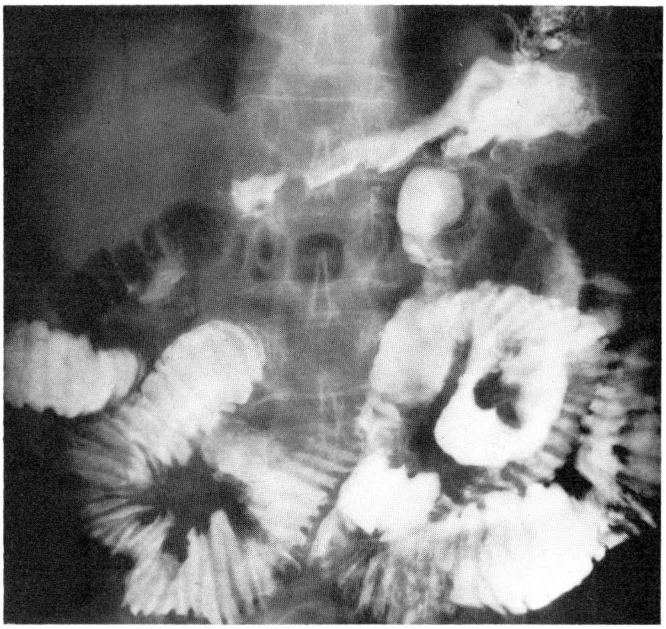

Figure 3–25. Small-bowel abnormalities in the Zollinger-Ellison syndrome. Note the dilatation and fold edema (thickening).

the barium to appear less dense and more finely granular than normal, and may also give the mucosal folds a blurred and indistinct appearance. All of these changes are most pronounced in the proximal jejunum and become less evident distally. This distribution is attributed to the large volume of highly acidic gastric secretion that reaches the proximal jejunum, and to its progressive neutralization as it passes through the small bowel. The resulting chemical enteritis is most severe proximally.

Ectopic ulceration occurs in 25 to 35 per cent of the patients with Zollinger-Ellison syndrome. One of the more common sites for such ulceration is at the duodenojejunal junction (Nelson, 1968). Unfortunately, ulcers at this junction or in the proximal jejunum proper are difficult to recognize and may be mistaken for ulcerating neoplasms. However, when ulcers in this region are associated with jejunal fold edema, dilatation, and excessive fluid content, the diagnosis of Zollinger-Ellison syndrome can be made with assurance. Stomal ulceration after hemigastrectomy and gastrojejunostomy is, of course, another common manifestation of this condition. Such ulcers often appear shortly after surgery, are frequently large, and are usually associated with the other findings (fold edema, jejunal dilatation, and so forth) seen in preoperative patients (Fig. 3–26). Like most stomal ulcers, those that develop in patients with Zollinger-Ellison syndrome are usually on the jejunal side of the anastomosis.

COLON

The transverse mesocolon is attached to the anterior surface of the head of the pancreas and to the inferior aspect of the body and tail. Furthermore, the tail of the pancreas is connected via the lienorenal and phrenicocolic ligaments to the splenic flexure of the colon. These peritoneal reflections constitute potential pathways which allow pancreatic disease to produce secondary changes in the transverse colon and splenic flexure. Their significance in relation to abnormalities of the transverse colonic gas pattern on plain film study of acute pancreatitis (the colon cut-off sign; Stuart, 1956) has already been described (Chapters 1 and 2), but the same anatomic relationships also form the basis for colonic findings demonstrable by barium enema

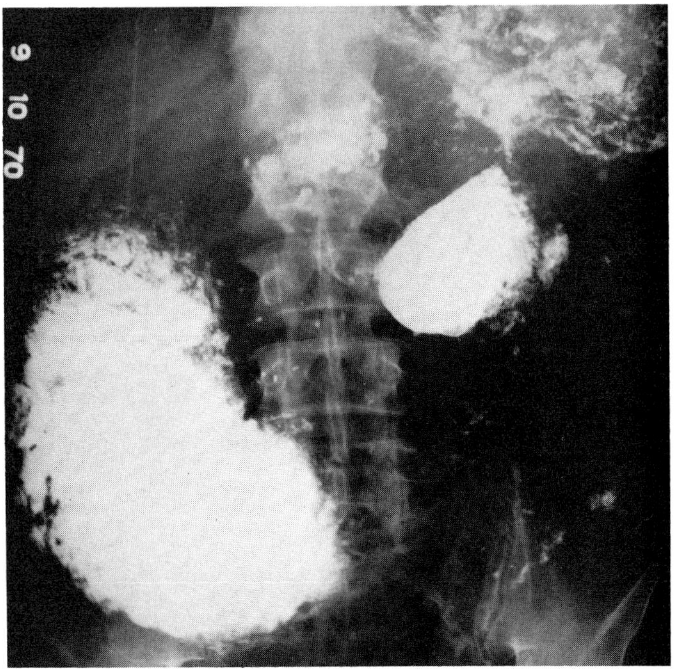

Figure 3–26. Huge stomal ulcer in the Zollinger-Ellison syndrome. Note the dilatation of the afferent loop. The generalized poor coating and granular barium texture indicate the presence of excessive intraluminal fluid.

in certain patients with pancreatic inflammation or neoplasia.

A wide variety of colonic abnormalities have been reported in patients with pancreatic disease. These include simple displacement (usually inferiorly and anteriorly) (Fig. 3–27), extrinsic indentation (Fig. 3–28), and "spiculation" (Fig. 3–29). Strictures suggesting colonic carcinoma may also develop (Fig. 3–30) although, in other instances, associated abnormalities may lead the radiologist to suspect an extracolonic etiology (Fig. 3–31). Mohiuddin (1971) described a total of 12 cases of colonic stenosis associated with pancreatitis. Eleven of the 12 cases involved the splenic flexure and, in five instances, a radiologic diagnosis of colonic cancer was made. Mani (1966) found colonic abnormalities in nine of 24 patients with cancer arising in the body or tail of the pancreas. In two cases, the findings simulated primary carcinoma of the splenic flexure. In some instances, colonic involvement may be so advanced that the clinical presentation is that of complete colonic obstruction (Schwartz, 1957).

Abnormalities of the splenic flexure and/or distal transverse colon can arise from pancreatitis, pancreatic abscess, pseudocyst, or pancreatic cancer (pancreatitis has been the most common cause of such changes in our experience); however, only pancreatic inflammation is likely to produce right colonic findings. Secondary involvement of the right colon and/or hepatic flexure by pancreatic disease has been described by Baylin (1944), Kent (1963), and Lukash (1967). In all instances, acute pancreatitis was the underlying disorder. Stenosis, mucosal irregularity, and extrinsic indentation were the findings noted in these reports, and similar findings were encountered in one case of pancreatic abscess studied by the authors of this monograph (Fig. 3–32).

URINARY TRACT

The tail of the pancreas ordinarily lies just anterior to the upper pole of the left kidney. In this location, the two organs are separated only by Gerota's fascia and a variable amount of perinephric fat. The head of the pancreas is frequently in contact with the medial aspect of the

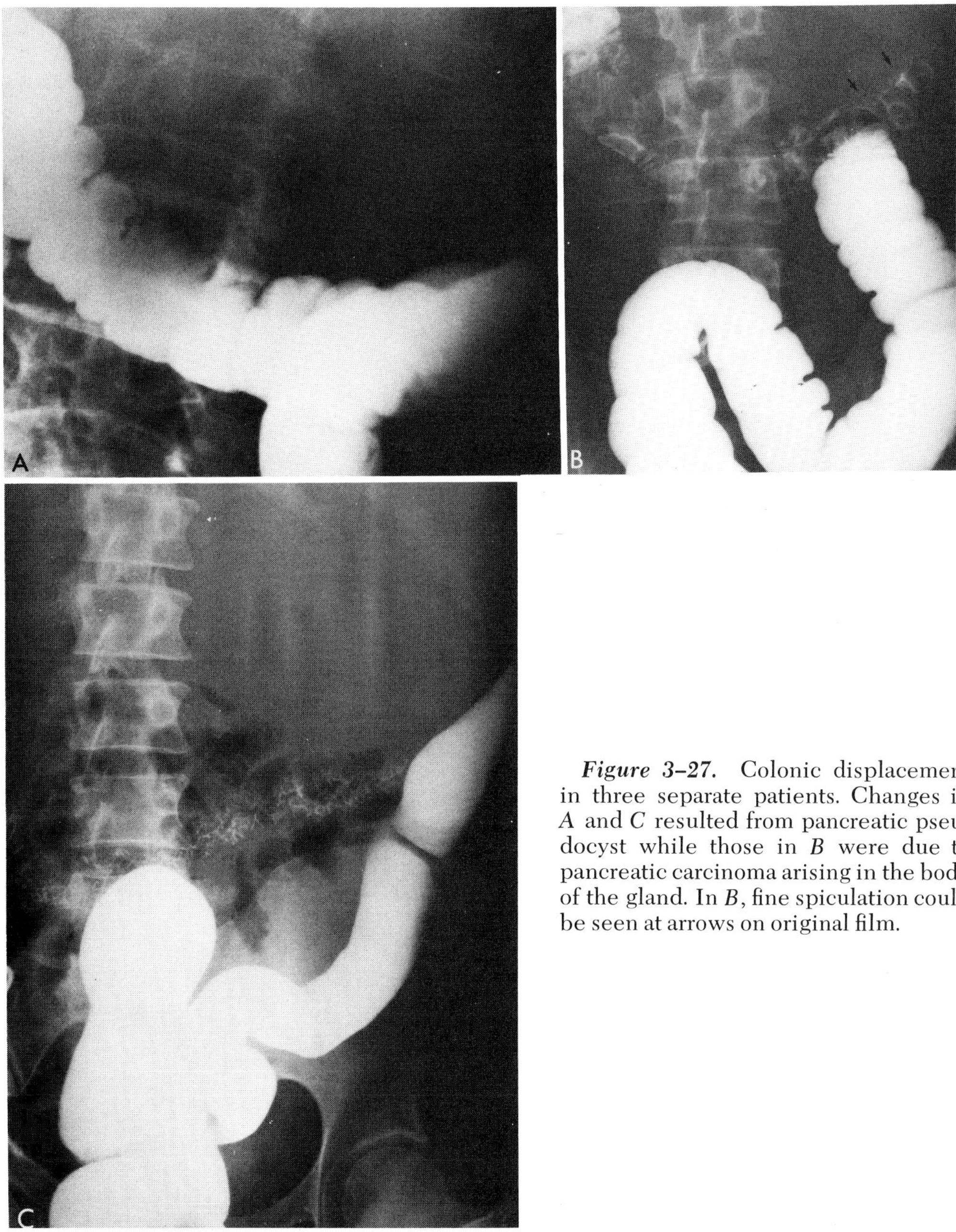

Figure 3–27. Colonic displacement in three separate patients. Changes in *A* and *C* resulted from pancreatic pseudocyst while those in *B* were due to pancreatic carcinoma arising in the body of the gland. In *B*, fine spiculation could be seen at arrows on original film.

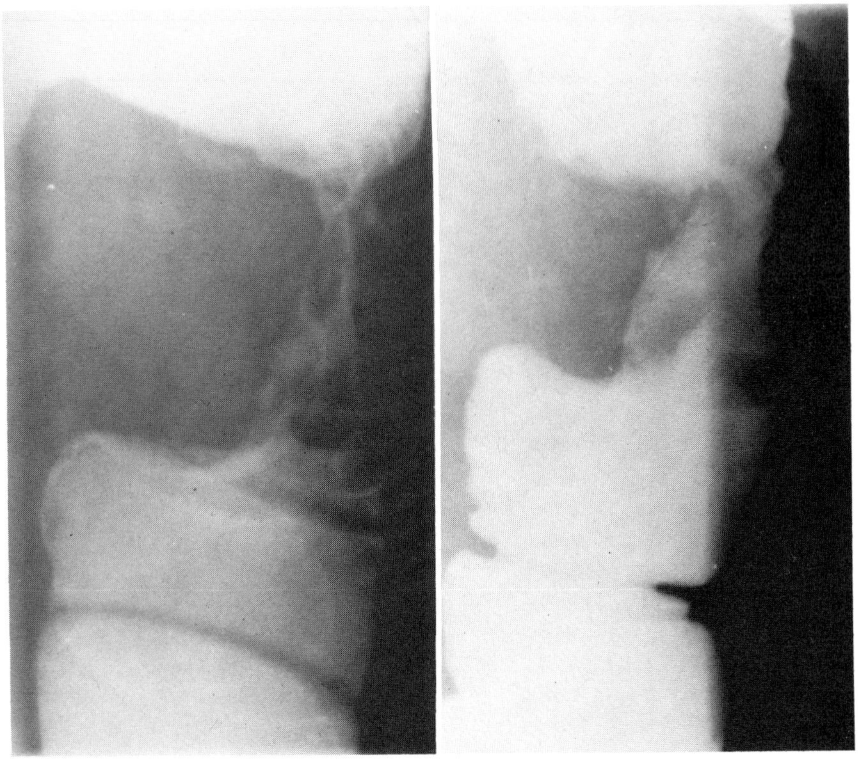

Figure 3–28. Pancreatic pseudocyst produces a localized extrinsic indentation defect near the anatomic splenic flexure of the colon. Note the edema of the colonic mucosal folds.

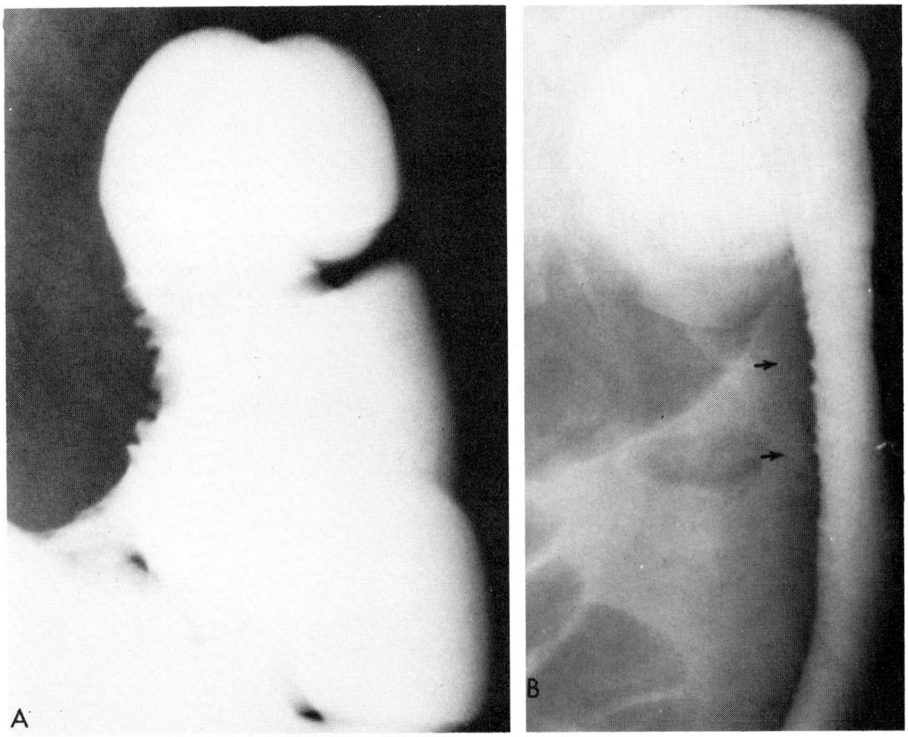

Figure 3–29. Colonic "spiculation" in two patients with pancreatic inflammation. *A*, Acute pancreatitis, and *B*, pancreatic abscess.

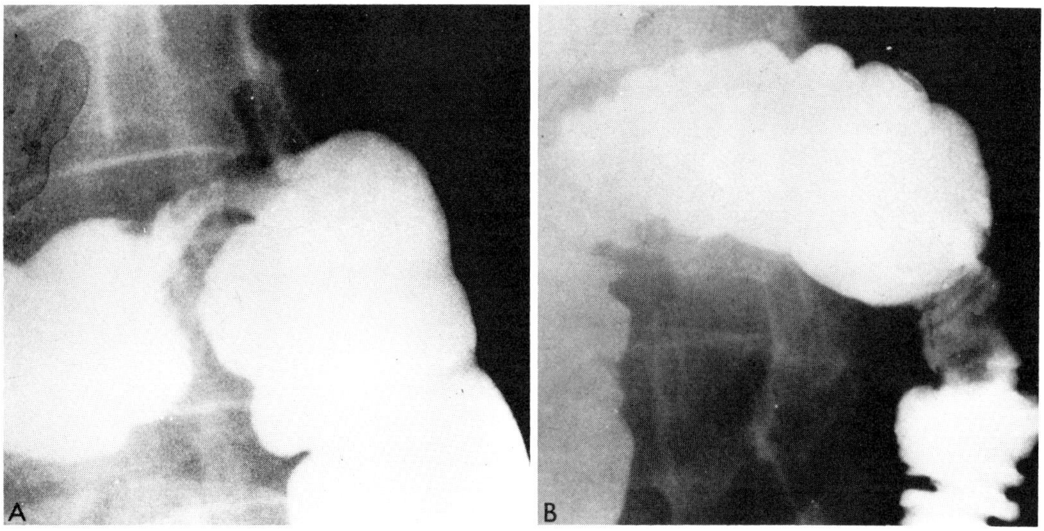

Figure 3–30. Colonic strictures in two separate patients. Cancer arising in the body of the pancreas produced *A*, while *B* resulted from pancreatic pseudocyst.

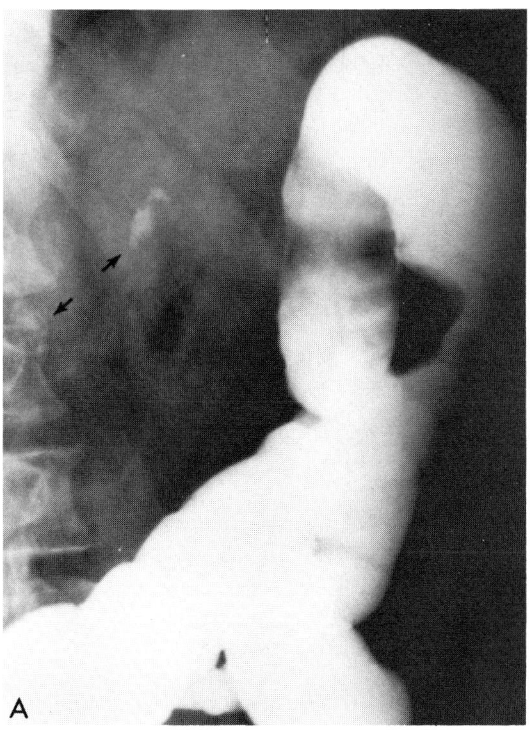

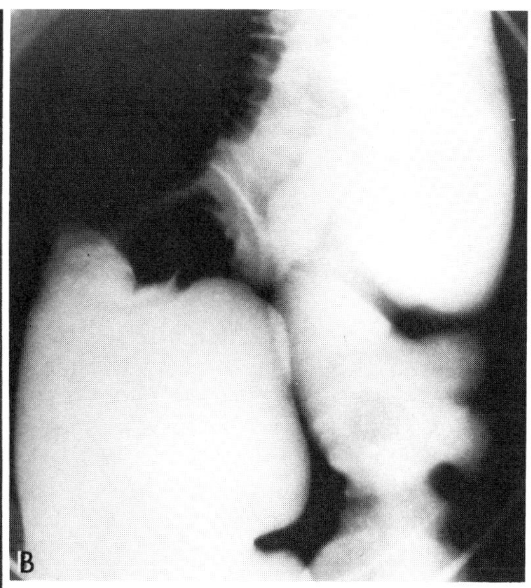

Figure 3–31. Colonic strictures in two separate patients. Pancreatic calcification (*arrows*) suggests a pancreatic cause for the colonic lesion (*A*) which resulted from a pancreatic pseudocyst. Associated spiculation (see also Fig. 29, *A*) indicates that inflammation is a possible cause for *B* which resulted from acute pancreatitis.

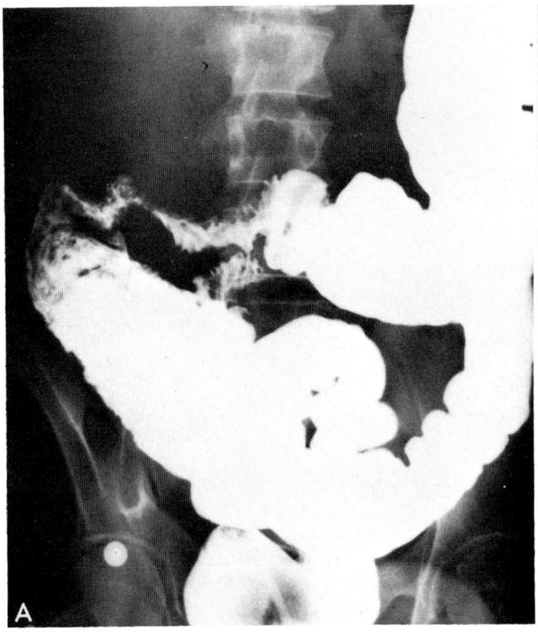

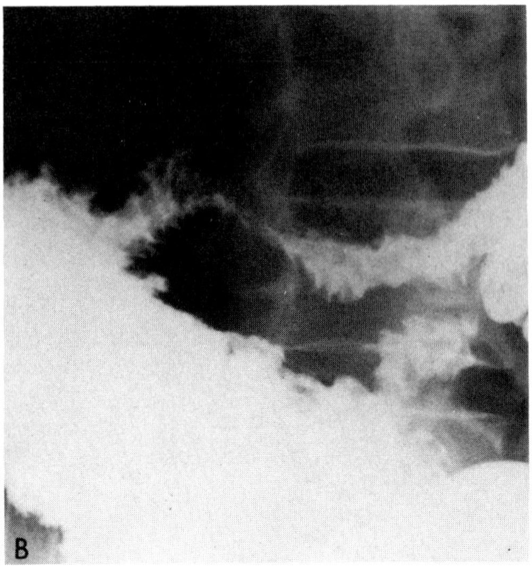

Figure 3–32. Persistent spasm, extrinsic indentation and mucosal edema of the hepatic flexure all resulting from a pancreatic abscess. Full overhead and detail views.

hilum of the right kidney, and the right and left renal veins are both ordinarily adjacent to pancreatic tissue. The close anatomic proximity of these retroperitoneal viscera accounts for the fact that pancreatic mass lesions not infrequently produce urinary tract abnormalities easily demonstrable by excretory urography.

The most common abnormal urographic finding in patients with pancreatic disease is inferior displacement of the left kidney, often with an associated lateral displacement of the upper pole which produces an unusually vertical renal axis (Fig. 3–33). The renal contour is typically normal and there is usually no distortion of the calyces (Mani, 1966). Another common finding which can be produced by pancreatic masses is an extrinsic compression effect on the pelvicalyceal system, with elongation and thinning of the major calyces (Chamberlin, 1954).

In occasional instances, pancreatic carcinomas or pseudocysts may become intimately adherent to or actually invade the kidney, producing the urographic appearance of an intrarenal mass lesion (Marshall, 1965; Gorder, 1969). In such cases, the major calyces are usually displaced and splayed rather than actually destroyed (Fig. 3–34). As might be expected, the upper pole is affected much more frequently than is the lower. The radiographic findings are most often thought to represent a renal cyst (rather than renal carcinoma) in cases of this sort.

Pancreatic mass lesions involve the left kidney far more often than the right; the left kidney was involved in 40 of 43 cases pooled from the literature (Poppel, 1951; Chamberlin, 1954; Marshall, 1965; Mani, 1966; Hellebusch, 1969; Gorder, 1969; Guerrier, 1970; and Atkinson, 1973). Of the 43 cases, urinary tract changes were produced by pancreatic cancers in 27, by pancreatic pseudocysts in 14, and by pancreatitis alone in two. The incidence of renal involvement by some forms of pancreatic disease is higher than might be expected. Of 20 patients with carcinoma involving the body or tail of the pancreas and who were studied by intravenous pyelography, urinary tract abnormalities were noted in ten (50 per cent) (Mani, 1966).

The propensity of pancreatic inflammatory collections to migrate along tissue planes occasionally results in bizzare urinary tract manifestations. Poppel

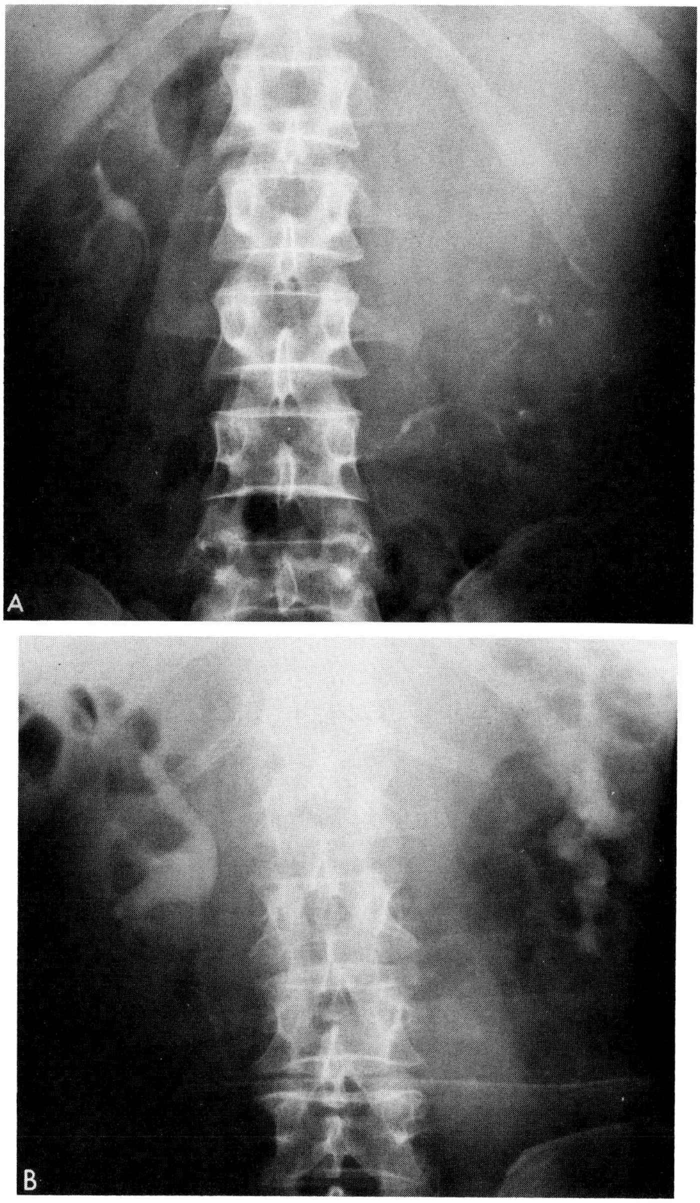

Figure 3–33. Inferior displacement of the left kidney is demonstrated by excretory urography in two separate patients with carcinomas arising in the body of the pancreas. Note the relatively vertical axis in both instances.

(1959) notes that pseudocysts may spread downward along the spine, ultimately producing ureteral compression and secondary hydronephrosis. The authors of this monograph have encountered a somewhat similar case in which comparable inferior extension occurred and the pseudocyst presented as a pelvic mass with lateral splaying of the ureters (Fig. 3–35). Ureteral abnormalities may also occur when metastatic lymphadenopathy from pancreatic carcinoma produces localized indentation and irregularity (Fig. 3–36) and, theoretically, in patients in whom pancreatic tumors have produced renal vein obstruction (Cope, 1969), with resulting ureteral impression by dilated collateral veins.

(*Text continued on page 80*)

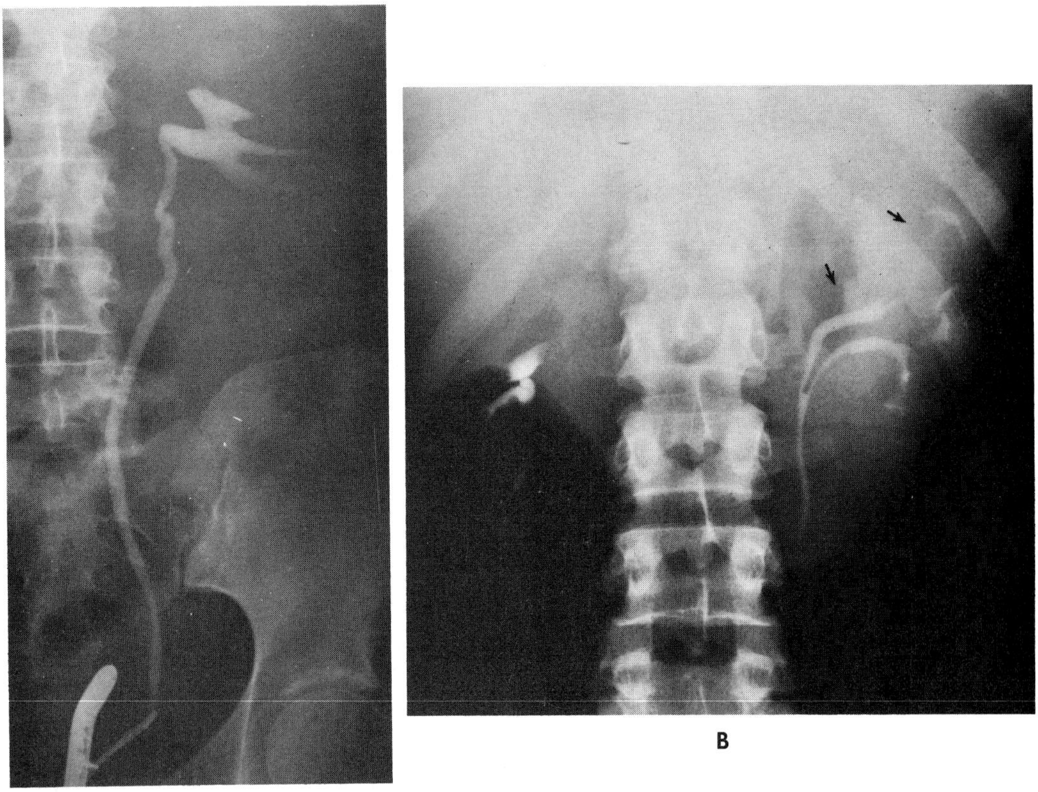

A B

Figure 3-34. Calyceal splaying and displacement produced by pancreatic disease.
A, Retrograde pyelogram in a patient with carcinoma arising in the body of the pancreas.
B, Excretory urogram in a patient with a pancreatic pseudocyst. *B*, From Atkinson, G. O., Clements, J. L., Milledge, R. D., and Weens, H. S.: Pancreatic disease simulating urinary tract disease. Clin. Radiol. (In press, 1973.)

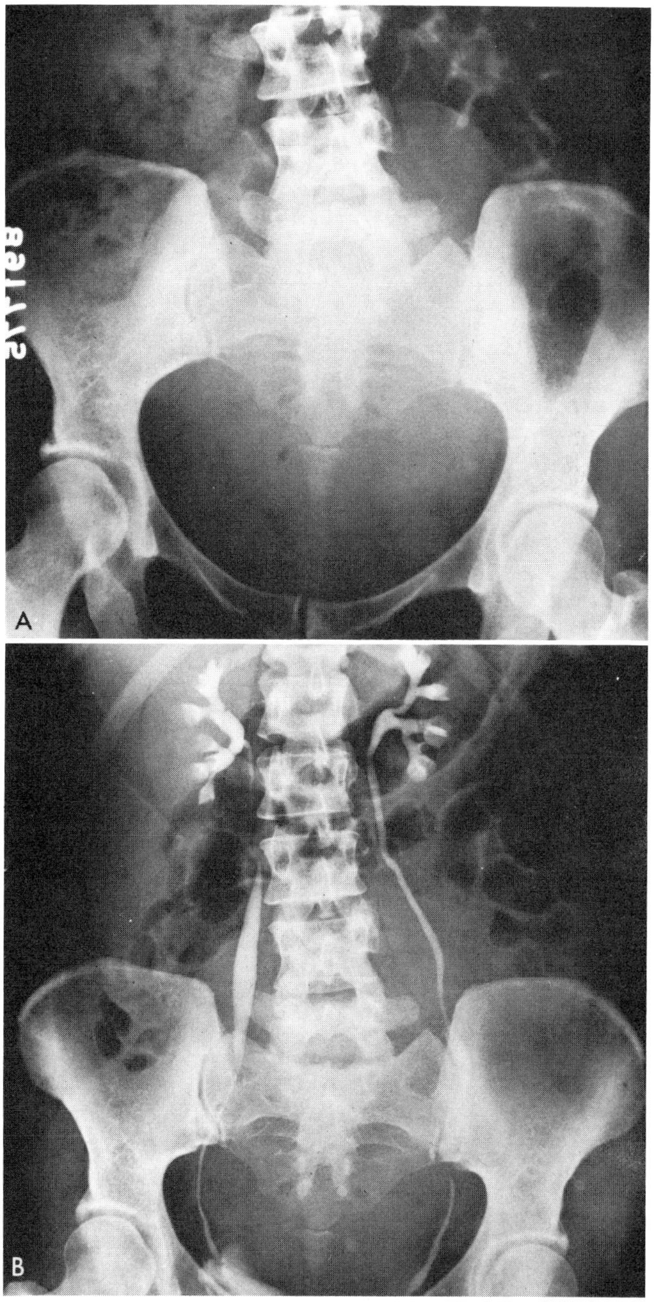

Figure 3–35. Pancreatic pseudocyst presenting as a pelvic mass (*A*). Excretory urography reveals ureteral displacement around the mass (*B*).

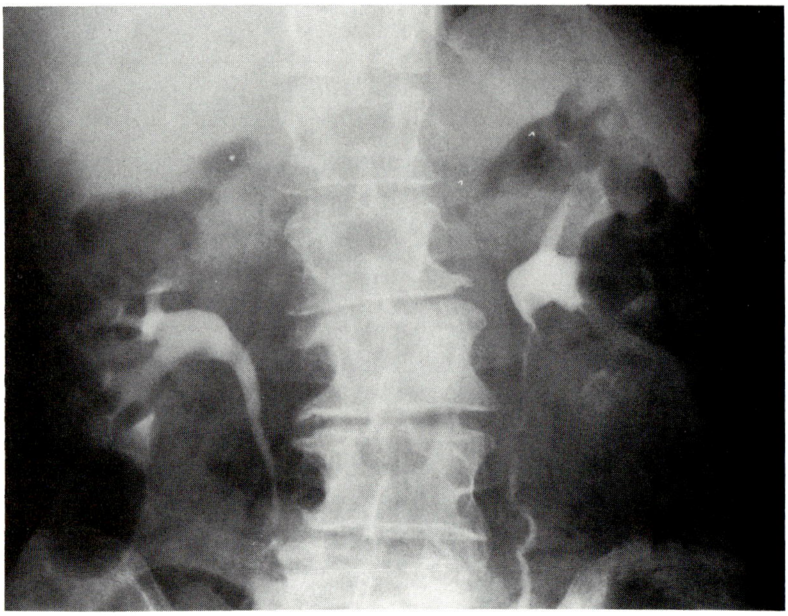

Figure 3-36. Excretory urogram reveals irregularity and indentation of the proximal left ureter. These changes, persistent throughout the examination, were found at surgery to result from adjacent lymphadenopathy resulting from pancreatic carcinoma.

BILIARY TRACT

Radiologic evaluation of the biliary tract is often of major significance in patients suspected of having inflammatory or neoplastic disease of the pancreas. The application of such studies to patients who present clinically with jaundice is discussed separately (Chapter 5); in this section, consideration is given to biliary tract abnormalities that can be encountered in patients with pancreatic disease which has not produced jaundice.

Oral Cholecystography

Properly timed radiologic evaluation of the gallbladder is of considerable importance in differentiating pancreatitis associated with biliary tract disease from that due to other causes (such as alcoholism). In the former condition, correction of the underlying biliary disorder frequently prevents further relapses of pancreatitis, whereas in other forms of pancreatic inflammation, biliary tract surgery is of little or no benefit in preventing repeated acute episodes (Howard, 1960; Dixon, 1970) (Fig. 3-37).

Oral cholecystography, performed during an acute episode of pancreatitis, may exclude cholelithiasis by demonstrating a normal gallbladder. However, in as many as 50 per cent of the patients with pancreatitis whose gallbladders are subsequently proven to be normal, oral cholecystography attempted in the acute period results in nonopacification (Kaden, 1955). Such failure of gallbladder visualization in the absence of intrinsic cholecystic disease may be due to the transient impairment of liver function which accompanies many acute abdominal disorders (Bockus, 1955), or to an accumulation of viscid bile in a gallbladder which has not been stimulated to contract because of a fat-free diet. In view of these considerations, Stein (1959) recommends that oral cholecystography be carried out only after BSP retention has become normal and the gallbladder has been stimulated to empty itself after the patient has been given one or more fatty meals.

Oral cholecystograms, performed in accordance with the criteria outlined above, were obtained by Stein and his

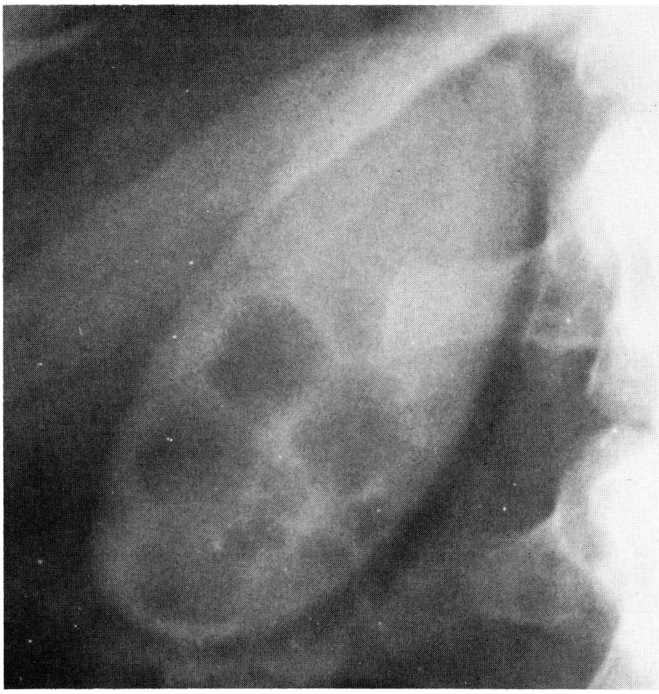

Figure 3–37. Oral cholecystogram reveals cholecystolithiasis in a patient who had experienced an attack of acute pancreatitis one month previously. A cholecystectomy was performed, and there have been no further episodes of pancreatitis to date.

co-authors in 51 patients who had suffered attacks of acute pancreatitis. Cholecystolithiasis was demonstrated in 15 and, in an additional four, there was failure of gallbladder opacification despite administration of a repeat dose of contrast material. In 31 patients, normal gallbladders were demonstrated. Of interest is the fact that all the patients considered to have alcoholic pancreatitis belonged to this latter category. This result is in keeping with the observations of Howard (1960) and Sarles (1965) that the incidence of cholelithiasis in patients with alcoholic pancreatitis is low.

Intravenous Cholangiography

Acute pancreatitis may present in a clinically unmistakable fashion but, in a fair number of instances, the symptoms and signs may suggest acute cholecystitis instead. In other cases, distinction between the two conditions may be unclear and, in still others, patients who actually have acute cholecystitis may have clinical findings which simulate pancreatitis. In circumstances of this sort, intravenous cholangiography may play an important role by demonstrating the presence or absence of cystic duct patency; the great majority of cases of acute cholecystitis are associated with mechanical or functional obstruction of the cystic duct (Weens, 1964).

Weens and his associates (Johnson, 1960; Weens, 1964) have described three major patterns which can be observed when intravenous cholangiography is performed in patients with upper abdominal inflammatory disease (Fig. 3–38; Table 3–2). In the first, opacification of both the biliary ducts and the gallbladder occurs (Fig. 3–39). This result effectively excludes acute cholecystitis. In the second pattern, the bile ducts become opacified, but the gallbladder is never visualized (Fig. 3–40). This pattern, indicating cystic duct obstruction, is highly sugges-

(Text continued on page 85)

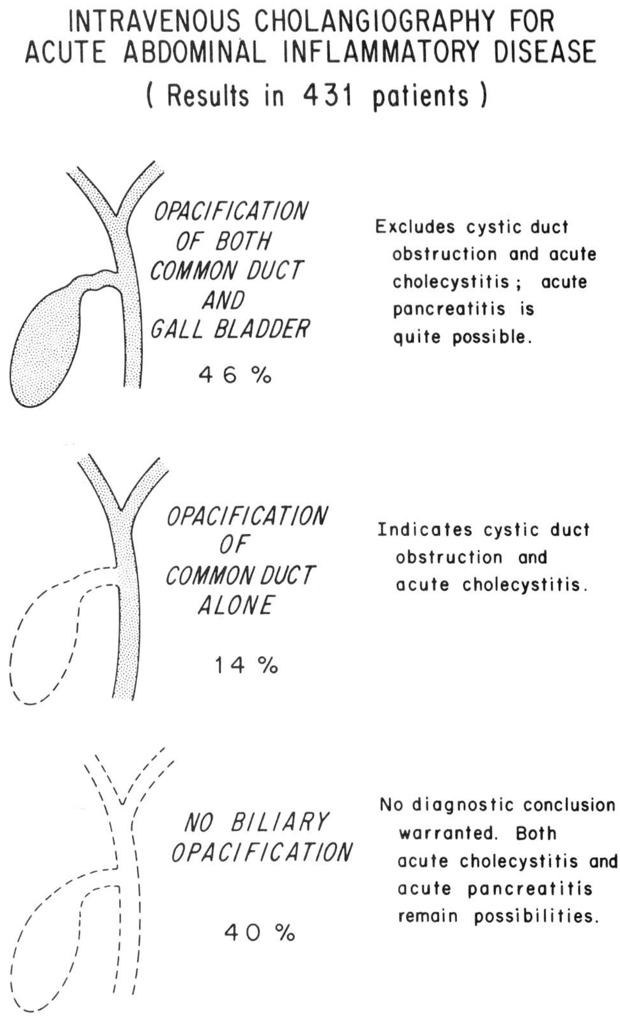

Figure 3–38.

TABLE 3–2. Intravenous Cholangiography in Patients with Acute Upper Abdominal Distress

STRUCTURES OPACIFIED	NO. OF PATIENTS	%	COMMENT
Gallbladder and common duct	198	46	None had acute cholecystitis
Common duct only	59	14	All but one had acute cholecystitis
Neither	174	40	Many different final diagnoses, especially that of acute pancreatitis, but just over 50% had acute cholecystitis

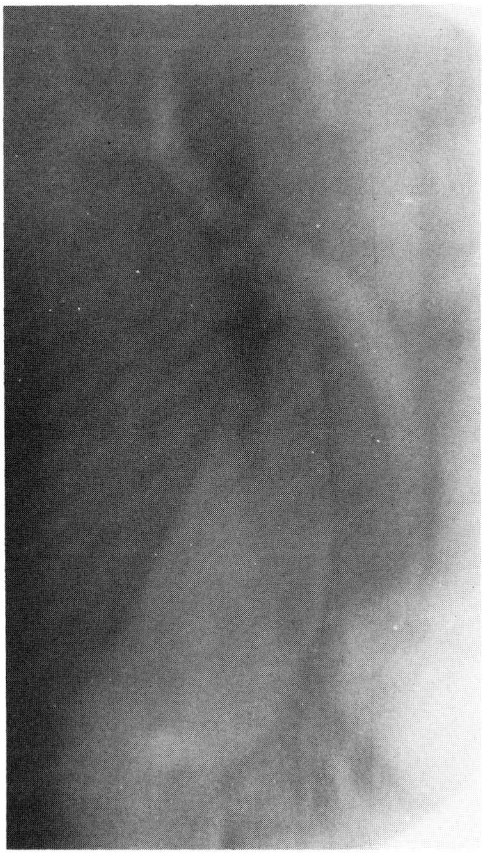

Figure 3–39. Intravenous cholangiography in a patient with acute pancreatitis. Both the common bile duct and the gallbladder opacify, thus excluding acute cholecystitis from diagnostic consideration.

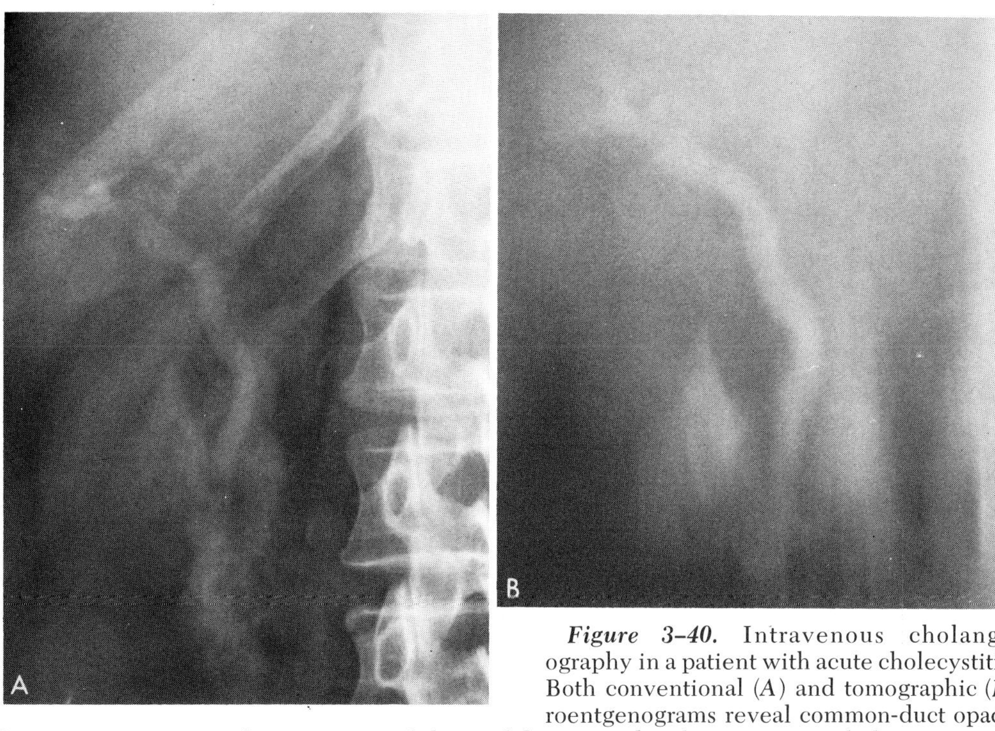

Figure 3–40. Intravenous cholangiography in a patient with acute cholecystitis. Both conventional (*A*) and tomographic (*B*) roentgenograms reveal common-duct opacification. In patients with acute upper abdominal distress and without previous cholecystectomy, this pattern indicates acute cholecystitis.

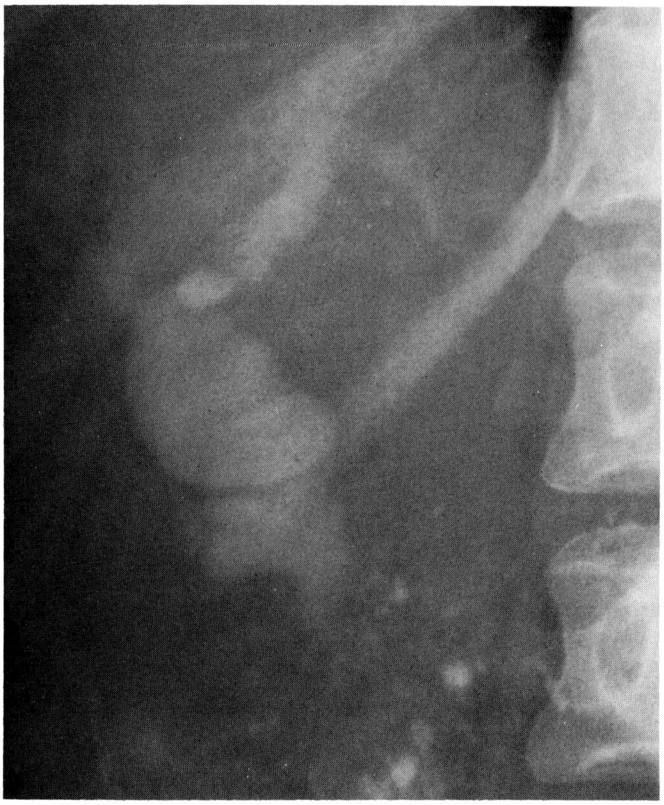

Figure 3–41. Incomplete common bile duct obstruction in chronic pancreatitis as demonstrated by intravenous cholangiography. The distal common bile duct is deformed, and the presence of pancreatic calcification indicates the cause of cholangiographic abnormalities.

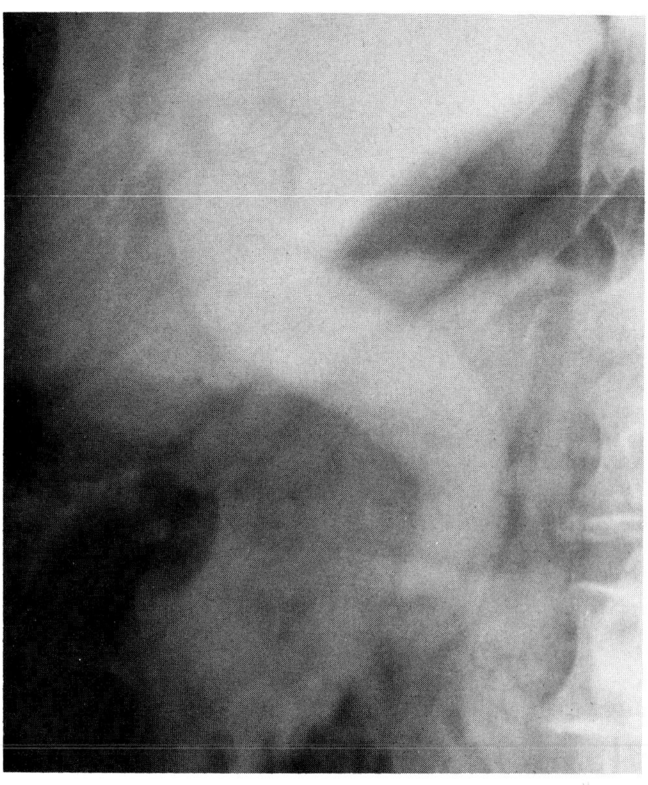

Figure 3–42. Incomplete common bile duct obstruction in chronic pancreatitis as demonstrated by intravenous cholangiography. The common bile duct is dilated, but the cause is not radiographically apparent.

tive of acute cholecystitis. In order to avoid false-positive diagnoses, it is important to extend the examination to two hours when common-duct opacification is of good quality, and to four hours when ductal visualization is faint. The third pattern occurs when neither the common duct nor the gallbladder can be identified after injection of Cholografin. In instances of complete nonopacification, specific diagnostic conclusions are usually unwarranted although, occasionally, the appearance of contrast in the colon is delayed (12 to 24 hours) while the gallbladder remains unopacified. This subpattern is considered to indicate cystic duct obstruction.

In two series (Johnson, 1960; Harrington, 1964) including a total of 431 cases, there was not one instance of gallbladder opacification in a patient subsequently found to have acute cholecystitis. Conversely, in every case but one, in which the common duct was seen and the gallbladder was not, acute cholecystitis was found (the exception was a patient with gallbladder carcinoma). There was a sizable number of patients in whom no biliary opacification occurred. Numerous different final diagnoses were made in this group but, in just over 50 per cent, acute cholecystitis was present (Table 3–2).

It is apparent that the diagnosis of acute pancreatitis cannot be established by intravenous cholangiography. The diagnosis can be excluded, for practical purposes, when the common duct is opacified and the gallbladder fails to be visualized. If both structures opacify, acute cholecystitis can be excluded and acute pancreatitis becomes that much more likely. About two-thirds of the patients with acute pancreatic inflammation follow this intravenous cholangiographic pattern. If neither the common bile duct nor the gallbladder is seen, then both cholecystitis and pancreatitis (as well as other conditions such as appendicitis, peptic ulcer, and so forth) must still be considered. About a third of the patients with acute pancreatitis will be included in this category (Weens, 1964).

Conventional Biliary Tract Contrast Studies in Nonacute Pancreatic Disease

In rare instances, oral or intravenous study of the biliary tree can demonstrate partial common bile duct obstruction in patients with chronic pancreatitis or carcinoma of the head of the pancreas (Levene, 1957; Wise, 1962; and Clemett, 1967). Although specific diagnoses have sometimes been made (Fig. 3–41), the findings seldom allow differentiation from incomplete obstruction produced by choledocholithiasis (Fig. 3–42).

REFERENCES

Atkinson, G. O., Clements, J. L., Milledge, R. D., and Weens, H. S.: Pancreatic disease simulating urinary tract disease. Clin. Radiol. (In press, 1973.)

Baylin, G. J., and Weeks, K. D.: Some roentgen aspects of pancreatic necrosis. Radiology, *42*: 466–470, 1944.

Beranbaum, S. L.: Carcinoma of the pancreas. A bi-directional roentgen approach. Amer. J. Roentgen., *96*:447–467, 1966.

Bergkvist, A., and Seldinger, S. I.: Contrast roentgenography in differential diagnosis between perforated ulcer and acute pancreatitis. Acta Chir. Scand., *118*:137–145, 1959.

Bockus, H. L., Kalser, M. H., Roth, J. L. A., Bogoch, A. L. and Stein, G.: Clinical features of acute inflammation of pancreas. Arch. Intern. Med., *96*:308–321, 1955.

Bolooki, H., Jaffe, B., and Gliedman, M. L.: Pancreatic abscesses and lesser omental sac collections. Surg. Gynec. Obstet., *126*:1301–1308, 1968.

Bowden, L.: Pancreatic carcinoma. Arch. Surg., *76*:559–563, 1958.

Broadbent, T. R., and Kerman, H. D.: One hundred cases of carcinoma of the pancreas: a clinical and roentgenologic analysis. Gastroenterology, *17*:163–177, 1951.

Brown, S.: Differential diagnosis of abdominal tumors by the roentgenological method. Radiology, *10*:48–56, 1928.

Buranasiri, S., and Baum, S.: The significance of the venous phase of celiac and superior mesenteric arteriography in evaluating pancreatic carcinoma. Radiology, *102*:11–20, 1972.

Caravati, C. M., Ashworth, J. S., and Frederick, P.: Pancreatic pseudocysts: a medical evaluation. J.A.M.A., *197*:572–576, 1966.

Case, J. T.: Roentgenology of pancreatic disease. Amer. J. Roentgen., *44*:485–518, 1940.

Chait, A., Matasar, K. W., Fabian, C. E., and Mellins, H. Z.: Vascular impressions on the ureters. Amer. J. Roentgen., *11*:729–749, 1971.

Chait, H., and Faegenburg, D. H.: Illusory neoplasms of the stomach and duodenum as a manifestation of carcinoma of the pancreas. Radiology, *74*:771–777, 1960.

Chamberlin, G. W., and Imber, I.: Pyelography for the diagnosis of lesions of the body and tail of the pancreas. Radiology, *63*:722–729, 1954.

Child, C. G.: The Liver and Portal Hypertension. Philadelphia, W. B. Saunders Company, 1964.

Clemett, A. R.: Nonneoplastic disease of the pancreas. *In* Alimentary Tract Roentgenology. Edited by A. R. Margulis and H. J. Burhenne. St. Louis, C. V. Mosby Company, 1967, pp. 874–895.

Cope, C., and Isard, H. J.: Left renal vein entrapment. Radiology, *92*:867–872, 1969.

Dixon, J. A., and Hillam, J. D.: Surgical treatment of biliary tract disease associated with acute pancreatitis. Amer. J. Surg., *120*:371–375, 1970.

Engel, H., and Lysholm, E.: New roentgenologic method of pancreas examination and its practical results. Acta Radiol., *15*:635–651, 1934.

Eyler, W. R., Clark, M. D., and Rian, R. L.: An evaluation of roentgen signs of pancreatic enlargement. J.A.M.A., *181*:967–971, 1962.

Gorder, J. L., and Stargardter, F. L.: Pancreatic pseudocysts simulating intrarenal masses. Amer. J. Roentgen., *107*:65–68, 1969.

Guerrier, K., and Persky, L.: Pancreatic disease simulating renal abnormality. Amer. J. Surg., *120*:46–49, 1970.

Harrington, O. B., Beall, A. C., Noon, G., and DeBakey, M. E.: Intravenous cholangiography in acute cholecystitis. Arch. Surg., *88*:585–589, 1964.

Hellebusch, A. A., Walton, K. N., and Griffen, W. O.: Perinephric pancreatic pseudocyst in a child. J. Urol., *102*:633–634, 1969.

Herbert, W. W., and Margulis, A. R.: Diagnosis of retroperitoneal masses by gastrointestinal roentgenographic measurements: a computer study. Radiology, *84*:52–57, 1965.

Hershenson, M. A.: Carcinoma of the tail and body of the pancreas: roentgenologic technique for its demonstration. Amer. J. Dig. Dis., *3*:835–839, 1937.

Howard, J. M.: Pancreatitis associated with gallstones. *In* Surgical Diseases of the Pancreas. Edited by J. M. Howard and G. L. Jordan. Philadelphia, J. B. Lippincott Company, 1960, p. 169.

Isbell, R. G., Carlson, H. C., and Hoffman, H. N.: Roentgenologic-pathologic correlation in malabsorption syndromes. Amer. J. Roentgen., *107*:158–169, 1969.

Johnson, H. C., McLaren, J. R., and Weens, H. S.: Intravenous cholangiography in the differential diagnosis of acute cholecystitis. Radiology, *74*:790–797, 1960.

Kaden, V. G., Howard, J. M., and Doubleday, L. C.: Cholecystographic studies during and immediately following acute pancreatitis. Surgery, *38*:1082–1086, 1955.

Kent, K. H.: Extrinsic lesions affecting the transverse colon. Amer. J. Roentgen., *89*:779–786, 1963.

Levene, G., and Scheff, S.: Intravenous cholangiography as an aid in diagnosis of carcinoma of the head of the pancreas. Radiology, *68*:714–717, 1957.

Lobsenz, H., and Jauernig, R. H.: The retrogastric space, roentgenographically considered. Radiology, *52*:701–704, 1949.

Lukash, W. M.: Complications of acute pancreatitis: unusual sequelae in 100 cases. Arch. Surg., *94*:848–852, 1967.

Mani, J. R., Zboralske, F. F., and Margulis, A. R.: Carcinoma of the body and tail of the pancreas. Amer. J. Roentgen., *96*:429–446, 1966.

Margulis, A. R., and Burhenne, H. J.: Alimentary Tract Roentgenology. St. Louis, Mo., The C. V. Mosby Company, 1967, p. 908.

Marks, L. J., Weingarten, B., and Gerst, G. R.: Carcinoma of the tail of the pancreas associated with bleeding gastric varices and hypersplenism. Intern. Med., *37*:1077–1084, 1952.

Marshak, R. H., and Lindner, A. E.: Malabsorption syndrome. Seminars Roentgen., *1*:138–177, 1966.

Marshall, S., Lapp, M., Schulte, J. W.: Lesions of the pancreas mimicking renal disease. J. Urol., *93*:41–45, 1965.

McGlone, F. B., Robertson, D., and Grogan, J. M.: The roentgenologic manifestations of pancreatic tumors. Gastroenterology, *31*:551–565, 1956.

Meschan, I., Landsman, H., Regnier, G., Ward, H. W., Brogdon, B. G., and Pool, C. S.: The "normal" radiographic adult stomach and duodenum. A study of their contour and size and their critical relationships to the spine in both symptomatic and asymptomatic individuals. Southern Med. J., *46*:878–887, 1953.

Mohiuddin, S., Sakiyalak, P., Gullick, H. D., et al: Stenosing lesions of the colon secondary to pancreatitis. Arch. Surg., *102*:229–231, 1971.

Nelson, S. W., and Christoforidis, A. J.: Roentgenologic features of the Zollinger-Ellison syndrome – ulcerogenic tumor of the pancreas. Seminars Roengten., *3*:254–266, 1968.

Poole, J. G.: A new roentgenographic method of measuring the retrogastric and retroduodenal spaces: statistical evaluation of reliability and diagnostic utility. Radiology, *97*:71–81, 1970.

Poppel, M. H.: Roentgen Manifestations of Pancreatic Disease. Springfield, Ill., Charles C Thomas, Publisher, 1951.

Poppel, M. H.: Some migratory aspects of inflammatory collections of pancreatic origin. Radiology, *72*:323–329, 1959.

Poppel, M. H., Sheinmel, A., and Mednick, E.: The procurement and critical appraisal of the width diameter of the midline retrogastric soft tissues. Amer. J. Roentgen., *61*:56–60, 1949.

Rigler, L. G.: Diagnosis of extra-gastrointestinal abdominal masses. Radiology, *21*:229–238, 1933.

Rosch, J.: Roentgenologic diagnosis of pancreatic disease. Amer. J. Roentgen., *100*:664–672, 1967.

Rosch, J., and Herfort, K.: Splenoportographic diagnosis of pancreatic diseases. Geriatrics, *19*: 725–734, 1964.

Sarles, H., Sarles, J. C., Camatte, R., Muratore, R., Gaini, M., Guien, C., Pastor, J., and LeRoy, F.: Observations on 205 confirmed cases of acute pancreatitis, recurring pancreatitis, and chronic pancreatitis. Gut, 6:545–559, 1965.

Schultz, E. H.: Aids to diagnosis of acute pancreatitis by roentgenologic studies. Amer. J. Roentgen., *89*:825–836, 1963.

Schwartz, S., and Nadelhaft, J.: Simulation of colonic obstruction at the splenic flexure by pancreatitis: roentgen features. Amer. J. Roentgen., *78*:607–616, 1957.

Shockman, A. T., and Marasco, J. A.: Pseudocysts of the pancreas. Amer. J. Roentgen., *101*:628–638, 1967.

Steedman, R. A., Doering, R., and Carter, R.: Surgical aspects of pancreatic abscess. Surg. Gynec. Obstet., *125*:757–762, 1967.

Stein, G. N., Kalser, M. H., Sarian, N. N., and Finkelstein, A.: An evaluation of the roentgen changes in acute pancreatitis: correlation with clinical findings. Gastroenterology, *36*:354–361, 1959.

Strang, C., and Walton, J. N.: Carcinoma of body and tail of pancreas. Ann. Intern. Med., *39*: 15–37, 1953.

Stuart, C.: Acute pancreatitis: new radiodiagnostic sign. J. Fac. Radiol., *8*:50–58, 1956.

Sutton, J. P., Yarborough, D. Y., and Richards, J. T.: Isolated splenic vein occlusion. Arch. Surg., *100*:623–626, 1970.

Tomford, N. R., and Jesseph, J. E.: Pseudocyst of the pancreas. A review of fifty cases. Amer. J. Surg., *118*:86–94, 1969.

Tucker, D. H., and Moore, I. B.: Vanishing pancreatic calcification in chronic pancreatitis. New Eng. J. Med., *268*:31–33, 1963.

Weens, H. S., and Walker, L. A.: The radiologic diagnosis of acute cholecystitis and pancreatitis. Radiol. Clin. N. Amer., *2*:89–106, 1964.

Yale, C. E., and Crummy, A. B.: Splenic vein thrombosis and bleeding esophageal varices. J.A.M.A., *217*:317–320, 1971.

Zboralske, F. F., and Amberg, J. R.: Detection of the Zollinger-Ellison syndrome: the radiologist's responsibility. Amer. J. Roengten., *104*:529–543, 1968.

Chapter 4

ROENTGENOLOGY OF THE DUODENUM

GENERAL CONSIDERATIONS

Despite the introduction of sophisticated radiologic techniques to evaluate the pancreaticoduodenal area (such as angiography, radionuclide imaging, and ultrasound), the barium meal examination continues to be the principal method for the recognition of pancreatic enlargement, extension of pancreatic disease into the peripancreatic space and, of course, primary duodenal disorders. Diagnostic difficulty is increased by the fact that peptic ulcer disease and disorders of the biliary tract may present clinical and radiographic findings which closely resemble primary disorders of the pancreas and duodenum. Furthermore, the duodenum itself may become involved with a variety of unusual inflammatory and neoplastic disorders, many of which are unique for this segment of the small bowel.

In general, roentgen signs of disease in structures contiguous to the duodenum are mediated through changes in the duodenal wall and thus may lack specificity. To complicate the problem further, most disease states tend to heighten duodenal peristalsis which, even under normal conditions, is quite active. In a normal patient, duodenal motor activity frequently produces a totally different roentgen image on each of several films. Interpretation becomes difficult in patients with high gastric acidity because the acid-barium mixture leaving the stomach produces poor coating of the duodenal surface (Kreel, 1967). These factors may obscure the nature of the underlying pathologic condition, or may suggest an abnormality where none in truth exists. Understandably, radiologists until recently have had limited success in correctly identifying the nature of duodenal abnormalities unless heavy emphasis was placed on clinical findings. Lacking an appropriate history of pancreatic or duodenal disease, one is tempted to dismiss all but the grossest abnormalities of the duodenal contour as being within the limits of normal variability. Although this chapter stresses roentgen pathology, the importance of clinical correlation cannot be overemphasized.

One of the most important indications for barium study of the duodenum is clinical suspicion of pancreatic cancer. Unfortunately, such tumors produce very few specific clinical or radiographic signs until the disease is far advanced, and are often found at surgery to be unresectable. Nonetheless, because of the universally poor prognosis in pancreaticoduodenal cancer, there has been persistent interest in a radical surgical approach to this disease in the form of the pancreaticoduodenal resection pioneered by Whipple. Although great effort was expended by radiologists to discover early signs of pancreaticoduodenal cancer on barium studies, the returns were disappointing; widely divergent results were recorded by highly qualified radiologists. In many series, the films on patients with proven cancer were reviewed retrospectively and abnormal findings consistent with cancer were considered sufficient for the diagnosis. Yet the illustrations of the roentgen findings in these older publications demonstrate a doubtful specificity. As Coe has aptly stated, "The early diagnosis of carcinoma of the head of the pancreas is best made with the 'retrospectoscope'; i.e., having found at exploratory operation an early carcinoma, go back and look at the films of the duodenal loop and see or imagine you see changes which are due to carcinoma. No roentgenologic diagnosis is more reprehensible and only tends to make referring physicians have less faith in radiologic studies" (Coe, 1963).

In recent years, hypotonic duodenography has become rather widely accepted as an important method in the evaluation of pancreaticoduodenal disease. Since we have been personally interested in this procedure for a number of years, the emphasis in this chapter will be based on our experience with hypotonic duodenography.

CONVENTIONAL BARIUM EXAMINATION

Technique

The requirements for optimal barium evaluation of duodenal morphology usually include the following:

1. Adequate filling of the duodenal lumen.
2. Positioning for radiography based on an understanding of the anatomic relationship between the pancreas and duodenum.
3. Usually, multiple films.

While motor abnormalities may be documented early in the course of an examination, detailed spot or overhead filming prior to complete filling is premature and often futile. The sine qua non for demonstrating duodenal pathologic conditions is adequate filling of the duodenum. This requires ingestion of a minimum of 6 to 8 ounces of barium, following which the patient is placed in the right decubitus position to promote gravity emptying of the stomach into the duodenum. Because of the retroperitoneal location of the descending duodenum, films made in the supine or supine right posterior oblique projection will maintain optimal barium filling of the duodenal loop while retaining close apposition of the pancreaticoduodenal surfaces (Salik, 1961). Contour changes on the inner aspect of the duodenal loop are best appreciated in this fashion.

On the other hand, films made in the prone oblique projection usually demonstrate excellent filling of the duodenum but may allow barium within the lumen to fall forward from the portion of the duodenal wall in contact with the pancreas, thus reducing the degree of extrinsic deformity of the duodenal wall. Radiographs made in the horizontal right lateral decubitus position with a vertical beam allow assessment of the retroduodenal space. Radiographs made in the supine position with a horizontal cross table beam have also been advocated for evaluation of the retroduodenal space (Poppel, 1951). However, these are technically less reliable unless one of the newer C-arm fluoroscopic units for horizontal radiography is available. Finally, the active peristaltic activity in the duodenum, which is often accentuated in the presence of a local pathologic condition, may produce misleading images unless multiple films are utilized. Hyperactive peristaltic contractions may obscure the presence of a genuine pathologic condition (such as an ulcer crater or filling defect) or may suggest the presence of disease where none in fact exists. It is in this context that the abolition of peristaltic activity achieved in hypotonic duodenography is of value.

Diagnostic Criteria

Few new signs have been added to the classic descriptions of barium meal alterations in diseases of the duodenum and pancreas recorded by Rigler (1933), Case (1940), Poppel (1951), Hodes (1954), Salik (1961), and Beranbaum (1966). Most of these can be conveniently included in the diagnostic criteria demonstrable by hypotonic duodenography, discussed later.

Motor Abnormalities

In the older literature dealing with the conventional barium meal examination, considerable emphasis was placed on alterations in duodenal motor activity as a sign of pancreaticoduodenal disease. A variety of motor abnormalities have been described in both benign and malignant disease of the duodenal region. None of these is entirely specific or particularly useful when the clinical findings are unclear. Marked hyperperistalsis, with frequent muscular contractions and to-and-fro motion of the barium, may occur in inflammatory diseases such as peptic ulcer or pancreatitis. Partial or complete smooth-muscle atony is more common than hyperperistalsis in patients with severe pancreatitis. The resulting duodenal ileus may be a useful plain film finding, as noted in Chapter 2. Less marked motor abnormalities may occur in malignant disorders, either because of direct irritation of duodenal musculature by tumor or because of associated inflammtory reaction. While motor changes may indeed be the sole early sign of malignancy (Salik, 1961), they lack diagnostic specificity and merely indicate the need for further study. Thus, while motor alterations may signify early evidence of pancreatic disease, the overlap with normal peristaltic variation is so great that even cineradiographic studies with detailed recording for interpretation of these patterns have not proved exceptionally rewarding (Adler, 1967; Jorgens, 1962).

Mucosal Changes

Focal alteration of the mucosal fold configuration along the inner duodenal margin has long been recognized as an early and important sign of an expanding lesion in the head of the pancreas (Salik, 1961). Barium-filled crevices between the plical folds of the duodenum may become blunted, deflected, stretched and sharpened into spicules or obliterated as a result of pressure from enlargement in the head of the pancreas. Typically, the density of the barium filling the medial portion of the duodenal loop is also reduced by extrinsic pressure from the pancreas. A finely tapered stretching of barium-filled crevices along the inner duodenal wall has been designated the "brush effect" and is associated with carcinoma of the head of the pancreas (Salik, 1961) (Fig. 4–1). Unfortunately, however, such subtle

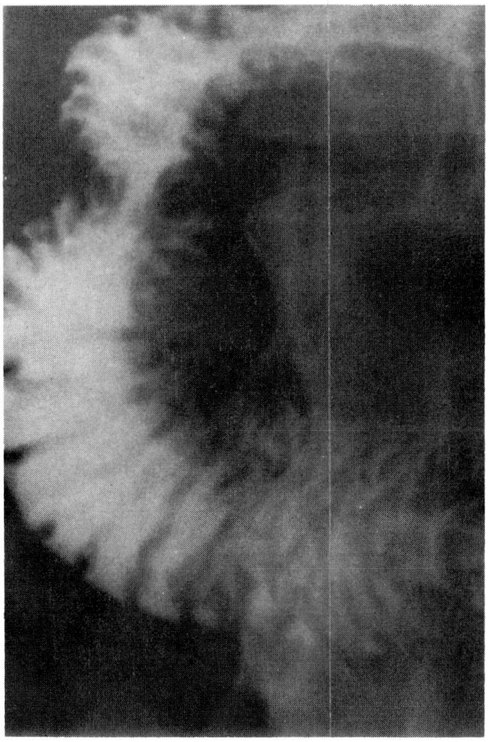

Figure 4–1. "Brush sign" in carcinoma of the head of the pancreas. Folds along the medial border are elongated and tapered (resembling the bristles of a brush). This sign is identical to spiculation described on duodenograms (see Figs. 4–29 and 4–40). A double-contour mass impression is also visible. (Courtesy of Dr. J. R. Dreyfuss.)

changes are not specific for cancer, nor do they invariably indicate the presence of a pathologic condition. Because of the active duodenal peristalsis, minor mucosal alterations are not uncommonly noted in apparently normal subjects, and even the so-called brush sign of pancreatic cancer has been encountered in normals (Fig. 4–2). Stein, writing in Bockus (1965), agrees that such subtle changes occur "frequently in patients in whom there is no clinical suspicion of pancreatic cancer making it extremely difficult to detect the abnormal on the basis of objective roentgen criteria." This judgment, of course, refers exclusively to conventional barium meal examination rather than to duodenography.

Displacement of the Duodenum

This is an important sign of periduodenal mass lesions. However, as in the case of retrogastric masses (Chapter 3), apparent alteration in the position or course of the duodenum must be accompanied by local compression or indentation to be certain that a pathologic process exists (Beranbaum, 1966). Although the literature contains elaborate protocols for measuring the retrogastroduodenal space (Poole, 1970) or for determining the position of the duodenal-jejunal flexure (Sifre, 1953), we feel that measurements alone are neither convenient nor reliable (Herbert, 1965). Widening of the retroduodenal soft tissues may occur without visible impression on the posterior duodenal wall, but it is difficult to recognize unless it is gross or is associated with obvious forward displacement of the stomach (Fig. 4–3). Forward displacement of a limited portion of the duodenum (e.g., the cap) is considered somewhat more reliable (Fig. 4–4).

The duodenal-jejunal junction at the ligament of Treitz approximates the junction of the body and tail of the pancreas; abnormalities of this segment may be the result of enlargement of the distal pancreas or of masses arising in the retroperitoneum. The duodenal-jejunal flexure is often projected behind the stomach above the lesser curvature, and the jejunum typically descends at an acute angle from the fourth portion of the duodenum. Loss of this acute angle has been reported as an early sign of enlargement of the body of the pancreas (Sifre, 1953), but we and others have found that considerable variation occurs (Eaton, 1972; Coe, 1963).

Substantial separation between the distal duodenum and greater curvature may be encountered in normal endomorphic males, as illustrated in Figure 4–5. This patient underwent a cholecystectomy for cholelithiasis but no local cause was found for the low position of the distal duodenum. Careful evaluation of the distal duodenum in patients with suspected pancreatic disease is important; however, the significant abnormalities are not positional but structural

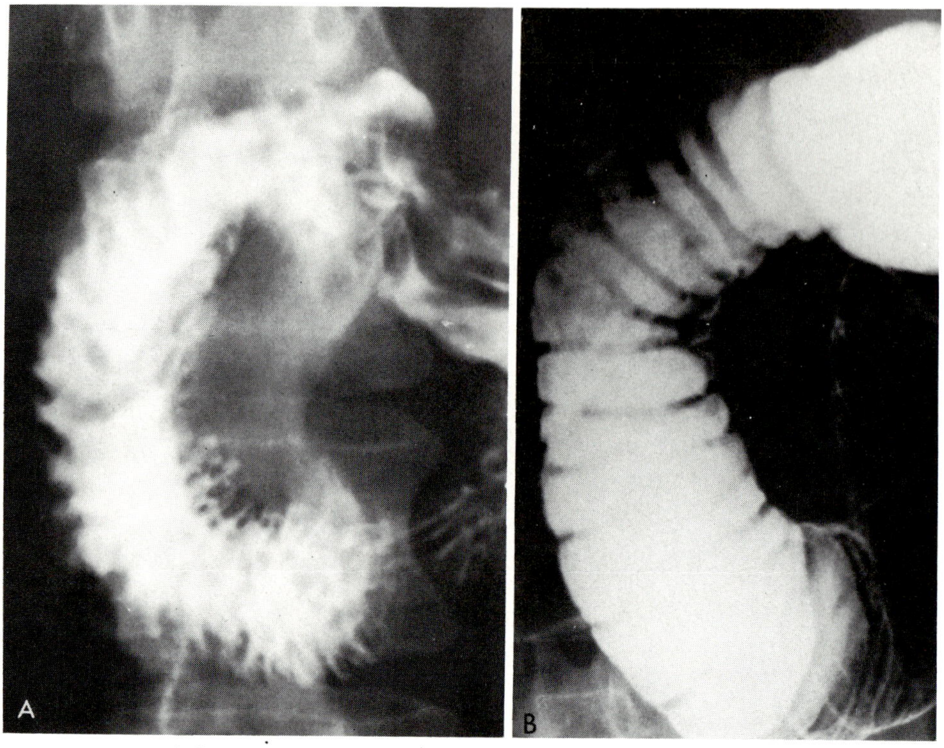

Figure 4–2. Brush-like appearance of the mucosal folds in a normal patient.

A, Standard barium meal study shows an apparent brush sign along the lower inner duodenal border. The appearance is indistinguishable from that of the pancreatic cancer illustrated in Figure 4–1.

B, Hypotonic duodenogram showing a normal inner duodenal margin. The configuration on the conventional study is a commonly encountered false-positive appearance.

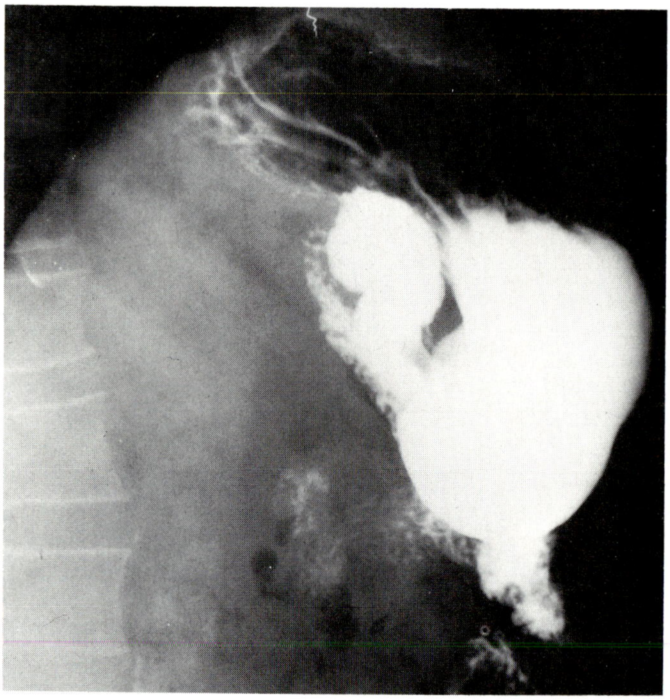

Figure 4–3. Widening of the retroduodenal space resulting from a large hypernephroma of the right kidney. Anterior displacement of the descending duodenum and distal antrum is apparent.

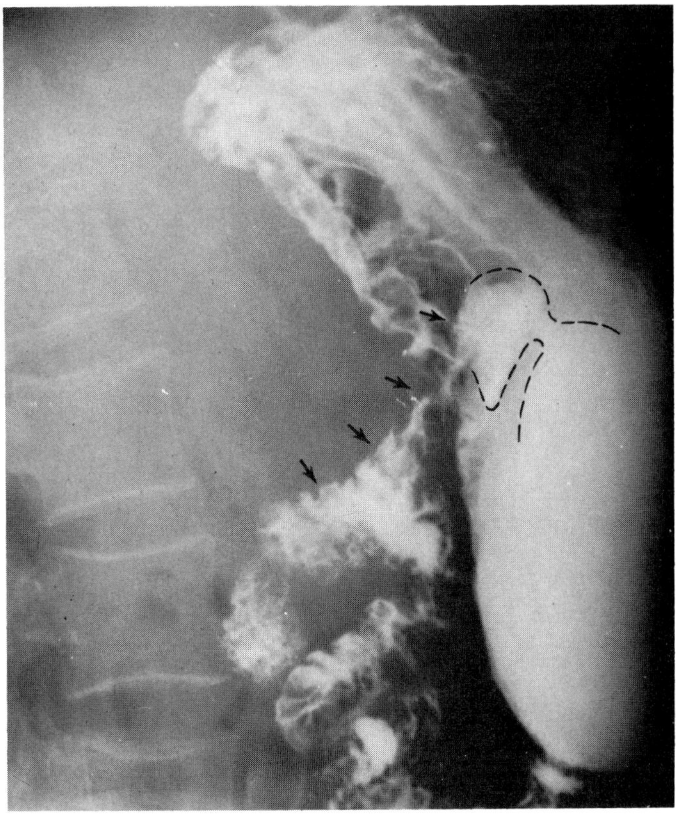

Figure 4–4. Forward displacement of the duodenal cap and upper descending duodenum resulting from a pancreatic pseudocyst. Local indentation of a portion of the duodenum is a more reliable sign of a retroduodenal mass than generalized widening of the prevertebral space. (Courtesy of Dr. M. G. Glickman.)

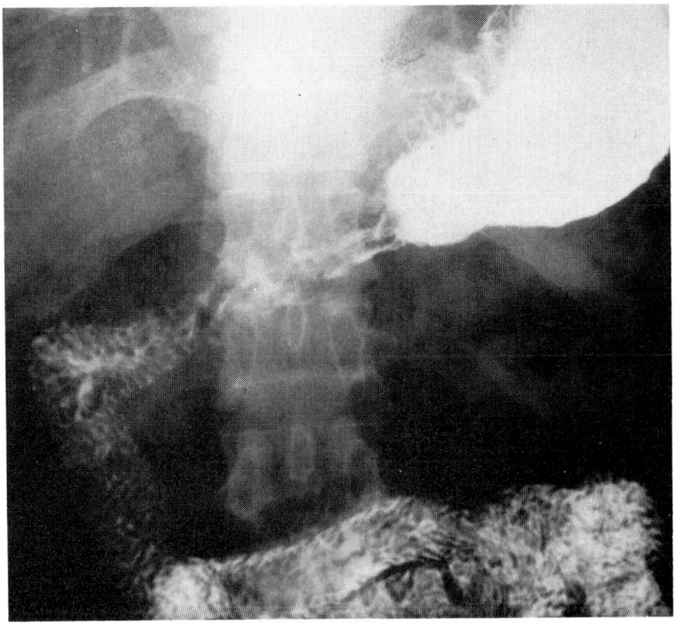

Figure 4–5. Normal low-lying duodenojejunal flexure. The patient was operated upon for cholelithiasis. The pancreas was normal at exploration. (Reproduced by permission of *American Journal of Roentgenology.*)

changes, such as indentation, mucosal splaying, elongation, and fixation of folds or frank ulceration (Fig. 4–6). These usually occur along the upper margin of the distal duodenum and vary from the obvious to the subtle (Fig. 4–7); they are important signs of disease in the distal pancreas. Such changes can be noted in up to 75 per cent of patients with cancer of the body or tail of the pancreas (Mani, 1966). Similar and often very minor fold abnormalities are common in pancreatitis, as illustrated in Figure 4–7. In general, fold abnormalities associated with pancreatitis demonstrate wider distribution and more edema than in cases of

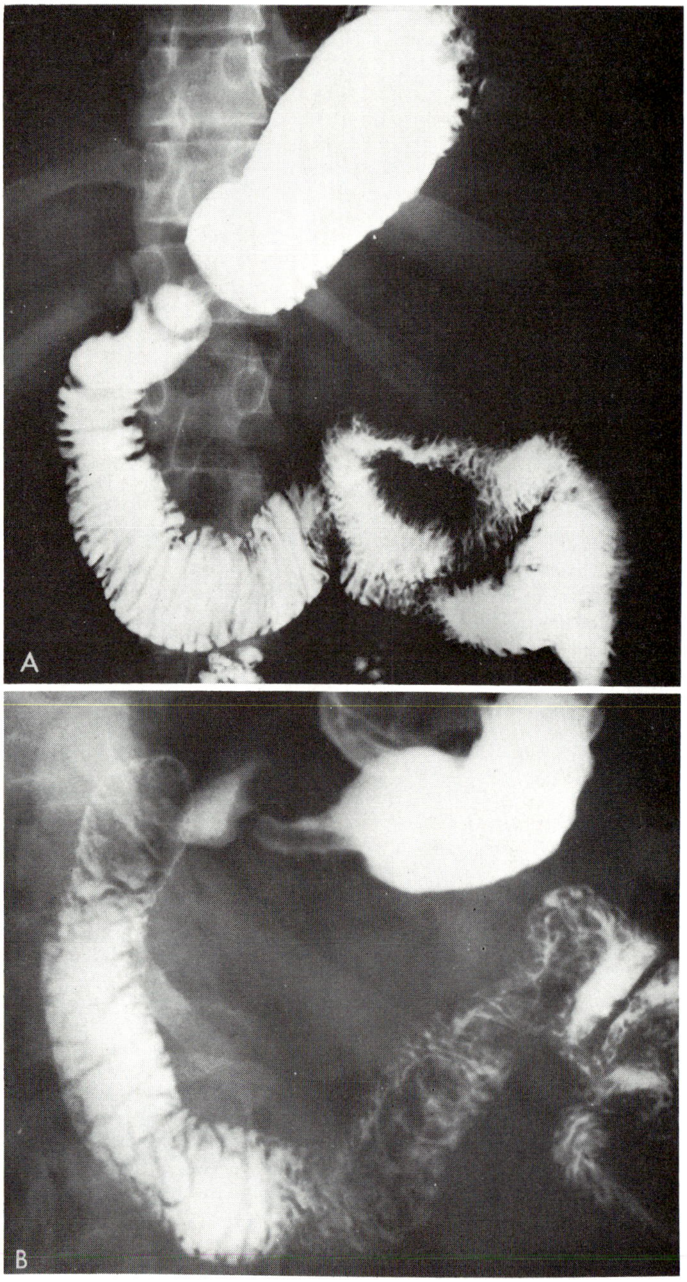

Figure 4–6. Pathologic depression of the duodenojejunal flexure.

A, Pancreatic abscess.

B, Carcinoma of the body of the pancreas. Note the focal indentation and splaying of folds along the superior duodenal border.

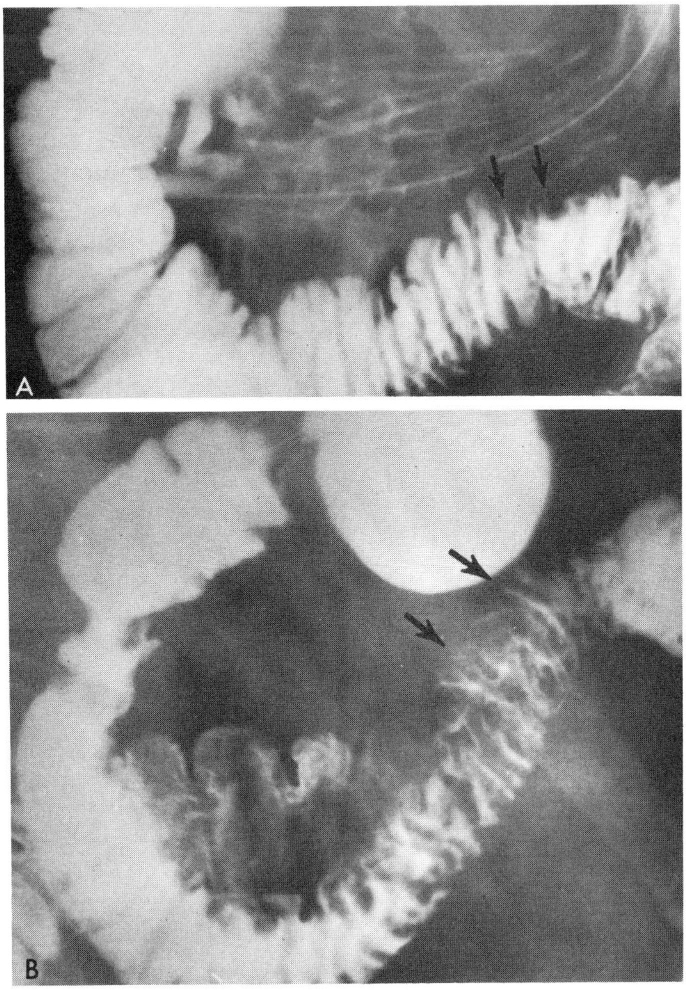

Figure 4–7. Subtle fold abnormalities along the upper margin of the duodenojejunal flexure in two patients with pancreatitis. Depression of the duodenum is minimal.

tumor, but these are not reliable differential features.

HYPOTONIC DUODENOGRAPHY: PRINCIPLES AND APPLICATIONS

Modern radiologists accept the fact that a precise delineation of duodenal morphology is frequently impossible with an ordinary barium meal study. Because of the vigorous peristaltic activity in the duodenum, roentgen findings vary from film to film and early changes are difficult to demonstrate.

Hypotonic duodenography is radiologic study of the duodenum rendered aperistaltic by anticholinergic drugs. Introduced by Liotta in 1955 as a method of evaluating the head of the pancreas, it became an established procedure in Europe over the next decade and more recently has achieved wide popularity elsewhere (Bilbao, 1968; Eaton, 1968; Martel, 1969; Eaton, 1970; and Ferrucci, 1971). The largest and most thoroughly analyzed series of hypotonic duodenograms (500 cases) is reported in an excellent monograph by Jacquemet and his associates (1965).

Hypotonic duodenography involves the induction of temporary paralysis of smooth muscle tone and peristaltic activity by the parenteral administration of high doses of an anticholinergic drug. The duodenum becomes flaccid and relaxes against the head of the pancreas so that pressure effects on the duodenal wall are clearly disclosed. The distention thus created causes the plical folds of the duodenum to be arranged in an orderly transverse fashion and allows intrinsic duodenal disease to be demonstrated more clearly. Figure 4–8 shows a normal hypotonic duodenogram.

The major indications for hypotonic duodenography are indicated in Table 4–1. When a conventional barium meal study clearly shows the duodenum to be normal, or demonstrates an abnormality readily correlated with clinical findings (e.g., acute pancreatitis), there is little need for performing duodenography. However, when pancreatic or periduodenal disease is suspected, and the duodenum is poorly shown or is apparently abnormal, hypotonic examination is a logical follow-up. When a lesion in the head of the pancreas or ampulla of Vater is strongly suspected (e.g., in obstructive jaundice), we believe the radiologic investigation should begin with duodenography. This approach will yield maximum diagnostic information with a minimum of cost and patient morbidity.

TABLE 4–1. Indications for Hypotonic Duodenography

Follow-up After Standard UGI Series If:
Duodenal abnormality is apparent
Duodenum is poorly shown – pancreaticoduodenal disease is suspected clinically
Primary Study for Obstructive Jaundice

The clinical applications of duodenography have been brought into focus by several recent investigators (Bilbao, 1968; Eaton, 1968; Martel, 1969; Eaton, 1970; and Ferrucci, 1971). Duodenography was originally intended as a method for the early detection of carcinoma of the head of the pancreas. Not surprisingly, there has been little success in this regard. When used as a search procedure in patients with epigastric or midback complaints, the yield of duodenography has been essentially nil. On the other hand, duodenography is now widely accepted

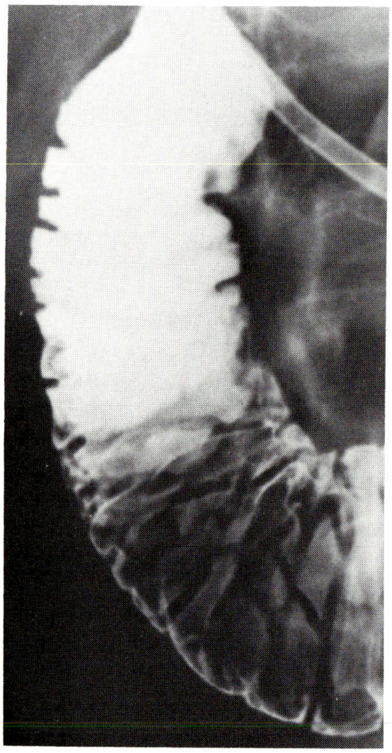

Figure 4–8. Normal hypotonic duodenogram. The plical folds assume a regular transverse arrangement. The duodenal walls demonstrate gently arcuate parallel contours.

by practicing radiologists as an important method for evaluating the questionable duodenum in daily work.

Frequently radiographic findings suggesting duodenal disease on a conventional barium study disappear completely during duodenography performed minutes later. Patients with apparent masses, pancreatic enlargement, or circumferential narrowing of the duodenum are commonly shown to have a distensible duodenal lumen on the hypotonic study (Figs. 4–9 to 4–11). Such "non-lesions" presumably represent the random effect of peristaltic activity and smooth muscle spasm. These are common occurrences in daily practice and their recognition by duodenography reduces the rate of false-positive diagnoses, thus avoiding further unnecessary studies or even an occasionally negative laparotomy.

A vivid example of the role of spasm in the production of a non-lesion is illustrated in Figure 4–12. In this case, an apparent mass in the head of the pancreas was shown to be a non-lesion at duodenography the following day. Reexamination by conventional barium study on the third day disclosed reappearance of the mass-like configuration, confirming the role of smooth muscle tonus.

More important, the duodenogram may confirm and clarify an abnormality previously suggested on the conventional study (Figs. 4–13 to 4–15). When the confusing images of peristalsis and spasm are eliminated, the true contours of an organic lesion emerge more clearly, and a more accurate differential diagnosis can be made.

The technical reasons for the superiority of duodenography are clear. When hyperperistalsis prevents adequate demonstration of the duodenum by conventional methods, anticholinergic-induced duodenal paralysis almost invariably circumvents this problem. Furthermore, hypotonia allows the fluoroscopist to obtain views of suspicious areas in

(Text continued on page 102)

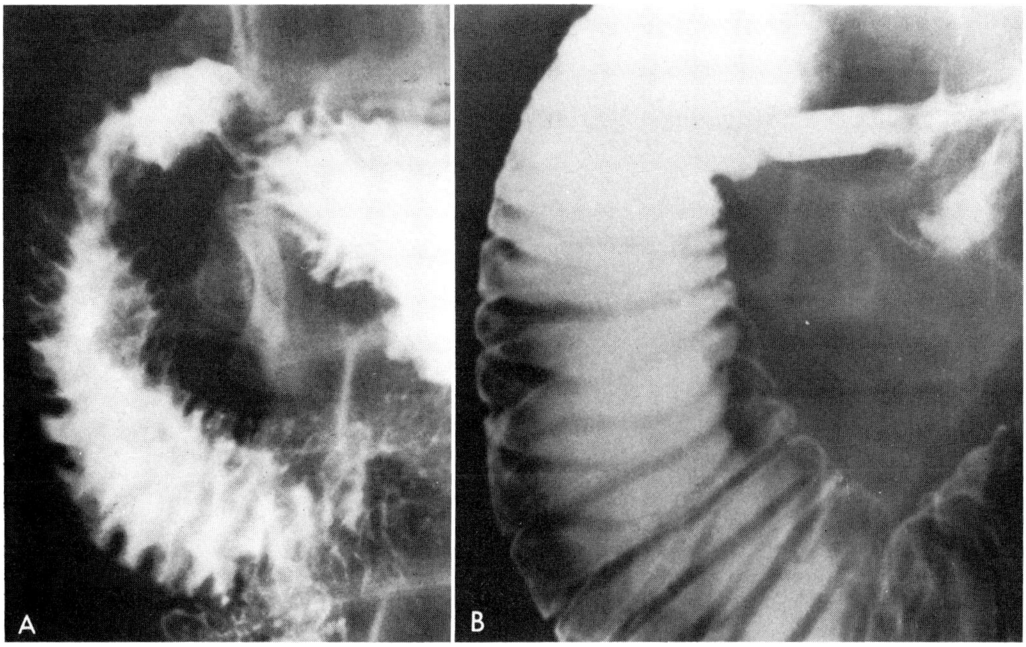

Figure 4–9. Duodenal "non-lesion" in a 60-year-old male with epigastric distress.

A, Upper gastrointestinal study suggests a nodular indentation along the inner margin of the duodenal loop.

B, Duodenogram reveals a normal inner duodenal contour with no evidence of a mass. The initial appearance was attributed to the effects of random peristaltic activity.

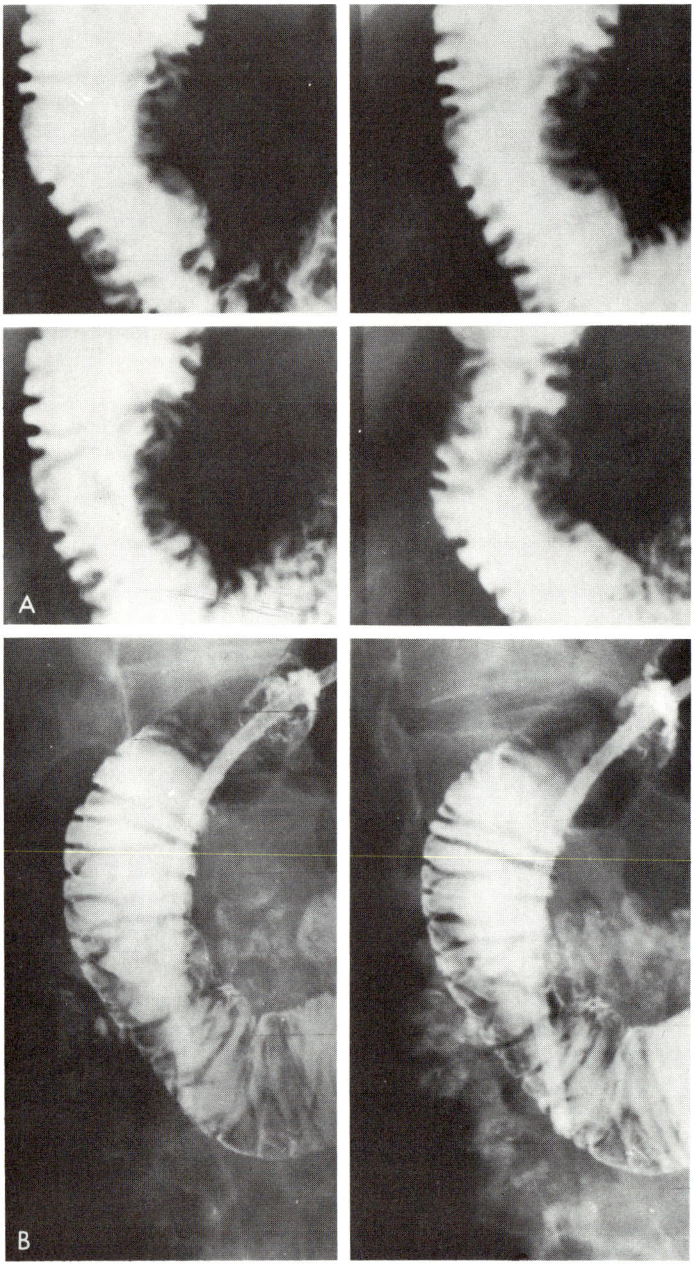

Figure 4–10. Duodenal "non-lesion" in a 45-year-old male with malaise and epigastric distress.

A, Multiple spot films from a conventional upper gastrointestinal study suggest a constant indentation on the medial aspect of the duodenal loop. Serum amylase was within normal limits.

B, Hypotonic duodenogram three days later reveals no abnormality. The patient was followed conservatively, with no further symptoms. The initial appearance was attributed to spasm.

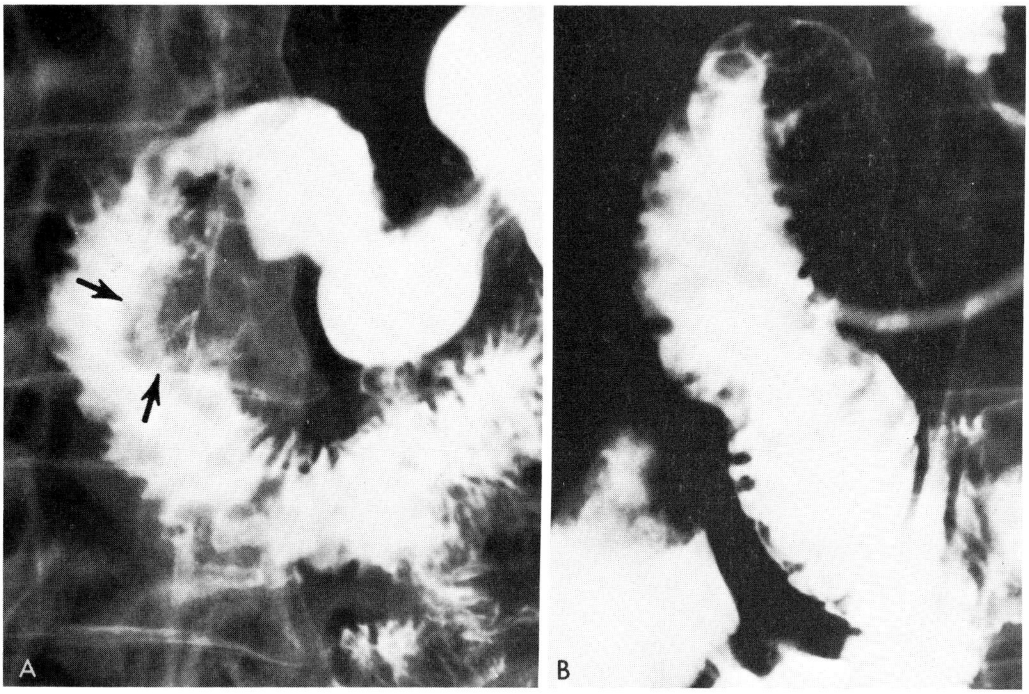

Figure 4–11. Duodenal "non-lesion."
A, Standard barium meal suggests a nodular mass in the region of the ampulla.
B, Duodenogram one day later reveals a normal inner duodenal margin.

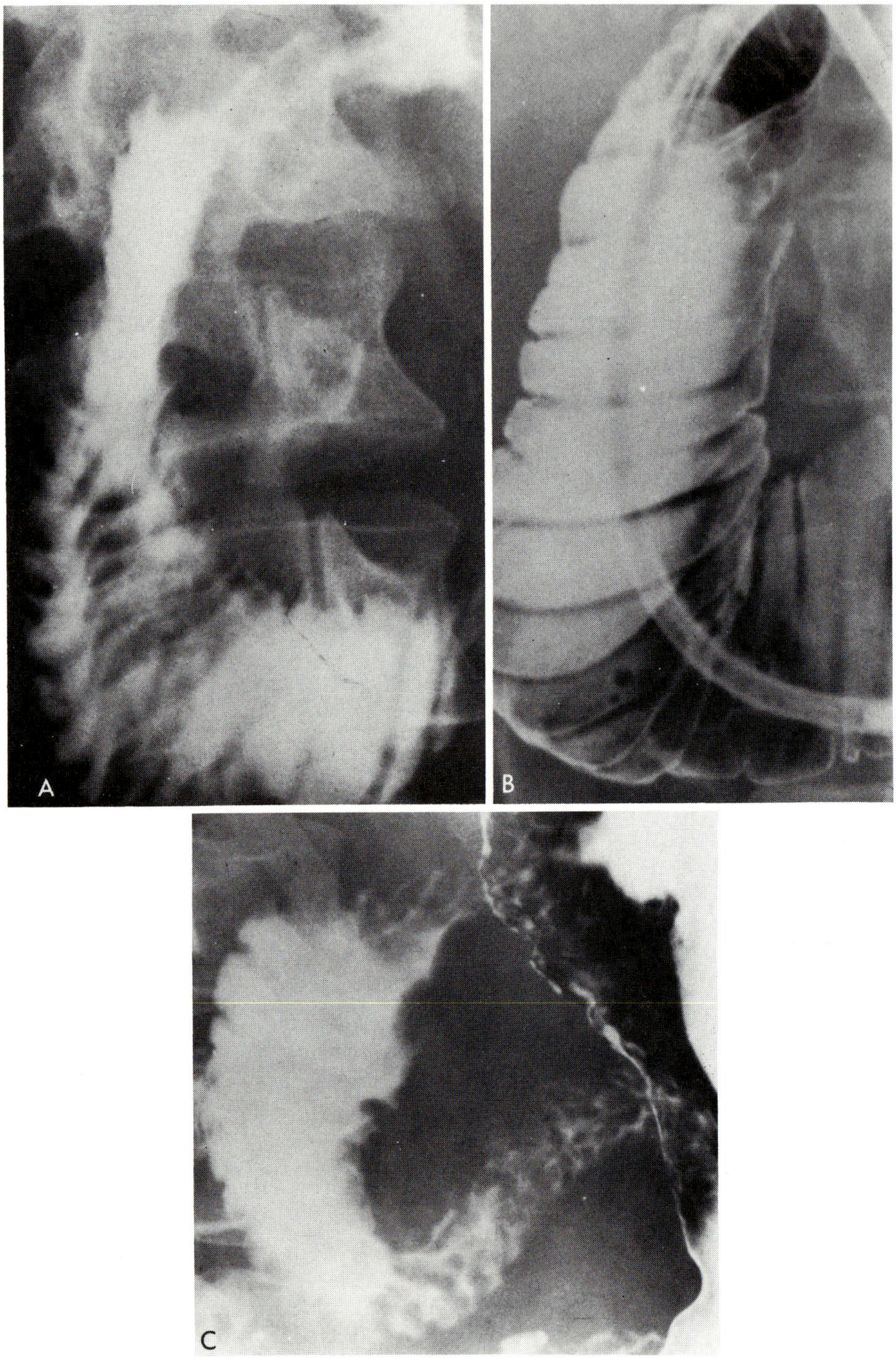

Figure 4–12. The role of spasm in the "non-lesion" effect. A 32-year-old alcoholic male with jaundice.

A, Standard upper gastrointestinal study suggests a mass in the head of the pancreas.

B, Hypotonic duodenogram one day later shows no evidence of a mass.

C, Repeat conventional barium study on the third day again suggests a mass impression. Final diagnosis: acute alcoholic hepatitis. The reappearance of the mass after negative duodenography emphasizes the role of muscular spasm in producing spurious images.

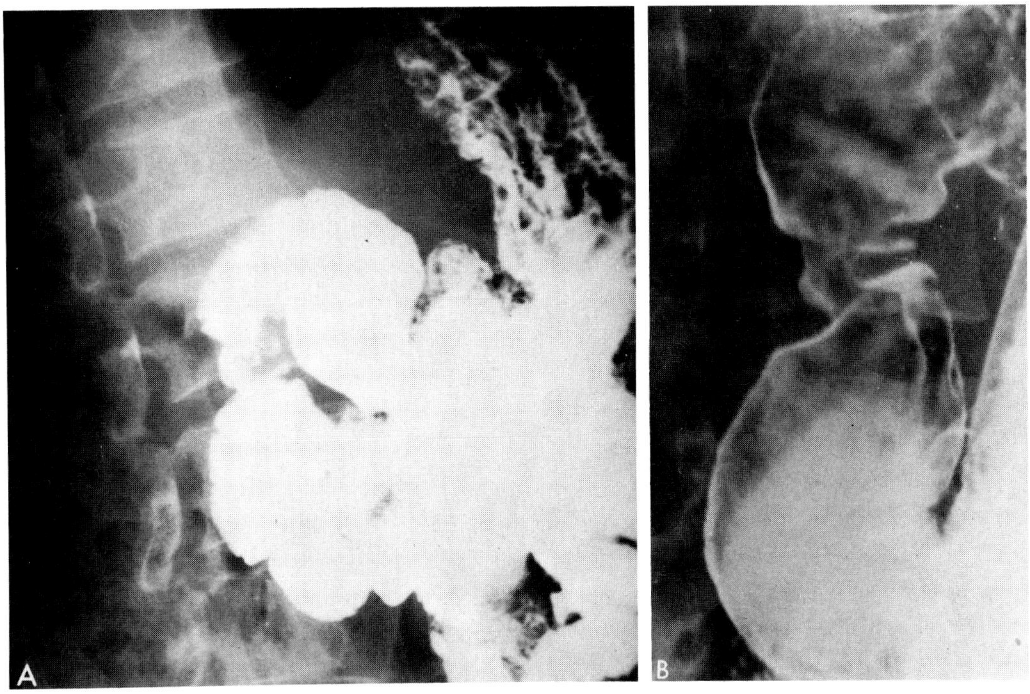

Figure 4–13. Duodenography clarifies the abnormality.

A, Conventional barium meal study shows a constricting lesion in the mid-descending duodenum suggesting the possibility of a neoplasm.

B, Duodenography shows a smooth ring-like stricture with intact mucosa. Diagnosis: post-peptic stricture.

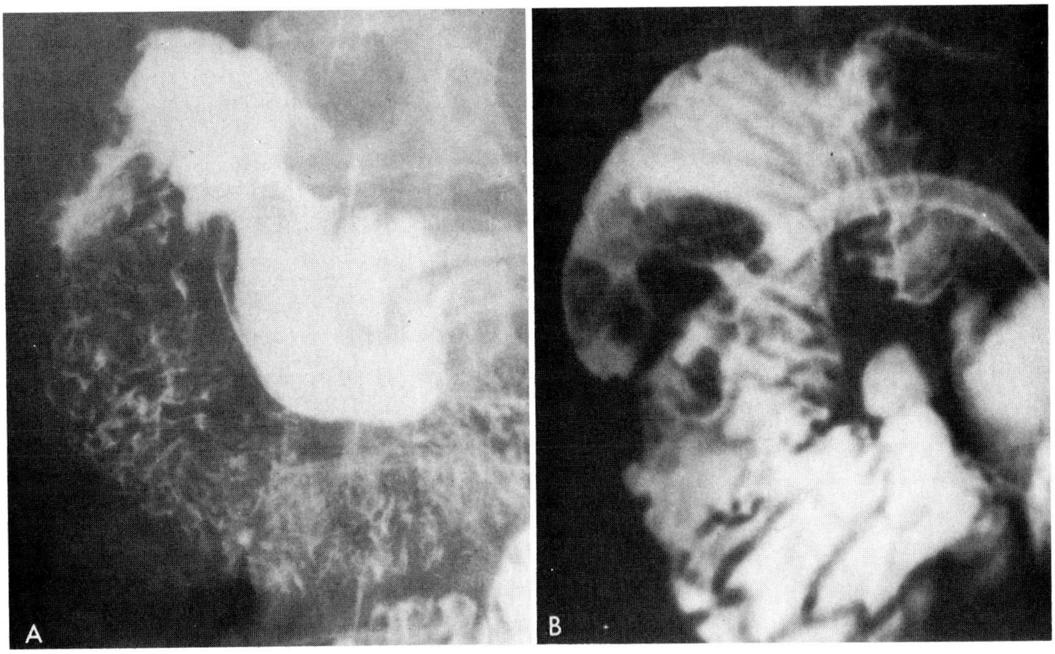

Figure 4–14. Duodenal tumor revealed by duodenography. A 65-year-old woman with occult blood in the stool.

A, Initial barium meal study disclosed only irregular thickening of folds in the descending duodenum. The original interpretation was negative.

B, Duodenography demonstrates a discrete lobulated mass proven at surgery to be a benign adenomatous polyp.

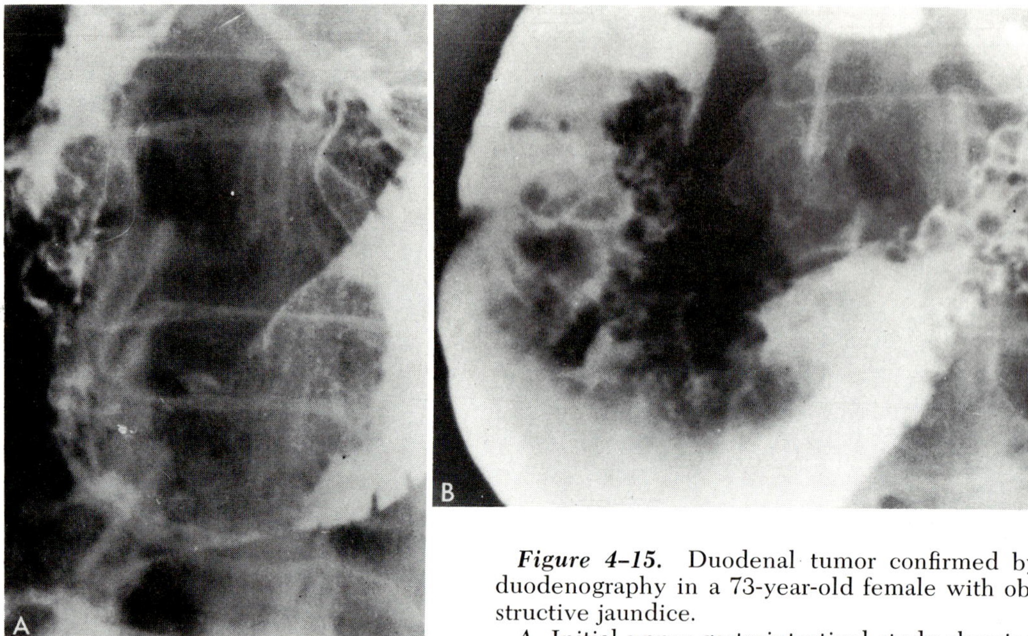

Figure 4-15. Duodenal tumor confirmed by duodenography in a 73-year-old female with obstructive jaundice.

A, Initial upper gastrointestinal study showing an apparent filling defect involving the second and third portions of the duodenum.

B, Hypotonic duodenography clearly shows a multinodular intraluminal mass. Final diagnosis: malignant villous adenoma. (Courtesy of Dr. R. Seidler.)

multiple projections more easily and reproducibly than can be accomplished by conventional study. The distention produced by duodenography demonstrates a larger pancreaticoduodenal interface and increases the chances for detecting subtle pancreatic pathologic conditions. Finally, air contrast views generally add to diagnostic accuracy and are more easily obtained via duodenography.

Admittedly, anticholinergic studies have a theoretical disadvantage in that significant functional changes, particularly irritability, and abnormal fold patterns could become obscured in a flaccid hypotonic viscus (Martel, 1969; Ferrucci, 1971). For this reason, the configuration of the gross anatomy in the hypotonic state should be carefully correlated with that seen on conventional studies for final interpretation (Ferrucci, 1971; Kikkawa, 1972). However, in practice, we have seldom found this to be a real problem.

ACCURACY OF HYPOTONIC DUODENOGRAPHY: COMPARISON WITH CONVENTIONAL BARIUM STUDY

The weight of evidence in the literature indicates that hypotonic duodenography permits a correct diagnosis of periduodenal disorders with approximately twice the frequency of conventional barium studies. Statistics on the reliability of conventional barium examination in nonmalignant periduodenal disease have been published infrequently. However, in the specific instance of pancreaticoduodenal cancer, the results of the standard barium study recorded in the literature are poor to indifferent, ranging from 19 to 77 per cent prospective accuracy. When the figures from five major modern series are combined, the preoperative diagnosis of cancer of the head of the pancreas was made in 41 per cent of the cases (Table 4–2). This figure, in one sense, represents the best results possible, coming from workers interested in pancreatic disease, but it has been estimated that in routine work, preoperative accuracy hovers at 25 per cent (Kreel, 1967). In one well-documented study of 100 proven cases of pancreatic cancer, only 24 per cent were correctly diagnosed preoperatively (Eyler, 1962). Innumerable retrospective reports of conventional studies in patients with proven peri-Vaterian cancer have described "abnormalities consistent with tumor" in 40 to 70 per cent of the cases (Broadbent, 1951; Beeler, 1952;

TABLE 4–2. Preoperative Accuracy in Carcinoma of the Pancreaticoduodenal Area: Conventional Barium Meal

AUTHOR	NO. OF CASES STUDIED	NO. CORRECTLY DIAGNOSED	PER CENT CORRECTLY DIAGNOSED
Broadbent (1951)	33	6	19
Hodes (1954)	102	51	50
Larsen (1956)	31	8	25
Salik (1961)	64	49	77
Eyler (1962)	100	24	24
TOTAL	330	138	41

and Perez, 1965). These studies are also somewhat misleading since, in most cases, they refer to a restricted group of patients, all of whom actually did have pancreatic carcinoma; accordingly, no false-positive diagnoses were possible. Strictly speaking, the results of such studies cannot be applied to patients merely suspected of having pancreatic carcinoma.

The accuracy of duodenography in detecting pancreaticoduodenal disease has varied from 76 to 97 per cent, according to published series (Table 4–3). In a group of 194 patients with pancreaticoduodenal disease, a correct duodenographic diagnosis was obtained in 84 per cent of the cases (Bilbao, 1968). Conventional studies of the same patients yielded a correct or equivocal diagnosis in 57 per cent and were falsely negative in 43 per cent. In another series of 150 proven cases studied by duodenography, the authors reported 76 per cent accuracy for pancreatic head tumors and 92 per cent for malignancy of the ampulla of Vater (Jacquemet, 1965). In two other series of 30 and 22 proven cases, one incorrect diagnosis occurred in each group (Baum, 1968; Martel, 1969). In a recent British series of 29 proven cases of cancer of the ampulla and pancreatic head, duodenography was correct in 22 (73 per cent) of the cases (Bourke, 1972). An initial report from the Massachusetts General Hospital noted 76 per cent accuracy in 26 proven cases of pancreatic cancer (Eaton, 1968). In a subsequent review of cases studied more recently, prospective accuracy in a variety of pancreaticoduodenal disorders was about 90 per cent (Novelline, in preparation).

These statistics warrant several general conclusions. False-positive duodenographic diagnoses are extremely uncommon—on the order of a few per cent (Benedict, 1970). In part, this is due to the elimination of "non-lesions" (see

TABLE 4–3. Preoperative Accuracy of Hypotonic Duodenography

AUTHOR	NO. OF CASES	PER CENT ACCURACY	COMMENT
Jacquemet (1965)	150	76 92	Pancreatic cancer Ampullary cancer
Baum and Howe (1968)	30	97	Pancreaticoduodenal disease
Bilbao (1968)	194	84	Pancreaticoduodenal disease
Eaton (1968)	26	76	Pancreatic cancer
Martel (1969)	22	95	Pancreaticoduodenal disease
MGH (1972)	300 (approx.)	90 (approx.)	Pancreaticoduodenal disease

text above). The incidence of false-negative diagnoses is slightly higher, ranging from 15 to 25 per cent. Nonetheless, the duodenogram remains considerably more sensitive than the conventional study in which false-negative diagnoses in good hands are reported as 43 per cent (Jacquemet, 1965) (Fig. 4–16). Lesions of the head of the pancreas are missed more often than those of the papilla of Vater. The lower incidence of positive findings in tumors of the head of the pancreas confirms the importance of location as a factor which determines whether a tumor of any given size will produce abnormality of the duodenum. This observation has been graphically documented in experimental models (Russell, 1965). The farther a tumor lies from the duodenal loop, the larger it must be to produce radiologically demonstrable changes. Finally, statistics on the reliability of hypotonic techniques in the evaluation of nonmalignant disease in this area are rarely encountered in the literature.

Rubinstein and his associates (1971) have recently reported abnormal duodenograms in 80 per cent of 40 patients with chronic pancreatitis, whereas conventional barium studies failed to reveal conclusive mucosal abnormalities in any instance. However, in four of six patients, extrinsic pressure defects were shown by both standard barium meal and duodenography. These authors emphasized the increased accuracy and sensitivity of duodenography but questioned the specificity of the findings in distinguishing carcinoma from chronic pancreatitis. As yet, an attempt to differentiate chronic pancreatitis from pancreatic cancer in a double-blind setting has yet to be reported.

HYPOTONIC DUODENOGRAPHY: TECHNICAL CONSIDERATIONS

The usual method for performing hypotonic duodenography combines the effects of the antispasmodic drugs and the benefits of direct duodenal intubation (Ferrucci, 1971). An indwelling catheter permits instillation of barium and air directly into the duodenal lumen, providing maximal distention and clear documentation of the anatomy without superimposition of overlying stomach or small-bowel loops.

The procedure can be simplified by

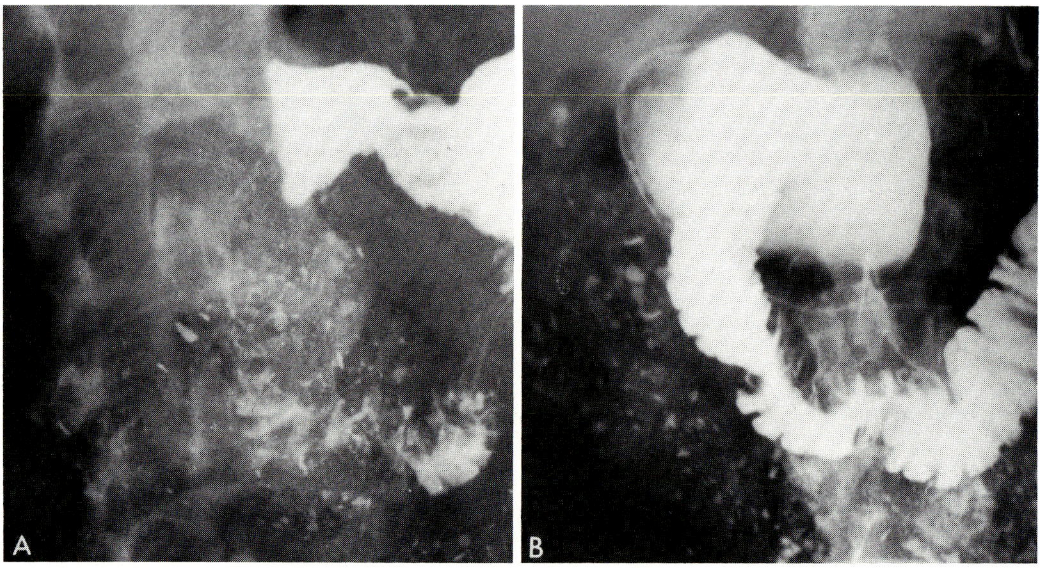

Figure 4–16. False-negative upper gastrointestinal study in a pancreatic malignancy.
A, Standard barium meal was technically suboptimal because of poor duodenal filling.
B, Hypotonic duodenogram (tubeless method) one day later disclosing an extrinsic mass with a nodular indentation of the inner duodenal margin. Spiculation of folds and a lateral incisura defect are also visible.

omitting duodenal intubation, a modification known as "tubeless duodenography" (Martel, 1969; Goldstein, 1969; Lawson, 1969). The simpler tubeless method is more convenient for the radiologist, and obviously more acceptable to the patient. However, we prefer the tube method when the patient is specifically referred for hypotonic duodenography because of suggestive roentgen findings on previous studies, because of jaundice, or when there is strong clinical suspicion of pancreatic or duodenal disease for some other reason. In such cases, the indwelling tube permits the operator to overcome incomplete hypotonia by direct air insufflation, thus also permitting optimally distended air contrast views. The simpler tubeless method is usually employed in conjunction with a conventional gastrointestinal study when an unusual duodenal configuration is encountered on the initial films, and particularly when a tumor is not suspected. Studies of adequate quality can be obtained by the tubeless method in many instances (Fig. 4–16). However, the tube method gives uniformly better results. In a teaching institution, residents often prefer the tube method in order to master the technique of rapid duodenal intubation which is useful in procedures involving other structures—e.g., decompression of acute small-bowel obstruction, diagnostic duodenal drainage and cytology studies, and small-bowel biopsy procedures (Gianturco, 1967; Sargent, 1969).

Tube Method

Duodenal intubation is accomplished with the aid of a specially designed radiopaque catheter and guide wire assembly which is commercially available* (Fig. 4–17). A thin-walled, soft polyvinyl catheter is equipped with a fitted guide wire which provides sufficient stiffness and torque to direct the catheter through the pylorus.

With the patient in the sitting position, the catheter is passed transnasally into the fundus of the stomach as the patient is given sips of water. The patient is placed in the supine position and the guide wire is inserted into the tip of the tube. The whole unit is then advanced into the duodenum under fluoroscopic control.

Two simple maneuvers insure rapid and successful intubation in nearly all cases. As the tube and guidewire assembly passes through the gastric cardia it is naturally directed toward the lateral gastric wall. The first maneuver is simply

*Cook Inc., 925 S. Corry Pike, Bloomington, Ind.

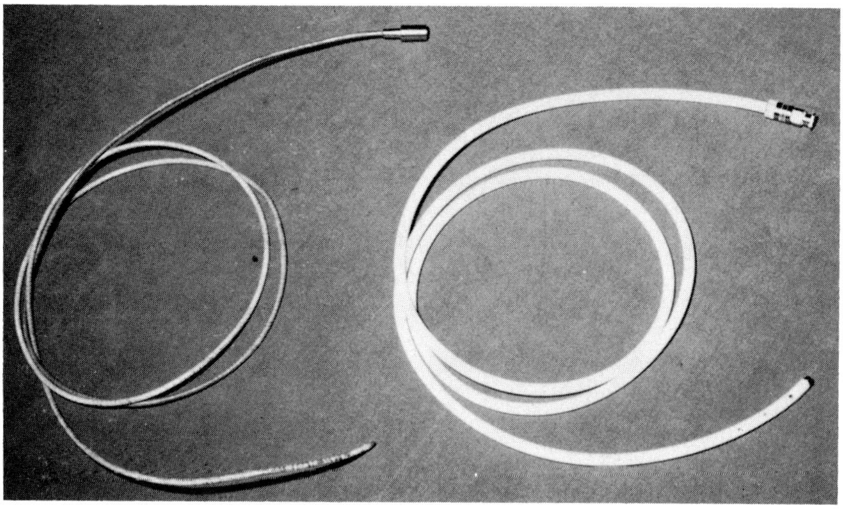

Figure 4–17. Duodenography catheter (*right*) and flexible inner guide wire (*left*). The guide wire provides stiffness and torque, facilitating rapid duodenal intubation.

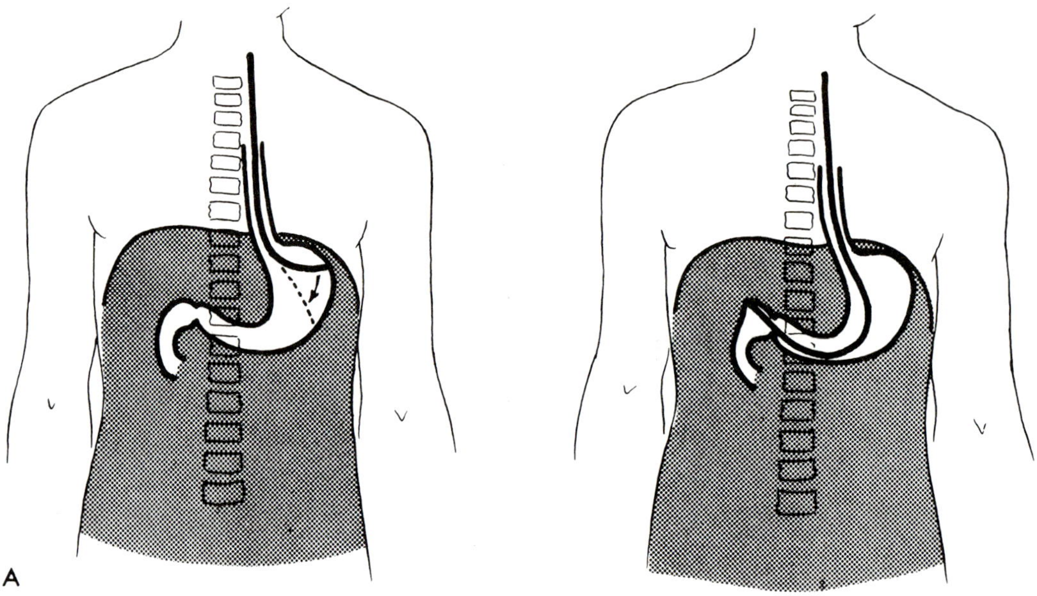

A

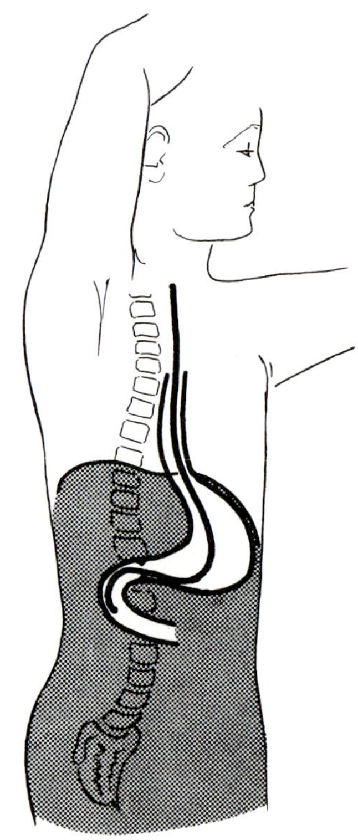

B

Figure 4–18. Two steps for rapid guided duodenal intubation.

A, The tube-guide wire assembly is deflected away from the greater curvature toward the anterior or posterior gastric wall (*left*) and pushed distally toward the pylorus (*right*).

B, The patient is turned into the supine left oblique position, allowing the cap to fill with air, and the tube is then advanced into the duodenum under direct fluoroscopic vision. In this position, the acute angle between the first and second portions of the duodenum diminishes, facilitating passage into the descending duodenum.

to twist the external hub of the guidewire, thus deflecting the tip of the tube to the anterior or posterior gastric wall (Fig. 4–18). The assembly is then readily pushed distally toward the antrum.

With the patient still in the supine position, the second maneuver is initiated by turning the patient into the left supine oblique position, so that air fills the antrum and bulb, making these structures visible fluoroscopically. The tube wire assembly is then pushed under direct vision through the pyloric canal into the descending duodenum. Before this maneuver, the guide wire is usually withdrawn several centimeters so that only the flexible tube itself engages the postbulbar turn and thus negotiates it more easily. It is noteworthy that in the supine oblique position, the acute axis change between the first and second portions of the duodenum diminishes, thus facilitating intubation (Fig. 4–18, *B*). In difficult cases, moving the patient to the prone oblique position or injecting small amounts of barium to localize the pyloric canal may be of value.

The tube is then advanced to the junction of the second and third portions of the duodenum, the guide wire is withdrawn completely, and a small amount of barium is instilled to confirm position. Next, 30 to 60 mg. of Pro-Banthine (propantheline bromide) is given intramuscularly, and test injections of barium are made. Within five minutes, duodenal peristalsis diminishes, and barium appears to puddle within the duodenal lumen.

It is advisable to proceed after five minutes, even though some peristaltic action persists, since hypotonia is often incomplete and may be brief in duration. Approximately 100 ml. of barium is then introduced through the catheter, and multiple spot radiographs are made in the anterior-posterior and left posterior oblique positions. Excess barium is aspirated, and air is introduced for double-contrast filming. Excellent air contrast studies can be obtained by attaching an Ambu bag* to the indwelling duodenography tube; a large volume of air can be delivered rapidly, resulting in optimal duodenal distention. The patient is then turned to the prone position for a similar sequence of spot filming. Air contrast films in both the prone and supine positions are of great value in detecting intrinsic duodenal masses and minor changes along the medial duodenal wall.

Inadvertent withdrawal of the tube during turning can be prevented if the patient is turned via the duodenum-dependent right decubitus position. It is also advisable to advance the tube slightly before turning in order to provide slack in the dilated hypotonic stomach. Should duodenal intubation fail, the tube can be left at the pylorus, and a modified study carried out.

*A. R. Shields Inc., Hatboro, Pa.

Tubeless Method

If a tubeless duodenogram is desired at the the completion of a standard upper gastrointestinal study, or as a primary procedure, the patient is given an additional 8 to 12 ounces of barium and placed in the right decubitus position in order to fill the duodenum. Pro-Banthine is then administered intramuscularly, and the patient is monitored fluoroscopically for the onset of duodenal hypotonia. The duodenum should be well filled with barium before the administration of Pro-Banthine, since any further gastric emptying is inhibited once hypotonia occurs. Multiple spot films in prone and supine projections are obtained. Air contrast studies are accomplished by turning the patient to the standard left posterior oblique position. Administration of Seidlitz powders or effervescent granules improves the quality of the air contrast (Hanelin, 1971). The use of a straw prepared with side holes is also an effective means of introducing air into the duodenum (Sear, 1972).

Pharmacology

A number of drugs with spasmolytic properties have been utilized for roentgen evaluation of gastrointestinal disorders, particularly of the duodenum. A considerable amount of clinical radiographic experience with the anticholinergic drugs has now been recorded, much of it the work of European and Oriental investigators. In this country, atropine, amyl nitrate, and propantheline bromide (Pro-Banthine) have all been employed. Of these, propantheline bromide (Pro-Banthine) is widely used in peptic ulcer therapy and as an antispasmodic in other gastrointestinal disturbances. At present, it is commonly used for hypotonic duodenography.

The anticholinergic drugs belong to the belladonna alkaloid family, of which atropine and scopolamine are natural derivatives. There are several synthetic preparations with specific therapeutic properties and fewer undesirable side effects. Pro-Banthine is the best known of these.

Pro-Banthine blocks neural impulses at autonomic ganglia and at parasympathetic effector sites in tissue by interfering with acetylcholine which normally conducts impulses across cell walls. Its specific therapeutic effect derives from the blockage of acetylcholine released by parasympathetic postganglionic autonomic nerves at effector cells. Pro-Banthine also exerts a direct spasmolytic action on smooth muscle, as well as a vagolytic effect. Important effects on organ systems include diminished tone and motility of smooth muscle in the alimentary and urinary tracts; decreased gastric acid output, as well as decreased salivary and upper respiratory tract secretions; and vagolytic effects on the heart which result in tachycardia. In the eye, paresis of the pupillary constrictors and ciliary muscles of the lens results in mydriasis (dilatation of the pupil) and cycloplegia (paralysis of accommodation). In combination, these two effects may increase intraocular pressure to aggravate or precipitate glaucoma.

Although a variety of cholinergic blocking agents have been used by diagnostic radiologists in Europe and elsewhere, Pro-Banthine has been the most widely used in this country (Bilbao, 1968; Martel, 1969; Eaton, 1970; and Ferrucci, 1970).

In examining the duodenum, intramuscular injections of 30 to 60 mg. (depending on body weight) are used. At these dose levels, hypotonia is adequate and anticholinergic side effects are minimal. Some workers have employed Pro-Banthine intravenously in doses of 15 mg., claiming that a more rapid onset of hypotonia is achieved by this route, and that pharmacologic side effects are fewer because the drug is more rapidly cleared from the blood stream. However, we prefer the intramuscular route because it is simpler and avoids the slightly greater risk associated with intravenous injection of parasympathetic blocking agents. The attending physician should be consulted before Pro-Banthine is administered.

When the drug is injected intramuscularly, onset of hypotonia occurs within three to eight minutes; usually the hypotonic state lasts for ten to 20 minutes, which allows ample time for spot filming and overhead radiography. The degree of hypotonia varies from patient to patient and is not predictable beforehand. At present, no adjustment in dosage is made when examining patients currently on anticholinergic drug therapy.

Precautions

Expected side effects are dose-related, and after parenteral injection of 60 mg. of Pro-Banthine, almost all patients experience a dry mouth and dilated pupils; some develop tachycardia and blurring of near vision. Some patients develop urinary hesitancy or gastric fullness. These effects subside within six to eight hours and are satisfactorily tolerated, provided the patient is advised ahead of time of their nature.

Urinary retention can be prevented by instructing all male patients to void immediately prior to the procedure. In a recent report, three cases of symptomatic abdominal distention occurred, requiring nasogastric intubation (Gelfand, 1970). Postprocedural aspiration of insufflated gastric air has prevented this complication in our experience.

A number of medical conditions are relative contraindications to the use of cholinergic blocking agents. These include glaucoma, significant cardiac disease (particularly when arrhythmia or severe angina pectoris is present), and prostatism. To date, we have not precipitated a case of glaucoma; however, a prior history of glaucoma is considered an absolute contraindication to the use of Pro-Banthine, unless ophthalmologic consultation has been obtained.

A Pro-Banthine study can be performed safely on outpatients, although it is helpful to prescribe a semisolid or liquid diet for the next meal, in view of the xerostomia. However, patients should not be allowed to drive for several hours after the procedure because of the effect of the drug on visual accommodation.

DIAGNOSTIC CRITERIA

Regardless of whether a conventional or hypotonic method has been employed to achieve a satisfactory barium study of the duodenum, interpretation is based on standard criteria. However, because duodenal hypotonia allows more accurate radiographic analysis of anatomic features and increased potential for detecting pancreatic pathologic conditions, the bulk of the illustrative material that follows is taken from hypotonic studies.

Normal Anatomy

The anatomy of the duodenum is customarily described in terms of its gross relationships to other upper abdominal or retroperitoneal structures (Lockwood, 1954; Coe, 1963). The salient features of these relations are highlighted in Chapter 1. Yet, until recently, the duodenum itself has remained a somewhat faceless structure. It has been termed a "symmetrical tube," its inner wall being "a mirror image of the outer." The current popularity of duodenography, however, necessitates more detailed knowledge of the contours of the inner duodenal wall if accurate interpretation of pancreaticoduodenal disorders is to be achieved.

Duodenal Contours

The normal duodenum, particularly as shown by duodenography, is fairly even in caliber, with gently arcuate borders and a regular fold pattern (see Fig. 4–2). When seen in profile, the folds along the duodenal walls are fairly uniform in depth and appearance. Areas of sphincter-like activity have been described at several levels along the course of the duodenum, and the shape of the descending portion has been analyzed according to a series of longitudinal axes (Jacquemet, 1965). The clinical value of these features is doubtful, however.

Of more value is a recently described constellation of radiographic features occurring along the inner margin of the descending duodenum (Ferrucci, 1970). This consists of a triad of findings termed the promontory, the straight segment, and the longitudinal fold. This configuration, schematically illustrated in Figure 4–19, can be recognized in the majority of normal duodenograms, and frequently on conventional studies as well. These anatomic features have been confirmed by the authors on analysis of normal postmortem "distention duodenograms."

The promontory (Fig. 4–20) is a localized bulging or projection of the lumen along the inner aspect of the mid-descending duodenum. The duodenal wall above the promontory usually demonstrates a deep notch-like indentation; occasionally, the axis of the duodenum tilts medially at this point, and the diameter of the lumen below the promontory appears widened. The promontory is of considerable importance as a landmark because the duodenal papilla (of Vater) usually sits on, or within a centimeter below, it.

The straight segment (Fig. 4–21) is a flat, smooth portion of the inner duodenal wall extending 2 to 3 cm. inferiorly and immediately distal to the promontory. Generally, the regular interfold indentations visible along the lateral wall at this level are not present within the zone of the straight segment.

The longitudinal fold (Fig. 4–22) is a vertically oriented ridge of mucosa and

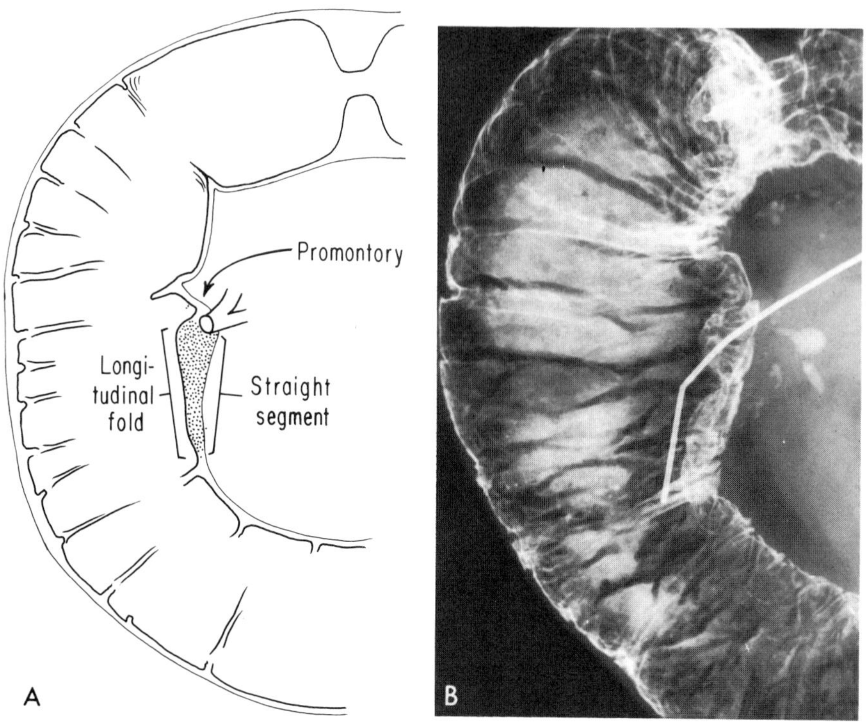

Figure 4–19. Normal anatomy of the inner duodenal margin.

A, Schematic representation of the descending duodenum showing the typical arrangement of the promontory, straight segment, longitudinal fold, and papilla.

B, Radiograph of a cadaver specimen demonstrating the characteristic physiognomy. A wire has been passed through the common duct into the duodenal lumen. Note the relationship of the papilla to the promontory, and the position of the longitudinal fold along the straight segment. (Reproduced by permission of *Radiology*.)

submucosa arising as a mucosal hood over the papilla of Vater and extending distally from the papilla for 2 to 3 cm. parallel to the straight segment (Fig. 4–23). The longitudinal fold runs perpendicular to the transverse plical folds of the duodenum. The structure is well known to anatomists (Sobotta, 1957). Poppel notes that the original description of this fold was recorded by Santorini in the 18th century (Poppel, 1953). The roentgen appearance of the fold recently has been described in a series of 15 normal cadavers studied in an investigation

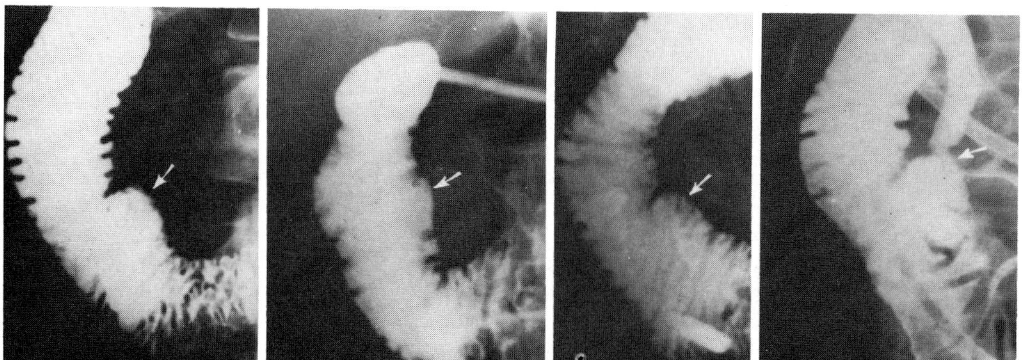

Figure 4–20. The promontory. Normal duodenograms in four different patients. A shoulder-like luminal projection (*arrow*) is visible along the medial border of the descending duodenum. (Reproduced by permission of *Radiology*.)

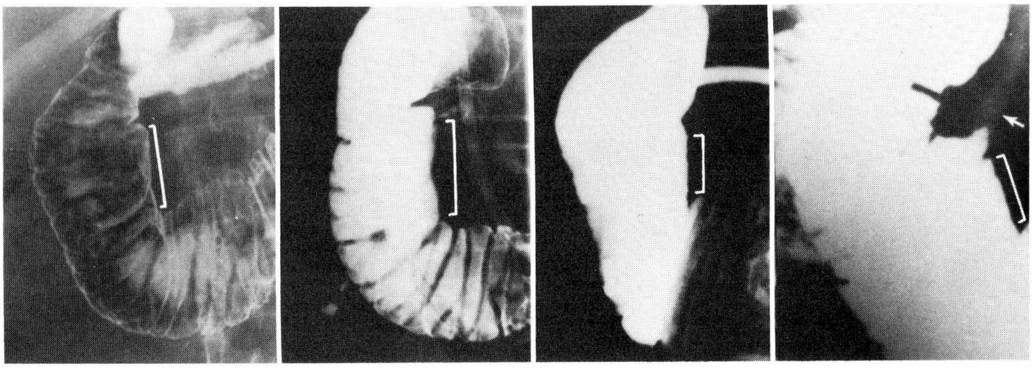

Figure 4–21. The straight segment. Normal duodenograms in four different patients. The medial wall of the descending duodenum just below the promontory shows a normal, smooth, straight contour as opposed to the fold projections visible on the corresponding lateral margin. (Reproduced by permission of *Radiology*.)

of normal duodenal anatomy (Ferrucci, 1970). Radiographically, it may be seen on air contrast study as a double-contour linear defect inferior to the promontory along the straight segment, and should not be confused with a mass lesion (Fig. 4–24).

The value of this triad of features—promontory, straight segment, and longitudinal fold—derives from their value in locating the papilla of Vater and thus permitting differentiation of duodenal filling defects as either papillary or nonpapillary (see Figs. 4–25 and 4–26).

The Papilla of Vater

The distinction between the terms "papilla" and "ampulla" is worthy of emphasis. The duodenal papilla is an elevated mound of tissue projecting into the duodenal lumen. The ampulla of Vater is that segment of the duct system within the papilla; this segment may be slightly dilated.

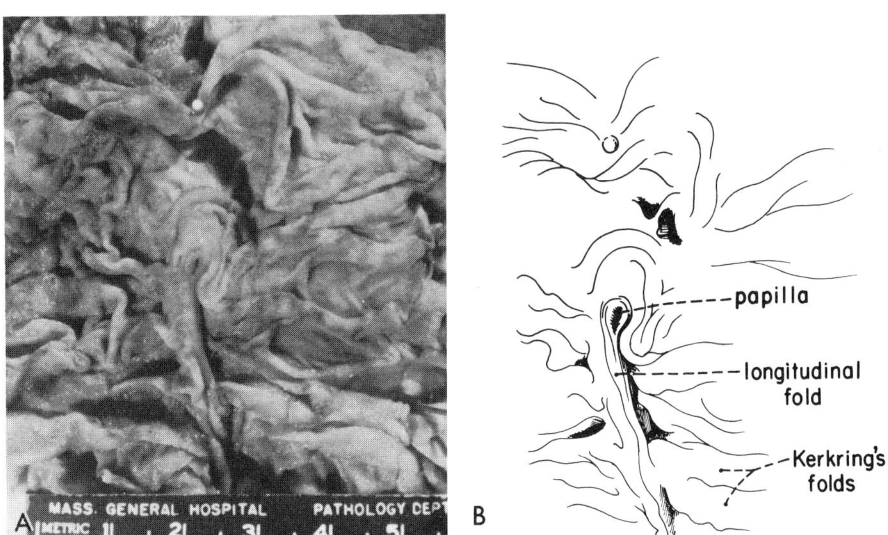

Figure 4–22. Gross appearance of the longitudinal fold.

A, Photograph of a cadaver specimen showing the duodenum opened longitudinally. A raised ridge of mucosa extends inferiorly from the papilla and terminates in several small subdivisions. Superiorly, the fold encompasses the papilla and merges above it much like a hood.

B, Schematic diagram. (Reproduced by permission of *Radiology*.)

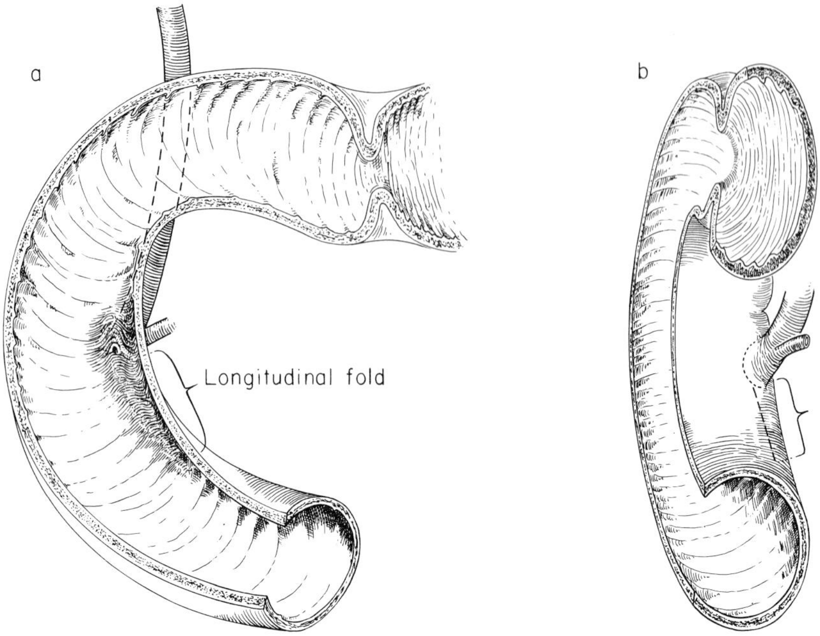

Figure 4–23. Artist's concept of the longitudinal fold. This structure is regularly visible at duodenoscopy, and aids in identifying the papilla of Vater.

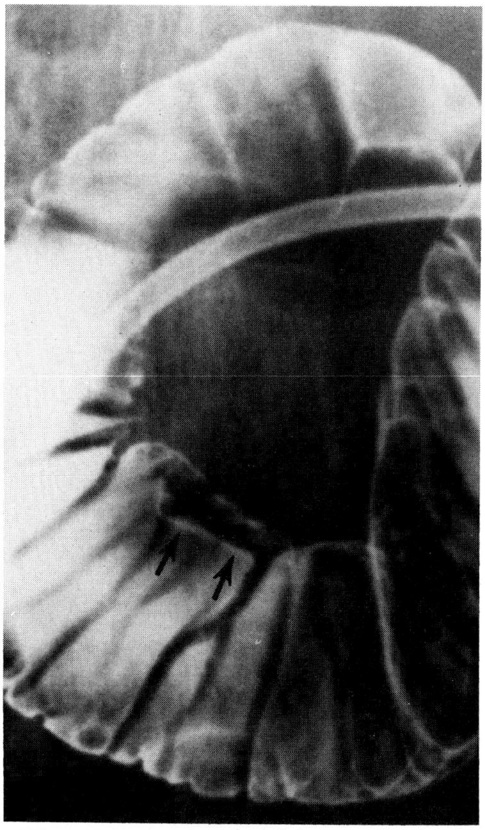

Figure 4–24. A normal longitudinal fold. A linear structure is visible parallel to the straight segment below the promontory, producing a double-contour image which should not be mistaken for a mass in the pancreatic head.

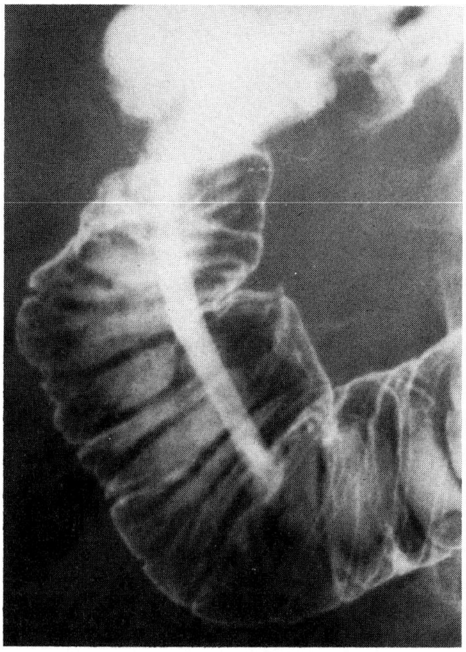

Figure 4–25. Triad of normal duodenographic features. Note the promontory, straight segment, and papilla. The longitudinal fold extends inferiorly from the papilla as a linear contour parallel to the straight segment.

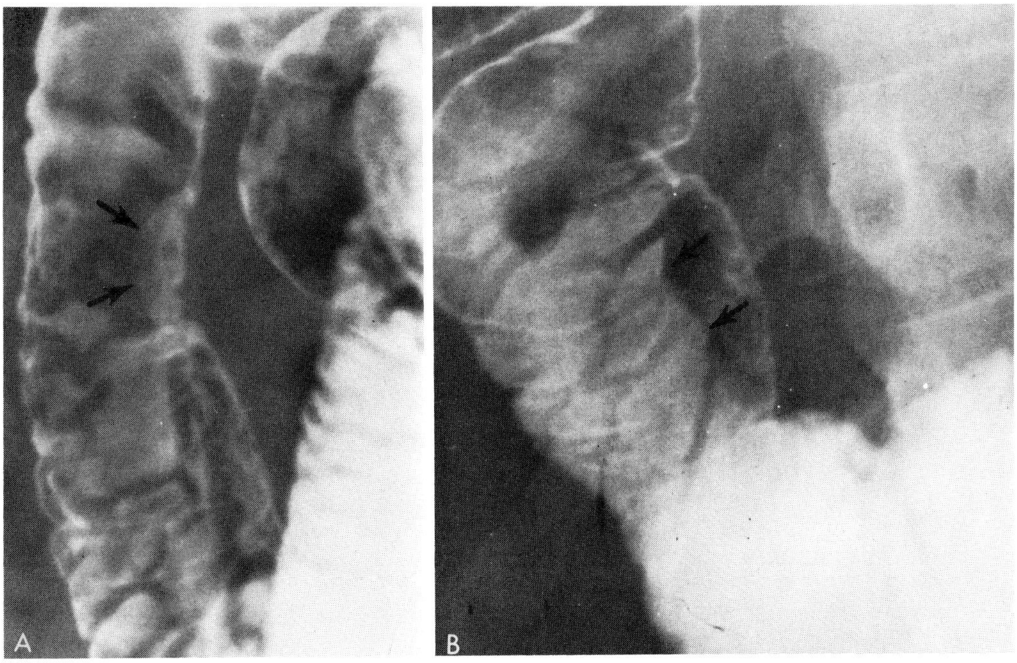

Figure 4–26. Use of the triad of landmarks for differential diagnosis of duodenal filling defects.

A, An oval lesion (*arrows*) situated above the promontory can be distinguished from an enlarged papilla by its location. It was correctly diagnosed preoperatively as ectopic pancreas. (Reproduced by permission of *Radiology*.)

B, In this case, a rounded filling defect situated opposite the promontory and longitudinal fold was considered a benign lesion and has been followed nonoperatively without change for two years. Arrows indicate longitudinal fold. (Courtesy of Dr. Ann Lewicki.)

The major papilla averages 8 to 10 mm. in length and presents as a rounded or oval filling defect blending with the normal mucosa along the posterior medial wall of the descending duodenum (Fig. 4–27). The minor papilla averages 2 to 3 mm. in size and is rarely identified radiographically. The older literature indicates that the major papilla can be recognized frequently (in 49 per cent of normal barium meal studies), and that it varies considerably in its location along the axis of the duodenum (Poppel, 1953; Schwartz, 1962). Modern studies of duodenographic anatomy indicate that a normal papilla is visible in only 20 to 30 per cent of the cases and is usually seen in relatively constant relation to the triad of landmarks noted above (Ferrucci, 1970; Eaton, 1972). The reason for this discrepancy is unclear but it may be due to differences in criteria. Published illustrations in which early authors claimed to have seen the papilla frequently leave one unconvinced. Often only a small notch, fleck, or oblique fold is said to represent the papilla. An example of such a falsely localized papilla is illustrated in Figure 4–28.

On radiographic study, most authorities accept 1.5 cm. in length as the upper limit of normal size of the major papilla (Ferrucci, 1970; Eaton, 1972), although normal papillae as large as 3.0 cm in length have been reported (Poppel, 1953). Papillary enlargement, in addition to carcinoma of the ampulla of Vater, accompanies a variety of inflammatory conditions and will be discussed below in the differential diagnosis of duodenal filling defects, under the heading Intrinsic Duodenal Mass Lesions.

Abnormalities Affecting the Inner Duodenal Border

Changes along the inner border of the duodenum generally implicate the pancreas as the prime diagnostic suspect.

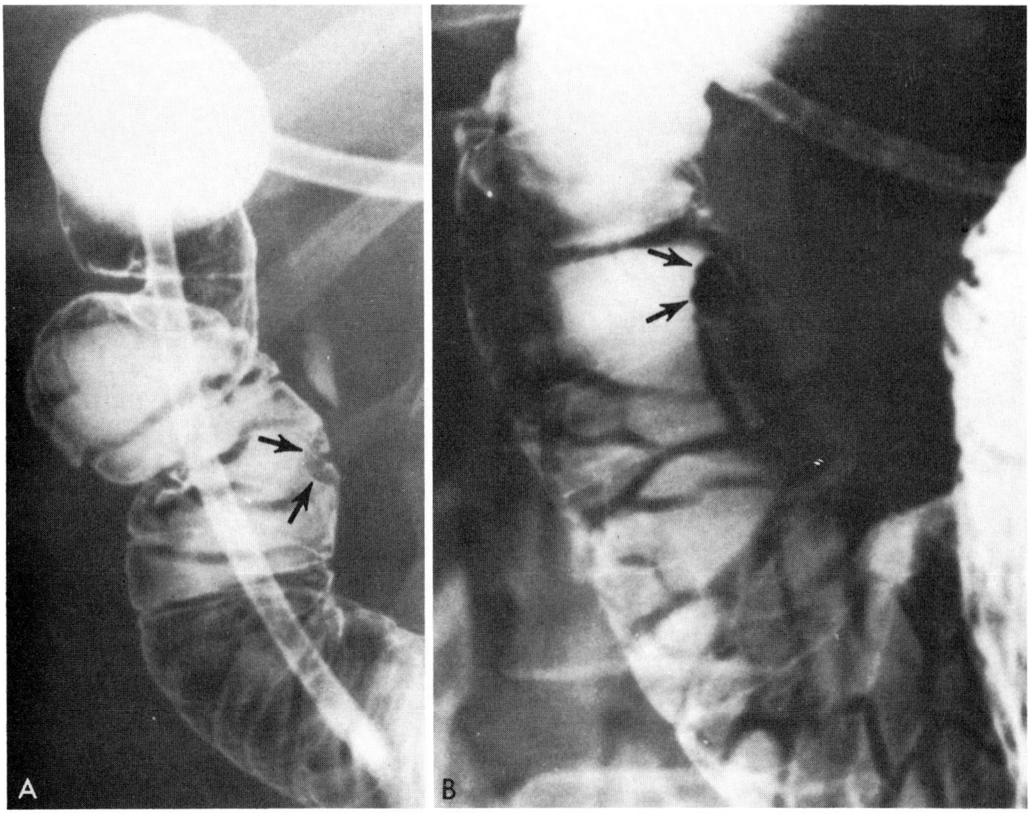

Figure 4–27. Normal papilla of Vater in two patients. A spherical or oval-shaped defect along the medial wall of the descending duodenum is the usual appearance (*arrows*).

A, Reflux into the common duct occurs as a result of previous sphincterotomy.

B, The longitudinal fold is visible *en face* as a linear lucent image extending inferiorly from the papilla.

However, disorders arising primarily in the duodenum or the vaterian structures should also be considered.

Signs of a Mass in the Head of the Pancreas

These include the following:

1. Mucosal fold changes.
2. Concave pressure defect (double-contour image).
3. Widened loop.
4. Displaced loop.
5. Distorted diverticulum.
6. Frostberg's inverted "3" sign.

MUCOSAL FOLD CHANGES. The earliest sign of pancreatic enlargement is alteration of the fold pattern along the concavity of the duodenum (Salik, 1961). Incomplete or poor filling of the interfold projections along the inner margin, as contrasted to the outer margin, is a very subtle finding. Folds may appear thinned, tapered, or sharpened, producing the so-called "brush effect" (Fig. 4–29). (This sign is related to spiculation of folds —a sign which will be discussed on p. 121.) In some cases, fold projections may appear blunted and ironed out, forming a smooth, continuous line when contrasted to the appearance of the opposite wall. As noted earlier, such minor fold alterations are often seen on conventional barium meal studies, but may be easily confused with spurious images due to peristalsis.

CONCAVE PRESSURE DEFECT. A local concave pressure defect indicates greater enlargement of the pancreatic head and is a more reliable sign. Frequently, such

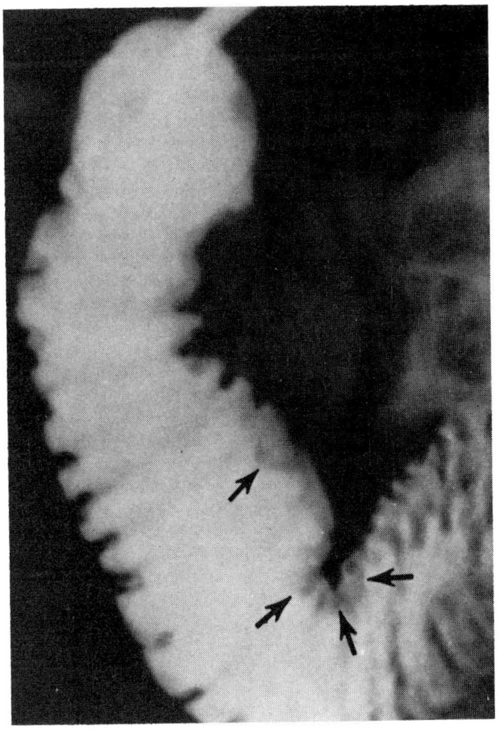

Figure 4-28. "False" papilla. The inferior filling defect at the junction of the second and third portions of the duodenum (*three arrows*) could be mistaken for the papilla. However, it merely represents a buckling effect as the duodenum sharply changes axis at this point. The true papilla is visible more proximally (*single arrow*). Note its relation to the promontory and straight segment.

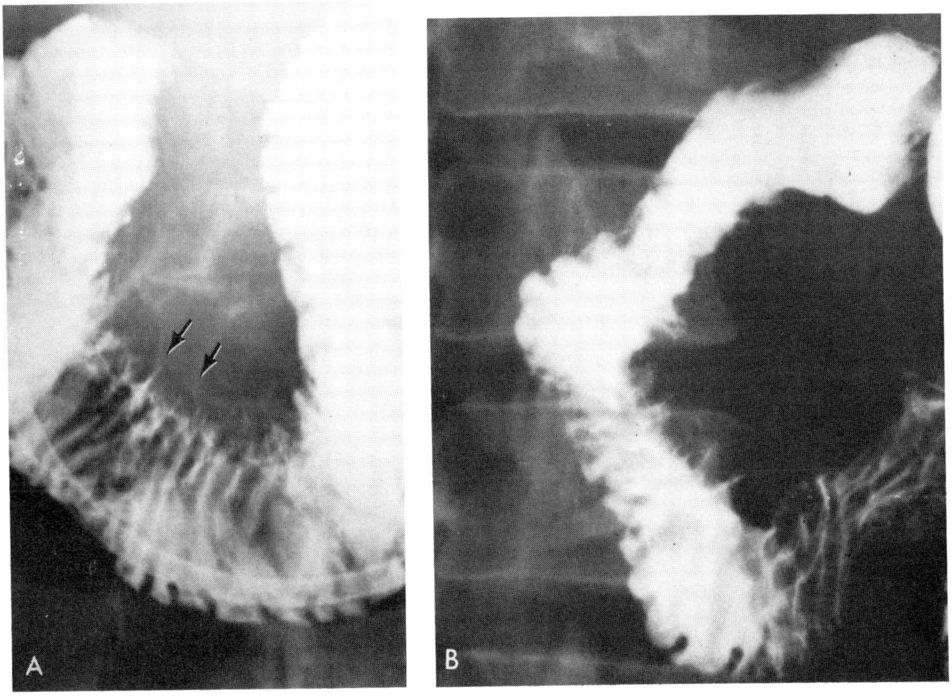

Figure 4-29. Brush effect in pancreatic cancer in two patients. Note the tapered, sharpened appearance of folds along the inner duodenal border. This sign is more reliable when shown by duodenography. (See also Figs. 4-1 and 4-40.)

pressure indentations are sufficient to cause actual narrowing of the duodenal lumen (Fig. 4–30). When extrinsic impression affects only a portion of the duodenal tube, the unaffected wall distends normally, producing a *double-contour* image (Fig. 4–31). The mechanism of the double-contour image is schematically illustrated in Figure 4–32. For the reason mentioned before

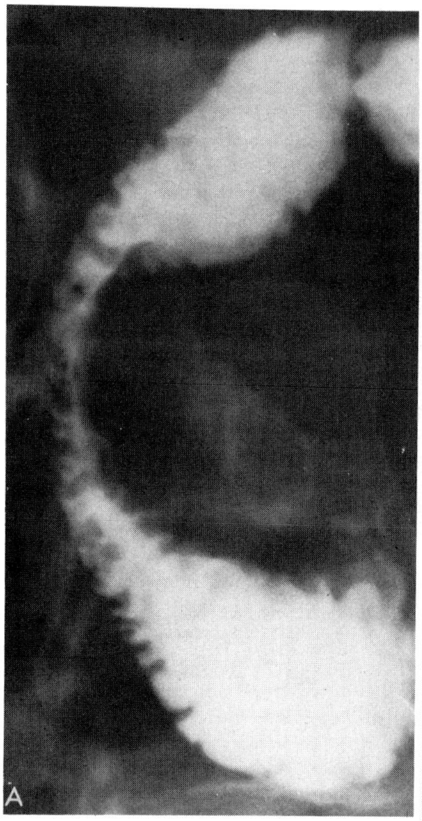

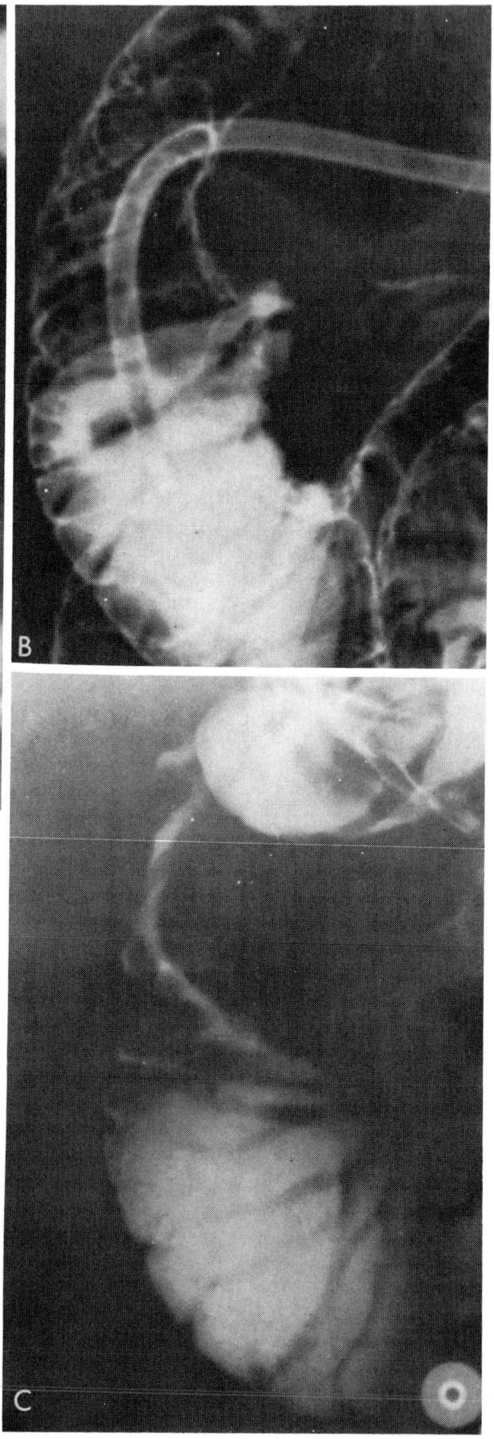

Figure 4–30. Local concave duodenal pressure defect indicating enlargement of the pancreatic head in acute pancreatitis (*A*), chronic pancreatitis (*B*), and a pseudocyst (*C*).

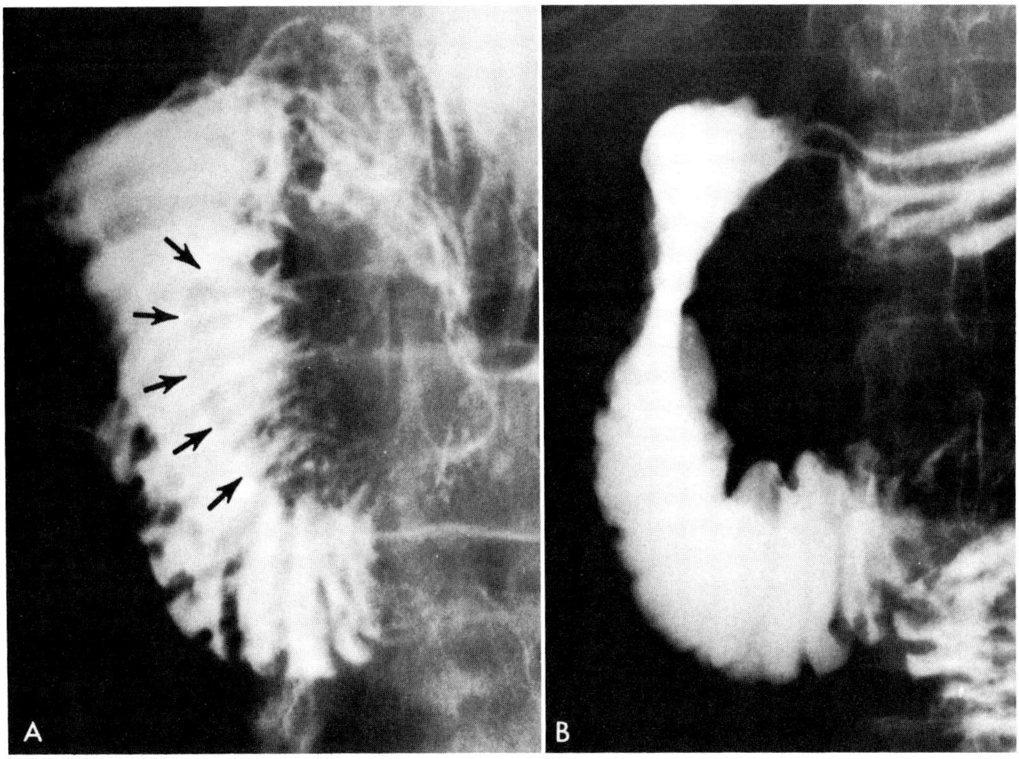

Figure 4–31. Double-contour image in carcinoma of the head of the pancreas in two patients.
A, A mass affecting only one wall allows the opposite wall to distend, producing a double contour (*arrows*). Also note the sharpened, spiculated mucosal folds along the medial duodenal margin.
B, A smoothly marginated double contour is

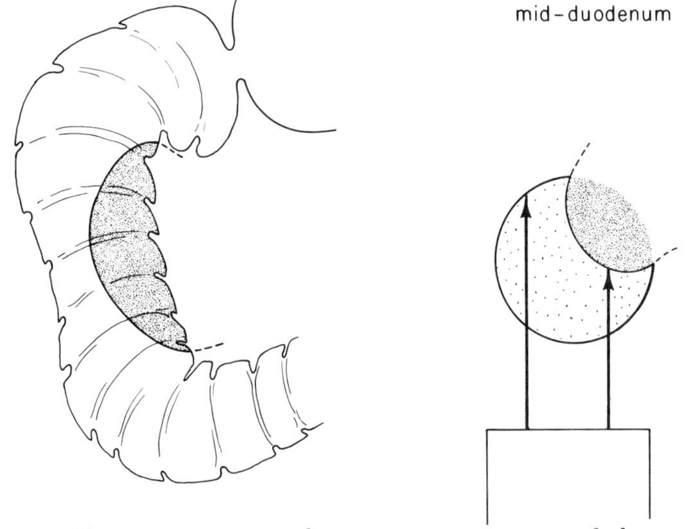

Figure 4–32. Double-contour sign. Schematic representation of the mechanism. Mass defect affecting a single wall allows normal distention of the opposite wall, producing a double-contour image.

(i.e., active peristaltic motor activity), a double contour seen on a standard barium meal study may occasionally be a spurious finding and should be confirmed with a hypotonic study.

Widened loop. Widening of the duodenal loop (Fig. 4–33) is often questioned by clinicians when pancreatic disease is suspected, but it is a sign that must be interpreted with caution. It is well recognized that the size of the duodenal loop is at best a poor indication of the size of the pancreatic head, irrespective of the presence or absence of pancreatic disease (Beranbaum, 1966). It is true, of course, that an enlarging mass may widen the duodenal sweep, but there is great variation in the configuration of the duodenal loop among normal patients. Typically, in mesomorphic males, the distal antrum is high and horizontal, and the descending duodenum has a long vertical course leading to an impression of a widened sweep. The concept of a widened loop is also better appreciated if we consider that upward pressure on the duodenal cap and downward impression on the horizontal duodenum are often important components (Fig. 4–34). Furthermore, it is worth emphasizing that marked enlargement of the duodenal loop is often an indication of benign disease such as pancreatitis or pseudocyst. In such cases, the inner contour of the loop may be quite smooth and regular. On the other hand, significant enlargement of the loop in malignant disease generally indicates an advanced lesion. Obviously, expanding lesions in the area of the pancreatic head may arise in structures other than the pancreas—e.g., enlarged lymph nodes, retroperitoneal masses, and aortic aneurysms. Conditions producing real or apparent enlargement of the pancreatic head are listed in Table 4–4.

Displaced loop. Displacement of the duodenal loop, usually to the right and inferiorly, occurs with greater enlargement of the pancreas (Fig. 4–35). Marked displacement is often a sign of a pancreatic pseudocyst or an unusual

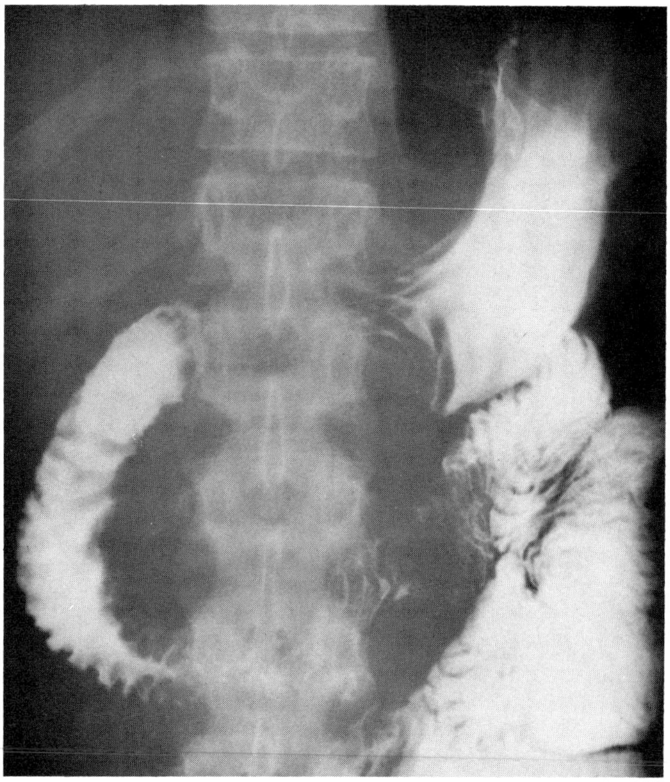

Figure 4–33. Widening of the duodenal loop in lymphosarcoma of the peripancreatic lymph nodes.

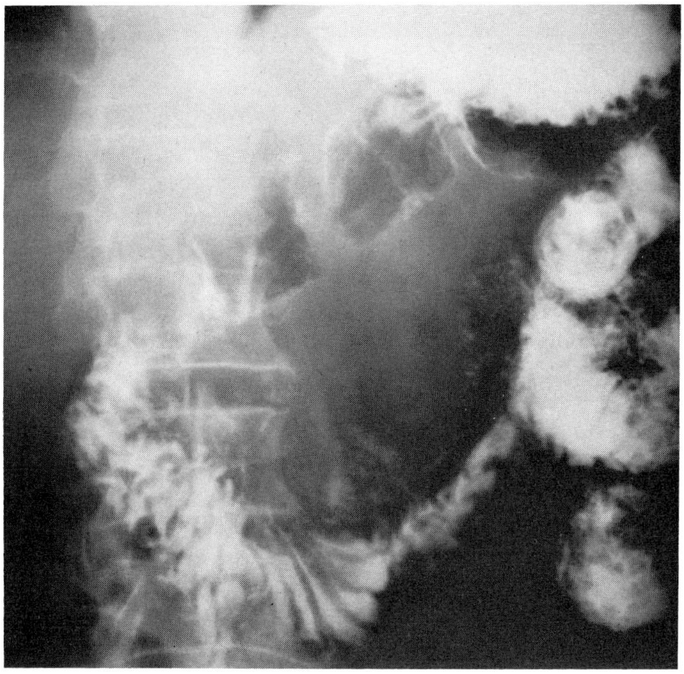

Figure 4–34. Widening of the duodenal loop resulting from a leaking abdominal aortic aneurysm.

tumor such as a sarcoma or cystadenoma rather than pancreatic cancer.

DISTORTED DIVERTICULUM. Distortion of a duodenal diverticulum is an infrequent but valid indication of an enlarging mass in the pancreas (Hodes, 1954; Beranbaum, 1966) (Fig. 4–36). Although distorted diverticula are usually mentioned in association with pancreatic cancer, they are obviously not specific and occur with any expanding process arising in the pancreas or peripancreatic area. Because of the variable position and size of duodenal diverticula, rotation and displacement are less useful findings than are changes in shape such as flattening, indentation, or other contour distortion (Eaton, 1972). Rarely considered is the fact that diverticula of the distal duodenum may become deformed by lesions in the body and tail of the pancreas (Fig. 4–37).

FROSTBERG'S INVERTED "3" SIGN. The epsilon or inverted "3" sign of Frostberg (Fig. 4–38) has long been recognized as a sign of disease along the pancreaticoduodenal interface. Although in his original article, Frostberg (1938) recognized that this configuration could be the result of pancreatitis as well as cancer, for many years subsequent teaching among non-radiologists implied an association with pancreatic cancer. Presently, there is no longer any debate that the sign is quite nonspecific, and, overall, it is probably more common in inflammatory disorders than in cancer. Actually, the sign is rather uncommon in pancreatic cancer, with a frequency in large series reported to be 4 per cent (Eyler, 1962) and 10 per cent (Broadbent, 1951), respectively.

Still open to debate, however, is the

TABLE 4–4. Disorders Causing Enlargement of the Duodenal Loop

Pancreas
- Pancreatitis
- Pseudocyst
- Pancreatic cancer
- Metastatic replacement of the pancreas
- Cystadenoma
- Pancreatic sarcoma

Lymph Node Enlargement
- Metastases
- Lymphoma
- Inflammation

Retroperitoneal Masses
- Aortic aneurysm
- Tumor
- Cysts

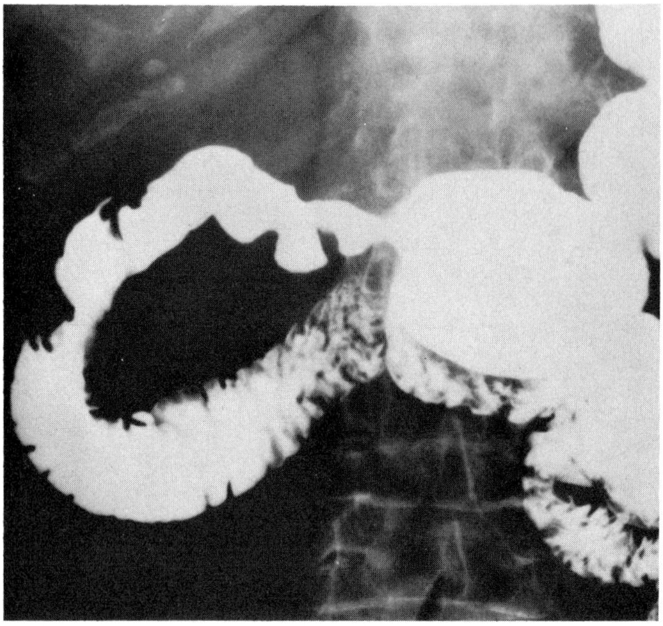

Figure 4–35. Lateral displacement of the duodenal loop resulting from carcinoma of the head of the pancreas. Extrinsic mass indentation and spiculation of folds are also visible along the inner duodenal border.

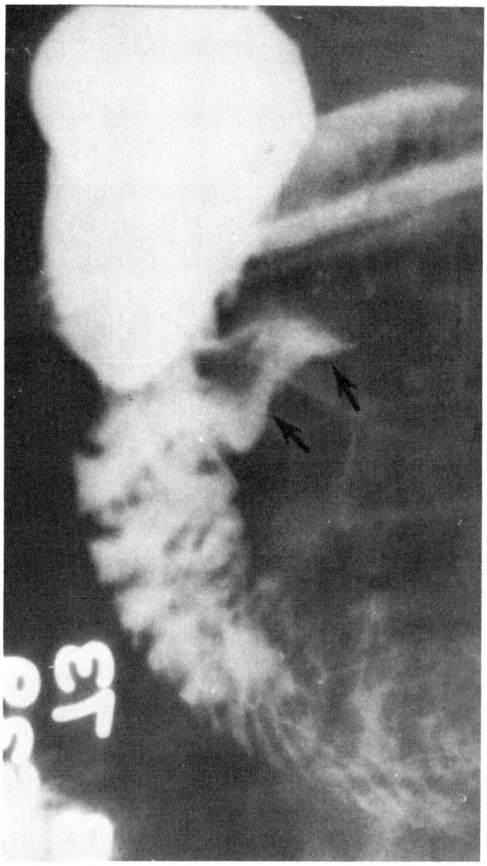

Figure 4–36. Distorted duodenal diverticulum. Pancreatic pseudocyst. The pancreatic surface of the diverticulum is elevated and flattened *(arrows).*

cause of the characteristic inverted "3" deformity. Most authorities agree that the central limb of the "3" represents a point of fixation of the duodenal wall where the pancreatic and common bile ducts are inserted. It has been suggested also that edema of the minor and major papillae accounts for the superior and inferior concavities (Stiennon, 1956). However, it seems more likely that smooth muscle spasm and edema in the duodenal wall play an important role in producing this deformity, whether the cause is pancreatitis or cancer. This is supported by the frequency of mass-like non-lesions that may accompany pancreaticoduodenal inflammation, as well as by an instance of recurrence of Frostberg's sign during clinical re-exacerbation in a case of pancreaticoduodenal inflammatory disease (Stiennon, 1956).

Having established the existence of pancreatic enlargement, there are several other signs of abnormality along the inner duodenal border which further the differential diagnosis. These include: (1) nodularity; (2) spiculation; and (3) flattening with fold effacement.

Nodularity

This is characterized by irregular nodular defects along the duodenal wall and

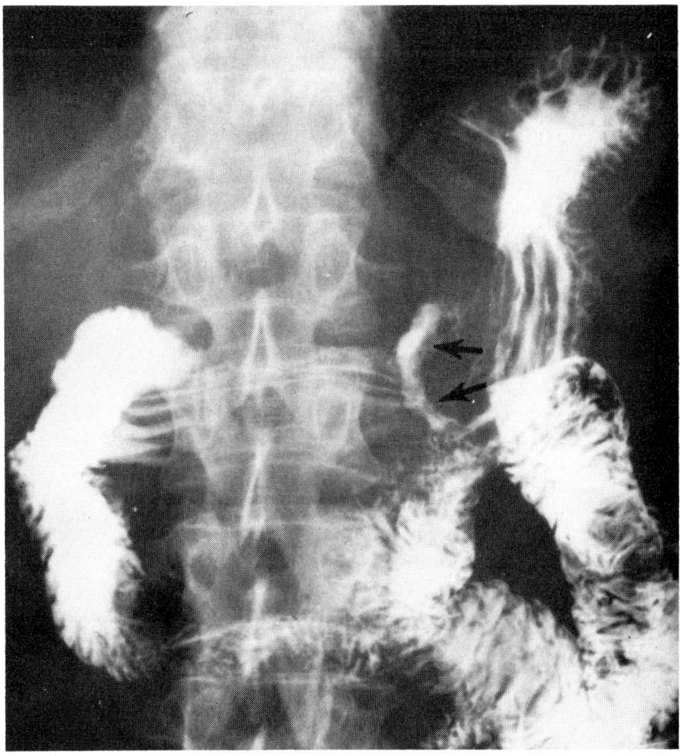

Figure 4–37. Distorted diverticulum of the duodenojejunal flexure secondary to carcinoma of the body of the pancreas. The lateral aspect of the diverticulum demonstrates a curvilinear deformity (*arrows*). (Courtesy of Dr. J. L. Williams. Reproduced by permission of *American Journal of Roentgenology.*)

may occur with or without an associated mass effect (Fig. 4–39). The sign is more vivid and reliable when demonstrated by duodenography. Generally, the finding of nodular impressions indicates the presence of a malignant process, although exceptions do occur. For instance, nodular impression defects along the proximal postbulbar duodenum may occur in pancreatitis, whereas more distal nodularity strongly suggests a tumor.

Spiculation

This refers to fine or coarse sharpening and elongation of the barium-filled crevices between plical folds (Fig. 4–40). Such spicules can be either short and numerous or few in number and longer. They have been variously described as "rose-thorns," "saw-toothing," and "spike-like" (Benedict, 1970). Mass lesions in the pancreatic head are frequently accompanied by spiculation of folds, but the sign is not entirely specific and is present in pancreatitis and pancreaticoduodenal cancer (Bilbao, 1968; Eaton, 1970; and Rubinstein, 1971).

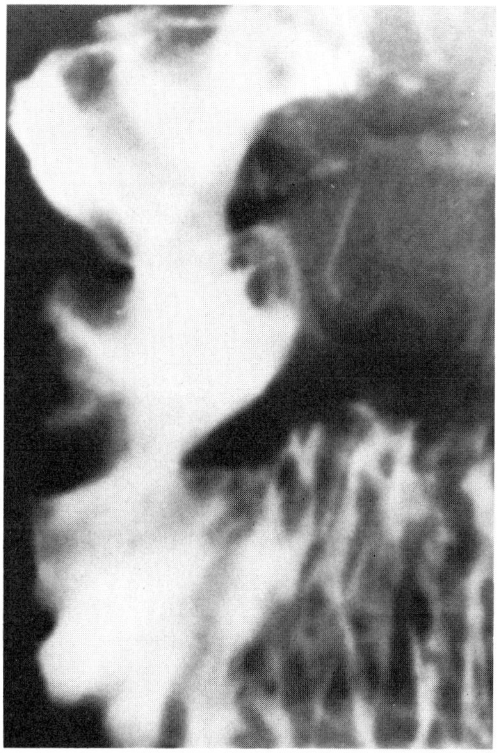

Figure 4–38. Frostberg's inverted "3" sign. Acute pancreatitis. Note the swollen mucosal folds. This configuration is not specific and simply indicates an expanding process in the head of the pancreas.

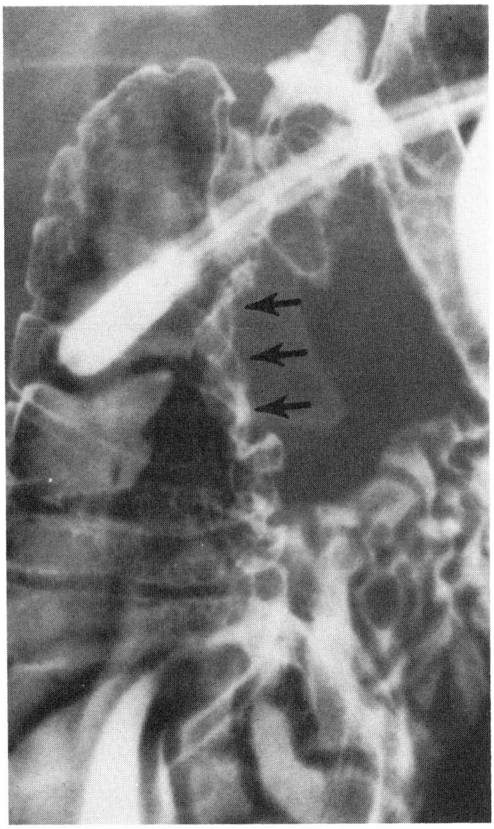

Figure 4–39. Nodularity. Carcinoma of the pancreas. The presence of irregular nodular defects along the inner duodenal wall usually indicates malignancy, although occasionally such findings occur in benign disease. (Reproduced by permission of *New England Journal of Medicine.*)

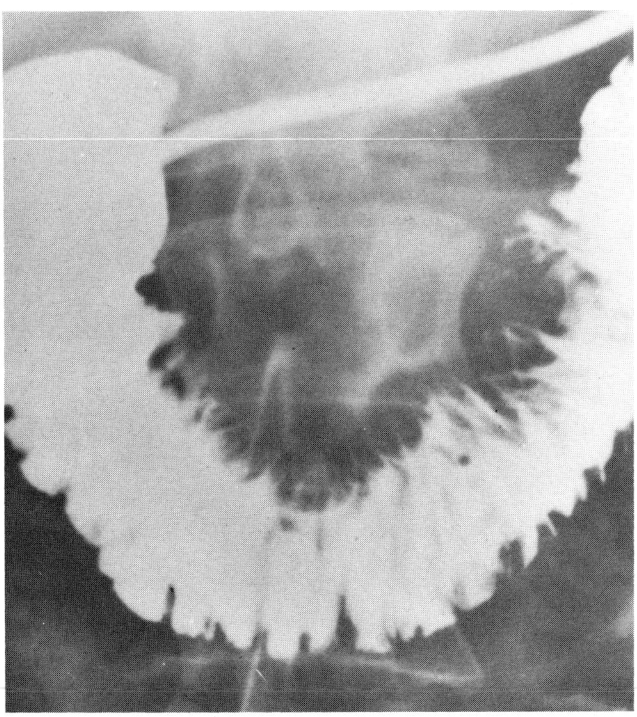

Figure 4–40. Spiculation of folds along the concavity of the duodenal loop. Carcinoma of the pancreas. The folds are sharpened and elongated. Extrinsic mass impression is also visible. (Courtesy of Dr. M. K. Bilbao. From Bilbao, M. K., et al.: Hypotonic duodenography. Radiology, 89: 438–443, 1967.)

The exact pathologic basis for spiculation is unclear. Neuromuscular irritability probably plays some role. Mucosal edema presumably accounts for the broad, widely separated spikes which frequently occur in pancreatitis (Fig. 4–41). However, when such spikes are displaced or frankly splayed, tumor should be considered. A plausible mechanism in cases of tumor would be neoplastic infiltration of the wall with traction and fixation of the folds. In addition to splayed and displaced spikes, numerous fine spicules, crowded together and clearly unrelated to mucosal folds, create the "fringed" effect described by Jacquemet (1965), and also suggest neoplasm. This is probably a variation of the "brush effect" mentioned earlier. In general, however, it would be hazardous to attempt to make a differential diagnosis from the appearance of spiculations alone.

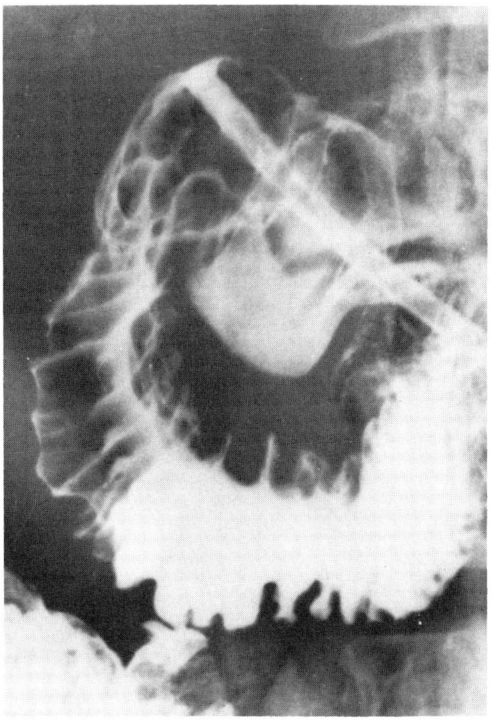

Figure 4–41. Widely separated spiculation caused by mucosal fold edema in relapsing pancreatitis. An extrinsic mass effect is also visible.

Flattening with Fold Effacement

This consists of undue straightening of the inner duodenal border accompanied by flattening or planing-off of the interfold crevices (Fig. 4–42). Usually, there is slight associated reduction in lumen caliber. Unless flattening of the wall is accompanied by fold effacement,

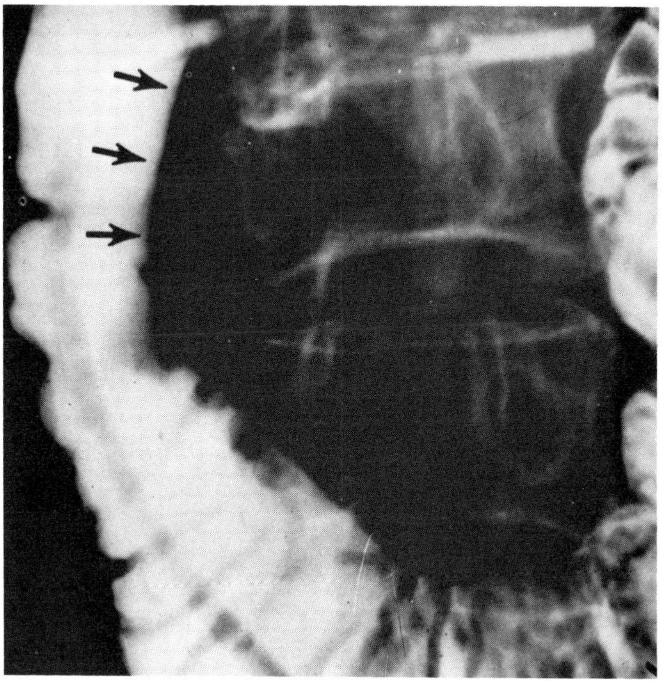

Figure 4–42. Flattening with fold effacement in chronic pancreatitis. The upper medial duodenal margin (*arrows*) appears flattened, and mucosal fold indentations are planed off (i.e., effaced). This is a highly reliable sign of chronic pancreatitis.

however, it should not be considered abnormal. Flattening with fold effacement is one of the more specific abnormalities of the duodenum and is a very reliable indicator of chronic pancreatitis (Jacquemet, 1965).

Flattening with fold effacement is usually detected along the proximal aspect of the descending duodenum where the pancreas and duodenum are most closely applied; it should be differentiated from the normal straight segment which is situated more inferiorly along the distal duodenum below the promontory. The cause of flattening with fold effacement is not known but possibly reflects chronic inflammatory change with fibrosis and rigidity of the duodenal wall.

Abnormalities Suggesting Intrinsic Duodenal Disease

Roentgen signs suggesting intrinsic duodenal disease may be grouped under the following headings:

1. Fold thickening.
2. Intrinsic duodenal mass lesions.
3. Biliary reflux.
4. Ulceration of the postbulbar duodenum.
5. Fistulous lesions of the duodenum.
6. Stenotic or obstructive lesions of the postbulbar duodenum.
7. Duodenal dilatation.

Fold Thickening

This occurs in a variety of disorders as indicated in Table 4–5. During conventional barium meal study, thickening of the mucosal folds usually produces a nodular pattern, whereas distention duodenography in the same case may display a regular, uniform pattern of fold thickening involving inner and outer duodenal margins equally. Peptic ulcer disease (duodenitis, Zollinger-Ellison syndrome) and pancreatitis are the commonest causes of fold thickening; the changes are generally attributed to inflammatory edema in the mucosa and in the submucosal layers (Fraser, 1964) (Fig. 4–43). When pancreatitis produces enlargement of the head of the pancreas, duodenal fold thickening is usually present as well, and aids in identifying the process as being inflammatory rather than neoplastic (see Fig. 4–41). Thickened folds occurring in a predominantly nodular pattern may be quite uniform in appearance, producing a "cobblestone" pattern. This finding may be associated with duodenitis, but is more commonly associated with diffuse hyperplasia of Brunner's glands, with or without lymphoid hyperplasia (Schulman, 1970) (Figs. 4–44 and 4–45).

In practical terms, these conditions are often lumped together as variations in the response of the duodenal mucosa

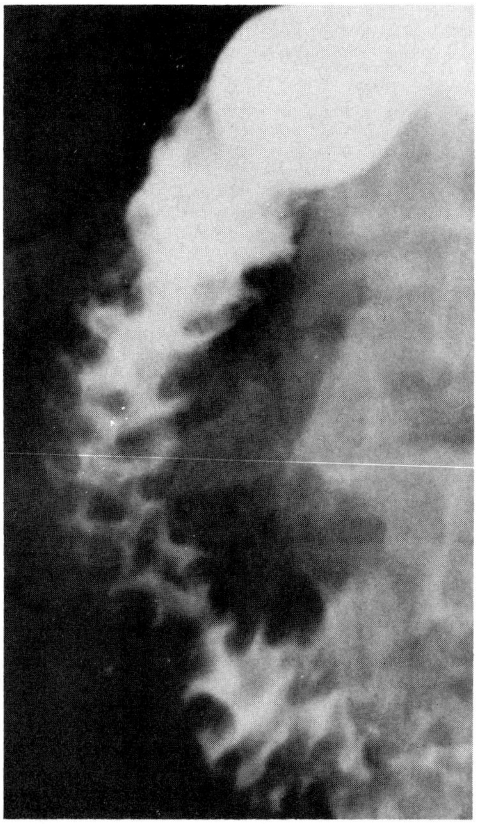

Figure 4–43. Fold thickening in nonspecific acid peptic disease. Such changes are generally attributed to inflammatory edema in the mucosal and submucosal layers of the bowel wall. However, diffuse hyperplasia of Brunner's glands may produce an identical appearance. Clinically, this distinction is of minor importance.

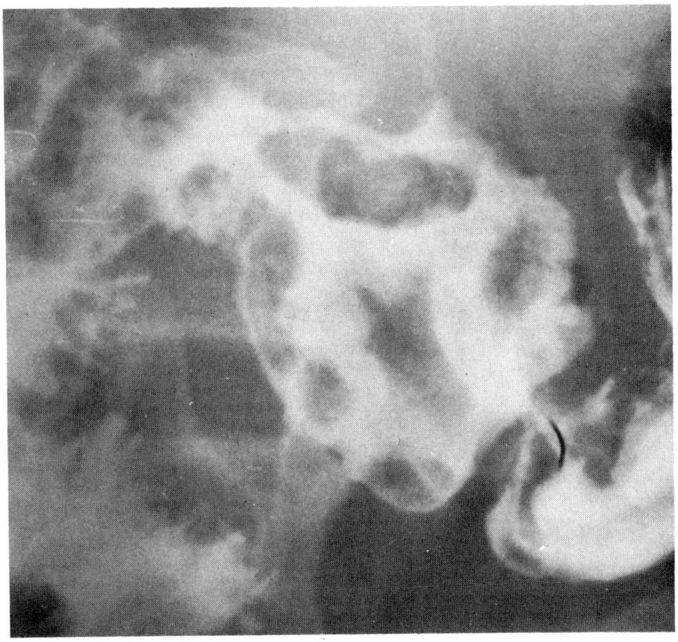

Figure 4–44. Brunner's gland hyperplasia. Nodular thickening of mucosal folds in a "cobblestone" pattern is the classic appearance. The usual location is the duodenal cap, since Brunner's glands decrease in number with increasing distance from the pylorus.

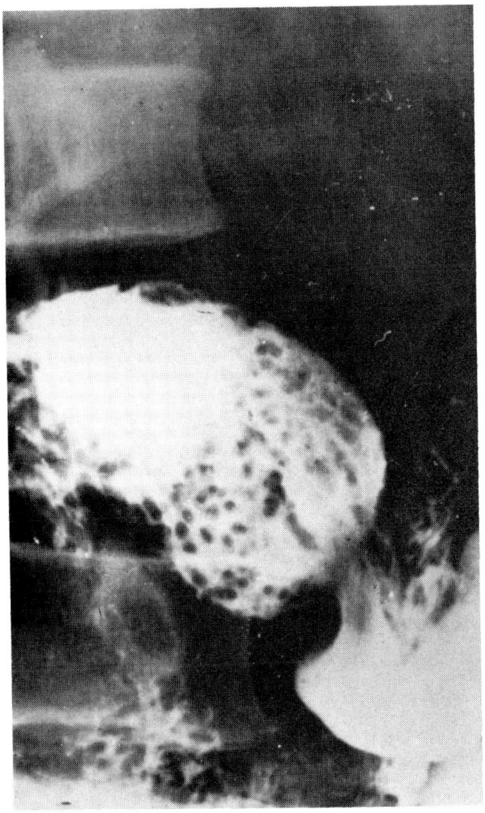

Figure 4–45. Nodular lymphoid hyperplasia. Multiple tiny nodular defects resemble the pattern which occurs when the terminal ileum is involved. The nodules here are smaller and more uniform than in cases of duodenitis or Brunner's gland hyperplasia.

to an ulcer diathesis (Perez, 1966). Patients with uremia undergoing chronic dialysis may develop nodular thickening of mucosal folds apparently unrelated to hyperacidity or peptic ulcer disease (Weiner, 1969). Nodular fold thickening in a nonuniform pattern occurs in a vari-

TABLE 4–5. Causes of Thickened Duodenal Folds

Inflammatory
Peptic ulcer disease (duodenitis)
Zollinger-Ellison syndrome
Pancreatitis
Uremia (chronic dialysis)
Brunner's gland hyperplasia (lymphoid hyperplasia)
Regional enteritis
Parasitic infestations (giardiasis, strongyloidiasis)
Neoplastic
Carcinoma of the duodenum
Lymphosarcoma
Metastases to peripancreatic lymph nodes
Related to the Vascular System
Duodenal varices
Mesenteric arterial collaterals (secondary to splanchnic arterial occlusion)
Intramural hemorrhage
Diffuse Infiltrative Disorders
Whipple's disease
Amyloidosis
Intestinal lymphangiectasia

ety of unrelated conditions, including infiltrating lymphosarcoma of the duodenum (Fig. 4–46) and peripancreatic lymph node metastasis (Fig. 4–47). In the latter condition, duodenal fold thickening may relate to lymphatic obstruction secondary to malignant replacement of normal nodal architecture.

Chronic inflammatory disorders such as the parasitic infestations (giardiasis, strongyloidiasis) as well as regional enteritis, tuberculosis, and sprue may produce bizarre nodular fold thickening in the early stages of the disease. Later, cicatrizing stenoses may ensue. These conditions will be considered in more detail in Chapter 10.

Intramural bleeding of the duodenum may thicken folds in a nodular fashion, occasionally producing a rigid "stacked coin" appearance. Mural hemorrhage in the duodenum often results from trauma; over-anticoagulation, hemophilia, and Henoch-Schönlein purpura are other uncommonly encountered causes (Handel, 1957; Dodds, 1970) (Fig. 4–48).

Duodenal varices may present as single or multiple lobulated filling defects simulating thickened folds in the duodenal cap or loop. They are usually associated with esophageal varices and are best demonstrated when the patient is prone, but they are rarely seen when he is in the erect position (Bateson, 1969). They may occur with supra- or intrahepatic portal obstruction but are more common with subhepatic portal vein occlusion and may be a major source of hemorrhage (Olson, 1963; Perchik, 1963; Fleming, 1968; and Bateson, 1969).

Multiple nodular defects in the duodenal loop have also been described in celiac and superior mesenteric arterial occlusion resulting from collateral flow through enlarged pancreaticoduodenal arterial arcades (Baum, 1965; Shimkin, 1972) (Fig. 4–49).

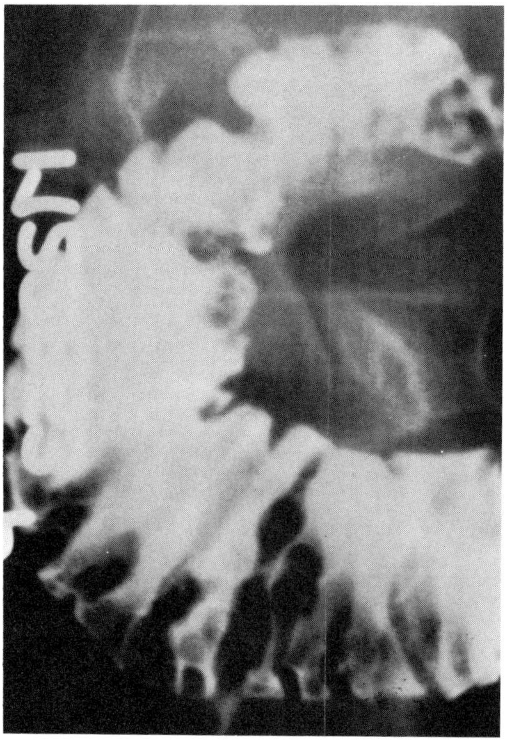

Figure 4–46. Fold thickening in lymphosarcoma. Note the multiple nodular filling defects in this patient with diffuse lymphomatous involvement of the gastrointestinal tract.

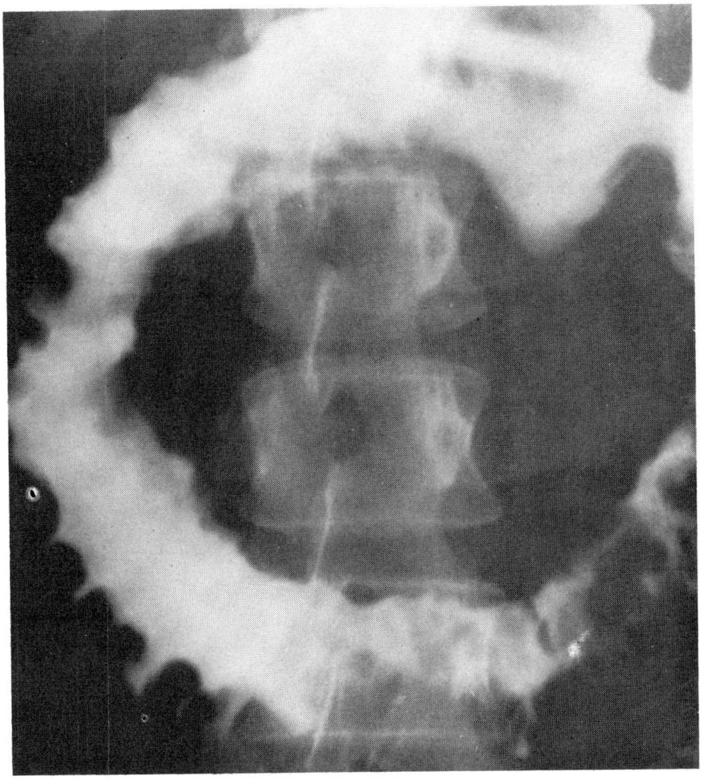

Figure 4–47. Thickened folds secondary to peripancreatic lymph node metastases from carcinoma of the breast. Impaired lymphatic drainage may account for the mucosal thickening.

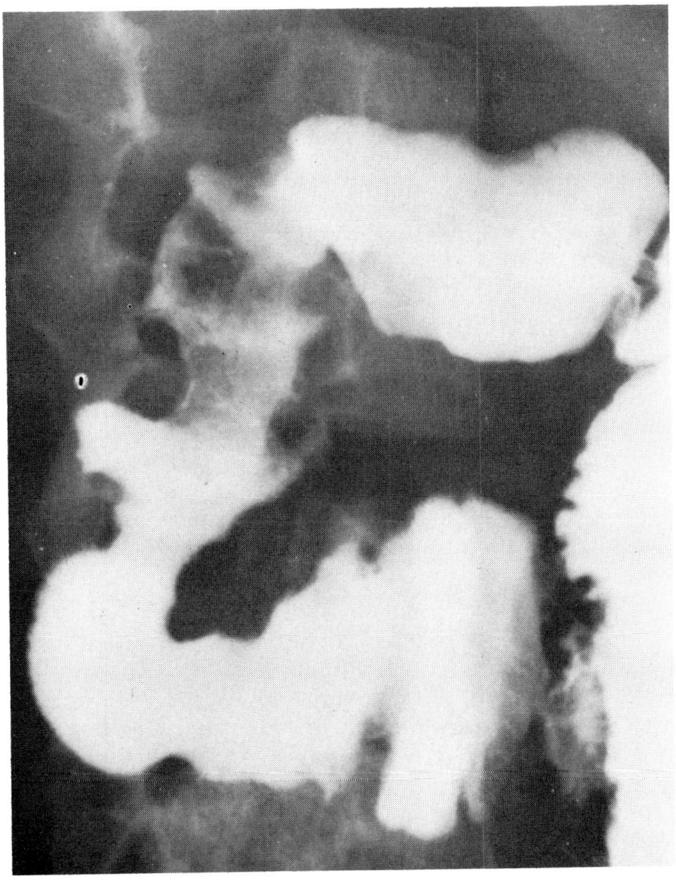

Figure 4–48. Fold thickening secondary to submucosal hemorrhage in Henoch-Schoenlein purpura. (Courtesy of Dr. Harry Newman.)

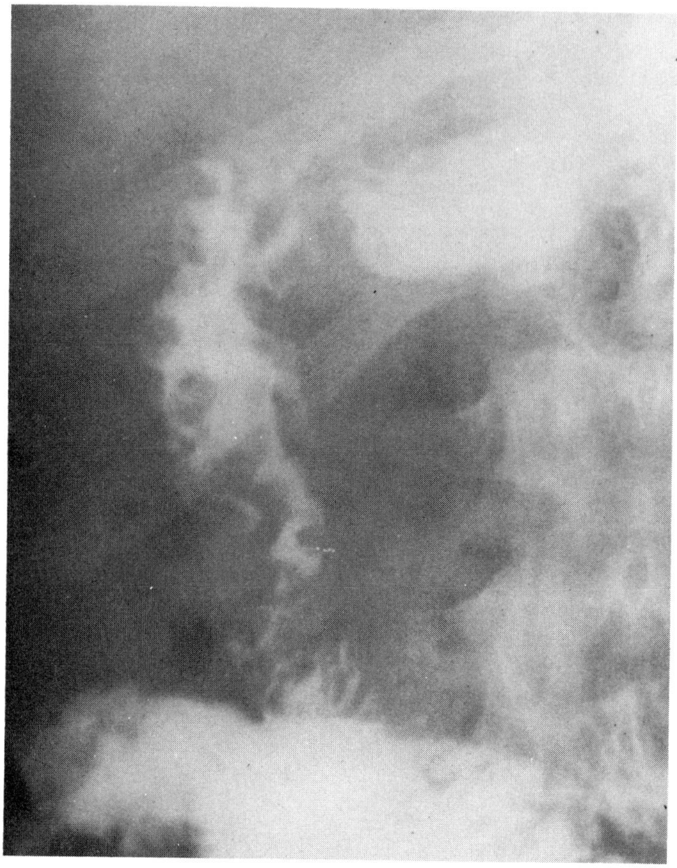

Figure 4–49. Nodular filling defects simulating mucosal fold thickening as a result of impression by enlarged pancreaticoduodenal arterial arcades in superior mesenteric and celiac artery occlusion. (From Shimkin, P. M., and Pearson, K. D.: Unusual arterial impressions on the duodenum. Radiology, *103*:295–297, 1972.)

Intrinsic Duodenal Mass Lesions

This designation includes discrete intraluminal filling defects which appear to be intrinsic to the duodenum (either mucosal or extramucosal) and which project intraluminally to a greater or lesser degree. These defects merge with the category of extrinsic indentations and, on occasion, may be difficult to distinguish from them, particularly when located in the peri-Vaterian region. In such instances, the term is of descriptive rather than diagnostic value.

Intrinsic duodenal masses ordinarily suggest the diagnosis of benign neoplasm. However, they may be the result of a remarkable variety of disorders, a number of which are non-neoplastic, as indicated in Table 4–6. Many of these conditions are rare and are not likely to be suspected by the referring physician. Usually, they are first discovered on barium meal examination; the radiologist therefore has an obligation to develop a knowledgeable approach to their differential diagnosis and management.

Appearances simulating duodenal masses occur with some frequency and have been termed "pseudotumors." For example, marked perifocal edema surrounding a small ulcer crater may simulate a mass lesion (Berger, 1955). Similarly, retained blood clot may present as a duodenal filling defect and occasionally has a central collection of barium on the surface, simulating an ulcerating tumor mass (Fig. 4–50). Foreign bodies enter the differential diagnosis since gallstones may erode into the duodenal lumen and present as a mass or produce frank obstruction. Fruit pits occasionally lodge in the duodenal cap, particularly in patients with chronic duodenal scarring from ulcer disease. Food particles at times produce bizarre

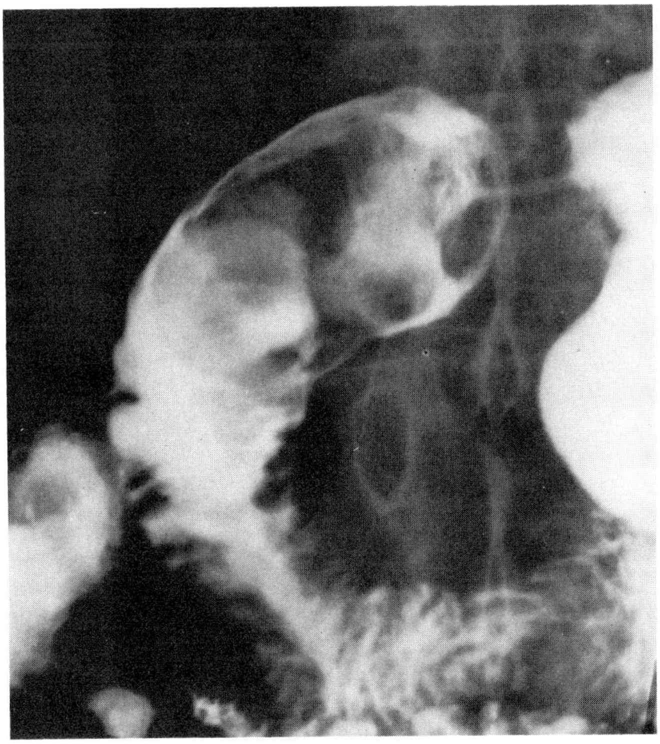

Figure 4–50. Blood clot in the duodenal cap simulating a tumor mass. Preoperative diagnosis was an ulcerating leiomyosarcoma. Site of bleeding was an acute duodenal ulcer.

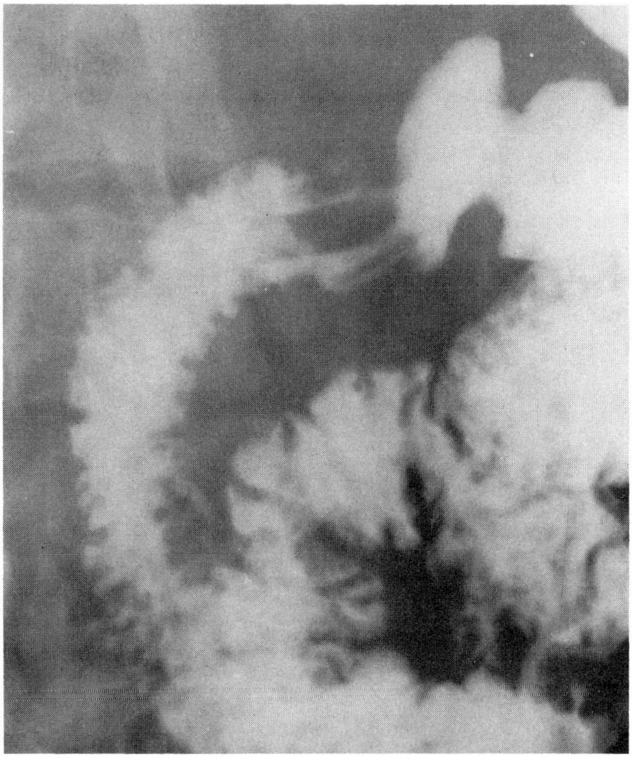

Figure 4–51. Foreign body in the duodenal cap. The patient had French fried potatoes for lunch.

filling defects in the stomach or duodenum (Fig. 4–51). Prolapsing adenomatous polyps of the stomach are also commonly encountered (Fig. 4–52). These are frequently multiple, and can be recognized by the presence of a stalk and changeable location on serial films (Short, 1968).

An arresting pseudotumoral appearance may occur at the flexure between the first and second portions of the duodenum, usually on the inner or inferior duodenal margin. This flexural pseudotumor is caused by an acute change in the duodenal axis at this point, which produces a "buckle" in the duodenal wall, thus creating an apparent filling defect (Fig. 4–53). Typically, the plical folds assume a circular or swirled configuration. Edematous thickening of duodenal folds sometimes accentuates this appearance, and a fleck of barium may become trapped between folds, simulating an ulcer crater (Fig. 4–54). The characteristic location, appearance, and changeability on serial films differentiate this from a real lesion.

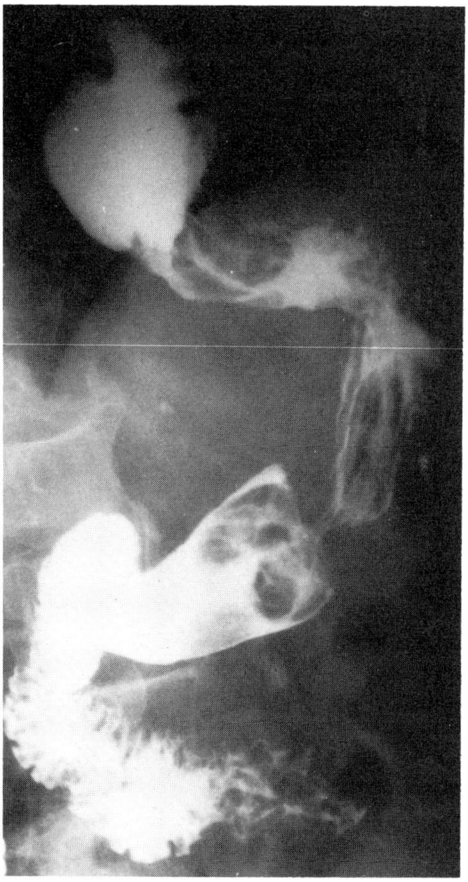

Figure 4–52. Prolapsing adenomatous polyps of the stomach presenting as filling defects in the duodenal cap.

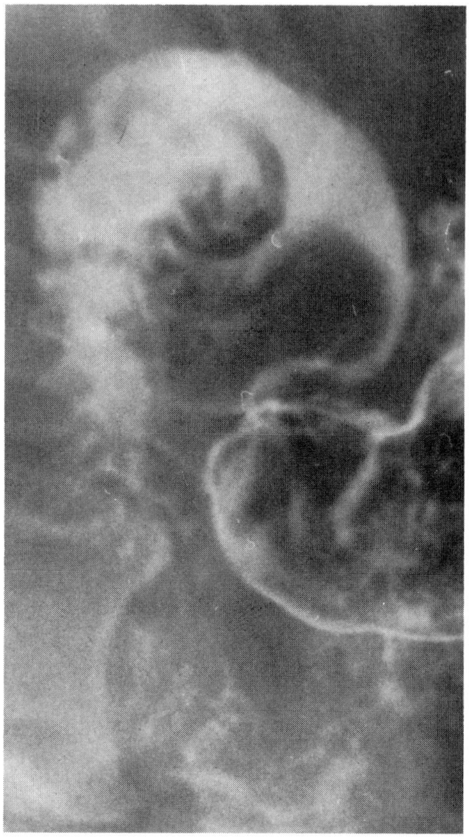

Figure 4–53. Duodenal pseudotumor at the apex of the cap. This is a commonly seen normal variant caused by the acute change in duodenal axis between the cap and the descending duodenum, which results in a buckling effect on the inner duodenal margin. Typical swirled mucosal folds are visible which may trap barium and simulate a centrally ulcerating tumor.

Analysis of many true duodenal filling defects begins with the critical question: Is the mass a duodenal papilla or something else? This distinction is facilitated by reference to the triad of landmarks described earlier in the discussion of normal anatomy. Examples of the value of these landmarks of normal anatomy are illustrated in Figure 4–26.

Enlargement of the papilla (e.g., greater than 1.5 cm. in length) as a result of edematous swelling accompanies a vari-

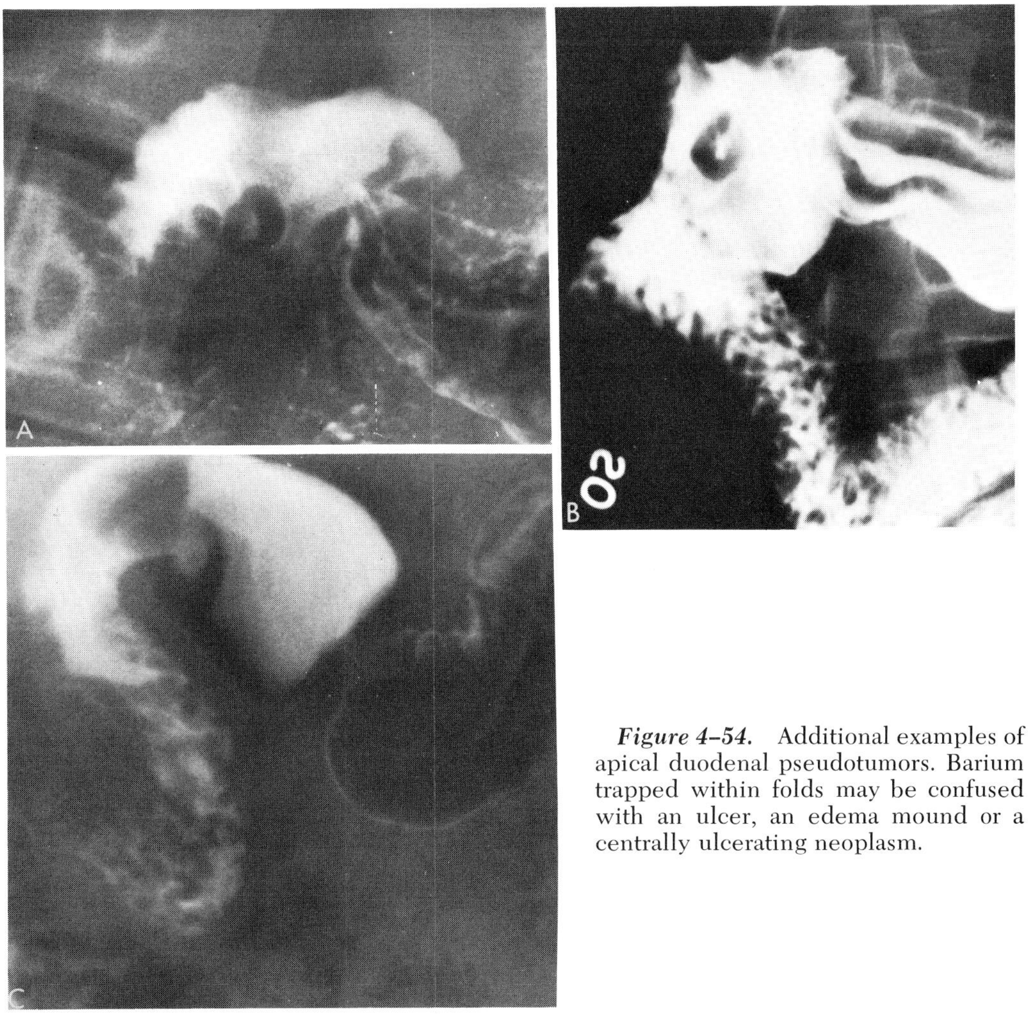

Figure 4–54. Additional examples of apical duodenal pseudotumors. Barium trapped within folds may be confused with an ulcer, an edema mound or a centrally ulcerating neoplasm.

ety of inflammatory disorders in addition to ampullary neoplasms (Table 4–7). Perhaps the best known cause of papillary edema is acute pancreatitis—the so-called Poppel's sign. When the papilla enlarges as a result of edema, it acquires a characteristic smooth, semilunar configuration (Fig. 4–55). The appearance is that of an intramural mass, and is identical whether the cause is pancreatitis (Poppel, 1954) (Fig. 4–56), acute duodenal ulcer (Jacobson, 1958) (Fig. 4–57), or impacted common duct stone (Eaton, 1972). Presumably, the enlarging papilla bulges forward into the longitudinal fold to produce the rather constant elliptical filling defect typical of a swollen papilla. When papillary swelling is severe (i.e., greater than 3 cm. in length), a more spherical configuration develops (Fig. 4–58).

Recently, attention has been drawn to the finding of papillary edema in impacted common duct stone (Eaton, 1972; Bree, 1972). This is a useful sign on conventional barium meal study and may be readily detected at duodenography in patients presenting with obstructive jaundice (Fig. 4–59). Apparently, papillary swelling occurs because of the reactive inflammatory changes around the distal common duct as it passes through the duodenal wall. This situation is analogous to swelling of the interureteric

TABLE 4–6. Intrinsic Duodenal Masses

Pseudotumors
- Acute ulcer mound
- Blood clot
- Foreign body (gallstones, fruit pit)
- Flexural pseudotumor

Non-Neoplastic Masses
- Edematous papilla
- Ectopic pancreas
- Prolapsed antral mucosa
- Duodenal varix
- Duplication cyst
- Retention cyst

Benign Neoplasms
- Prolapsed antral polyp
- Brunner's gland adenoma
- Adenomatous polyp
- Lipoma
- Fibroma
- Leiomyoma
- Carotid body tumor

Tumors of Variable Malignant Potential
- Villous adenoma
- Carcinoid (islet cell tumor)

Malignant Tumors
- Adenocarcinoma (duodenum or pancreas)
- Ampullary carcinoma
- Sarcoma
- Lymphosarcoma
- Metastases

ridge of the bladder, resulting from calculi lodged in the distal ureter (Wisoff, 1961). Benign swelling of the papilla of Vater may be differentiated from ampullary carcinoma, which generally produces an irregular, nodular, or frankly ulcerating filling defect. Uncommonly, however, carcinoma of the ampulla may present as a smooth-surfaced mass indistinguishable from benign papillary edema. Demonstration of an enlarged papilla in a patient with obstructive jaundice therefore indicates the presence of mechanical extrahepatic obstruction and localizes the level. In those cases in which greater diagnostic precision is required, percutaneous transhepatic cholangiography, described in Chapter 5, is the next logical examination. The significance of a large papilla (i.e., approximately 3 cm. in length) in an otherwise normal patient is uncertain. Possibly, some of these patients have asymptomatic papillitis (Griffen, 1968) or adenomatous polyps of the papilla (Oh, 1965) as described in Chapter 10.

Aberrant pancreas is a commonly encountered non-neoplastic duodenal filling defect, usually presenting in the

TABLE 4–7. Causes of Papillary Enlargement

Large but Normal Papilla

Papillary Edema
- Pancreatitis (Poppel's sign)
- Acute duodenal ulcer
- Impacted common duct stone

Ampullary Neoplasm
- Adenomatous polyp
- Carcinoma

R/O Ectopic Pancreas

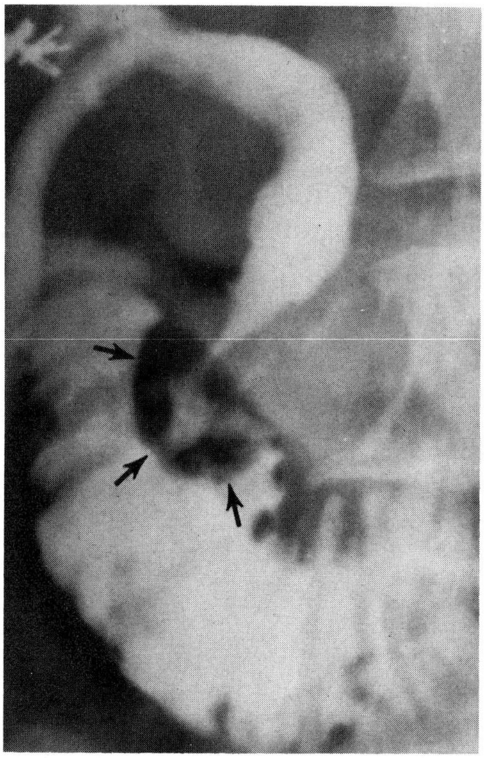

Figure 4–55. Papillary edema. T-tube cholangiogram after common duct exploration. Note the typical smooth semilunar filling defect. This configuration is probably produced by the swollen papilla–longitudinal fold complex.

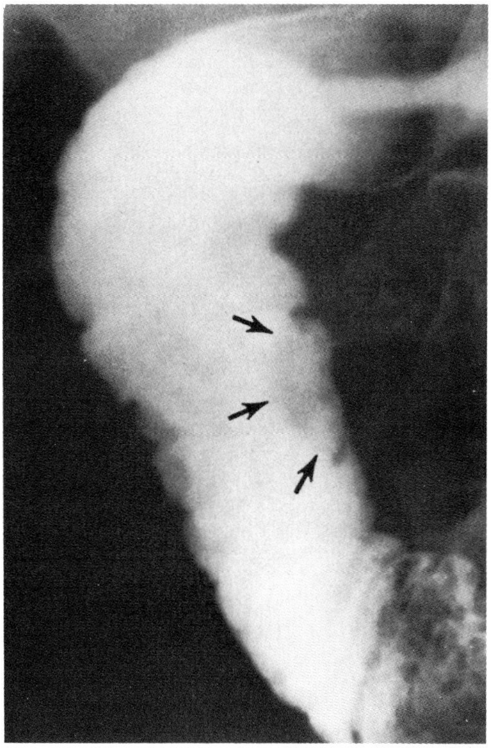

Figure 4–56. Papillary edema in subacute relapsing pancreatitis – Poppel's sign. The smooth elliptical configuration of an edematous papilla is constant regardless of the cause.

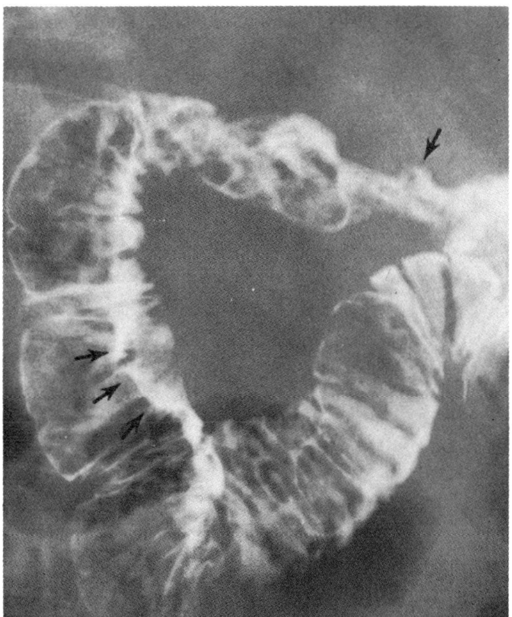

Figure 4–57. Swollen papilla associated with acute benign peptic ulcer of the pyloric canal.

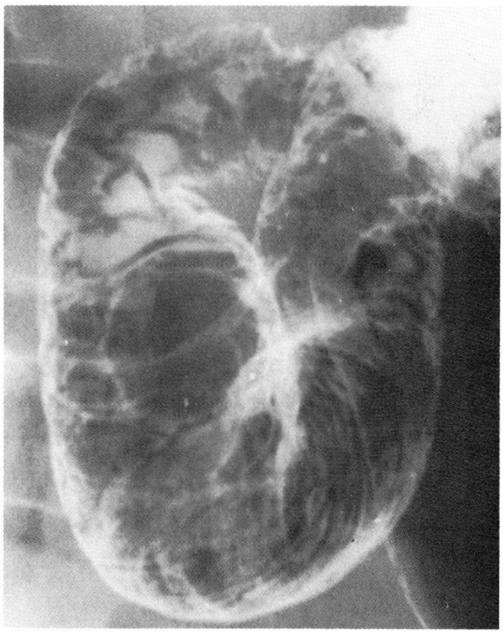

Figure 4–58. Marked papillary edema associated with impacted common-duct stone. With massive swelling, the papilla assumes a spherical shape resembling a neoplasm.

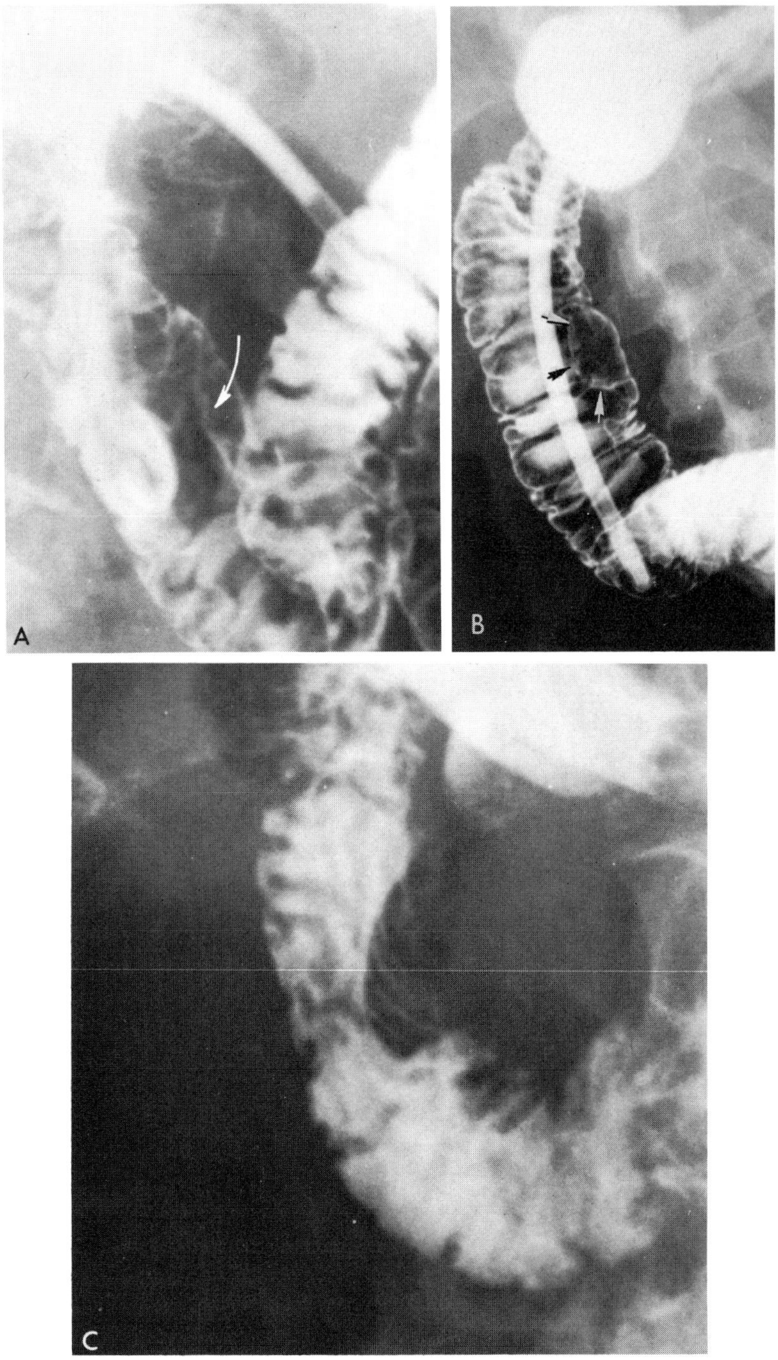

Figure 4–59. Edema of the papilla resulting from common-duct calculi in three patients. The smooth, elliptical defect is identical to that seen in pancreatitis and may permit the preoperative diagnosis of impacted common-duct stone in patients presenting with obstructive jaundice.

proximal descending duodenum as a discrete filling defect less than 1 cm. in diameter (Besemann, 1969). Gastric nodules are usually larger, up to 3 cm. in size, and are more readily diagnosed radiographically (see Chapter 3). The nodule of heterotopic tissue is commonly submucosal in location, and is often asymptomatic. Radiographically, the appearance is fairly constant and the characteristic roentgen finding is said to be a central niche or dimple of barium, representing filling of the ostium of miniature duct-like structures which are histologically present within the nodule of pancreatic tissue (Fig. 4–60). These minute ramifying ducts are much more often demonstrated pathologically than radiographically. In at least some instances, the central collection of barium is due to a simple ulceration, and, in others, it is found to be a blind diverticulum-like pit.

Duplication and retention cysts have few identifying features (Fig. 4–61). They usually have an intramural configuration and vary considerably in size, occasionally becoming large enough to obstruct the duodenal lumen. Because of their fluid content, they are soft and, like lipomas, may change contour on serial films. Rarely, such cysts may originate in Brunner's glands (Hately, 1968).

Filling defects representing true neoplasms will be considered in the discussion of duodenal tumors in Chapter 10.

Biliary Reflux

Reflux of barium into the biliary or pancreatic ducts is an unusual but dramatic roentgen finding, indicating local abnormality in the vaterian segment with a high degree of certainty. In clinical practice, the majority of cases are due to prior surgery (i.e., sphincterotomy).

A distinction should be made between barium visualization of the ampulla of Vater, which is a normal finding, and reflux filling of the biliary or pancreatic ducts proper, which is pathologic. Visualization of the ampulla is occasionally seen on conventional barium studies and more often on hypotonic examination, presumably because of the spasmolytic

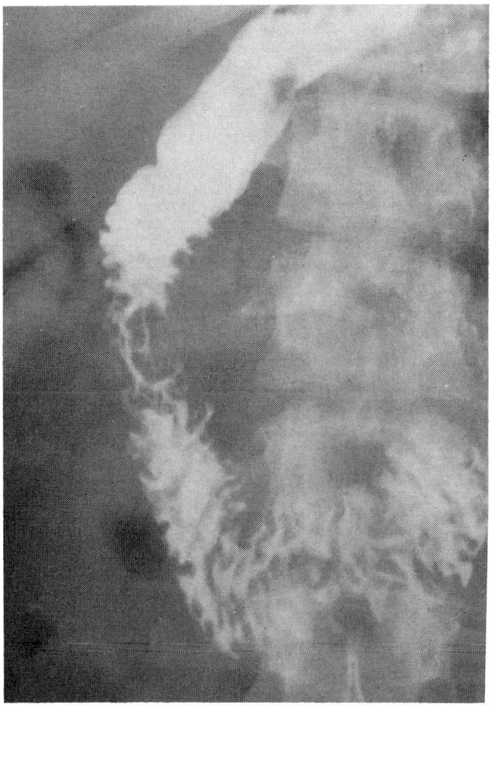

Figure 4–60. Ectopic pancreas. Note the central collection of barium with linear branch-like extensions. These are more often identified on pathologic study than by roentgenography (see also Fig. 9–10).

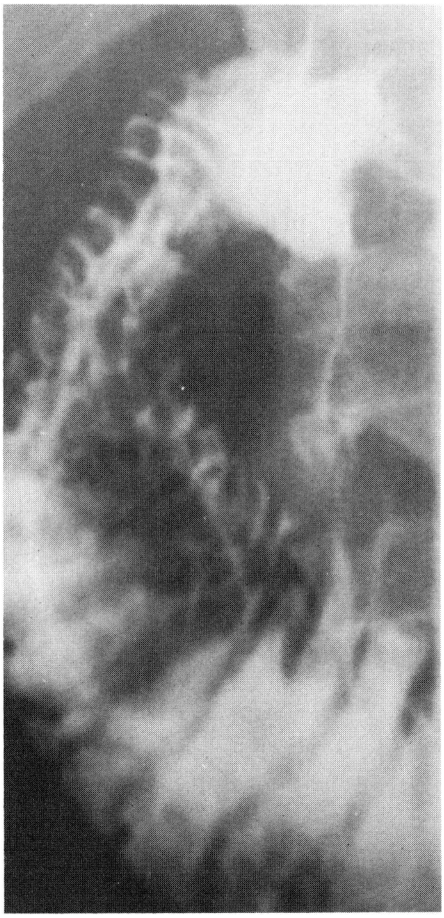

Figure 4–61. Duplication cyst. Retention and duplication cysts have the appearance of intramural filling defects and may reach a considerable size. These are fluid-filled cystic spaces and, like lipomas, may have a variable contour on serial films.

effect of the drug on fibers in the lower portion of the periampullary sphincter (sphincter of Oddi). As noted earlier, the ampulla is a slightly dilated segment of duct just below the mucosal opening on the papilla. Embryologically, it is universally present during prenatal life, but rapidly involutes so that only 2 per cent of adults have a demonstable ampulla (Royer, 1944). It is of interest that some surgical authorities dispute the existence of any intraduodenal dilatation of the common bile duct and consider the term ampulla anatomically incorrect (Hand, 1963). This discrepancy possibly reflects a sampling problem; these authors each selected only 50 postmortem cases for examination. Nonetheless, in nearly 400 duodenograms performed in the last four years, we have seen several cases which fulfill the criteria for roentgen appearance of the ampulla as described by Poppel (1953). Not infrequently, T-tube cholangiograms demonstrate what appears to be an ampullary configuration (see Fig. 4–55). Kasugai and his associates (1972) also report occasional visualization of the ampulla during pancreatography performed by perioral endoscopic cannulation of the papilla. Waldron (1972) has also demonstrated ampullary filling in normal patients by means of

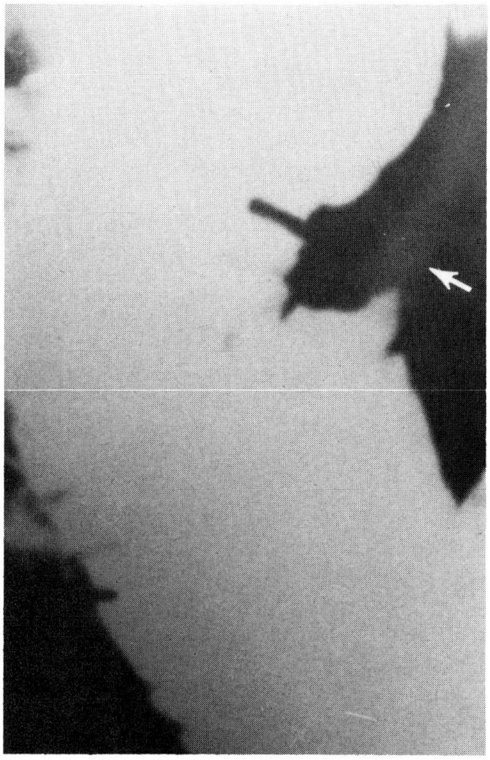

Figure 4–62. Ampullary filling demonstrated at hypotonic duodenography. A simultaneous intravenous cholangiogram (*arrow*) confirms the relationship between the common duct and ampulla. The ampulla is visible as a short, truncated cone arising from the promontory.

his double-balloon distention duodenography technique. Accordingly, we continue to believe that an ampulla is frequently present and occasionally demonstrable roentgenographically. The ampulla may be seen on duodenograms as a short, truncated, conical, or pyramidal projection often arising from the region of the promontory (Fig. 4–62). The average size is 7 to 10 mm. in length. It can be differentiated from perivaterian diverticula which are larger, usually more spherical, have a visible neck, and empty more slowly (Poppel, 1953) (Fig. 4–63).

Reflux of barium into the common bile or main pancreatic duct is definitely abnormal and indicates dysfunction of the sphincteric fibers in the duodenal wall or supraduodenal portions of the ducts and sometimes both. Surgical sphincterotomy is the commonest cause of pancreaticobiliary reflux (Fig. 4–64), but other causes have been recorded (Table 4–8). The mechanism of sphincteric incompetence involves anatomic distortion of the sphincter fibers by surgery, edema, tumor infiltration, or fibrosis. Several cases of ampullary and pancreaticoduodenal carcinoma with biliary reflux have been recorded in the recent literature (Eaton, 1970*b*) (Fig. 4–65). Legge (1970) has also reported three cases of regional enteritis of the duodenum with spontaneous reflux. However, biliary reflux occurring without a history of surgery or known regional enteritis makes peri-Vaterian malignancy the prime consideration.

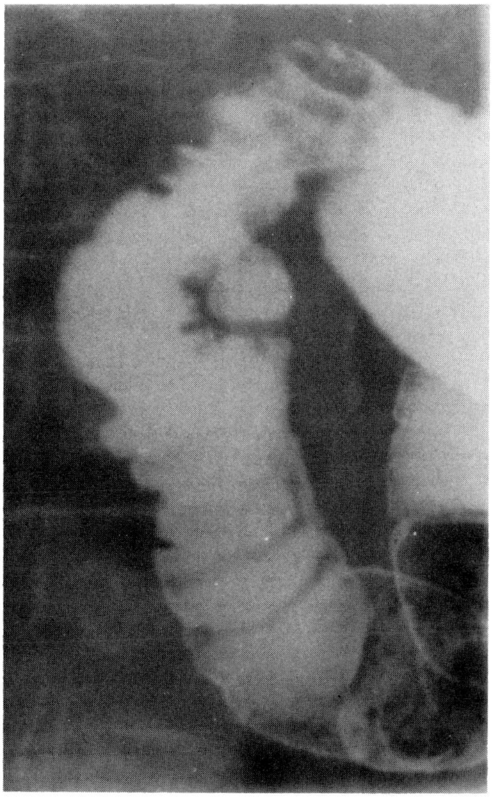

Figure 4–63. Diverticulum in area of ampulla of Vater. The spherical shape and definite neck of the diverticulum distinguish it from the ampulla. Note the relationship to the promontory and straight segment.

Ulceration of the Postbulbar Duodenum

Benign postbulbar ulcers usually occur on the medial side of the upper descending duodenum or on the concave side of the apex of the cap (Fig. 4–66). An important roentgenographic sign is an indentation defect (incisura) on the opposite duodenal margin at the level of

TABLE 4–8. Causes of Pancreaticobiliary Reflux

Surgery
Prior sphincterotomy
Biliary enteric anastomoses
Choledochoduodenostomy
Cholecystoduodenostomy
Cholecystojejunostomy
Inflammatory Edema and/or Fibrosis
Pancreatitis, duodenitis, perforated ulcer
Recently passed common duct stone
Cicatrizing chronic inflammation (regional enteritis, strongyloidiasis)
Neoplastic Infiltration
Carcinoma of ampulla, pancreas, or duodenum
Metastatic malignancy to Vaterian area
Anomalies
Anomalous insertion of common duct into duodenal diverticulum

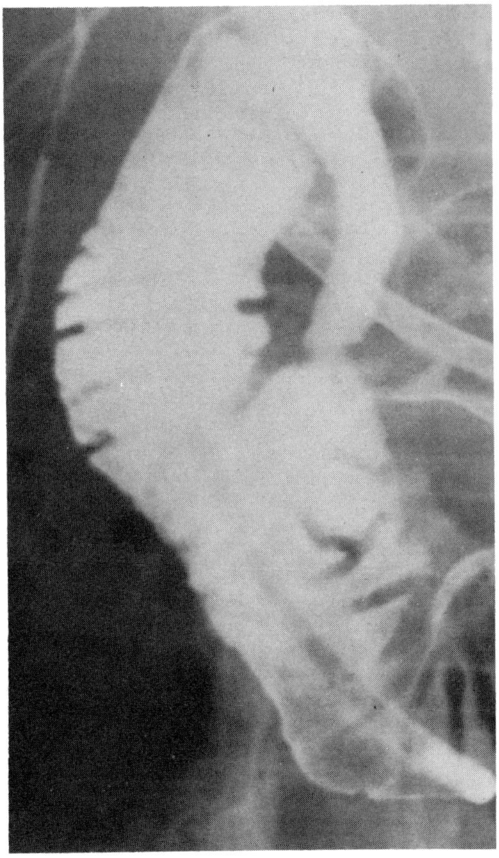

Figure 4–64. Biliary reflux secondary to prior sphincterotomy. The relaxation of muscle tone achieved during duodenography often increases the amount of reflux. Note the relationship of the papillary area to the promontory. (Reproduced by permission of *Radiology*.)

the crater. This indentation occurs in acute ulcers as a result of spasm and may persist during and after healing as a result of inflammatory fibrosis. Usually, an eccentric narrowing of lumen is visible as the ulcer crater burrows medially into the head of the pancreas (Fig. 4–67). An associated inflammatory mass in the head of the pancreas frequently coexists. Mucosal folds and valvulae conniventes may be thickened or distorted, but the absence of nodularity or frank destruction usually excludes a malignant lesion. Another differential diagnostic consideration is a partially filled or distorted duodenal diverticulum. Usually, however, mucosal folds can be seen passing into the neck of the diverticulum, as contrasted with the clear zone of edematous folds sometimes present around the margin of an ulcer crater. In addition, an ulcer niche usually retains a constant, rigid shape, whereas diverticula frequently can be seen to fill and empty with barium in successive films. Differential diagnosis from annular pancreas may be extremely difficult, particularly if the crater is poorly visualized.

Duodenal ulcers occurring in atypical locations distal to the cap are hallmarks of the Zollinger-Ellison syndrome. Distal duodenal ulcer occurred in six of 14 patients reported by Christoforidis (1966). These are usually benign-appearing ulcers with intact mucosal folds but may be multiple, and are usually associated with a dilated atonic duodenum, marked mucosal edema, and dilution of the barium mixture by high volumes of gastric secretion (Fig. 4–68). Characteristic associated changes of gastric hyperrugosity and an enteritis pattern in the small bowel confirm the diagnosis (see Chapter 10).

Ulcerations occurring on the surface of discrete filling defects frequently indicate benign tumors, especially the spindle cell types. Although these tumors arise from the submucosal coats of the duodenal wall, the mucosa over the summit of the tumor ulcerates, producing a characteristic rounded or oval central crater (Fig. 4–69). Ectopic pancreas may produce a similar appearance. Somewhat flatter filling defects with central craters occur in hematogenous metastases to the mucosal surface. The so-called target or bull's-eye sign may occur in melanoma, lymphosarcoma, or Kaposi's sarcoma as a result of endarterial tumor emboli which grow on the mucosal surface and then ulcerate centrally (Figs. 4–70 and 4–71). Occasionally, massively excavating mucosal ulcerations result in fatal hemorrhage in such patients (Fig. 4–72).

It is not widely recognized that, apart from ulcers of the duodenal apex, the majority of postbulbar ulcers are neoplastic lesions and are usually malignant.

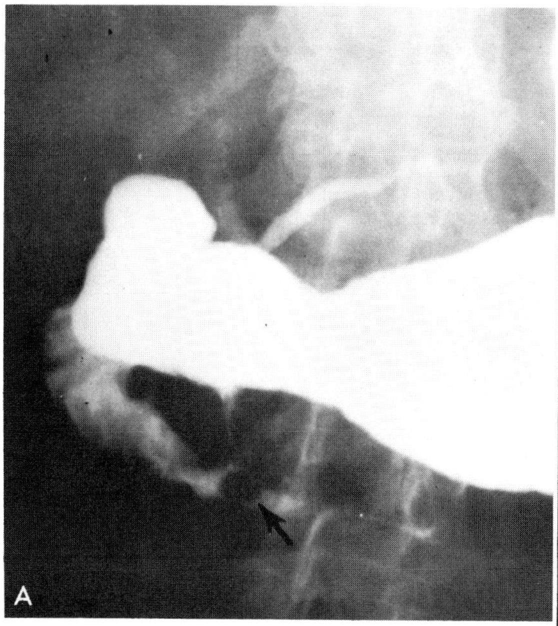

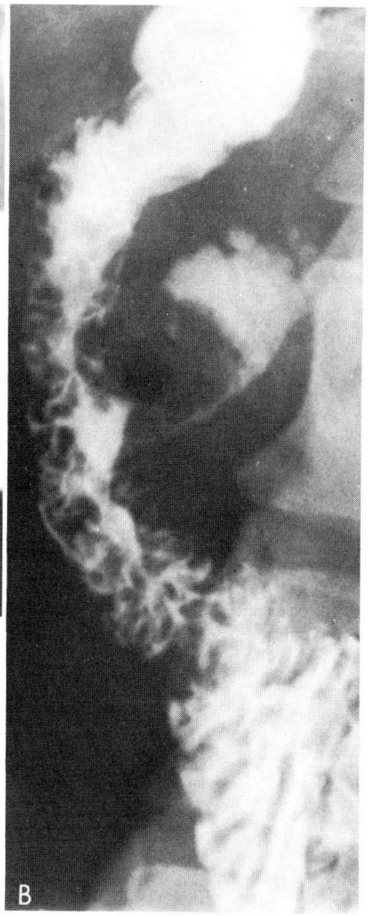

Figure 4–65. Spontaneous biliary reflux in two patients with carcinoma of the ampulla of Vater.

A, Note the smooth-appearing nodule involving the papillary region. Barium refluxes into the bile ducts as a result of neoplastic destruction of muscle fibers in the ampullary sphincter.

B, Barium fills a dilated common duct, demonstrating an intraluminal tumor nodule within the duct.

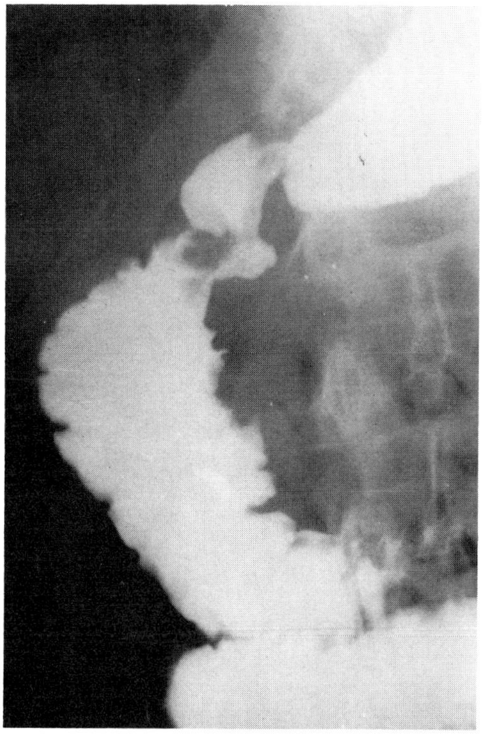

Figure 4–66. Benign postbulbar ulcer showing medial retraction of the lumen and a lateral incisura defect. Flattening of folds and nodular defects along the upper inner duodenal margin indicate penetration into the pancreas.

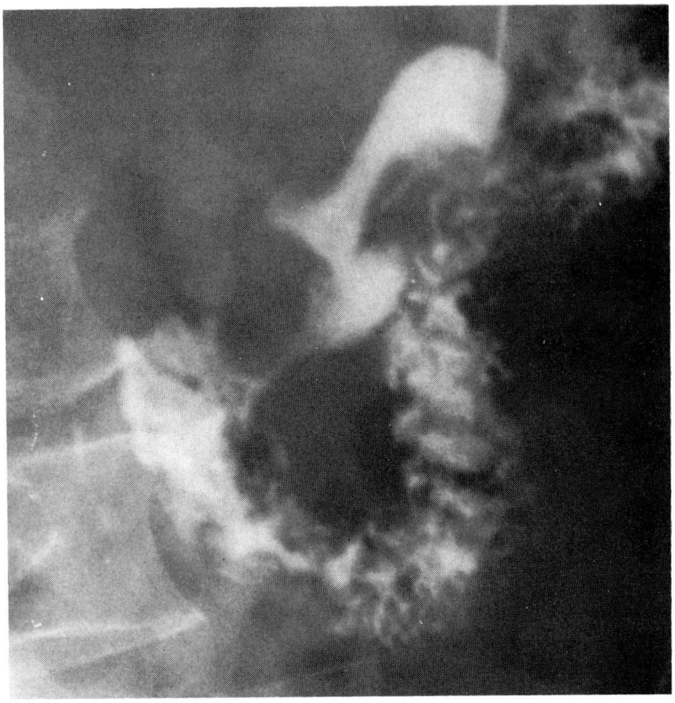

Figure 4–67. Benign postbulbar ulcer. Marked narrowing and medial retraction of the lumen are associated with a striking lateral nodular incisura defect.

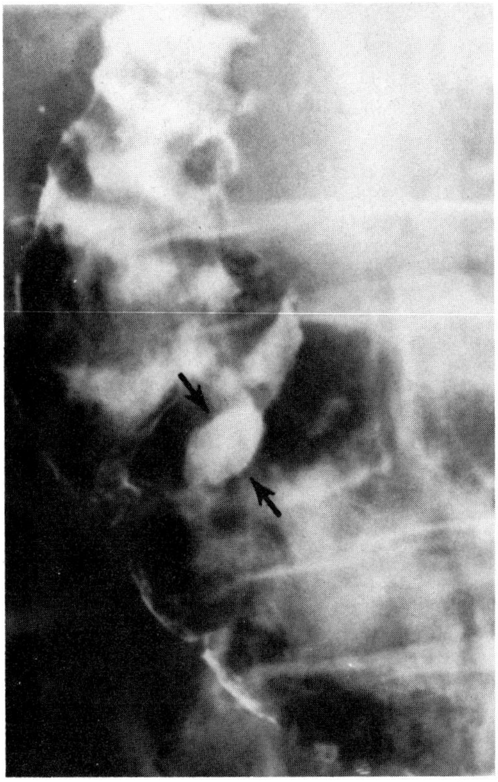

Figure 4–68. Postbulbar ulcer in the Zollinger-Ellison syndrome. Oval ulcer in the distal duodenal loop is associated with markedly thickened mucosal folds.

Irregular ulcerating lesions occur in both primary and metastatic duodenal malignancies. The latter occur by contiguous invasion of tumors arising in adjacent organs (e.g., pancreas, colon, gallbladder, and lymph nodes), or by hematogenous endarterial mucosal deposits (Table 4–9). A nodular mass or eccentric stricture may occur with any malignant ulceration (Fig. 4–73), but the roentgen appearance is not specific. In the descending duodenum, adenocarcinomas of the duodenum and ampulla

TABLE 4–9. Ulceration of the Postbulbar Duodenum

Benign Postbulbar Peptic Ulcer
Zollinger-Ellison Syndrome
Benign Neoplasms
R/O ectopic pancreas
Primary Duodenal Malignancy
Adenocarcinoma, lymphoma, sarcoma
Metastatic Malignancy
Contiguous invasion (pancreas, right colon, right kidney, gallbladder)
Invasion from metastases in lymph nodes
Hematogenous metastases (melanoma, Kaposi's)

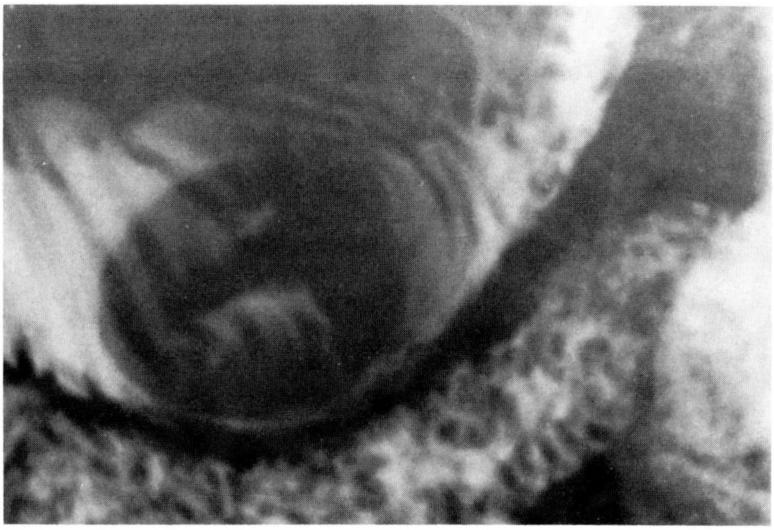

Figure 4–69. Surface ulceration occurring in an intramural tumor of the spindle cell variety.

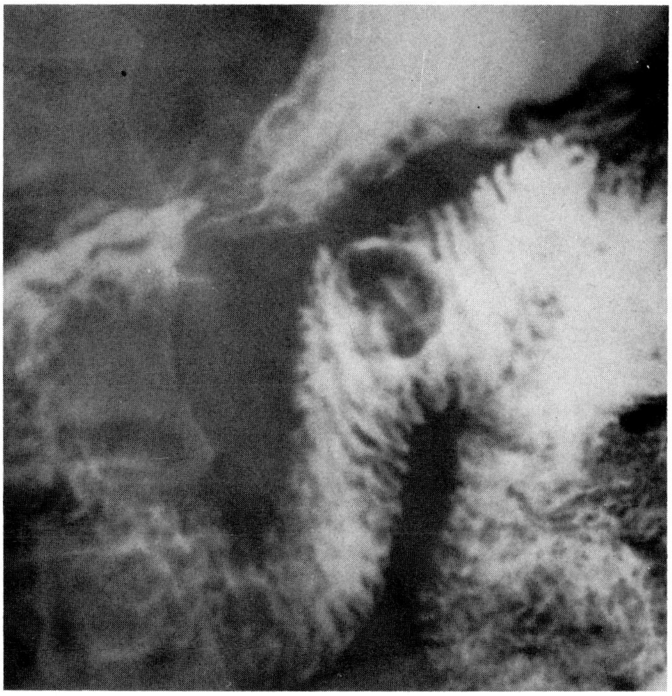

Figure 4–70. Target ulcer in metastatic melanoma. This results from central ulceration in a mucosal or intramural tumor mass.

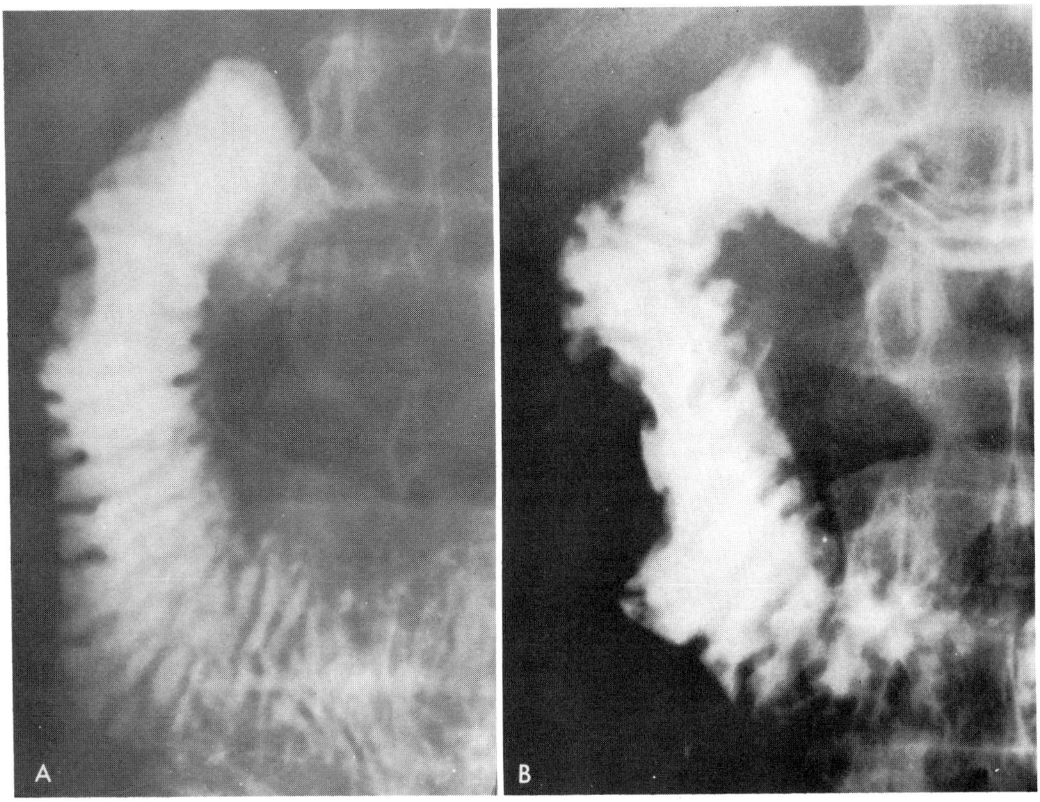

Figure 4–71. Target ulcers seen in profile in two patients with metastatic malignancy involving the duodenal wall. *A*, Malignant melanoma; *B*, reticulum cell sarcoma. (Courtesy of Dr. Ann Lewicki.)

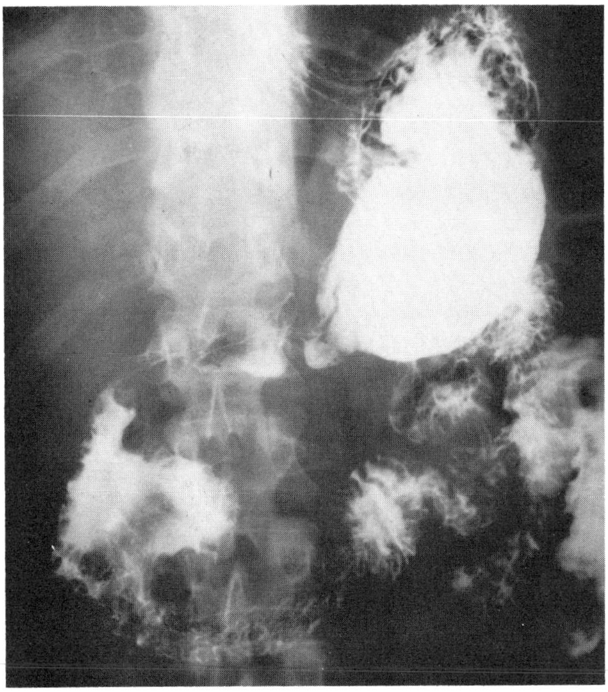

Figure 4–72. Large irregular excavating ulcer in the descending duodenum secondary to metastatic malignant melanoma.

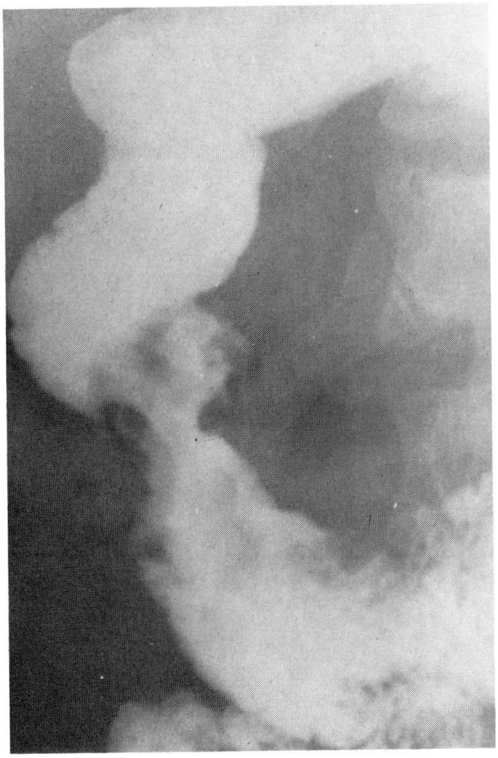

Figure 4–73. Nodular ulcerating lesion with eccentric narrowing of the lumen resulting from primary adenocarcinoma of the duodenum. Carcinoma of the ampulla or invading carcinoma of the pancreas may produce an identical appearance.

of Vater are often indistinguishable; more distally, adenocarcinoma predominates statistically over lymphomas and other sarcomas.

Contiguous invasion of the duodenum by cancer in adjacent structures may produce an ulcer-mass complex involving the intervening duodenal wall. Cancer of the right colon, right kidney, or gallbladder can invade the duodenal cap or outer border of the duodenal loop (Khilnani, 1962; Treitel, 1970) (Fig. 4–74); carcinoma of the pancreas may ulcerate into the concavity of the duodenum at any site from the cap to the duodenojejunal flexure (Blatt, 1971; Eaton, 1972) (Figs. 4–75 and 4–76). Similarly, metastatic malignancy in periduodenal lymph nodes may invade and ulcerate into the duodenal lumen (McCort, 1953) (Fig. 4–77).

Fistulous Lesions of the Duodenum

Duodenal fistulae are rare but dramatic findings involving a variety of adjacent hollow organs in a variety of different disorders (Table 4–10).

Biliary duodenal connections are the

Figure 4–74. Irregular ulceration of the descending duodenum secondary to invasion of the duodenum by carcinoma of the hepatic flexure.

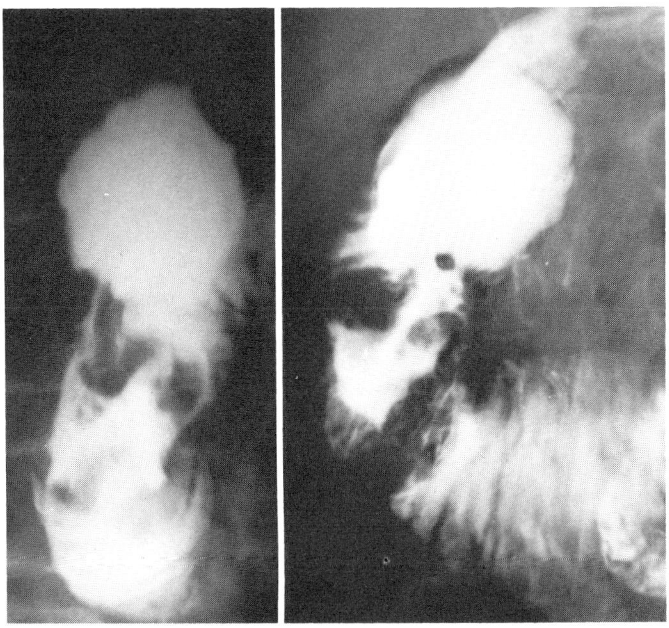

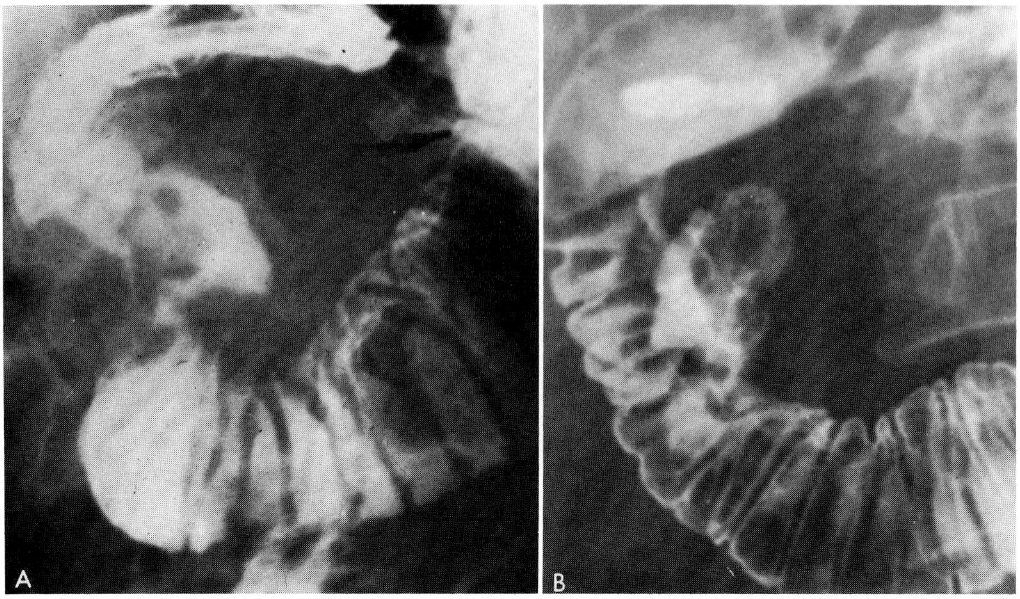

Figure 4–75. Irregular ulceration of the mid-descending duodenum secondary to carcinoma of the head of the pancreas in two patients. (Courtesy of Dr. M. K. Bilbao. *A*, From Bilbao, M. K., et al.: Hypotonic duodenography in the diagnosis of pancreatic diseases. Seminars Roentgen., *3*:280, 1968. By permission of Grune & Stratton, Inc. *B*, From Bilbao, M. K., et al.: Hypotonic duodenography. Radiology, *89*:438, 1967.)

commonest duodenal fistulae and are usually demonstrated by barium meal study as barium or air filling the gallbladder and biliary tree. Calculous disease of the gallbladder, as well as duodenal ulcer, account for the majority of cases (Constant, 1968), although carcinoma of the gallbladder may perforate into the duodenal lumen. Cholecystoduodenal fistula, which usually results from cholelithiasis, is more common in women in accordance with the incidence of calculous disease and may lead to gallstone ileus. Similarly, duodenal ulcer, which is more common in males, accounts for a higher incidence of choledochoduodenal fistula in men (Craighead, 1954; Constant, 1968; and Lewis, 1969) (Fig. 4–78).

TABLE 4–10. Fistulous Lesions of the Duodenum

Cholecystoduodenal	usually benign, occasionally malignant
Choledochoduodenal	mostly benign
Duodenocolic	malignant and benign
Renoduodenal	mostly benign
Aorticoduodenal	due to ruptured aneurysm

Duodenocolic fistulae are usually best shown by barium enema examination, and generally involve the descending duodenum (Fig. 4–79). Carcinoma of the right colon is the commonest cause (Hershenson, 1951; Medhurst, 1956), although benign conditions such as duodenal ulcer, regional enteritis, and perforated duodenal diverticulum may give rise to this finding (Clayton, 1953; Nash, 1956; and Winter, 1959) (Fig. 4–80).

Renoduodenal fistulae invariably involve the right kidney and are usually a sequel of pyelonephritis which is often tuberculous (King, 1950). A perirenal abscess usually develops first, followed by rupture into the duodenum. The communication is best shown by retrograde pyelography. Stock (1954) has also reported a case of renoduodenal fistula which was the result of a penetrating duodenal ulcer.

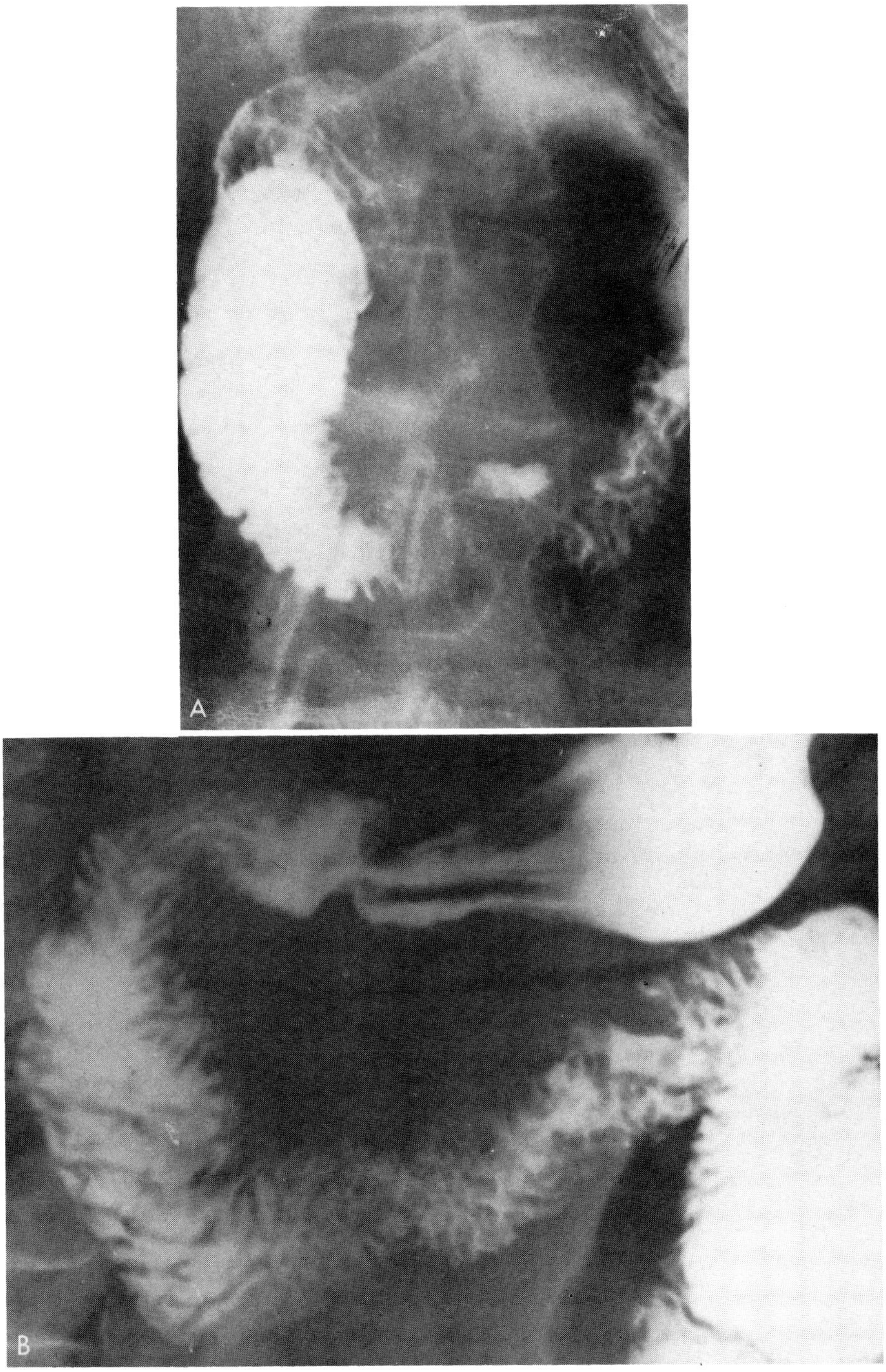

Figure 4–76. Ulceration of the horizontal portion of the duodenum resulting from contiguous invasion by carcinoma of the body of the pancreas in two patients. (*B*, Reproduced by permission of *American Journal of Roentgenology.*)

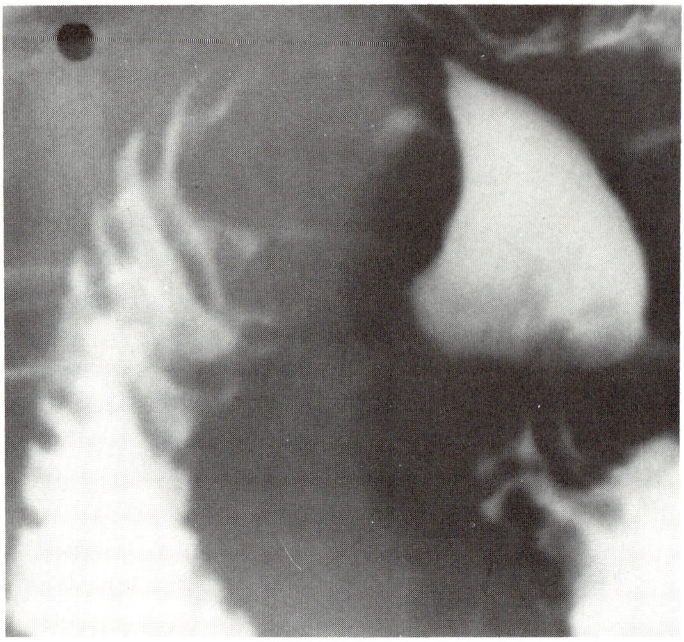

Figure 4–77. Postbulbar ulcer-mass complex resulting from periduodenal lymph node metastases. Primary lesion was in the sigmoid colon.

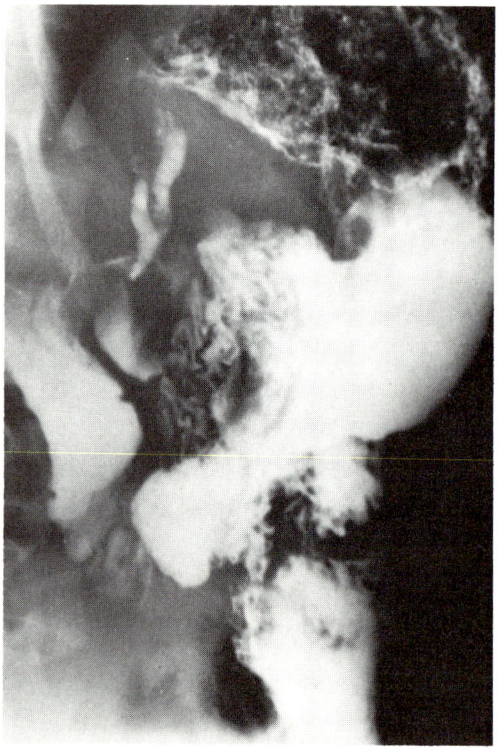

Figure 4–78. Choledochoduodenal fistula resulting from perforation of a peptic duodenal ulcer into the common bile duct. Cholecystoduodenal fistulae, usually the result of cholelithiasis, are more common in females and may result in gallstone ileus. (From Lewis, E. A., and Bohrer, S. P.: Choledochoduodenal fistula complicating chronic duodenal ulcer in Nigerians. Gut, *10*:146–149, 1969.)

Aorticoduodenal fistulae are the result of the rupture of an abdominal aortic aneurysm usually into the horizontal portion of the duodenum, which is closely fixed to the anterior aortic surface (Ferguson, 1966). This is a well-known complication of abdominal aneurysms and often occurs after prosthetic Dacron graft replacement (Baumler, 1961; Eadie, 1968). Radiographically, the third portion of the duodenum may be compressed or displaced by an extrinsic mass with visible central ulceration. Only rarely are the contours of the aortic wall outlined by barium (Fig. 4–81). Abdominal pain associated with a palpable mass and hematemesis is a characteristic feature. The outcome is often fatal, although prompt diagnosis and surgical intervention may be lifesaving.

Stenotic or Obstructive Lesions of the Postbulbar Duodenum

These also may be manifestations of a broad spectrum of diseases, as indicated in Table 4–11 (Deluca, 1973).

Except for annular pancreas, the majority of duodenal anomalies causing stenosis or obstruction are recognized in infancy. Occasionally, the anatomic characteristics are such that diagnosis

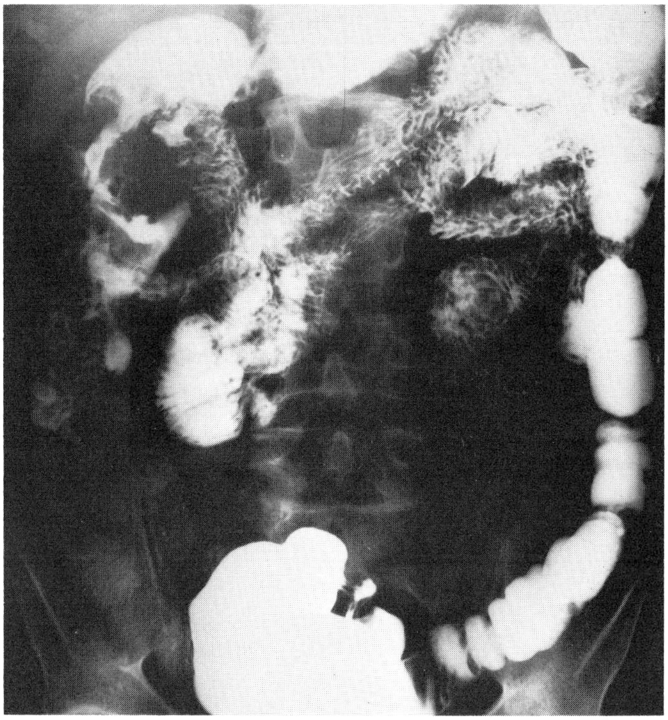

Figure 4–79. Duodenocolic fistula secondary to carcinoma of the hepatic flexure. Barium enema fills the duodenum, demonstrating a nodular constricting tumor mass.

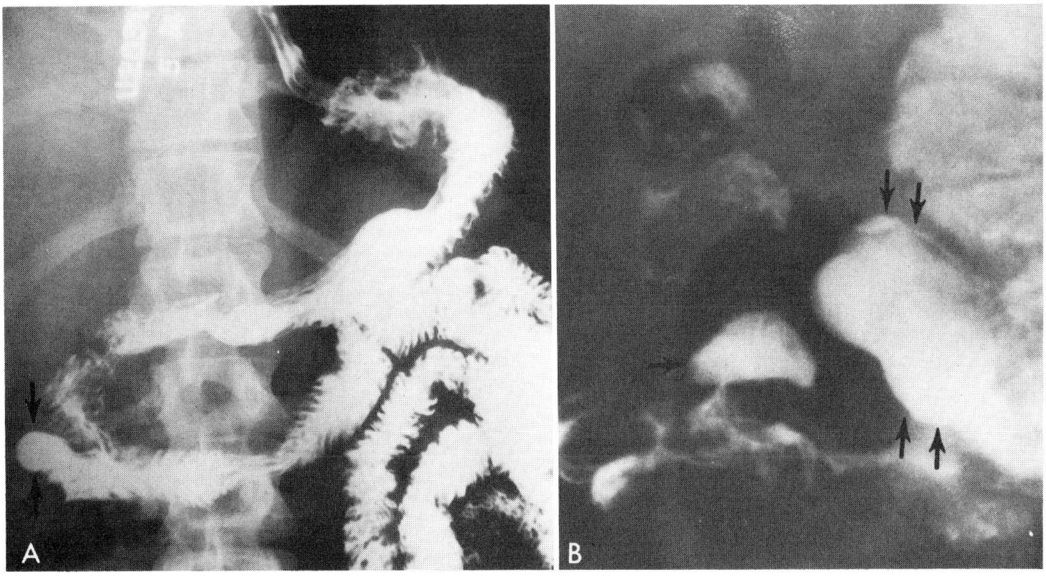

Figure 4–80. Duodenocolic fistula resulting from perforation of a lateral duodenal diverticulum.

A, Upper gastrointestinal study showing an asymptomatic lateral diverticulum arising from the lower descending duodenum (*arrows*).

B, Detailed view of the right upper quadrant several years later showing barium passing from the diverticulum (*double arrows*) into the right colon (*single arrow*). (Courtesy of Dr. L. L. Robbins. Reproduced by permission of *New England Journal of Medicine.*)

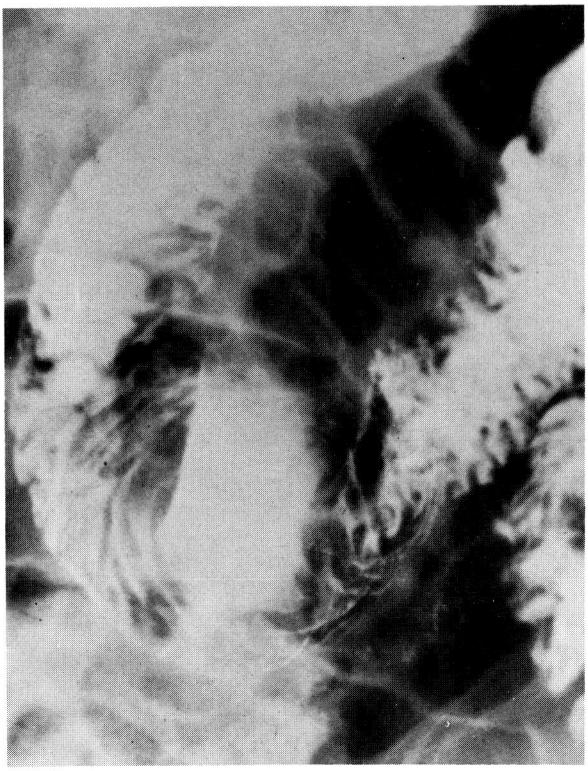

Figure 4–81. Aorticoduodenal fistula. Barium outlines the wall of the abdominal aorta, indicating the fistulous communication. In this patient, the fistula involved a previously placed prosthetic graft.

is delayed until adult life. These conditions have been summarized in an excellent review by Faegenburg and Bosniak (1962). Obstructing congenital webs usually occur in the second and third portions of the duodenum and may present as a thin radiolucent line extending across the lumen. On occasion, this thin diaphragm may balloon out aborally like a windsock, producing a rounded barium-filled sac—the so-called intraluminal diverticulum (Fig. 4–82). The appearance of the barium-filled diverticulum has also been referred to as a "comma sign" (Pratt, 1971; Heilbrun, 1964; and Laudan, 1963). Partially digested food particles may lodge within this sac, accentuating the degree of luminal obstruction.

Annular pancreas is a ring of normal pancreatic tissue encircling the duodenal lumen usually at or above the papilla of Vater. Symptoms vary but may indicate duodenal obstruction. In adult life, symptoms attributed to annular pancreas are often related to supervening disorders such as duodenal ulcer and pancreatitis, and one of these two conditions has been found in approximately one-fourth of the cases in which surgery was performed (Faegenburg, 1962). The cause of this association is not clear. The anomalous tissue may interfere with the normal flow of pancreatic secretions and gastric acid, which may predispose to both of these disorders. Conversely, radiographic study for epigastric complaints may draw attention to an asymptomatic annulus (Dodd, 1956).

Radiographically, the duodenum may be retracted medially toward the pancreas, with a notch-like defect on the lateral duodenal wall causing an eccentric hourglass narrowing of the lumen (Fig. 4–83). Duodenography accentuates these findings (Lieber, 1968). However, postbulbar ulcer may produce a similar deformity; the presence of a niche on the medial wall permits the differential diagnosis. Significant luminal narrowing

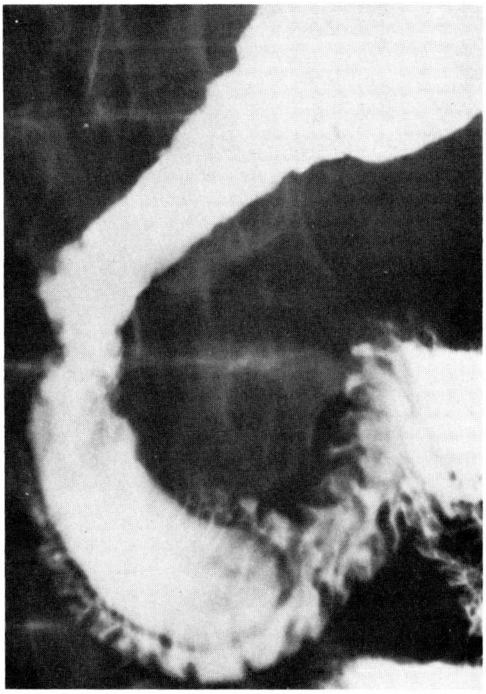

Figure 4–82. Intraluminal duodenal diverticulum. A barium-filled sac-like membrane is visible within the lumen of the horizontal duodenum, producing a "comma sign."

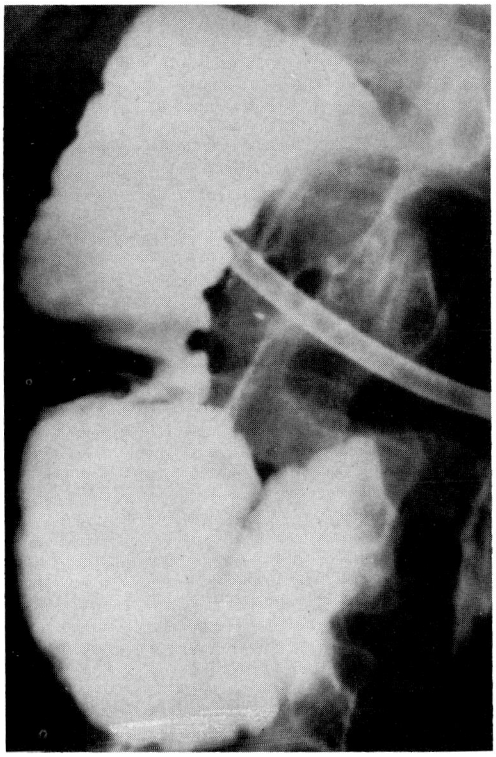

Figure 4–83. Annular pancreas. An area of narrowing, with medial retraction of the lumen and intact mucosal folds, is evident in the upper descending duodenum. A typical lateral notch-like indentation is visible. (Courtesy of Dr. A. Lewicki.)

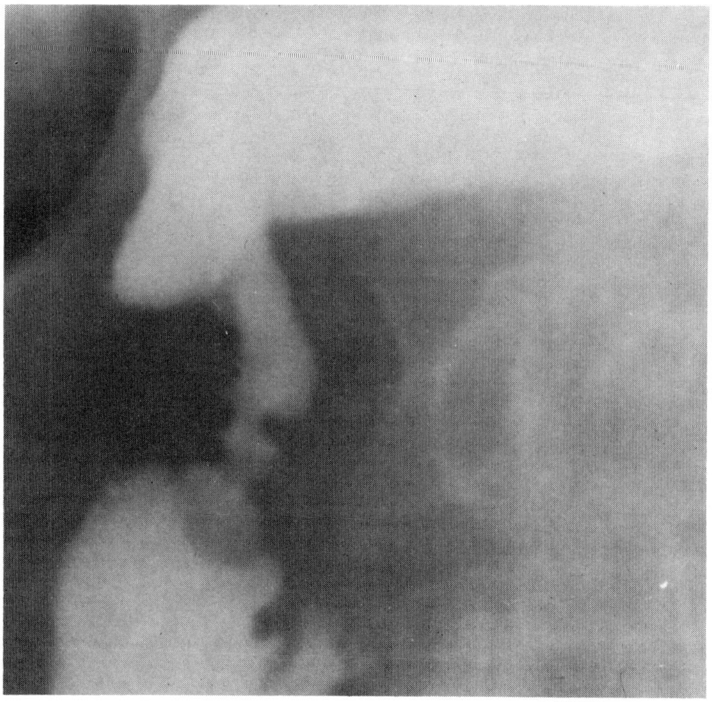

Figure 4–84. Annular pancreas. An elongated, irregular narrowing involves the upper descending duodenum. Associated peptic ulcer or pancreatitis may complicate the clinical and radiographic manifestations of the annular pancreas.

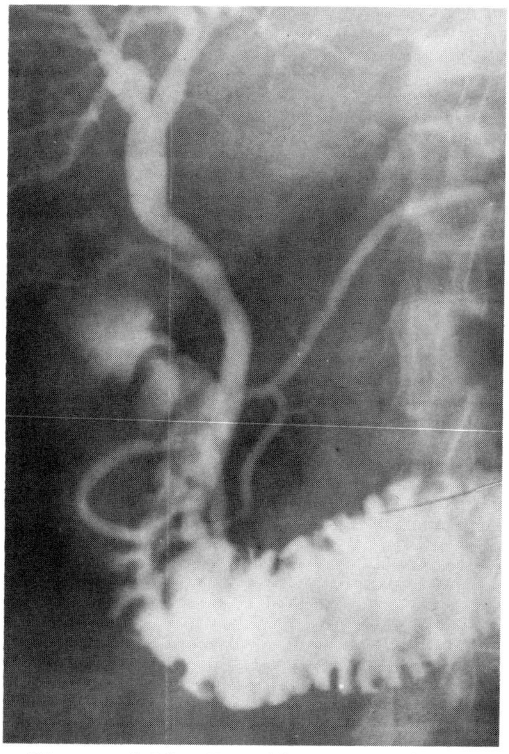

Figure 4–85. Ring-like circumferential ductal system in annular pancreas. Operative cholangiogram. Encircling pancreatic tissue encountered at surgery should be bypassed rather than divided. (From Heyman, R. L., and Whelan, T. J.: Annular pancreas: Demonstration of the annular duct on cholangiography. Ann. Surg., *165*:470–472, 1967.)

TABLE 4–11. Causes of Duodenal Obstruction or Stenosis

Developmental Anomalies
- Congenital atresia
- Congenital web or diaphragm
- Intraluminal diverticulum
- Reduplications
- Annular pancreas

Intrinsic Disorders
- Postbulbar ulcer-stricture
- Regional enteritis
- Tuberculosis
- Duodenal or ampullary malignancy
- Submucosal hemorrhage (anticoagulants, trauma, Henoch-Schoenlein)
- Sprue

Disease in Adjacent Structures
- Pancreatitis, acute or chronic
- Pseudocyst
- Pancreatic cancer
- Contiguous metastasis (gallbladder, right colon, right kidney)
- Contiguous abscess (perinephric, pericholecystic)
- Lymph node enlargement
- Aortic aneurysm
- Retroperitoneal masses

Superior Mesenteric Artery Syndrome

Trauma
- Duodenal rupture
- Duodenal hematoma

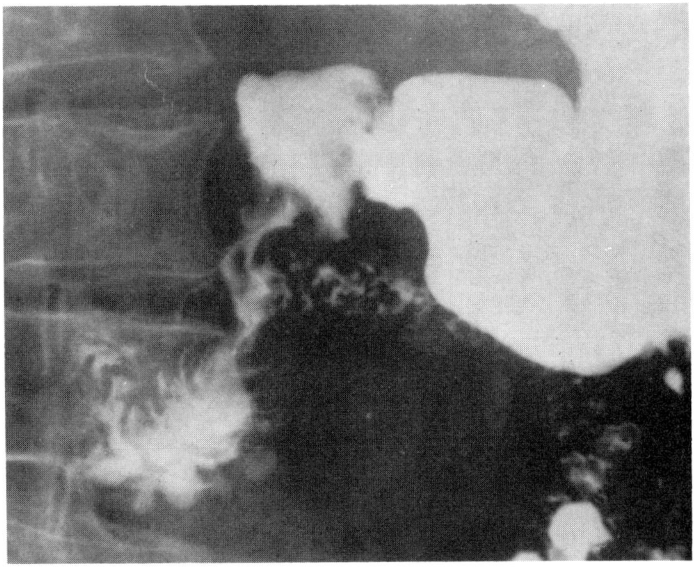

Figure 4–86. Carcinoma arising in annular pancreas. The appearance is similar to that of primary carcinoma of the duodenum. (Courtesy of Dr. Harry Newman.)

by the annulus may produce marked enlargement of the duodenal cap (Fig. 4–84). As a rule, a well-developed duct system is present within the annulus (Fig. 4–85). Thus, most authorities recommend that surgical management rely on bypass procedures rather than on division of the encircling pancreatic tissue (Hyden, 1963). Rarely, pancreatic cancer arises in the annulus and appears indistinguishable from intrinsic duodenal carcinoma (Fig. 4–86).

Inflammatory reaction from postbulbar ulcer may produce an eccentric medially retracted narrowing or a discrete 2 to 3 mm. ring-like stricture in the upper descending duodenum (Fig. 4–87; see also Fig. 10–25, Chapter 10). The latter configuration has recently been emphasized as a sign of probable active postbulbar ulcer, and is said to be as specific a sign of benign peptic ulcer disease as is the cloverleaf deformity in the duodenal cap (Bilbao, 1971). Demonstration of the ring-stricture configuration requires optimal duodenal distention above and below the lesion and is clearly seen only by duodenography; conventional barium meal studies usually yield incorrect diagnoses.

Regional enteritis may occur in the duodenum as an isolated finding but more often occurs after the disease is well established in the more distal small bowel (Legge, 1970). Diffuse narrowing of the third and fourth portions of the duodenum, with irregular nodular thickening of folds and visible skip areas in the upper jejunum, is a recognized pattern (Fig. 4–88) (Nelson, 1969). Alternatively, the disease may affect the proximal descending duodenum and, by contiguous extension in retrograde fashion across the pylorus into the antrum, may produce a tubular tapered narrowing termed the "pseudo-Billroth I appearance" (Nelson, 1969) (Fig. 4–89); (see also Fig. 10–34, Chapter 10).

Nontropical sprue may be complicated by intestinal ulcerations leading to multiple areas of stenosis, usually in the duodenum or jejunum (Bayless, 1967) (Fig. 4–90).

Duodenal stenosis or obstruction is an occasional finding in both acute and chronic pancreatitis, and occurs in two forms. In acute pancreatitis, the superior mesenteric artery syndrome may cause high-grade duodenal obstruction. Characteristically, this occurs at the third portion of the duodenum (Simon, 1962) (Fig. 4–91; see also Fig. 9–41, Chapter 9). Retroperitoneal edema narrows the angle between the aorta and superior mesenteric artery, constricting the duodenal lumen at this point. Primary duodenal atony is a contributing factor.

Another form of duodenal narrowing, occurring in both acute and chronic pancreatitis, may cause severe stenosis and deformity of the upper descending duodenum. This usually takes the form of tapered constriction with granular-appearing, flattened mucosal folds (Fig. 4–92). Postbulbar duodenal ulcer disease may coexist with chronic pancreatitis, and it may be difficult to determine which is the primary entity. Severe spasm is often present, even in periods of clinical remission; thus, hypotonic duodenography shows the anatomy to best advantage.

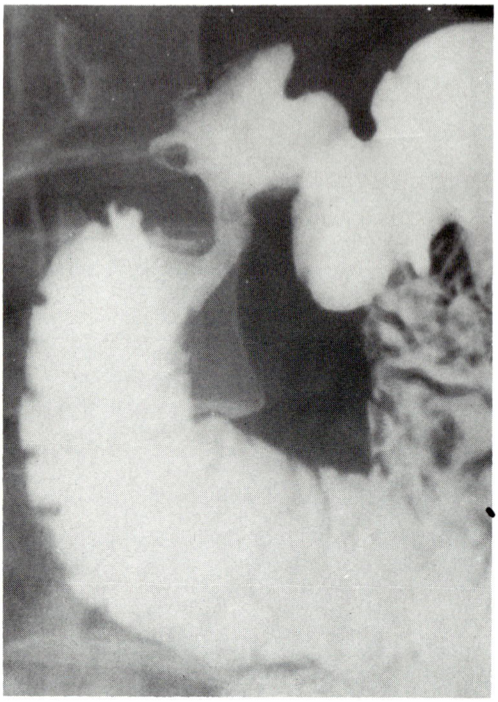

Figure 4–87. Postpeptic duodenal stricture. No definite ulcer is visible. The appearance closely resembles annular pancreas. Effaced granular-appearing mucosa in the narrowed segment suggests healed ulceration.

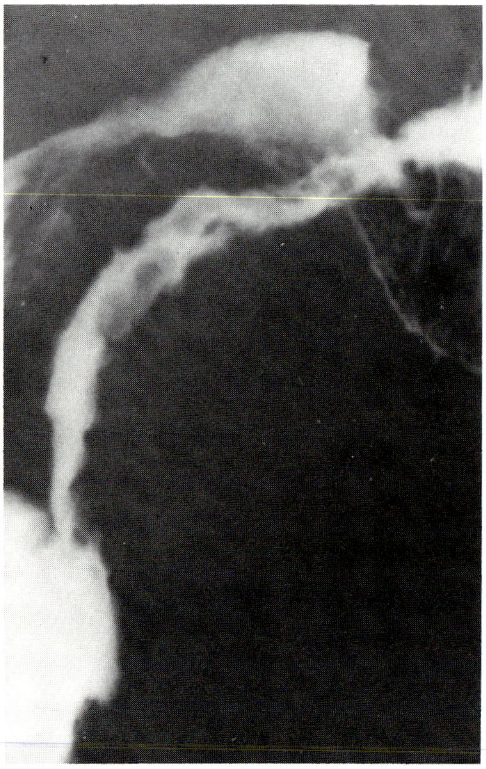

Figure 4–88. Regional enteritis of the duodenum. Stenotic areas involve the postbulbar duodenum and the horizontal duodenum in a "skip" fashion. Note the nodular hyperplastic mucosal changes.

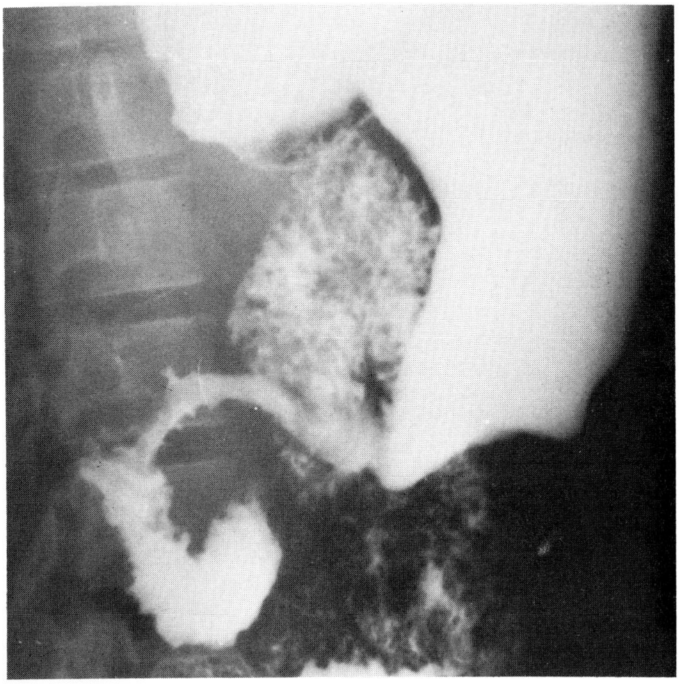

Figure 4–89. Regional enteritis of the proximal duodenum producing the "pseudo-Billroth I" appearance by contiguous retrograde involvement of the pyloric region.

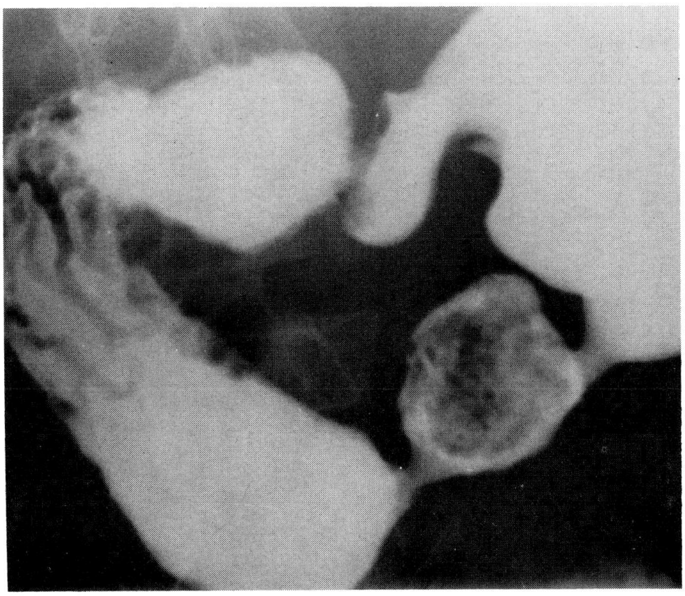

Figure 4–90. Duodenal strictures complicating long-standing nontropical sprue. Inspissated food particles are entrapped between two stenotic areas in the horizontal portion of the duodenum. (Courtesy of Dr. Robert E. Paul.)

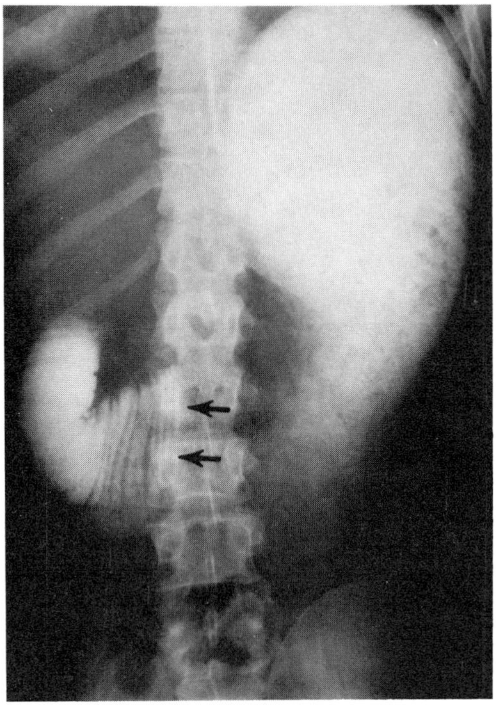

Figure 4–91. Duodenal obstruction due to superior mesenteric artery compression in acute pancreatitis. Periduodenal edema compresses the duodenum between the superior mesenteric artery and aorta, producing a characteristic linear termination of the barium column (*arrows*) and proximal dilatation of the duodenum and stomach.

Pseudocysts may become adherent to the duodenal wall and produce narrowing and displacement (Fig. 4–93). Generally in pancreatitis and pseudocyst, mucosal folds are thickened, splayed, and distorted, but not destroyed.

Pancreatic cancer, by contrast, may invade, narrow, and obstruct the duodenum at any level, from the pylorus to the duodenal jejunal flexure. Mucosal destruction is a helpful sign pointing to malignancy, but may not be present, since pancreatic tumors may produce submucosally infiltrating stenosis, especially along the horizontal duodenum (Fig. 4–94). In cancer of the pancreatic head, tumor infiltration may produce a fixed lateral defect which has been termed the "wraparound effect" (Beranbaum, 1966); this has recently been confirmed by Eaton (1972) as a frequent finding in pancreatic cancer (Fig. 4–95).

In primary malignancy of the duodenum, stenosis is usually accompanied by overhanging edges or mucosal destruction and ulceration, or both. The findings in duodenal neoplasm will be described in detail in Chapter 10.

Contiguous involvement of the duodenum by neoplasms or inflammatory lesions of the gallbladder, right colon, or kidney will be discussed in detail below. In general, roentgenographic differential diagnosis of masses affecting the lateral duodenal wall is based on evidence of mucosal destruction, ulceration, or frank intraluminal extension of tumor (Ngan, 1970).

Peripancreatic lymph node groups surround the descending duodenum, and the celiac and paraaortic nodes rest along the horizontal portion of the duodenum. Enlargement of these node groups, particularly due to metastatic deposits, may impinge upon the duodenal lumen, producing irregular pressure indentations, narrowing, or frank ulceration (McCort, 1953) (Fig. 4–96). The finding of a stenotic lesion in the horizontal duodenum of a patient with a history of previous abdominal malignancy should suggest celiac lymph node metastasis (Fig. 4–97).

Retroperitoneal masses, especially aortic aneurysms, may narrow and obstruct as well as displace the duodenum (Gay, 1953). Rupture of an abdominal aortic aneurysm into the transverse portion of the duodenum is a well-recognized clinical entity. This occurs with increased frequency after prior aneurysmectomy and prosthetic graft placement (see Fig. 4–81). In such a setting, radiologic recognition of a distal duodenal ulcer or aorticoduodenal fistula may prompt an effort at lifesaving surgery.

A detailed consideration of the superior mesenteric artery syndrome and duodenal trauma will be presented in Chapter 9.

Duodenal Dilatation

Dilatation of the duodenum unrelated to distal obstruction is termed "primary

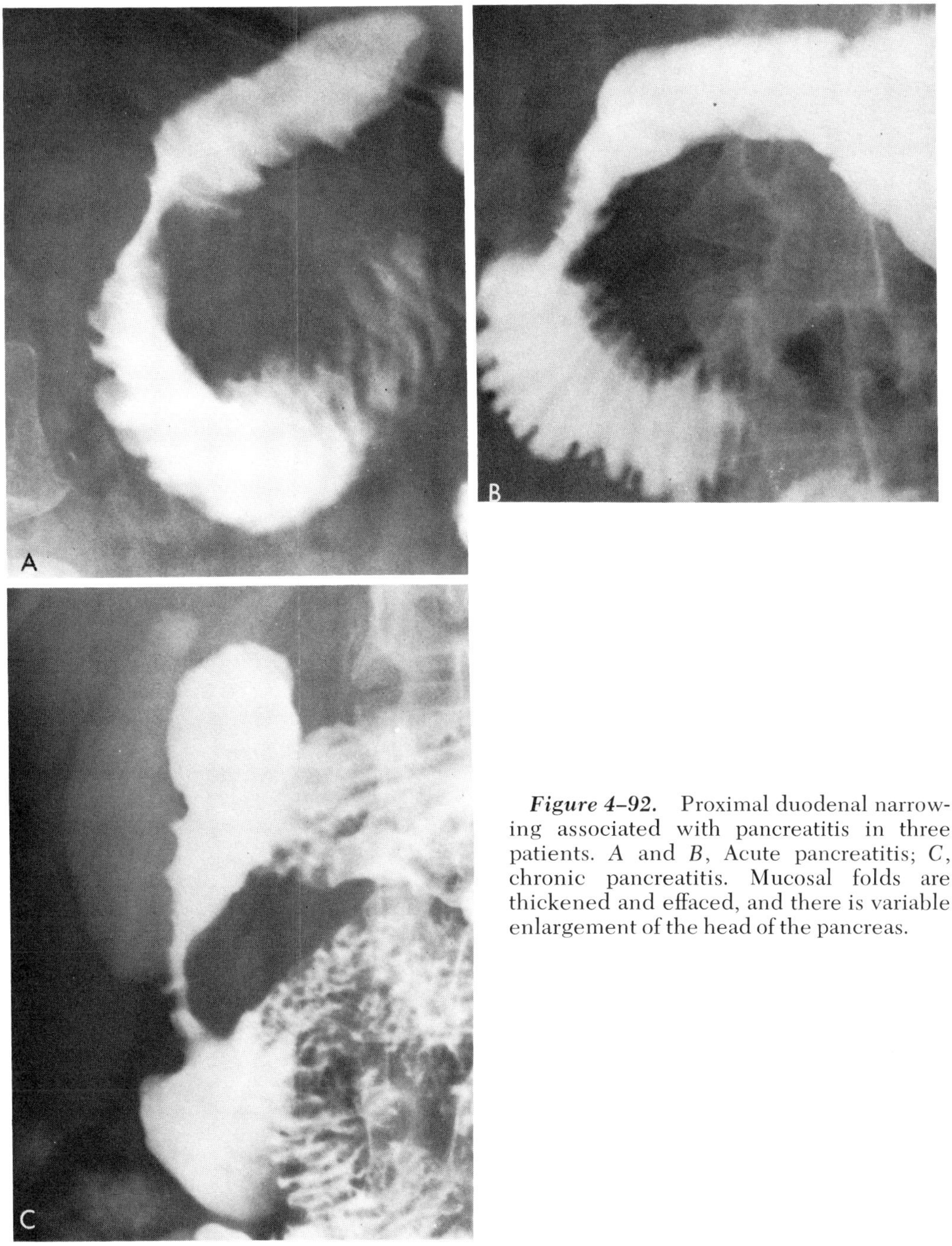

Figure 4–92. Proximal duodenal narrowing associated with pancreatitis in three patients. *A* and *B*, Acute pancreatitis; *C*, chronic pancreatitis. Mucosal folds are thickened and effaced, and there is variable enlargement of the head of the pancreas.

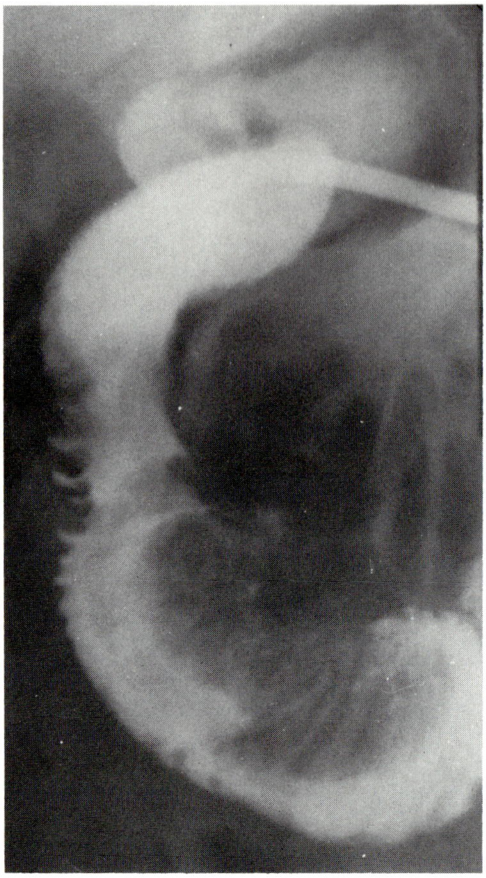

Figure 4–93. Pancreatic pseudocyst adherent to the duodenum. Proximally, the lumen is narrowed, with thick effaced folds. Distally, a mass impression is visible.

megaduodenum." Dilatation, elongation, and prolonged retention of barium in the absence of mechanical obstruction occur in a variety of acute and chronic disorders generally associated with some alteration in neuromuscular function (Fig. 4–98). In a comprehensive review of the etiologies of megaduodenum, Fischer (1960) recognized three major mechanisms (Table 4–12). Nonetheless, despite evident neuromuscular dysfunction in some of these disorders, it also seems likely that the midline barrier of normal structures—spine, aorta, and superior mesenteric artery—contributes to duodenal stasis in some instances.

Duodenal atony accompanying acute upper abdominal inflammatory processes is a form of the sentinel loop phenomenon, and is a useful plain film sign in acute pancreatitis (see Chapter 2). Duodenal ileus is also a recognized component of the Zollinger-Ellison syndrome (Christoforidis, 1966). Patients sustaining severe trauma or acute burns may develop duodenal as well as gastric ileus (Wallace, 1970). Collagen disease is also a common cause of chronic megaduodenum. In scleroderma, absence of ganglion cells, muscular atrophy, and fibrosis within intestinal walls lead to duodenal atony and dilatation, classic roentgen signs of this disorder (Fig. 4–99).

(*Text continued on page 161*)

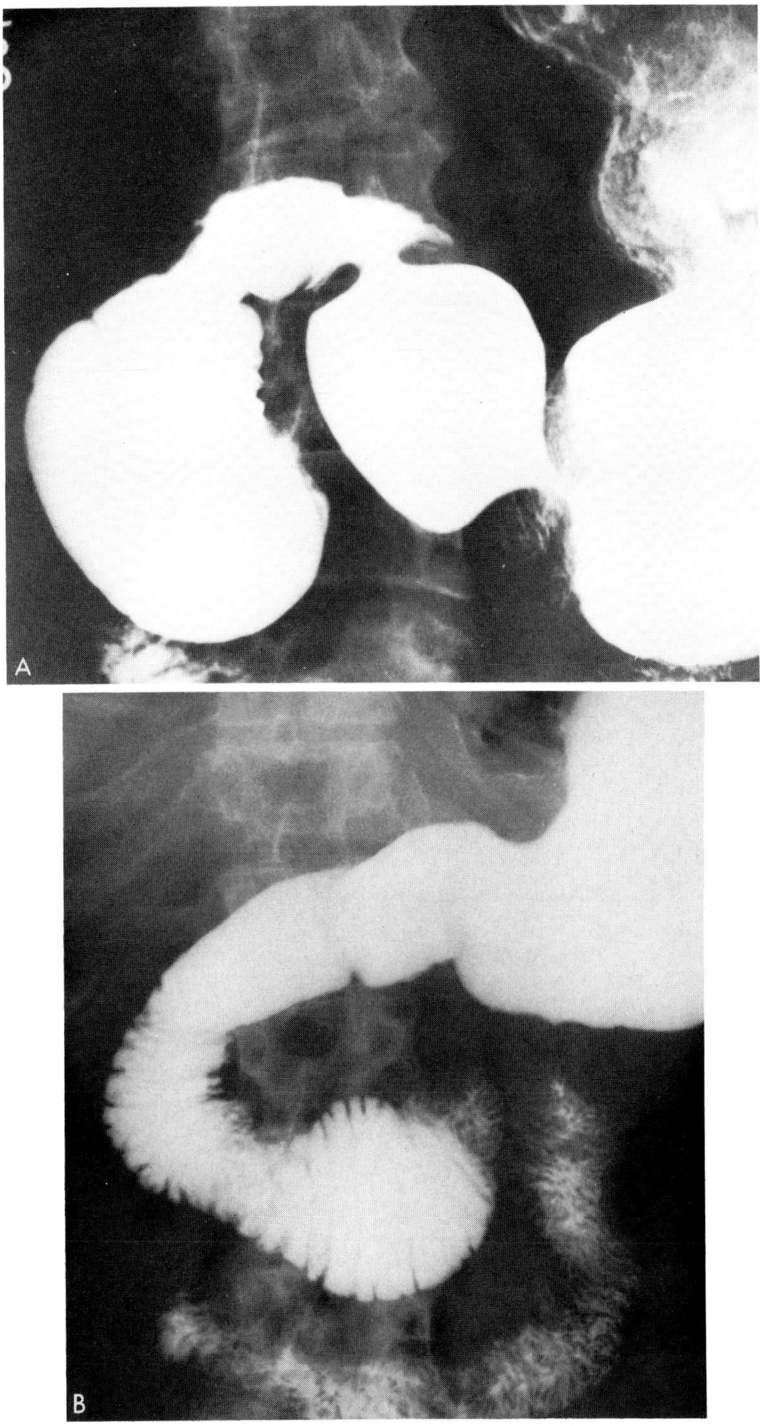

Figure 4–94. Stenosis and obstruction of the distal duodenum due to carcinoma of the body of the pancreas in two patients. The configuration suggests extrinsic circumferential constriction.

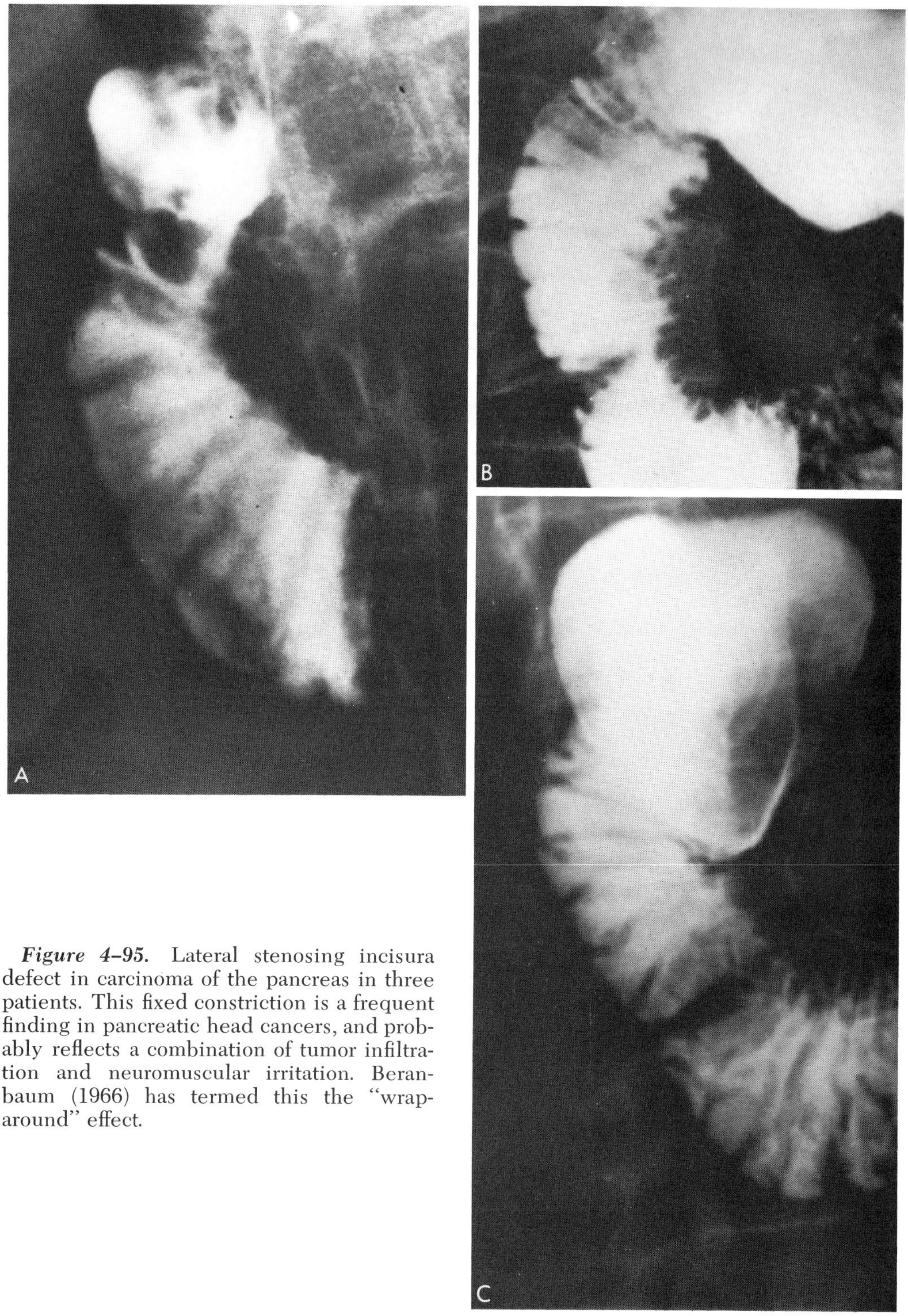

Figure 4–95. Lateral stenosing incisura defect in carcinoma of the pancreas in three patients. This fixed constriction is a frequent finding in pancreatic head cancers, and probably reflects a combination of tumor infiltration and neuromuscular irritation. Beranbaum (1966) has termed this the "wrap-around" effect.

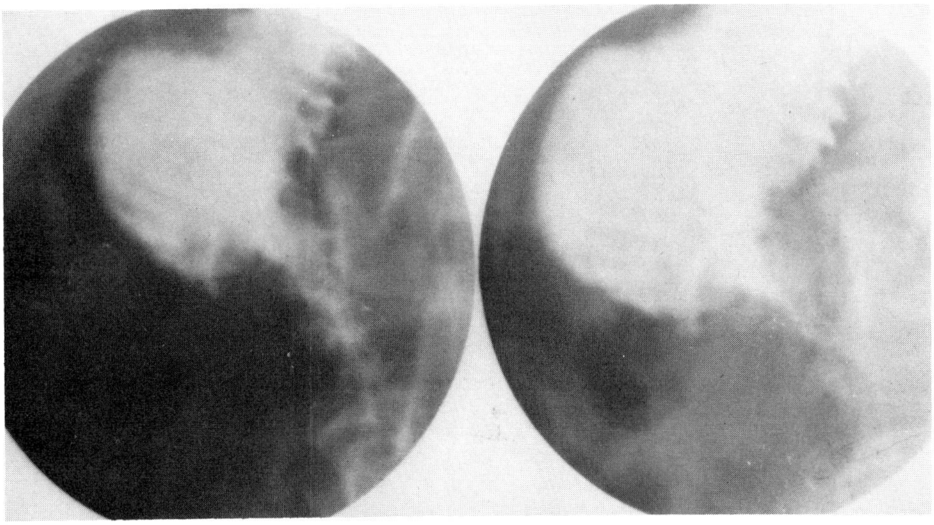

Figure 4–96. Metastatic adenocarcinoma of the breast to peripancreatic lymph nodes, producing circumferential constriction of the mid-descending duodenum.

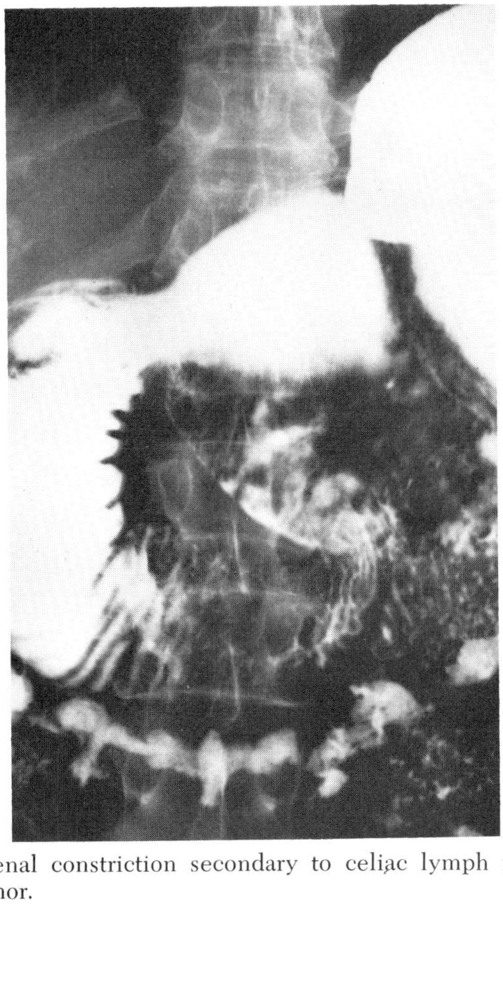

Figure 4–97. Duodenal constriction secondary to celiac lymph node replacement by a malignant carcinoid tumor.

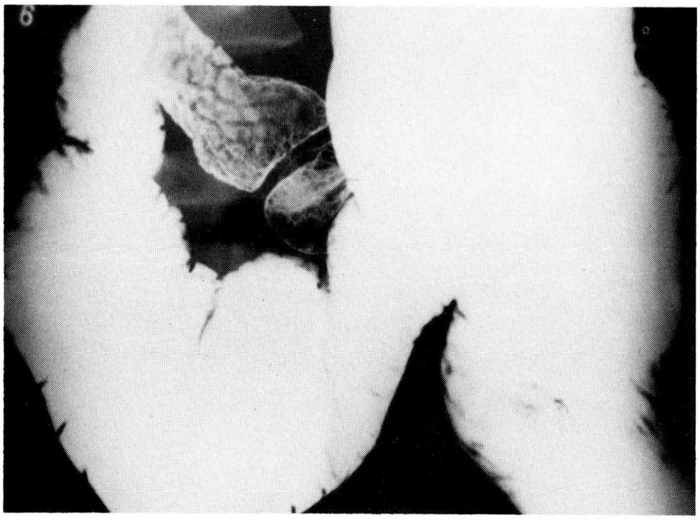

Figure 4–98. Megaduodenum in Chagas disease. (Courtesy of Dr. L. Mattoso.)

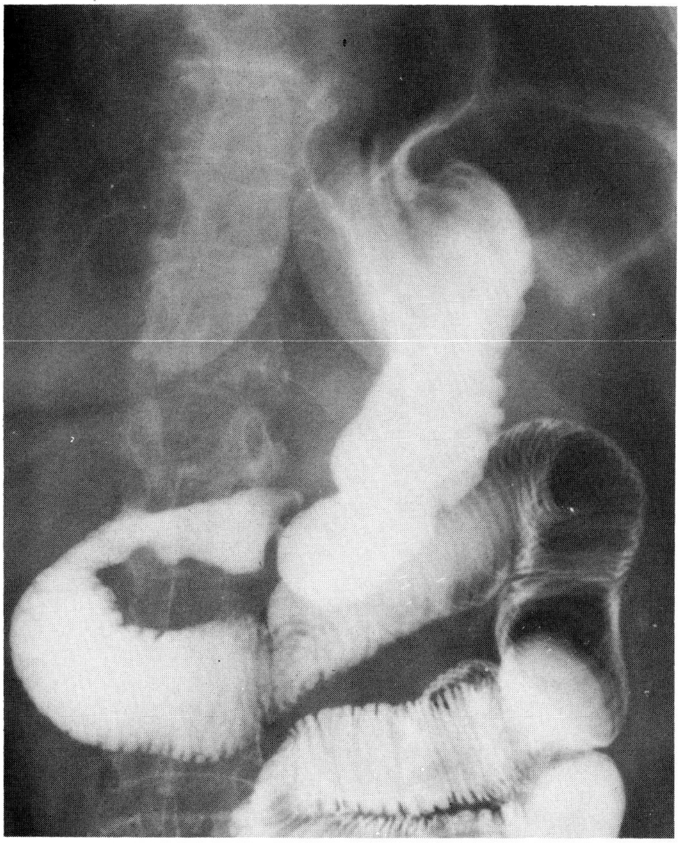

Figure 4–99. Megaduodenum in scleroderma. Note the generalized small intestinal dilatation which is a hallmark of this disorder.

TABLE 4–12. Primary Megaduodenum

Dilatation Mediated via the Central Nervous System (Paralytic Ileus)
- Pancreatitis
- Cholecystitis
- Peptic ulcer
- Zollinger-Ellison syndrome
- Trauma, acute burn
- Emotional states

Dysfunction of the Vagus or Splanchnic Nerves
- Postvagotomy
- Neuropathic (diabetes, porphyria, thiamine deficiency)

Neuromuscular Abnormality Within the Bowel Wall
- Aganglionosis
- Collagen diseases (scleroderma, lupus, dermatomyositis)
- Porphyria
- Local inflammation (sprue, regional enteritis)
- Anticholinergic drugs

Adapted from Fischer, H. W.: The Big Duodenum. Amer. J. Roentgen., 83:861–875, 1960.

Abnormalities Affecting the Outer Duodenal Border

Disease states arising in any of the structures of the right upper abdominal quadrant may produce roentgen findings indicating an extrinsic process along the convexity of the duodenal bulb or the descending duodenum. In general, the signs of extrinsic disease in this location recapitulate those described along the inner duodenal border and possess the same order of specificity. Roentgen abnormalities thus include mucosal fold changes, pressure deformities, narrowing and displacement of the duodenum, fixation of folds, rigidity of the wall and, finally, ulceration and frank fistula formation into other right upper quadrant viscera. The more common causes of lateral duodenal deformities are indicated in Table 4–13.

Enlargement of the gallbladder occurs in malignant obstruction of the common bile duct (Courvoisier phenomenon) as well as in calculous or noncalculous obstruction of the cystic duct (hydrops) and will be considered in Chapter 5. Occasionally, in cases of hepatic enlargement or low-lying diaphragm, a normal gallbladder indents the convexity of the duodenum. In either case, a smooth, rounded impression of the duodenum is demonstrated (Fig. 4–100). Rarely, discrete hepatic masses may indent the superior aspect of the duodenum. In one report, such an impression was caused by a nodule of regenerating liver tissue in the quadrate lobe of a patient with cirrhosis (Meyers, 1958).

Pericholecystic abscess may produce fold thickening, spiculation, and irregular indentations on the lateral duodenal wall. Carcinoma of the gallbladder may form a large mass indenting and displacing the duodenal cap and loop both inferiorly and medially (McConnell, 1957; Khilnani, 1962). In advanced cases, ulceration into the duodenum occurs and may permit air to enter the biliary tree (Fig. 4–101).

Enlargement of the right kidney or discrete right renal masses may indent

TABLE 4–13. Conditions Producing Alteration on the Outer Duodenal Wall

Gallbladder
- Enlarged gallbladder
  - Courvoisier phenomenon
  - Hydrops
- Carcinoma of the gallbladder
- Pericholecystic abscess
- Cholecystoduodenal fistula

Right Kidney
- Enlargement 2° to cyst, tumor, bifid collecting system
- Hypernephroma invading duodenum

Pancreas
- Annular pancreas
- Carcinoma of pancreas wrapped around duodenum

Liver
- Periportal lymphadenopathy, hepatic enlargement (especially quadrate lobe), hepatic cyst, or tumor

Colon
- Duodenocolic apposition
- Carcinoma of the hepatic flexure

Duodenum
- Hematoma, varices
- Postbulbar ulcer (lateral incisura)

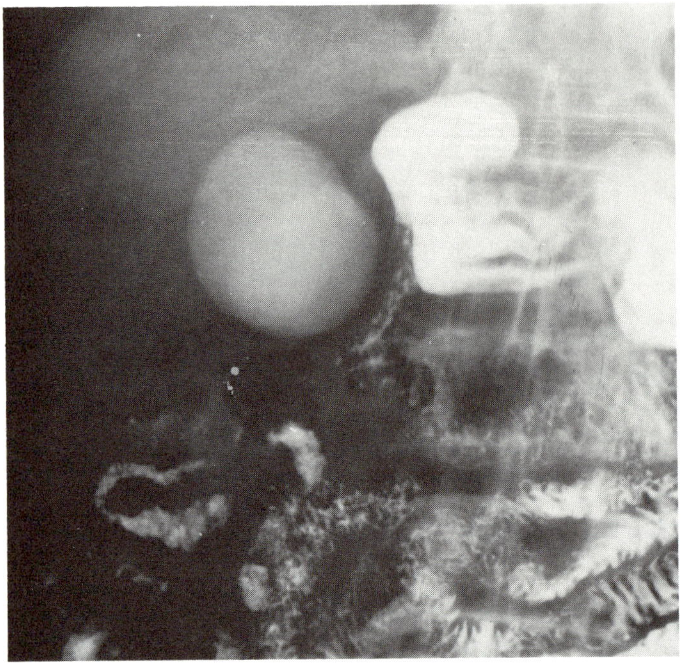

Figure 4–100. Impression on the lateral convexity of the descending duodenum by a normal gallbladder. Low-lying diaphragms or hepatic enlargement may contribute to this phenomenon.

the posterolateral aspect of the duodenum. Hydronephrosis, bifid kidney, polycystic kidney, simple cyst, and tumor have all been associated with duodenal

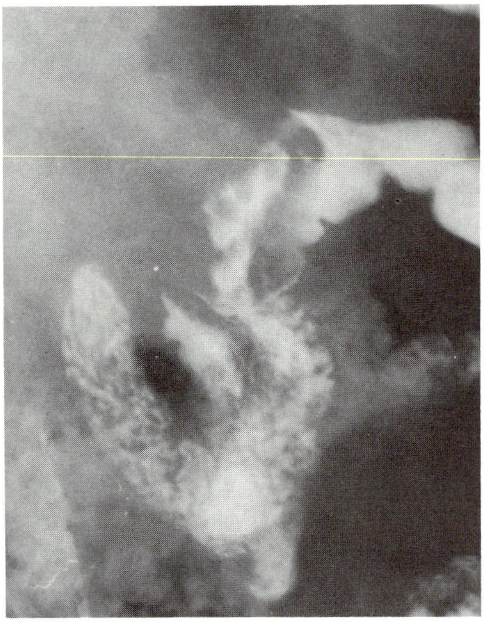

Figure 4–101. Carcinoma of the gallbladder invading the lateral aspect of the upper descending duodenum. Note the oval mass indentation with central ulceration.

deformities (Fig. 4–102). Hypernephroma may invade the duodenum by direct extension, producing irregular pressure defects, ulcerations, or a frank intraluminal duodenal mass (Bluth, 1961). Duodenal impression from right adrenal masses has also been observed.

A discrete single nodular defect in the midportion of the lateral descending duodenum may be a prominent feature of postbulbar peptic ulcer, annular pancreas, or carcinoma of the head of the pancreas. In annular pancreas, the lateral defect represents part of the constricting ring of pancreatic tissue (see Fig. 4–83); in postbulbar peptic ulcer, inflammatory spasm and fibrotic cicatrix account for the defect (see Fig. 4–87). In carcinoma of the pancreas, tumor infiltration produces a fixed lateral defect, which has been termed the "wraparound effect" (Beranbaum, 1966; Eaton, 1972) (see Fig. 4–95).

The hepatic flexure of the colon is also closely applied to the duodenal loop and, in some normal patients, produces a demonstrable convex impression on its lateral border (Fig. 4–103). This condition is an incidental finding in which the two viscera have a fixed, closer than

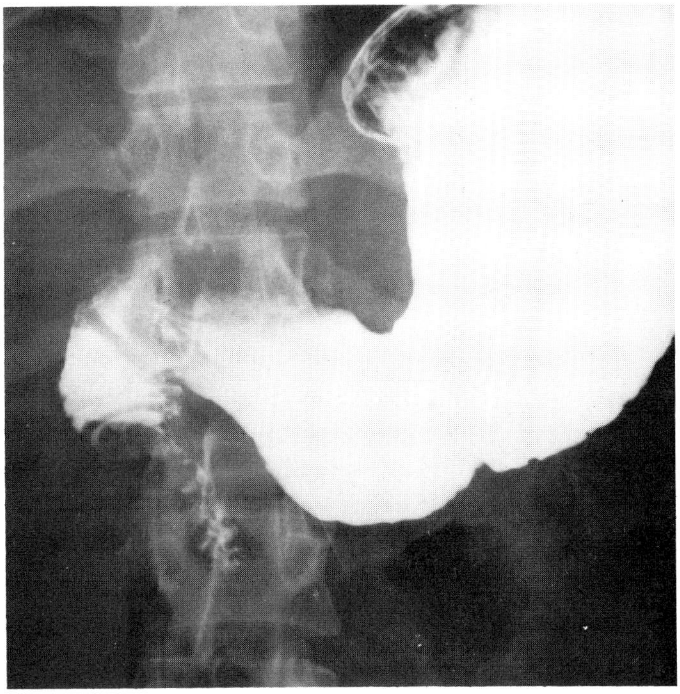

Figure 4–102. Hydronephrosis of the right kidney, producing compression and displacement along the lateral duodenal margin. Renal enlargement of any nature may produce similar deformity.

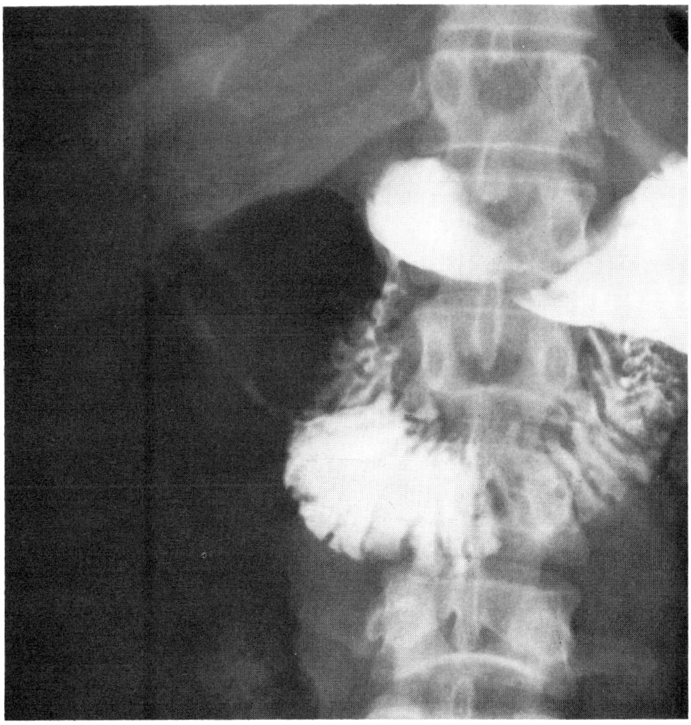

Figure 4–103. Duodenocolic apposition. The normal close relationship of the hepatic flexure and the descending duodenum allows the gas-filled colon to impress itself upon the lateral convexity of the duodenum. The condition is of no clinical importance.

normal relationship; it has been termed "duodenocolic apposition" (Poppel, 1960).

Carcinoma of the hepatic flexure of the colon may invade the duodenum via lymphatics or by direct extension (Treitel, 1970). Mucosal irregularities and mass indentations may lead to large, irregular ulceration as well as frank duodenal colic fistula (Fig. 4–104).

Duodenal varices may present as lobulated extrinsic filling defects involving the duodenal cap or loop (Fig. 4–105). As previously noted, they are usually associated with esophageal varices and may bleed. They occur in portal obstruction at all levels, but are most frequent with subhepatic portal vein occlusion (Olson, 1963; Perchik, 1963; Fleming, 1968; and Bateson, 1969).

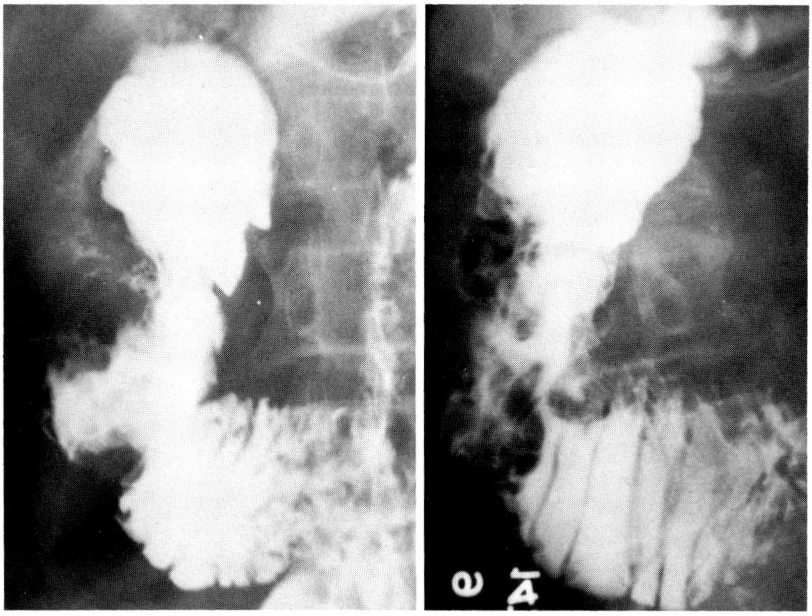

Figure 4–104. Nodular ulcerating mass indenting the lateral duodenal border as a result of carcinoma of the hepatic flexure.

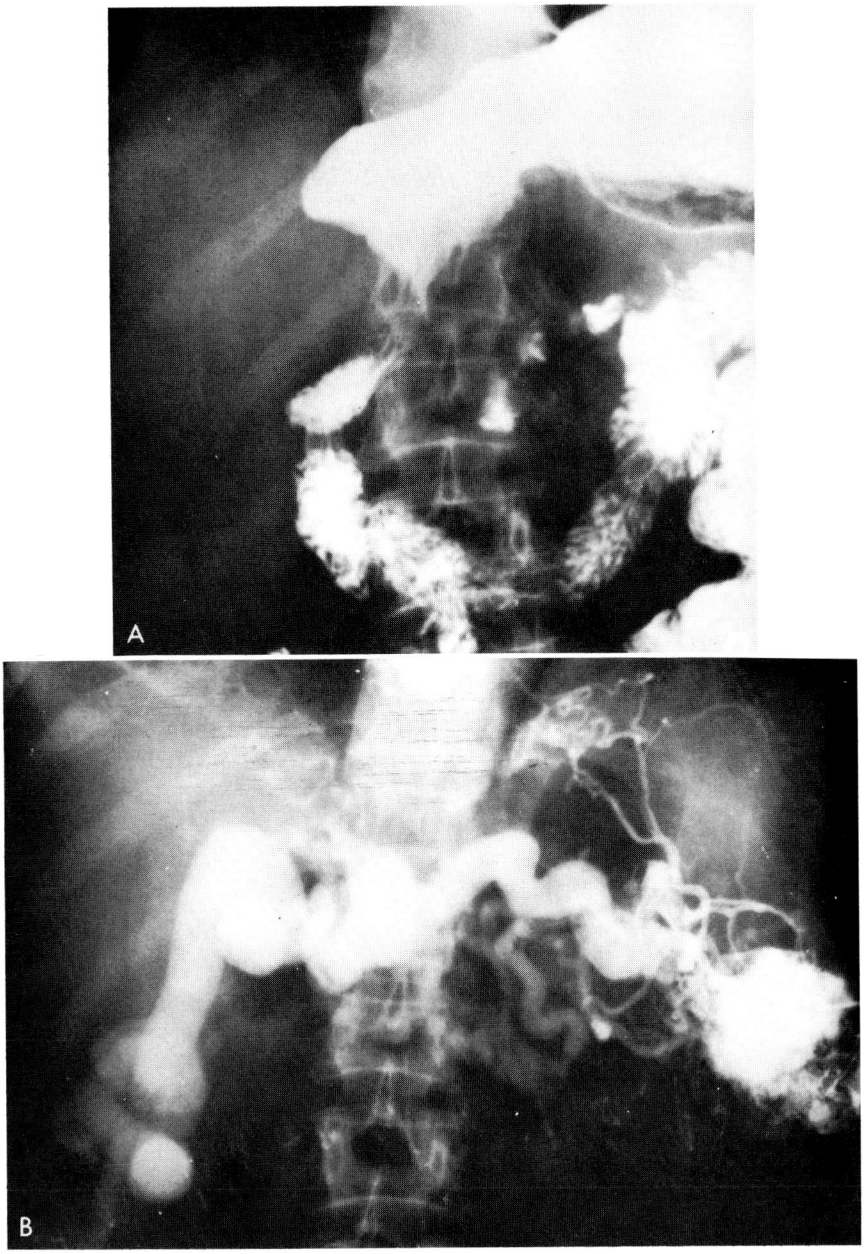

Figure 4–105. Paraduodenal varices producing lateral duodenal indentation.

A, Upper gastrointestinal study shows an extrinsic mass compressing the lateral aspect of the descending duodenum.

B, Percutaneous splenoportogram showing portal occlusion and large paraduodenal collateral channels in the porta hepatis. (Courtesy of Dr. Arch W. Templeton.)

REFERENCES

Adler, D. C., and Meyers, H. I.: Cineradiographic examination of the upper gastrointestinal tract in obstructive jaundice. J.A.M.A., *199*:709–713, 1967.
Bateson, E. M.: Duodenal and antral varices. Brit. J. Radiol., *42*:744–747, 1969.
Baum, M., and Howe, C. T.: Hypotonic duodenography in the diagnosis of carcinoma of the pancreas and its further use when combined with percutaneous cholangiography and pancreatic scintiscanning. Amer. J. Surg., *115*:519–525, 1968.
Baum, S., Stein, G. N., and Baue, A.: Extrinsic pressure defects on the duodenal loop in mesenteric occlusive disease. Radiology, *85*: 866–874, 1965.
Baumler, R. A.: Arteriosclerotic abdominal aortic aneurysm rupturing into the duodenum. J.A.M.A., *176*:146–147, 1961.
Bayless, T. M., Kapelowitz, R. F., Shelley, W. M., Ballinger, W. F., and Hendrix, T. R.: Intestinal ulceration: a complication of celiac disease. New Eng. J. Med., *276*:996–1002, 1967.
Beeler, J. W., and Kirklin, B. R.: Roentgenologic findings accompanying carcinoma of pancreas. Amer. J. Roentgen., *67*:576–584, 1952.
Benedict, K. T., Ferrucci, J. T., and Eaton, S. B.: Hypotonic duodenography: current concepts in technique, interpretation, and clinical usefulness. CRC Critical Reviews in Radiological Sciences, *1*:567–578, 1970.
Beranbaum, S. L.: Carcinoma of the pancreas: a bi-directional roentgen approach. Amer. J. Roentgen., *96*:447–467, 1966.
Berger, S. M.: Pseudotumors of the duodenal bulb. Amer. J. Roentgen., *74*:580–586, 1955.
Besemann, E. F., Auerbach, S. H., and Wolfe, W. W.: The importance of roentgenologic diagnosis of aberrant pancreatic tissue in the gastrointestinal tract. Amer. J. Roentgen., *107*: 71–76, 1969.
Bilbao, M. K., Frische, L. H., Dotter, C. T., and Rösch, J.: Hypotonic duodenography. Radiology, *89*:438–443, 1967.
Bilbao, M. K., Rösch, J., Frische, L. H., and Dotter, C. T.: Hypotonic duodenography in the diagnosis of pancreatic disease. Seminars Roentgen., *3*:280–287, 1968.
Bilbao, M. K., Frische, L. H., Rösch, J., Benson, J. A., and Dotter, C. T.: Postbulbar duodenal ulcer and ring-stricture. Radiology, *100*:27–35, 1971.
Blatt, C. J., Bernstein, R. G., and Lopez, F.: Uncommon roentgenologic manifestation of pancreatic carcinoma. Amer. J. Roentgen., *113*: 119–124, 1971.
Bluth, I., and Vitale, P.: Right renal enlargements causing alteration in the descending duodenum. A radiographic demonstration. Radiology, *76*:777–784, 1961.
Bockus, H. L.: Gastroenterology. Vol III. Philadelphia, W. B. Saunders Company, 1965, p. 921.
Bourke, J. B., Brown, C. L., Swann, J. C., and Ritchie, H. D.: Exocrine pancreatic function studies, duodenal cytology, and hypotonic duodenography in the diagnosis of surgical jaundice. Lancet, *1*:605–608, 1972.
Bree, R. L., and Flynn, R. E.: Hypotonic duodenography in the evaluation of choledocholithiasis and obstructive jaundice. Amer. J. Roentgen., *116*:309–319, 1972.
Broadbent, T. R., and Kerman, H. D.: One hundred cases of carcinoma of the pancreas: A clinical and roentgenologic analysis. Gastroenterology, *17*:163–177, 1951.
Case, J. T.: Roentgenology of pancreatic disease; Caldwell Lecture, 1939. Amer. J. Roentgen., *44*:485–518, 1940.
Christoforidis, A. J., and Nelson, S. W.: Radiological manifestations of ulcerogenic tumors of the pancreas. J.A.M.A., *198*:511–516, 1966.
Clayton, R. S., and Thornton, W. L.: Benign duodenocolic fistula: review of the literature and a case report. Radiology, *60*:832–835, 1953.
Coe, F. O., Bickham, C. E., Edwards, C.: The duodenal loop. Amer. J. Roentgen., *89*:819–824, 1963.
Constant, E., and Turcotte, J. G.: Choledochoduodenal fistula: the natural history and management of an unusual complication of peptic ulcer disease. Ann. Surg., *167*:220–228, 1968.
Craighead, C. C., and St. Raymond, A. H.: Duodenal fistula, with special reference to choledochoduodenal fistula complicating duodenal ulcer. Amer. J. Surg., *87*:523–533, 1954.
Deluca, S., Eaton, S. B., Ferrucci, J. T., and Dreyfuss, J. R.: The radiology of duodenal stricture in the adult. (In preparation.)
Dodd, G. D., and Nafis, W. A.: Annular pancreas in the adult. Amer. J. Roentgen., *75*:333–342, 1956.
Dodds, W. J., Spitzer, R. M., and Friedland, G. W.: Gastrointestinal roentgenographic manifestations of hemophilia. Amer. J. Roentgen., *110*: 413–416, 1970.
Eadie, D. G. A., and Pollock, D. J.: A complicated aortoduodenal fistula. Brit. J. Surg., *55*:314–317, 1968.
Eaton, S. B., Fleischli, D. J., Pollard, J. J., Nebesar, R. A., and Potsaid, M. S.: Comparison of current radiologic approaches to the diagnosis of pancreatic disease. New Eng. J. Med., *279*: 389–396, 1968.
Eaton, S. B., Ferrucci, J. T., and Benedict, K. T.: A comprehensive evaluation of radiologic exploration of the pancreas. CRC Critical Reviews in Radiological Sciences, *1*:165–202, 1970*a*.
Eaton, S. B., Benedict, K. T., Ferrucci, J. T., and Fleischli, D. J.: Hypotonic Duodenography. Radiol. Clin. N. Amer., *8*:125–137, 1970*b*.
Eaton, S. B., Ferrucci, J. T., Benedict, K. T., and Margulis, A. F.: Diagnosis of choledocholithiasis by barium duodenal examination. Radiology, *102*:267–274, 1972.
Eaton, S. B., Ferrucci, J. T., Margulis, A. R., and Weens, H. S.: Unfamiliar roentgen findings in pancreatic disease. Amer. J. Roentgen., *116*:396–405, 1972.
Eyler, W. R., Clark, M. D., and Rian, R. L.: An evaluation of roentgen signs of pancreatic enlargement. J.A.M.A., *181*:967–971, 1962.

Faegenburg, D., and Bosniak, M.: Duodenal anomalies in the adult. Amer. J. Roentgen., *88*:642–657, 1962.

Ferguson, M. J., and Arden, M. J.: Gastrointestinal hemorrhage secondary to rupture of aorta: a review of four duodenal and three esophageal cases. Arch. Intern Med., *117*:133–140, 1966.

Ferrucci, J. T., and Benedict, K. T.: Anticholinergic-aided study of the gastrointestinal tract. Radiol. Clin. N. Amer., 9:23–39, 1971.

Ferrucci, J. T., Benedict, K. T., Page, D. L., Fleischli, D. J., and Eaton, S. B.: Radiographic features of the normal hypotonic duodenogram. Radiology, *96*:401–408, 1970.

Fischer, H. W.: The big duodenum. Amer. J. Roentgen., *83*:861–875, 1960.

Fleming, R. J., and Seaman, W. B.: Roentgenographic demonstration of unusual extra-esophageal varices. Amer. J. Roentgen., *103*:281–290, 1968.

Fraser, G. M., Pitman, R. G., Lawrie, J. H., Smith, G. M. R., Forrest, A. P. M., and Rhodes, J.: The significance of the radiological finding of coarse mucosal folds in the duodenum. Lancet, *2*:979–982, 1964.

Frostberg, N.: Characteristic duodenal deformity in cases of different kinds of peri-Vaterial enlargement of pancreas. Acta Radiol. (Stockholm), *19*:164–173, 1938.

Gay, B. B., Leigh, T. F., and Rogers, J. V.: Abdominal aneurysm as an uncommon cause of duodenal loop widening. Radiology, *61*: 630–632, 1953.

Gelfand, D. W., and Moskowitz, M.: Massive gastric dilatation complicating hypotonic duodenography. Radiology, *97*:637–639, 1970.

Gianturco, C.: Rapid fluoroscopic duodenal intubation. Radiology, *88*:1165–1166, 1967.

Goldstein, H. M., and Zboralske, F. F.: Tubeless hypotonic duodenography. J.A.M.A., *210*: 2086–2088, 1969.

Griffen, W. O., Schaefer, J. W., Schindler, S., Hyde, G., and Bryant, L. R.: Ampullary obstruction by benign duodenal polyps. Arch. Surg., *97*:444–449, 1968.

Hand, B. H.: An anatomical study of the choledochoduodenal area. Brit. J. Surg., *50*:486–494, 1963.

Handel, J., and Schwartz, S.: Gastrointestinal manifestations of the Schönlein-Henoch syndrome: roentgenologic findings. Amer. J. Roentgen., *78*:643–652, 1957.

Hanelin, J.: Some technical aspects in the demonstration of gastric lesions. Seminars Roentgen., *6*:235–253, 1971.

Hately, W.: Cyst of Brunner's glands. Brit. J. Radiol., *11*:384–385, 1968.

Heilbrun, N., and Boyden, E. A.: Intraluminal duodenal diverticula. Radiology, *82*:887–894, 1964.

Herbert, W. W., and Margulis, A. R.: Diagnosis of retroperitoneal masses by gastrointestinal roentgenographic measurements: a computer study. Radiology, *84*:52–57, 1965.

Hershenson, L. M., and Kirsner, J. B.: Duodenocolic fistula. Gastroenterology, *19*:864–873, 1951.

Hodes, P. J., Pendergrass, E. P., and Winston, N. J.: Pancreatic, ductal, and Vaterian neoplasms: their roentgen manifestations. Radiology, *62*: 1–15, 1954.

Hyden, W. H.: The true nature of annular pancreas. Ann. Surg., *157*:71–77, 1963.

Jacobson, H. G., Shapiro, J. H., Pisano, D., and Poppel, M. H.: The Vaterian and peri-Vaterian segments in peptic ulcer. Amer. J. Roentgen., *79*:793–798, 1958.

Jacquemet, P., Liotta, D., and Mallet-Guy, P.: The Early Radiological Diagnosis of Diseases of the Pancreas and Ampulla of Vater: Elective Exploration of the Ampulla of Vater and the Head of the Pancreas by Hypotonic Duodenography. Springfield, Ill., Charles C Thomas, Publisher, 1965.

Jorgens, J., Kiesel, I. O., and Leonard, J. P.: A cinefluorographic study of the duodenum. Radiology, *79*:760–762, 1962.

Kasugai, T., Kuno, N., Kobayashi, S., and Hattori, K.: Endoscopic Pancreatocholangiography. I. The normal endoscopic pancreatocholangiogram. Gastroenterology, *63*:217–226, 1972.

Khilnani, M. T., Wolf, B. S., and Finkel, M.: Roentgen features of carcinoma of the gallbladder on barium-meal examination. Radiology, *79*: 264–273, 1962.

Kikkawa, K., and Littleton, J. T.: "Pseudotumor effect" in hypotonic duodenography: report of 2 cases. Radiology, *102*:527–530, 1972.

King, J. D.: Spontaneous renoduodenal fistulas. Radiology, *54*:82–85, 1950.

Kreel, L.: The pancreas: newer radiological methods of investigation. Postgrad. Med. J., *43*: 14–23, 1967.

Larson, K. A., and Pederson, A.: Roentgenologic findings in the stomach and duodenum in cancer of the pancreas. Acta Radiol., *45*:459, 1956.

Laudan, J. C. H., and Norton, G. I.: Intraluminal duodenal diverticulum. Amer. J. Roentgen., *90*:756–760, 1963.

Lawson, T. L., and Margulis, A. R.: A simplified tube control method of hypotonic duodenography. Radiology, *92*:1119–1120, 1969.

Legge, D. A., Carlson, H. C., and Judd, E. S.: Roentgenologic features of regional enteritis of the upper gastrointestinal tract. Amer. J. Roentgen., *110*:355–360, 1970.

Lewis, E. A., and Bohrer, S. P.: Choledochoduodenal fistula complicating chronic duodenal ulcer in Nigerians. Gut, *10*:146–149, 1969.

Lieber, A., Schaefer, J. W., and Belin, R. P.: Hypotonic duodenography. Diagnosis of annular pancreas in an adult. J.A.M.A., *203*:425–427, 1968.

Liotta, D.: Pour le diagnostic des tumeurs du pancreas: la duodenographie hypotonique. Lyon Chir., *50*:455, 1955.

Lockwood, I. H., Smith, A. B., and Shook, L. D.: Lesions in and about the second portion of the duodenum. Amer. J. Roentgen., *71*:573–580, 1954.

Mani, J. R., Zboralske, F. F., and Margulis, A. R.: Carcinoma of the body and tail of the pancreas. Amer. J. Roentgen., *96*:429–446, 1966.

Martel, W., Scholtens, P. A., and Lim, L. W.: "Tubeless" hypotonic duodenography: technique, value and limitations. Amer. J. Roentgen., *107*:119–130, 1969.

McConnell, F.: Malignant neoplasm of the gallbladder: roentgenological diagnosis. Radiology, *69*:720–725, 1957.

McCort, J. J.: Roentgenographic appearance of metastases to the central lymph nodes of the superior mesenteric artery in carcinoma of the right colon. Radiology, *60*:641–646, 1953.

Meyers, H. L., and Jacobson, G.: Displacements of stomach and duodenum by anomalous lobes of the liver. Amer. J. Roentgen., *79*:789–792, 1958.

Mudhurst, G. A.: Duodeno-colic fistula. Brit. J. Radiol., *29*:381–385, 1956.

Nash, H. E., and Daland, E. M.: Benign duodenocolic fistula. New Eng. J. Med., *254*:1032–1033, 1956.

Nelson, S. W.: Some interesting and unusual manifestations of Crohn's disease ("regional enteritis") of the stomach, duodenum and small intestine. Amer. J. Roentgen., *107*:86–101, 1969.

Ngan, H.: Involvement of the duodenum by metastases from tumours of the genital tract. Brit. J. Radiol., *43*:701–705, 1970.

Novelline, R., Ferrucci, J. T., and Eaton, S. B.: Hypotonic duodenography: prospective accuracy in 300 cases. (In preparation.)

Oh, C., and Jemerin, E. E.: Benign adenomatous polyps of the papilla of Vater. Surgery, *57*: 495–503, 1965.

Olson, R. W., Hodgson, J. R., and Adson, M. A.: The significance of duodenal deformity in patients with extrahepatic portal obstruction. Radiology, *80*:636–640, 1963.

Perchik, L., and Max, T. C.: Massive hemorrhage from varices of the duodenal loop in a cirrhotic patient. Radiology, *80*:641–644, 1963.

Perez, C. A., Powers, W. E., Holtz, S., and Spjut, H. J.: Roentgenologic-pathologic correlation of resectable carcinoma of the pancreaticoduodenal region. Amer. J. Roentgen., *94*: 438–448, 1965.

Perez, C. A., and Dorfman, R. F.: Benign lymphoid hyperplasia of the stomach and duodenum. Radiology, *87*:505–510, 1966.

Poole, G. J.: A new roentgenographic method of measuring the retrogastric and retroduodenal spaces: statistical evaluation of reliability and diagnosis utility. Radiology, *97*:71–81, 1970.

Poppel, M. H.: Duodenocolic apposition. Amer. J. Roentgen., *83*:851–856, 1960.

Poppel, M. H.: Roentgen Manifestations of Pancreatic Disease. Springfield, Ill., Charles C Thomas, Publisher, 1951.

Poppel, M. H.: The roentgen manifestations of relapsing pancreatitis. Radiology, *62*:514–521, 1954.

Poppel, M. H., Jacobson, H. G., and Smith, R. W.: The Roentgen Aspects of the Papilla and Ampulla of Vater. Springfield, Ill., Charles C Thomas, Publisher, 1953.

Pratt, A. D.: Current concepts of the obstructing duodenal diaphragm. Radiology, *100*:637–643, 1971.

Rigler, L. G.: Diagnosis of extra-gastro-intestinal abdominal masses. Radiology, *21*:229–238, 1933.

Royer, M., and Solari, A. V.: Radiological anatomy of normal terminal choledochus. Gastroenterology, *2*:180–185, 1944.

Rubinstein, Z. S., Bank, S., Marks, I. N., and Psillos, C.: Hypotonic duodenography in chronic pancreatitis. Brit. J. Radiol., *44*:142–149, 1971.

Russell, W. M., and Margulis, A. R.: Impression on the duodenal loop resulting from tumor of the pancreas: a roentgenographic evaluation. Amer. J. Roentgen., *94*:449–452, 1965.

Salik, J. O.: Pancreatic carcinoma and its early roentgenologic recognition. Amer. J. Roentgen., *86*:1–28, 1961.

Sargent, E. N., and Meyers, H. I.: Wire guide and technique for Cantor tube insertion. Amer. J. Roentgen., *107*:150–155, 1969.

Schulman, A.: The cobblestone appearance of the duodenal cap, duodenitis, and hyperplasia of Brunner's glands. Brit. J. Radiol., *43*:787–795, 1970.

Schwartz, A., and Birnbaum, D.: Roentgenologic study of the topography of the choledochoduodenal junction. Amer. J. Roentgen., *87*: 772–776, 1962.

Sear, H. S., and Friedenberg, M. J.: Simplified technique for tubeless hypotonic duodenography. Radiology, *103*:210, 1972.

Shimkin, P. M., and Pearson, K. D.: Unusual arterial impressions upon the duodenum. Radiology, *103*:295–297, 1972.

Short, W. F., and Young, B. R.: Roentgen demonstration of prolapse of benign polypoid gastric tumors into the duodenum, including a dumbbell-shaped leiomyoma. Amer. J. Roentgen., *103*:317–320, 1968.

Sifre, R. A., Stenberg, E. S., and Graybill, L. D.: Roentgen configuration of the duodenojejunal area in carcinoma of the pancreas. Geriatrics, *8*:486–493, 1953.

Simon, M., and Lerner, M. A.: Duodenal compression by the mesenteric root in acute pancreatitis and inflammatory conditions of the bowel. Radiology, *79*:75–81, 1962.

Sobotta, J., and Uhlenhuth, E.: Atlas of Descriptive Human Anatomy. New York, Hafner Co., 1957.

Stiennon, O. A.: The anatomical basis for the epsilon sign of frostberg. Amer. J. Roentgen., *75*:282–290, 1956.

Stock, F. E.: Duodenorenal fistula: a complication of peptic ulceration. Brit. J. Surg., *42*:330–331, 1954.

Treitel, H., Meyers, M. A., and Maya, V.: Changes in the duodenal loop secondary to carcinoma of the hepatic flexure of the colon. Brit. J. Radiol., *43*:209–213, 1970.

Waldron, R. L., Seaman, W. B., and Foster, S.: Reflux pancreatography and distension duodenography in humans. Radiology, *104*:295–300, 1972.

Wallace, R. G., and Howard, W. B.: Acute superior mesenteric artery syndrome in the severely burned patient. Radiology, *94*:307–310, 1970.

Weiner, S. N., Vertes, V., and Shapiro, H.: The upper gastro-intestinal tract in patients undergoing chronic dialysis. Radiology, *92*:110–114, 1969.

Winter, J.: Benign duodenocolic fistula. J. Fac. Radiol., *10*:221–222, 1959.

Wisoff, C. P., and Parsavand, R.: Edema of the interureteric ridge: a useful roentgen sign. Amer. J. Roentgen., *86*:1123–1126, 1961.

Chapter 5

THE RADIOLOGY OF JAUNDICE

The evaluation of jaundiced patients is often a difficult challenge. While most cases belong to well-defined diagnostic categories, the remainder frequently have confusing, inconclusive, or contradictory clinical and laboratory features which fail to identify the underlying disease process. The classically "medical" conditions such as cirrhosis or hepatitis may be complicated by intrahepatic bile stasis resulting from edema and inspissation of bile within biliary canaliculi so that chemical abnormalities normally associated with biliary obstruction develop (Phillips, 1957; Shaldon, 1957). Conversely, long-standing extrahepatic obstruction may produce secondary hepatic dysfunction and laboratory findings ordinarily considered to indicate hepatocellular disease (Culver, 1961). Finally, intrahepatic cholestasis such as that which can occur in patients undergoing therapy with phenothiazine derivatives may almost exactly mimic the clinical and laboratory findings of extrahepatic biliary tract obstruction (Datta, 1963).

Despite the inherent difficulties, it is of great importance to distinguish between those patients whose jaundice is due to surgically correctable extrahepatic biliary obstruction and those with purely intrahepatic conditions which must be treated medically. Patients with hepatocellular disease may be seriously and adversely affected by the general anesthesia and operative manipulation necessary during surgical exploration. Smith and Sherlock (1964) describe 12 patients with hepatitis who mistakenly underwent surgery for suspected obstruction. Five died within four weeks of operation and four others suffered marked exacerbation, developing ascites and recovering only after a prolonged illness. Harville (1963) and Davis (1962) report similar experiences.

While identification of extrahepatic obstruction is the most important single aim of diagnosis in jaundiced patients, significant additional benefit results if the exact site and specific nature of the obstructing process can be determined. Such preoperative knowledge enables the surgeon to plan his procedure beforehand. When malignant obstruction is present, the types of feasible bypasses can be considered and the possibility of resection assessed. A surgeon familiar with the complexities of cancer surgery in the pancreaticoduodenal area can be consulted and enlisted for operative assistance. General anesthesia time can be held to the minimum, thus reducing operative morbidity and mortality (Glenn, 1964; Sato, 1968).

Because of these important considerations, radiologic examination of jaundiced patients has assumed increasing significance. The procedures available vary broadly in terms of information provided, complexity, indications, and expense. It is the purpose of this chapter to present and evaluate the contributions of diagnostic radiology to the assessment of patients with clinically suspected obstructive jaundice.

PLAIN ABDOMINAL ROENTGENOGRAMS

Pancreatic Calcification

Plain abdominal roentgenograms can provide important, and even diagnostic, information in occasional patients with jaundice. For example, the presence of pancreatic calcification is of significance since it establishes the diagnosis of chronic pancreatitis (Sarles, 1965), a condition which can produce inflammatory stenosis of the intrapancreatic portion of the common bile duct, with resultant obstruction. Such obstruction is most commonly transient (mild jaundice occurs in 15 to 25 per cent of the patients with acute pancreatitis) (Weinstein, 1963), but can be persistent (as a result of progressive cicatricial narrowing or of pseudocyst formation in the head of the pancreas) (Weinstein, 1963). Since most of the pancreatic calcification in patients in the United States and Western Europe is the result of alcoholic pancreatitis (Howard, 1960), there is a high incidence of coexistent cirrhosis in these patients, so that both hepatocellular and extrahepatic obstructive causes for jaundice are suggested by the demonstration of pancreatic lithiasis.

Gallbladder Enlargement

Rarely, the gallbladder can be identified on plain abdominal films as a soft-tissue mass in the right upper abdominal quadrant (Fig. 5–1). It must be differentiated from the right kidney (i.e., both the kidney and the gallbladder should be visible as separate and discrete entities) and is usually seen only when sufficiently enlarged to indent adjacent air-containing viscera. Stringent criteria for determination of gallbladder enlarge-

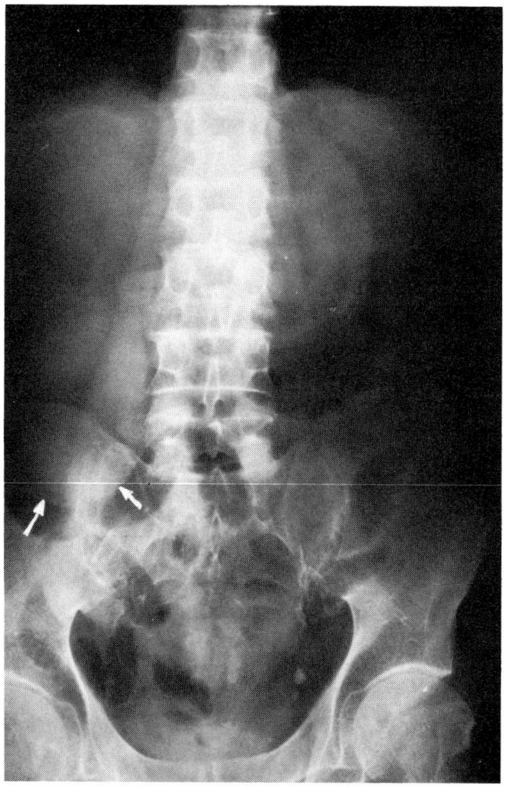

Figure 5–1. Plain abdominal roentgenogram. Courvoisier gallbladder due to carcinoma of the head of the pancreas. Note how the gallbladder (*arrows*) can be distinguished from the lower pole of the right kidney. (From Eaton, S. B., Ferrucci, J. T., Handmaker, H., and James, A. E.: Radiologic diagnosis of extrahepatic biliary obstruction in jaundiced patients. Amer. J. Gastroent., *58*:477–490, 1972.

ment are not firmly established, but a width greater than 5 cm. is probably enough to suggest abnormality (Redman, 1970*a*). Gallbladder enlargement in a patient with jaundice usually indicates malignant extrahepatic biliary obstruction. This relationship, initially emphasized by Courvoisier, results from the fact that most patients with malignant obstruction have intrinsically normal gallbladders which can be distended. Patients in whom jaundice is due to an impacted common duct calculus usually have scarred, chronically inflamed gallbladders. An enlarged gallbladder is found at surgery in about 87 per cent of the patients with cancer of the head of the pancreas, but is uncommon in patients with choledocholithiasis (Hess, 1965).

Choledocholithiasis

From 15 to 20 per cent of all gallstones are sufficiently calcified for identification on abdominal roentgenograms. The demonstration of calcific cholecystolithiasis alone is of only modest diagnostic significance but, when one or more stones of this type enter the common bile duct, a definite diagnosis of choledocholithiasis is possible (Sahler, 1944). When numerous calculi outline the entire course of the common duct, diagnosis is easy (Fig. 5–2). A more typical pattern, however, is observed when several stones can be identified in the gallbladder, while another is noted in a location consistent with the position of the common bile duct (Fig. 5–3). In such cases, one must exclude the coexistence of cholecystolithiasis and mesenteric lymphnodal calcification. This is best done by comparing the appearance of the individual calcifications. In choledocholithiasis, the common duct stone should closely resemble the gallbladder calculi; in most instances, a calcified mesenteric lymph node will have a different appearance (Fig. 5–4).

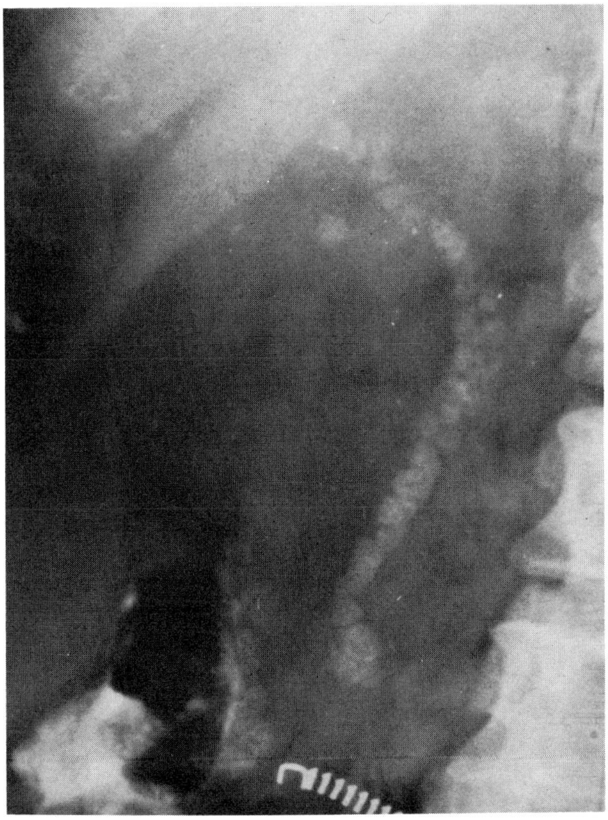

***Figure* 5–2.** Plain abdominal roentgenogram. Multiple calculi outline the common bile duct in a patient with jaundice resulting from choledocholithiasis. (From Eaton, S. B., Ferrucci, J. T., Handmaker, H., and James, A. E.: Radiologic diagnosis of extrahepatic biliary obstruction in jaundiced patients. Amer. J. Gastroent., 58:477–490, 1972.)

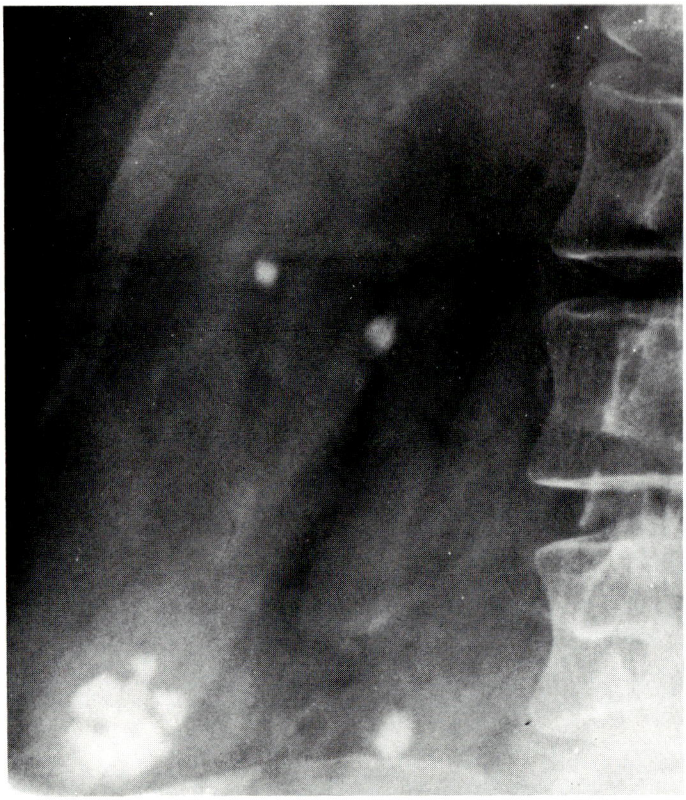

Figure 5–3. Plain abdominal roentgenogram. Several calculi are present in the gallbladder; two are located near the junction of the cystic and common ducts, and one is found in the distal common bile duct. Note that the calculi are all fairly similar in appearance.

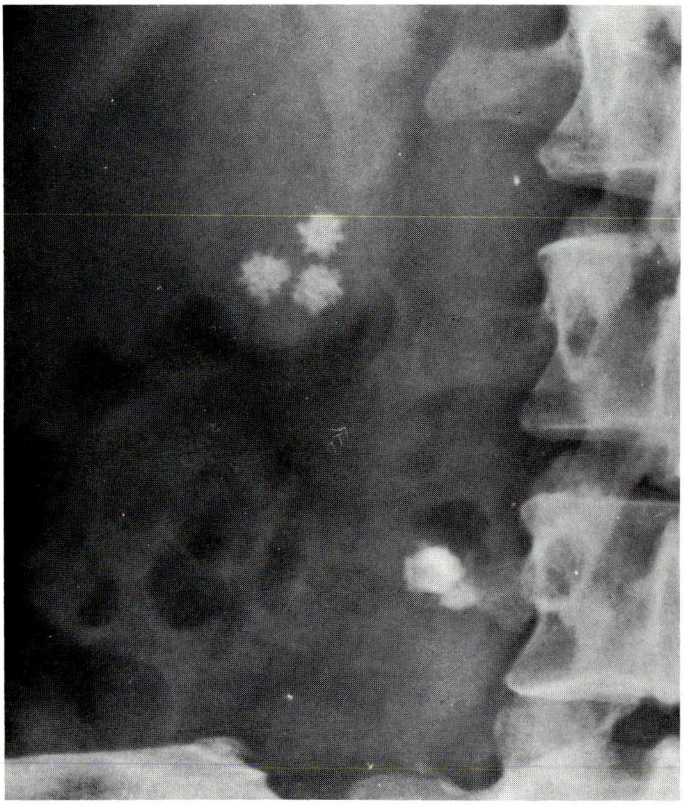

Figure 5–4. Plain abdominal roentgenogram. Three calculi are present in the gallbladder, while a calcified mesenteric lymph node simulates calculus in the distal common bile duct. Contrast the spiculated appearance of the gallstones with the amorphous lymph nodal calcification.

BARIUM UPPER GASTROINTESTINAL EXAMINATION

While plain abdominal roentgenograms only occasionally provide significant diagnostic information in patients with jaundice, barium examination of the upper gastrointestinal tract often makes valuable contributions. Close proximity of the gallbladder, common bile duct and pancreas to the duodenum forms the anatomic basis for most of these important findings (Fig. 5–5). The duodenal papilla (of Vater) is situated on the posteromedial aspect of the descending duodenum, and the common bile duct ascends behind the apical portion of the duodenal bulb. The cystic duct passes over the apical portion of the bulb to reach the gallbladder which lies adjacent to the anterolateral aspect of the upper descending duodenum. It can be seen that biliary structures thus form an incomplete ring around the duodenum and, when one or all portions enlarge, they create characteristic extrinsic indentations.

When jaundice results from obstruction of the distal common bile duct by *pancreatic or ampullary cancer,* barium examination of the duodenum will usually demonstrate a pathologic mass in the head of the pancreas. The characteristics of these lesions (and of inflammatory pancreatic masses) are described in Chapter 4 but, when present, the cause of jaundice can usually be clearly established.

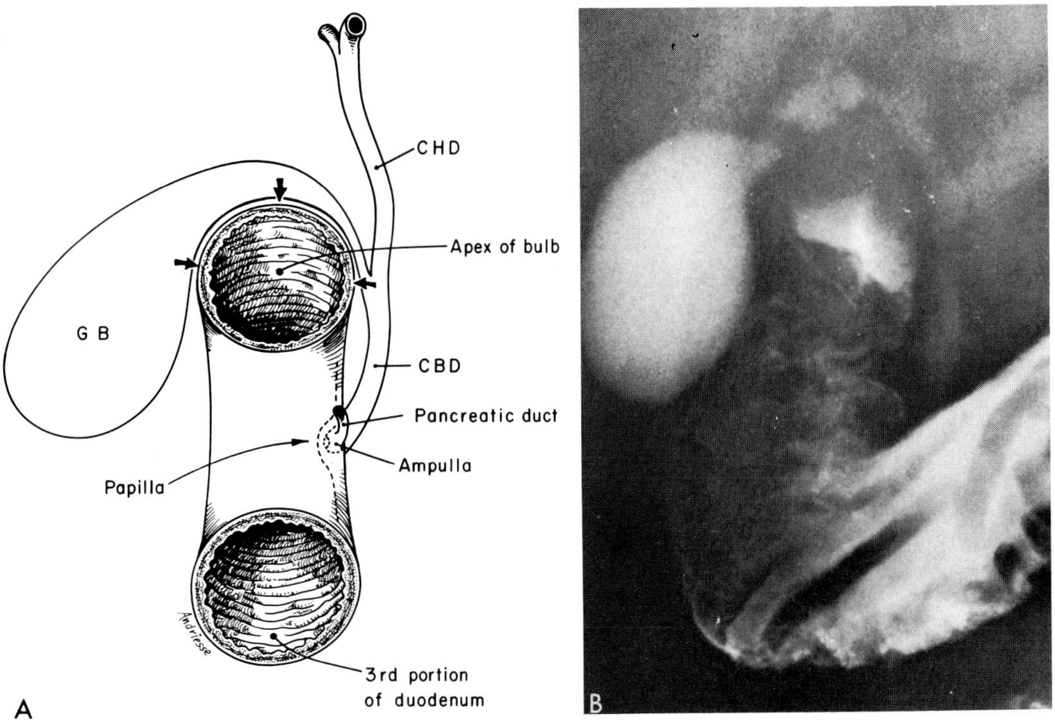

Figure 5–5. Relationship of the biliary tree to the duodenum in a right parasagittal section. *A,* Diagrammatic representation. The gallbladder, cystic duct, common bile duct, and duodenal papilla are observed to form an incomplete ring around the superior duodenal flexure. (From Eaton, S. B., Ferrucci, J. T., Handmaker, H., and James, A. E.: Radiologic diagnosis of extrahepatic biliary obstruction in jaundiced patients. Amer. J. Gastroent., 58:477–490, 1972.)

B, Oral cholecystogram obtained when a fatty meal was given after upper gastrointestinal barium examination. The gastric antrum is superimposed on the descending duodenum; otherwise, the anatomic details correspond to those of the diagrammatic representation (*A*).

Edema of the Duodenal Papilla

In contrast with the often dramatic findings indicating pancreaticoduodenal malignancy, evidence of *choledocholithiasis* is usually subtle (Eaton, 1972*a*). Gallstones arrested in the common bile duct tend to lodge in its distal end where the lumen abruptly narrows as the duct passes through the duodenal wall. Impacted calculi produce mechanical irritation of the ductal wall and the resulting inflammatory reaction commonly spreads to the duodenal papilla which becomes congested and swollen, with a diameter several times that of the impacted stone (Fig. 5–6). On barium examinations, papillary edema generally appears as a smoothly rounded indentation on the inner border of the second or proximal third portion of the duodenum (Fig. 5–7). The defect is typically between 1.5 and 4.0 cm. in its greatest dimension and is usually smooth-surfaced (Table 5–1).

An appearance similar to that of the edematous duodenal papilla which is the result of choledocholithiasis may be produced by periampullary carcinoma, papillary edema secondary to pancreatitis, benign tumors, and unusually large, but otherwise normal papillae (Table 5–2). The latter two possibilities are rarely associated with jaundice, but ampullary carcinoma and acute pancreatitis can present diagnostic difficulty. In most instances, peri-Vaterian malignancy has an irregular or even ulcerated appearance (Fig. 5–8), and acute pancreatitis associated with papillary edema (Poppel's sign) often produces edema of the duodenal folds and/or a pancreatic mass effect (Fig. 5–9). In certain cases, however, distinction between these entities and choledocholithiasis is impossible on purely radiographic grounds (Fig. 5–10). In these circumstances, the authors

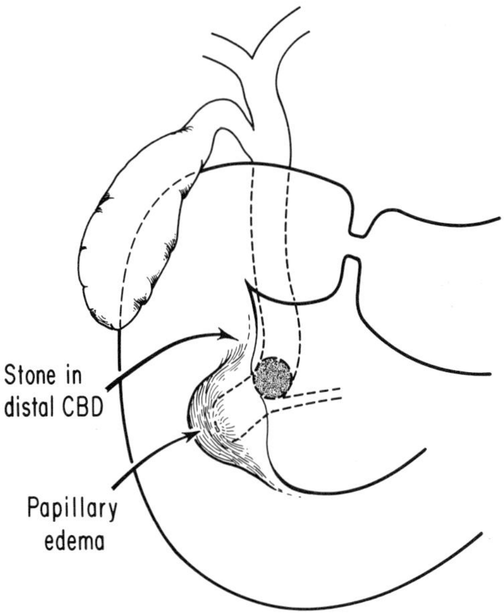

Figure 5–6. Diagrammatic representation of a gallstone impacted in the distal common bile duct, producing edema of the duodenal papilla. The edematous papilla is considerably larger than the stone itself.

TABLE 5–1. Appearance of Edematous Duodenal Papillae in 17 Patients with Choledocholithiasis

ROENTGEN FEATURE	NO. OF PATIENTS	%
Size (greatest dimension)*		
<1.5 cm.	2	12
1.5–2.5 cm.	8	47
2.5–3.5 cm.	6	35
3.5–4.5 cm.	1	6
Shape		
Rounded or semilunar	11	65
Other	6	35
Surface character		
Perfectly smooth	12	70.5
Almost perfectly smooth	2	12.0
Irregular	3	17.5

*Average of 17 patients = 2.4 cm.

From Eaton, S. B., Ferrucci, J. T., Benedict, K. T., and Margulis, A. F.: Diagnosis of choledocholithiasis by barium duodenal examination. Radiology, *102*:267–273, 1972.

TABLE 5–2. Duodenal Abnormalities Which Can Simulate Papillary Edema Resulting from Choledocholithiasis

Large normal papilla
Papillary edema resulting from pancreatitis (Poppel's sign)
Papillary edema resulting from duodenal ulceration
Ectopic pancreas
Lipoma
Spindle cell tumors
Periampullary carcinoma

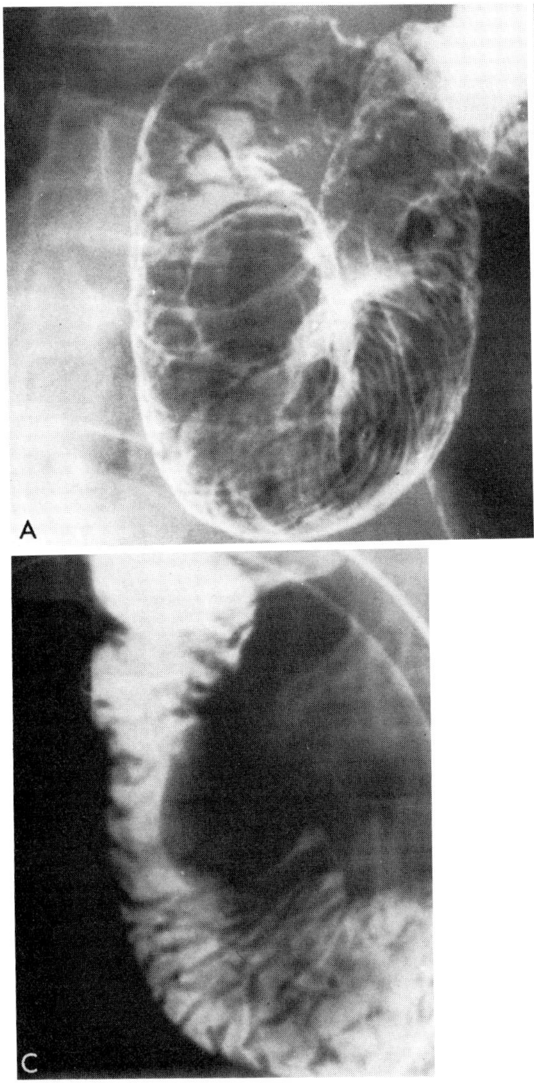

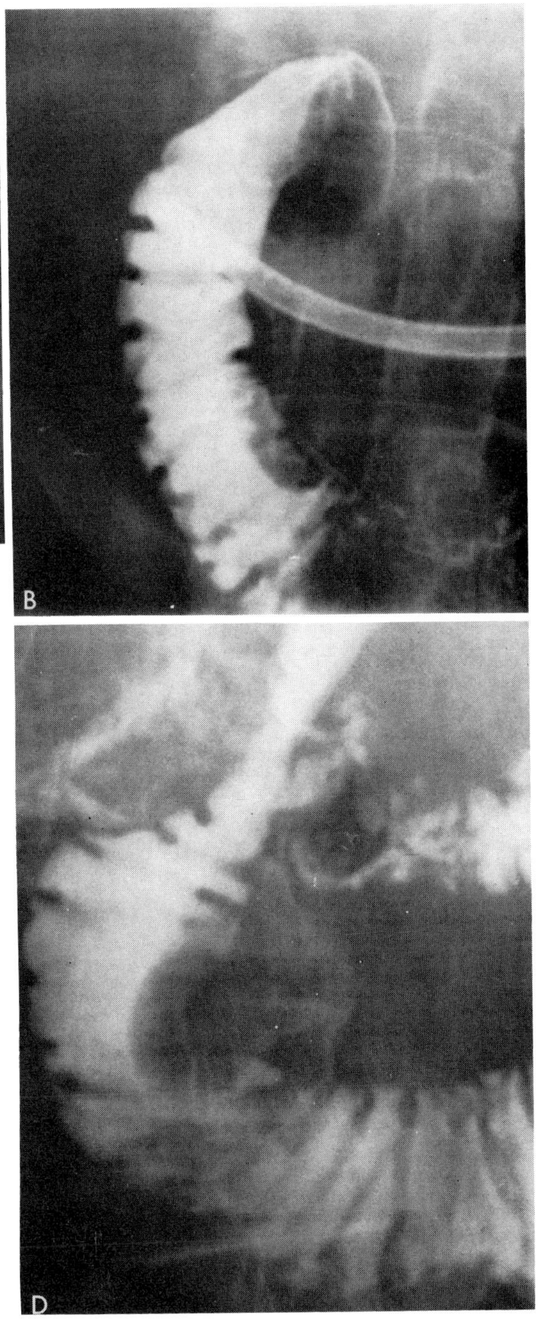

Figure 5–7. Duodenal barium examinations in four patients with papillary edema secondary to choledocholithiasis. Note the rounded, smooth-surfaced indentation in each instance. *A*, *B*, and *C* are hypotonic duodenograms; *D* is a conventional barium upper gastrointestinal examination. (*A*, From Eaton, S. B., Benedict, K. T., Ferrucci, J. T., and Fleischli, D. J.: Hypotonic duodenography. Radiol. Clin. N. Amer., *8*:125–137, 1970. *B*, *C*, and *D*, From Eaton, S. B., Ferrucci, J. T., Benedict, K. T., and Margulis, A. F.: Diagnosis of choledocholithiasis by barium duodenal examination. Radiology, *102*:267–273, 1972.)

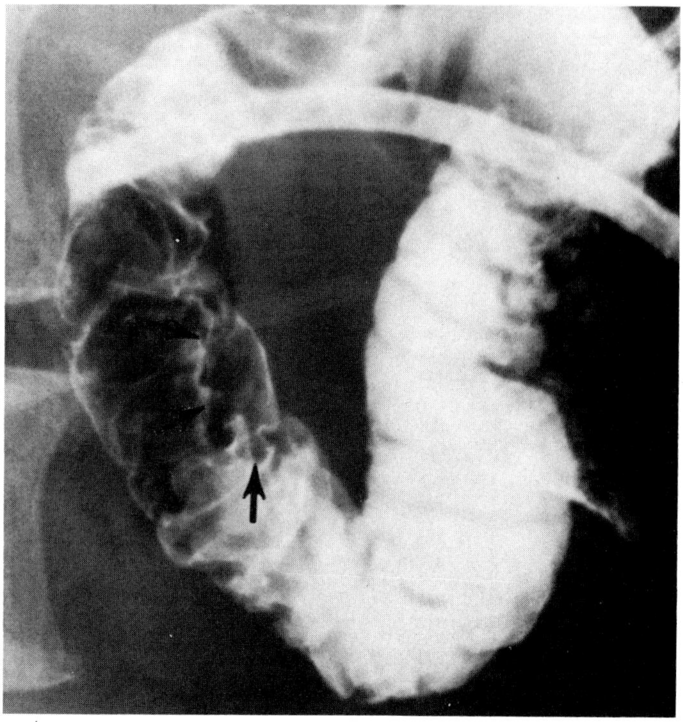

Figure 5–8. Hypotonic duodenogram. Irregular-surfaced indentation along the inner aspect of the descending duodenum. Ampullary carcinoma. Compare with the edematous papillae illustrated in Figure 5–7. (From Ferrucci, J. T., and Eaton, S. B.: Current concepts: Radiology of the pancreas. New Eng. J. Med., *288*:506–510, 1973.)

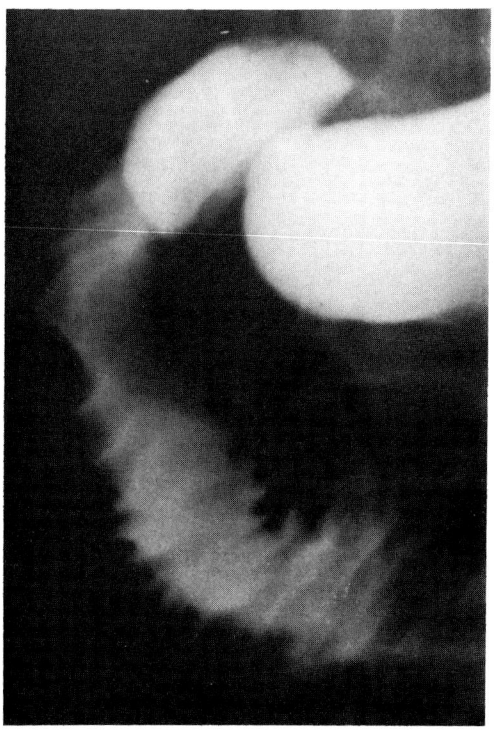

Figure 5–9. Upper gastrointestinal examination. Papillary edema secondary to acute pancreatitis (Poppel's sign). Note the associated edema of the duodenal folds.

have found clinical features to be helpful in arranging a logical order of diagnostic possibilities to explain the roentgen abnormalities (Table 5–3). Problems related to radiologic evaluation of peri-Vaterian mass lesions are discussed in greater detail in Chapter 4.

Enlargement of the Common Bile Duct

Both the common bile duct and the gallbladder can dilate secondary to distal biliary tract obstruction, and enlargement of these structures can be identified on barium examination of the duodenum. Over 50 per cent of the dilated common bile ducts can be detected by this means (Perez, 1965). The typical finding is an extrinsic indentation defect on the apical portion of the duodenal bulb. The defect is rather sharply defined and fairly tubular in appearance (Fig. 5–11). There is usually a smooth, rounded indentation on the superior aspect of the duodenum in the same area. There are three important considerations related to the employment of this radiographic sign. First, both benign and malignant extrahepatic obstruction can produce

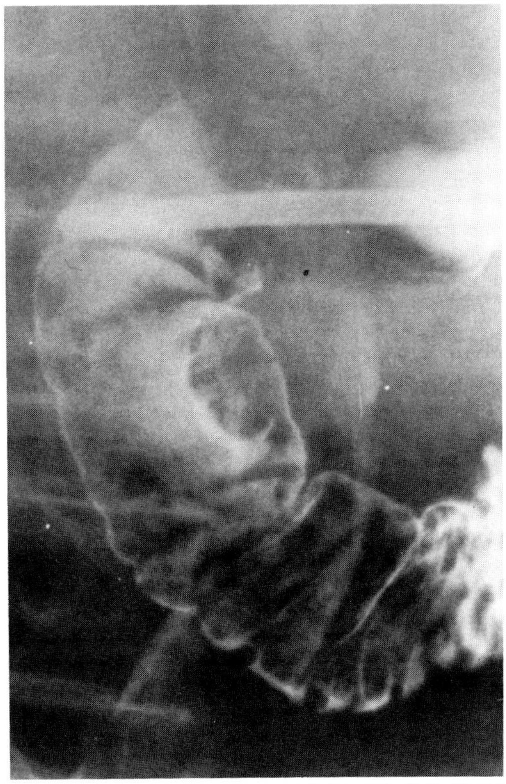

Figure 5-10. Hypotonic duodenogram. Relatively smooth-surfaced indentation due to cancer arising in the area around the ampulla of Vater. Distinction from papillary edema secondary to choledocholithiasis would be hazardous if based solely on radiographic criteria. (From Eaton, S. B., Benedict, K. T., Ferrucci, J. T., and Fleischli, D. J.: Hypotonic duodenography. Radiol. Clin. N. Amer., 8:125–137, 1970.)

TABLE 5-3. Differentiating Clinical Features

MANIFESTATIONS	CHOLEDOCHOLITHIASIS	PERIAMPULLARY TUMOR	PANCREATITIS
		History	
Past history	Cholelithiasis and/or biliary colic; not excluded by prior cholecystectomy	Nonspecific	Previous episodes of abdominal pain with hyperamylasemia; alcoholism; cholelithiasis
Onset	Usually abrupt	Insidious	Abrupt
Pain*	Occurs in most patients; usually intense, often colicky	Occurs in 50%; dull and steady when present	Occurs in most patients; generally constant and severe
Jaundice	Often fluctuates, can be constant	Usually progressive; rarely decreases temporarily	Usually mild; subsides promptly
Fever and chills	Common	Occasional	Fever fairly common; chills rare
Weight loss	Only occasionally significant	Usually prominent	Common in chronic disease
Pruritus	Common	Common	Uncommon
		Physical Examination	
Jaundice	Usually moderate	Usually intense	Usually faint
Epigastric tenderness	Common	Uncommon	Common
Palpable gallbladder	Rare	Occurs in 25% of cases	Rare
		Laboratory Findings	
Leukocytosis	Frequent	Uncommon	Frequent
Guaiac-positive stools ± anemia	Rare	Fairly common	Rare
Hyperbilirubinemia	Moderate	Usually marked	Minimal
Alkaline phosphatase	Moderately to markedly elevated	Usually markedly elevated	Minimally elevated
Hepatocellular chemistries†	Normal or slightly elevated	Normal or slightly elevated	Occasionally elevated by associated cirrhosis
Amylase and/or lipase	Elevated transiently in about 33% of cases	Occasionally elevated	Elevated early in nearly all cases

*Pain can radiate to the back in all three conditions.

†Include serum glutamic oxaloacetic transaminase, lactic dehydrogenase, albumin/globulin ratio, thymol turbidity, and so forth.

From Eaton, S. B., Ferrucci, J. T., Benedict, K. T., and Margulis, A. F.: Diagnosis of choledocholithiasis by barium duodenal examination. Radiology, *102*:267–273, 1972.

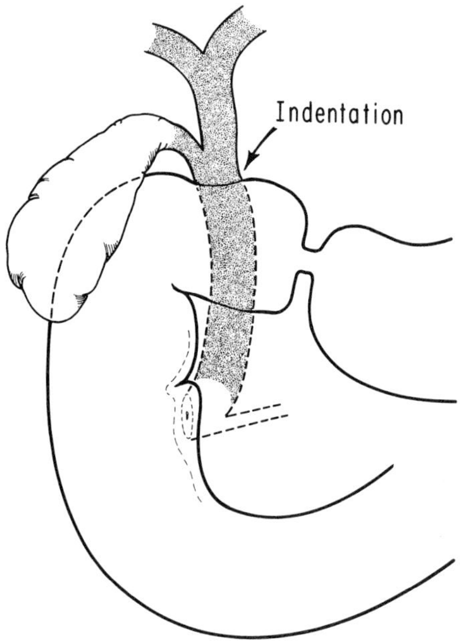

A

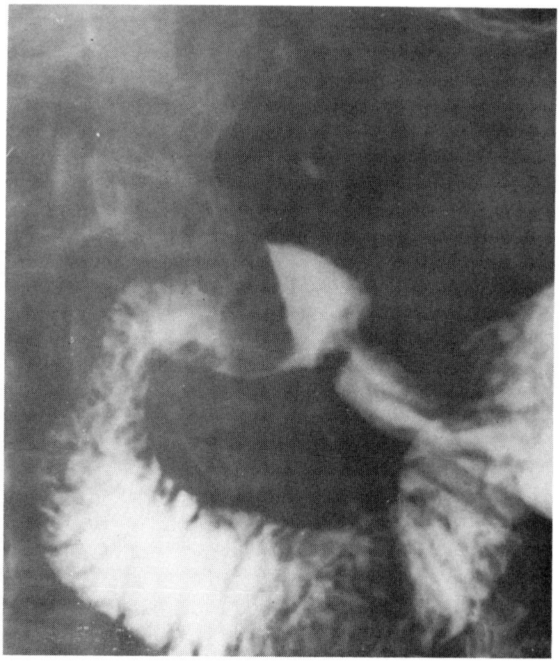

B

Figure 5–11. Dilated common bile duct produces a tubular, sharply defined indentation on the apex of the duodenal bulb.

A, Diagrammatic representation.

B, Upper gastrointestinal examination in a patient with dilatation of the common bile duct produced by impaction of a common duct stone. Note similarity to the diagram. (From Eaton, S. B., et al.: Radiologic diagnosis of extrahepatic biliary obstruction in jaundiced patients. Amer. J. Gastroent., *58*:396–405, 1972.)

dilatation of the common bile duct. Second, an appearance suggesting common duct enlargement can be seen in 12 per cent of the normal patients (i.e., where there is no clinical evidence of jaundice) (Eaton, 1972*b*). Such an appearance may represent angulation at the superior duodenal flexure, peristaltic activity, incomplete filling, the cystogastrocolic ligament (a broad, band-like peritoneal reflection present in a minority of the population) (Samuel, 1952), and a nondistended, nonpathologic gallbladder. Third, several pathologic processes unrelated to common bile duct obstruction can simulate its presence. These include duodenal varices, an enlarged quadrate lobe of the liver, a dilated hepatic artery, masses in the porta hepatis, duodenal ulcer disease, and hydrops of the gallbladder (Table 5–4).

The 12 per cent incidence of presumptive false positives and the broad differential requiring consideration abate the confidence with which a radiographic diagnosis of common bile duct enlargement can be based on barium gastrointestinal examination. On the other hand, when findings suggestive of a dilated common duct are noted in patients with jaundice, they should not be disregarded. They may best be considered as an indication for more refined examination by angiography, isotopic imaging, or percutaneous cholangiography.

Gallbladder Enlargement

Over 70 per cent of all dilated gallbladders can be detected by barium meal study (Eyler, 1962) and this accuracy compares favorably with that possible through physical examination. The most conclusive finding is a smooth extrinsic indentation defect on the outer aspect of the upper descending duodenum (Fig. 5–12). When present in a patient with jaundice, this is a very reliable sign,

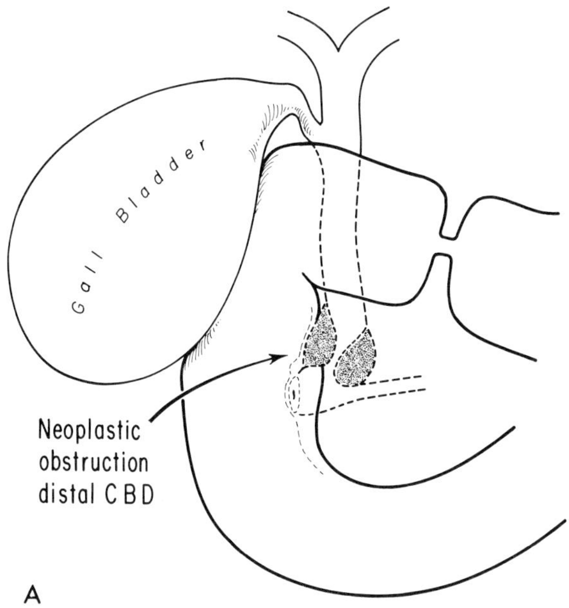

A

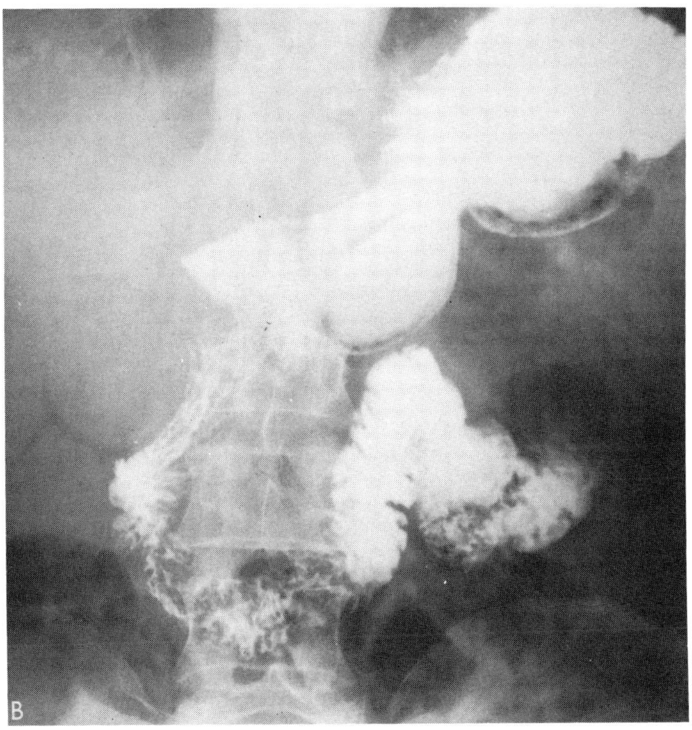

Figure 5–12. Gallbladder dilatation produces a smoothly rounded indentation on the outer aspect of the upper descending duodenum.

A, Diagrammatic representation.

B, Upper gastrointestinal examination. Note the similarity to the diagram. Courvoisier gallbladder results from ampullary carcinoma. (From Eaton, S. B., et al.: Radiologic diagnosis of extrahepatic biliary obstruction in jaundiced patients. Amer. J. Gastroent., 58:396–405, 1972.)

TABLE 5–4. Duodenal Indentations Suggesting Common Duct Dilatation

Normal	Present in 35 of 300 patients (12%)
Duodenal angulation	
Duodenal peristalsis	
Cystogastrocolic ligament	
"Neck" of gallbladder (whether dilated or not)	
Idiopathic	
Pathologic	
Duodenal ulcer disease	
Dilated pancreaticoduodenal and/or portal vein	
Enlarged quadrate lobe of liver	
Dilated hepatic artery	
Masses in porta hepatis	

being falsely positive in less than 1 per cent of instances (Eaton, 1972*b*). As previously noted, enlargement of the gallbladder in a jaundiced patient usually indicates malignant extrahepatic biliary obstruction. There are many exceptions to Courvoisier's law, but false negatives (i.e., a nonpalpable gallbladder in malignant obstruction) are much more common than are false positives. Accordingly, radiologic demonstration of gallbladder enlargement has considerable significance.

Conditions which can also produce a smooth indentation of the outer wall of the descending duodenum and thus simulate the radiographic appearance of a Courvoisier gallbladder include masses arising from the right kidney and liver, hydrops of the gallbladder, and duodenocolic apposition (an indentation produced by unusually close approximation of the hepatic flexure and duodenum and present in less than 3 per cent of normal persons) (Poppel, 1960) (Table 5–5). Since these conditions are rarely associated with jaundice, they should seldom cause diagnostic confusion.

TABLE 5–5. Extrinsic Indentations: Outer Duodenal Border

Enlarged gallbladder
Pericholecystic abscess
Hepatic cyst or tumor
Enlarged right kidney
Duodenocolic apposition
Carcinoma of the hepatic flexure
Duodenal hematoma
Duodenal varices

NONINVASIVE CONTRAST STUDIES OF THE BILIARY TRACT

Intravenous Cholangiography

The value of intravenous cholangiography in patients with jaundice is inversely related to the degree of hyperbilirubinemia present. Although satisfactory opacification of the biliary tree can sometimes be obtained in patients with serum bilirubin levels as high as 4 mg. per 100 ml., in most instances, it is impossible to achieve adequate visualization when the bilirubin level is as high as 3 mg. per 100 ml. (Wise, 1962). Since clinically evident icterus usually indicates a serum bilirubin value of at least 3 mg. per 100 ml., intravenous cholangiography is only occasionally a feasible technique for evaluation of jaundice. When the study can be employed, common bile duct stones can be directly demonstrated as *filling defects* in just over half of the cases in which they are present (Fig. 5–13).

In an additional group of patients with choledocholithiasis, partial obstruction can be inferred from an abnormal *time-density relationship* (Wise, 1962). This concept applies only in patients who have had a prior cholecystectomy or in whom the cystic duct is obstructed. Normally, in such patients, the density of contrast material in the common bile duct should be maximal at some time between 30 and 60 minutes after injection and distinctly less at two hours after injection (Fig. 5–14). If the density of opacified bile in the common duct is greater at 120 minutes than it was at one hour, partial common duct obstruction (e.g., choledocholithiasis or distal common bile duct stricture, and so forth) is considered to be present (Fig. 5–15). The value of *widening* alone as a sign of obstruction is a controversial topic, but if the common bile duct is greater than 15 mm. in width, partial obstruction is probably present. By employing both direct (i.e., actual demonstration of stones as filling defects) and indirect (time-density concept and common duct width)

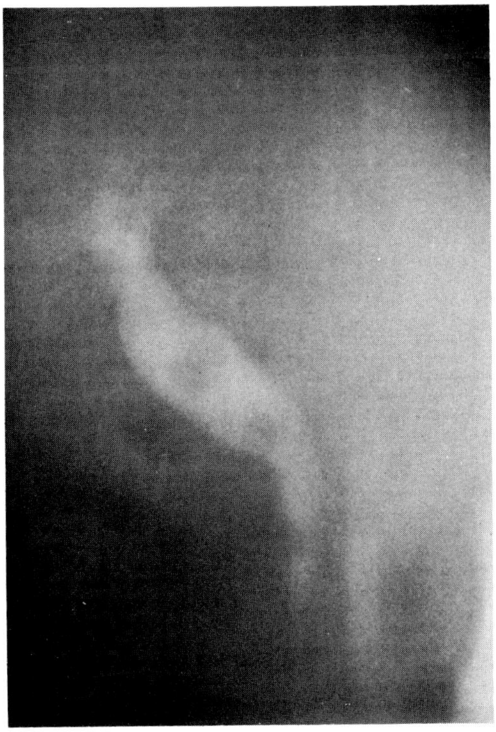

Figure 5-13. Intravenous cholangiogram (tomographic section). Three nonopaque calculi are present in the common bile duct. (From Sullivan, F. J., Eaton, S. B., Ferrucci, J. T., Dreyfuss, J. R., and Sloan, R. W.: Cholangiographic manifestations of acute biliary colic. New Eng. J. Med., *288*:33–35, 1973.

criteria for diagnosis, Wise (1962) was able to establish the diagnosis of choledocholithiasis in 64 per cent of the patients with an intact gallbladder and in 92 per cent of the patients after cholecystectomy in 116 cases in which satisfactory opacification could be achieved.

Salzman Test

Administration of iopanoic acid (Telepaque) for four successive days (i.e., the "four-day Telepaque" or "Salzman" test) may result in deposition of contrast material on the surface of the common bile duct stones (Fig. 5–16). In Salzman's series of 13 patients with choledocholithiasis, this technique demonstrated calculi in ten instances (77 per cent) (Salzman, 1966). Surface deposition of iopanoic acid occurs optimally when the calculi are pigment-surfaced. Common bile duct stones are usually of this type, but gallbladder stones are most often cholesterol or calcium-surfaced. For this reason, the Salzman technique has been more successful in demonstrating choledocholithiasis than cholecystolithiasis. The four-day Telepaque test has been

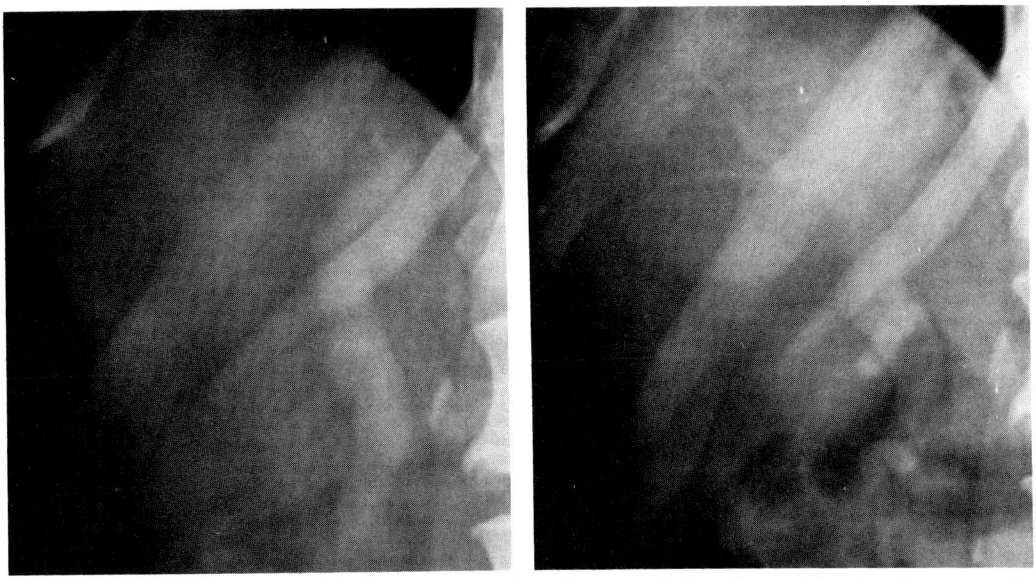

Figure 5-14. Intravenous cholangiogram. The density of ductal opacification is noticeably greater at 45 minutes (*left*) than at two hours (*right*). This is the normally expected time-density relationship in patients who have undergone a cholecystectomy or in whom the cystic duct is obstructed.

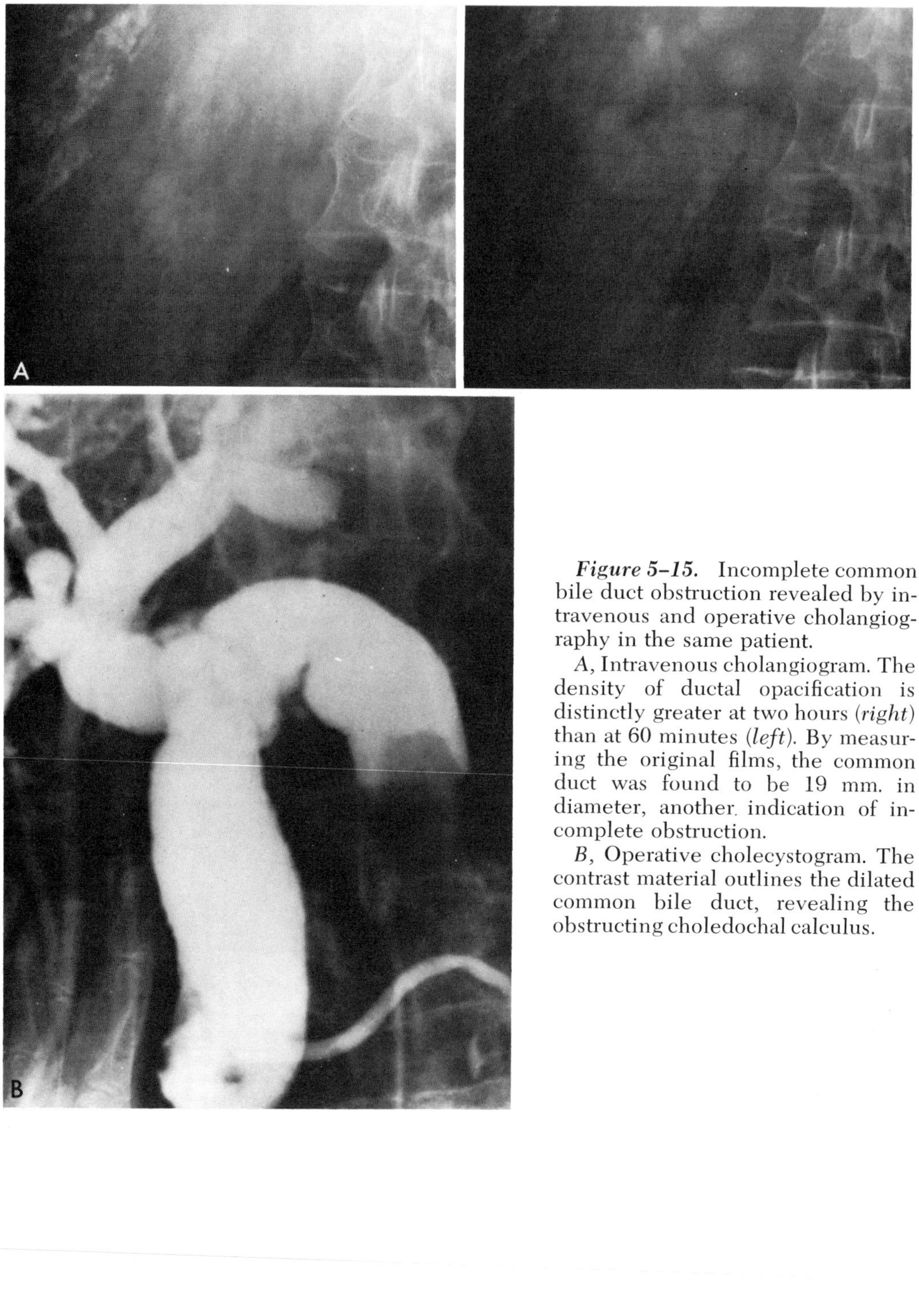

Figure 5–15. Incomplete common bile duct obstruction revealed by intravenous and operative cholangiography in the same patient.

A, Intravenous cholangiogram. The density of ductal opacification is distinctly greater at two hours (*right*) than at 60 minutes (*left*). By measuring the original films, the common duct was found to be 19 mm. in diameter, another indication of incomplete obstruction.

B, Operative cholecystogram. The contrast material outlines the dilated common bile duct, revealing the obstructing choledochal calculus.

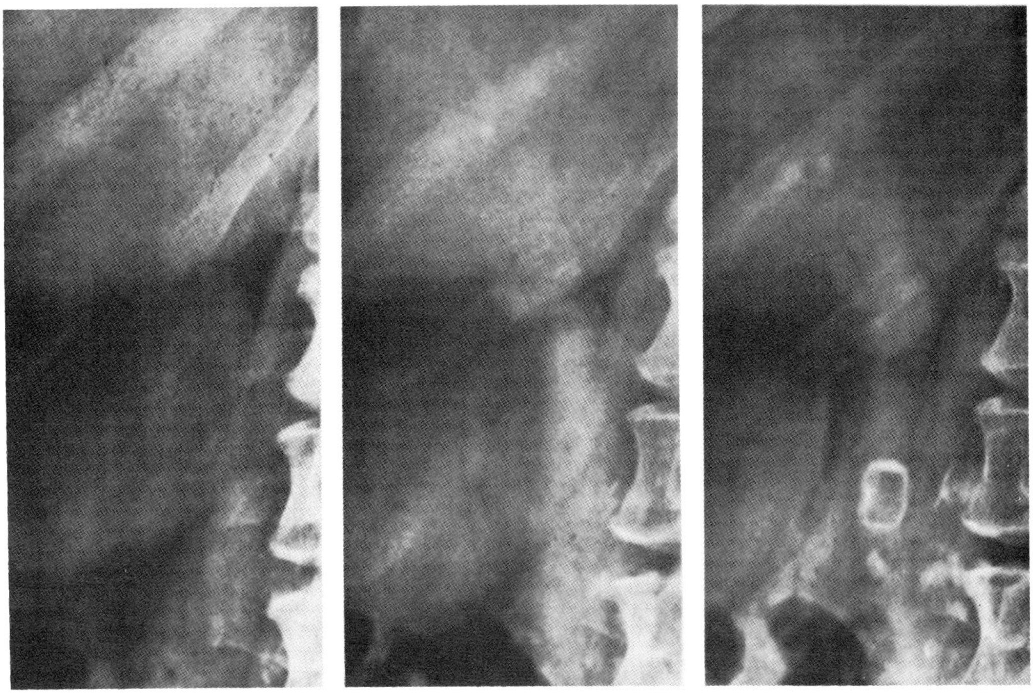

Figure 5–16. Salzman test. Administration of telepaque over four successive days results in deposition of contrast material on the surface of the common bile duct calculus. Roentgenograms were made on the first (*left*), second (*center*) and fourth (*right*) days of examination. (From Lloyd, G. A. S.: The four day telepaque test in the investigation of the post-cholecystectomy syndrome. Brit. J. Radiol., 33:522–523, 1960.)

used successfully in patients with serum bilirubin levels as high as 5 mg. per 100 ml., but not in those with more severe jaundice. The examination is contraindicated if significant hepatocellular disease is present and, particularly, in the hepatorenal syndrome.

RADIOISOTOPIC EXAMINATIONS

Two different types of radiopharmaceuticals can be utilized for evaluation of jaundiced patients by isotopic imaging techniques. The first, radioiodinated rose bengal, is cleared from the blood by hepatic parenchymal (polygonal) cells and excreted through the biliary tree into the intestinal tract. The second type consists of colloidal agents (such as ^{99m}Tc sulfur colloid) which are phagocytized by Kupffer cells of the liver's reticulo endothelial system.

Radioiodinated Rose Bengal Examination

In normal patients, maximum hepatic uptake of ^{131}I rose bengal occurs 20 to 30 minutes after intravenous administration, and abdominal scintiscans made at this time delineate the liver image. Detectable intestinal radioactivity typically becomes apparent 30 to 60 minutes after injection and the gallbladder can usually be identified shortly thereafter (Fig. 5–17). When no radioactivity can be detected in the intestines 90 minutes after administration, follow-up images are obtained over the ensuing 24 hours. If, during this period, no radioactivity has appeared in the gut, the diagnosis of biliary obstruction can be considered established (Fig. 5–18).

In practice, this statement must be carefully qualified. Failure of radioiodinated rose bengal to appear in the

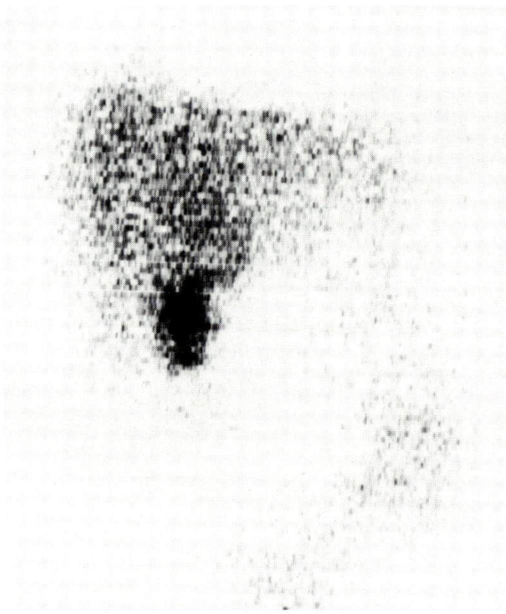

Figure 5–17. ^{131}I rose bengal abdominal scintiscan. The distribution of abdominal radioactivity, scanned 90 minutes after intravenous administration of radioiodinated rose bengal, reveals a normal pattern of activity in the liver, gallbladder, and gut.

intestines after intravenous administration cannot, by itself, distinguish between intra- and extrahepatic obstruction. For this reason, an external blood clearance determination has now been made an integral part of the procedure. The clearance rate is determined by placing a probe (scintillation detector) over the patient's head (which is used as a convenient nonhepatic blood pool). Count rates are recorded for a 20-minute period after injection; the five- and 20-minute count rates are utilized for calculation of ^{131}I rose bengal blood clearance. Under normal circumstances, the 20-minute count rate should be no greater than 55 per cent of the five-minute value (Nordyke, 1965). Blood clearance of ^{131}I rose bengal can be slowed by both hepatocellular and extrahepatic obstructive disease, but marked reductions in clearance are considered to indicate hepatocellular disease (Fig. 5–19).

The findings considered most reliable in identifying "medical" jaundice are blood retention of 90 per cent or more at 20 minutes and/or definite passage of radioactivity into the intestines. (Such passage may be considerably delayed by intrahepatic cholestasis, hence the need for delayed imaging (at four and 24 hours) when no intestinal radioactivity can be detected at 90 minutes.) In approximately 5 per cent of instances, surgical lesions allow passage of rose bengal into the intestines; in most cases of this kind, "ball-valve" common duct calculi are ultimately found (Greene, 1972). The most conclusive evidence of extrahepatic

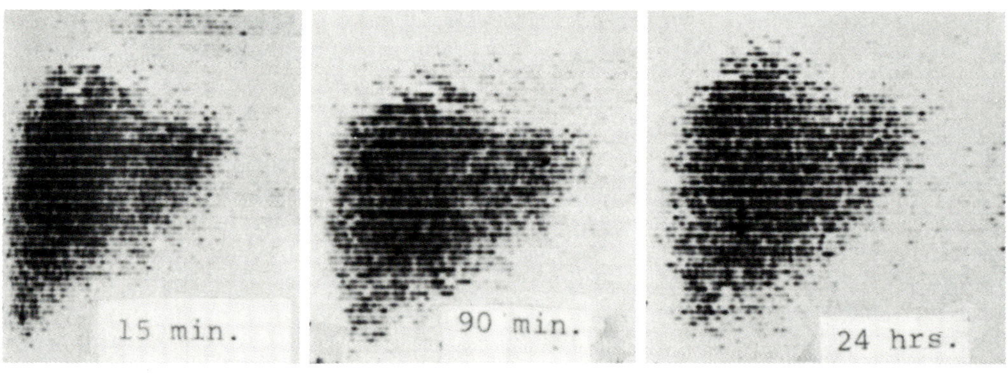

Figure 5–18. ^{131}I rose bengal abdominal scintiscans. Scans made up to 24 hours after administration of rose bengal reveal no passage of activity into the gut or gallbladder. This pattern establishes the presence of biliary obstruction but does not, by itself, distinguish between an intrahepatic (i.e., cholestatic) and an extrahepatic (i.e., surgical) pathologic condition. (From Eyler, W. R., Schuman, B. M., Du Sault, L. A., et al.: The radioiodinated rose bengal liver scan as an aid in the differential diagnosis of jaundice. Amer. J. Roentgen., *94*:469–476, 1965.)

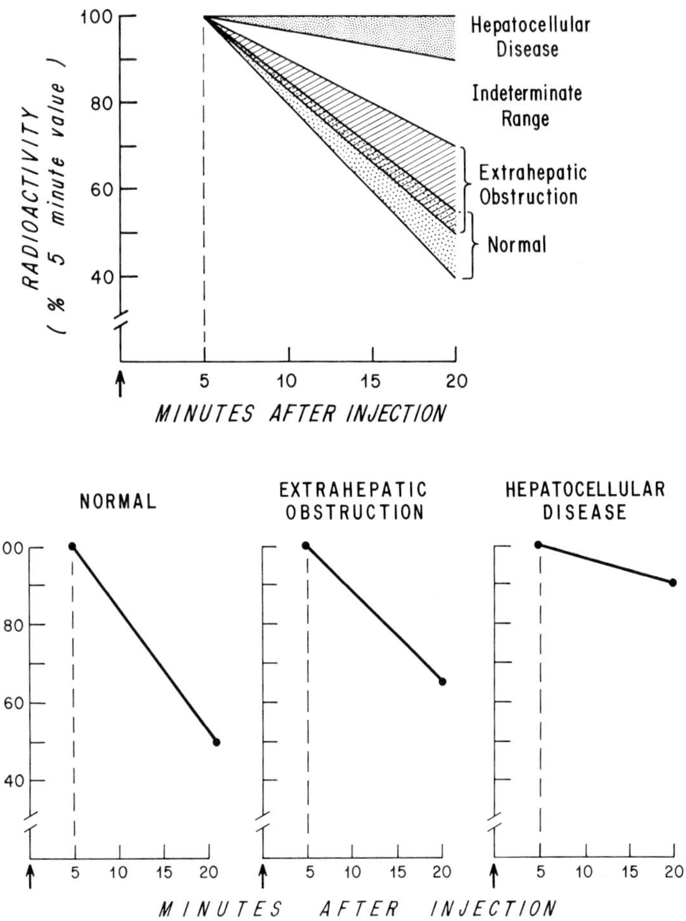

Figure 5–19. Rose bengal blood clearance rate.

A, Detector positioned over the patient's head measures the disappearance of radioactivity from the blood; hepatic uptake is the main determinant of this rate. The 20-minute value is compared with the five-minute value. If 90 per cent or more remains at 20 minutes, hepatocellular disease is most likely; if 70 per cent or less remains, extrahepatic obstruction is strongly suggested. Values that are between 70 and 90 per cent are indeterminate.

Since definite passage of radioactivity into the gut excludes surgical jaundice with 95 per cent reliability, determination of the rose bengal blood clearance rate is chiefly valuable in patients with an obstructive pattern on abdominal rose bengal imaging.

B, Typical pattern as determined in normal patients and in those with extrahepatic obstruction and hepatocellular disease.

obstruction is failure of intestinal activity to appear over 24 hours, coupled with a blood retention of 70 per cent or less. When there is elevated blood retention (e.g., 70 to 90 per cent), together with failure of ^{131}I rose bengal passage into the intestines, the pattern is considered indeterminate. Such a result may be due to "medical" diseases such as acute hepatitis, severe postnecrotic cirrhosis, or drug-induced cholestasis, but long-standing extrahepatic obstruction can produce a similar pattern (Nordyke, 1965). In a few patients who otherwise would belong to this indeterminate category, the gallbladder or extrahepatic duct system can be identified, although no passage into the intestines occurs (Fig. 5–20). This appearance is considered pathognomonic of distal common

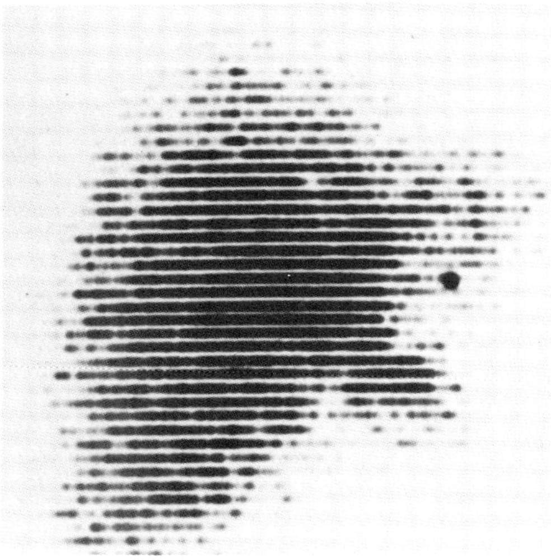

Figure 5–20. Rose bengal hepatic scintiscan. In the extrahepatic duct system or gallbladder, extension of radioactivity from the inferior margin of the liver indicates extrahepatic (surgical) obstruction, regardless of the rose bengal blood clearance rate. (From Eyler, W. R., Schuman, B. M., Du Sault, L. A., et al.: The radioiodinated rose bengal liver scan as an aid in the differential diagnosis of jaundice. Amer. J. Roentgen., *94*:469–476, 1965.)

duct obstruction, regardless of the ^{131}I rose bengal blood clearance (Freeman, 1966).

In some patients with impaired hepatic function (whether or not due to extrahepatic biliary obstruction), renal excretion of ^{131}I rose bengal occurs. The resulting appearance of radioactivity in the kidneys may be mistaken for intestinal accumulation on anterior abdominal scintiscans. In such cases, posterior imaging to reveal the degree of renal radioactivity or a delayed study (i.e., at 24 hours) to check for colonic activity should resolve the issue (Freeman, 1968).

Recent clinical studies have suggested that when a combination of serial abdominal imaging together with external blood clearance measurement is employed, remarkable diagnostic accuracy (e.g., 94 to 98 per cent) can be achieved (Freeman, 1968; Whiting, 1968; and Greene, 1972). Our own results have been less spectacular. As many as one-third of the cases seem to belong to the indeterminate category previously described (i.e., blood retention of ^{131}I rose bengal between 70 and 90 per cent, together with failure of excretion into the intestinal tract). In these instances, a confident diagnosis is not possible and further radiologic evaluation is indicated.

The degree of hepatic radiation exposure resulting from examination with radioiodinated rose bengal (1 μCi/kg.) had been calculated at 2.1 m rads when the liver was normal, and 19.8 m rads with complete biliary obstruction (Sharp, 1967). Since 150 μCi ^{131}I rose bengal is the most commonly administered dosage, the actual exposure received in a clinical setting will be roughly twice that estimated above (i.e., from 4 to 40 m rads). These values are not excessive when compared with other standard roentgen diagnostic procedures (e.g., barium enema, excretory urogram, and so forth). Oral ingestion of Lugol's solution to block thyroidal uptake of any free radioiodine is recommended.

Examination with Colloidal Radiopharmaceuticals

While radioiodinated rose bengal has been recognized as a valuable agent for examination of jaundiced patients for over a decade, the use of colloidal radiopharmaceuticals in such cases has only recently been advocated. Agents of this type (of which ^{99m}Tc sulfur colloid is currently the most popular) make a diagnostic contribution by virtue of their ability to depict dilated intrahepatic bile ducts near the porta hepatis in patients with extrahepatic biliary obstruction. In most instances, nonspecific enlargement of the zone of decreased radioactivity at the porta hepatis is observed but, occasionally, a branching pattern suggesting dilated right and left hepatic ducts can be identified (Fig. 5–21). This appearance is considered characteristic of extrahepatic obstruction. Breath-holding techniques and imaging equipment capable of tomography and/or respiratory gating increase the percentage of cases in

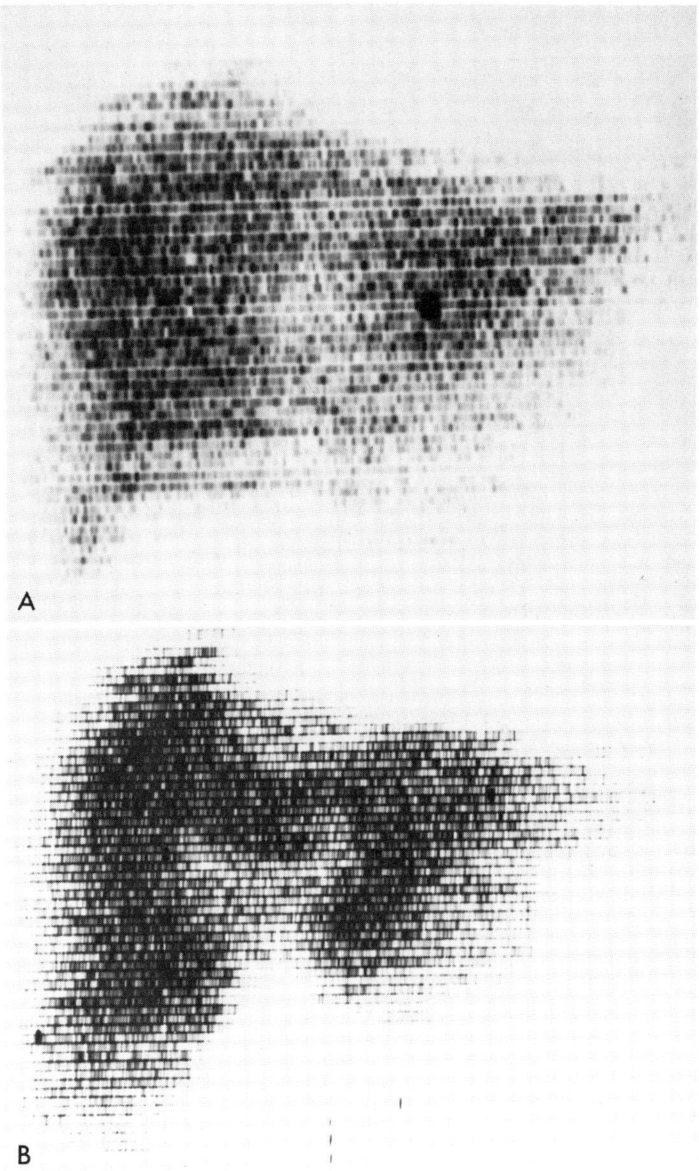

Figure 5–21. ^{99m}Tc sulfur colloid hepatic scintiscan.

A, Enlargement of the porta hepatis area. This nonspecific pattern could result from tumor in this area (either primary or secondary) or from dilated bile ducts. This patient had periampullary cancer, with dilated bile ducts in the porta hepatis and no evidence of hepatic or nodal metastasis at surgery.

B, Branching pattern characteristic of the dilated bile ducts. Extrahepatic obstruction is due to pancreatic cancer. (From DeLand, F. H., and Wagner, H. N.: Reticuloendothelial System, Liver, Spleen and Thyroid. Philadelphia, W. B. Saunders Company, 1972, p. 117.)

which the more specific branching pattern can be demonstrated.

No prospective evaluation of the accuracy of colloidal radionuclide hepatic imaging in identifying extrahepatic biliary obstruction has appeared as yet, but one carefully controlled retrospective analysis suggests that the technique is approximately 80 per cent accurate in distinguishing between hepatocellular and extrahepatic obstructive jaundice (Heck, 1971).

Discrete hepatic metastases (Fig. 5–22) and a pattern indicating hepatocellular disease (i.e., diffuse decrease in hepatic radioactivity, together with increased uptake by spleen and bone marrow) (Fig. 5–23) are additional findings which are demonstrable by ^{99m}Tc sulfur colloid hepatic imaging capable of pro-

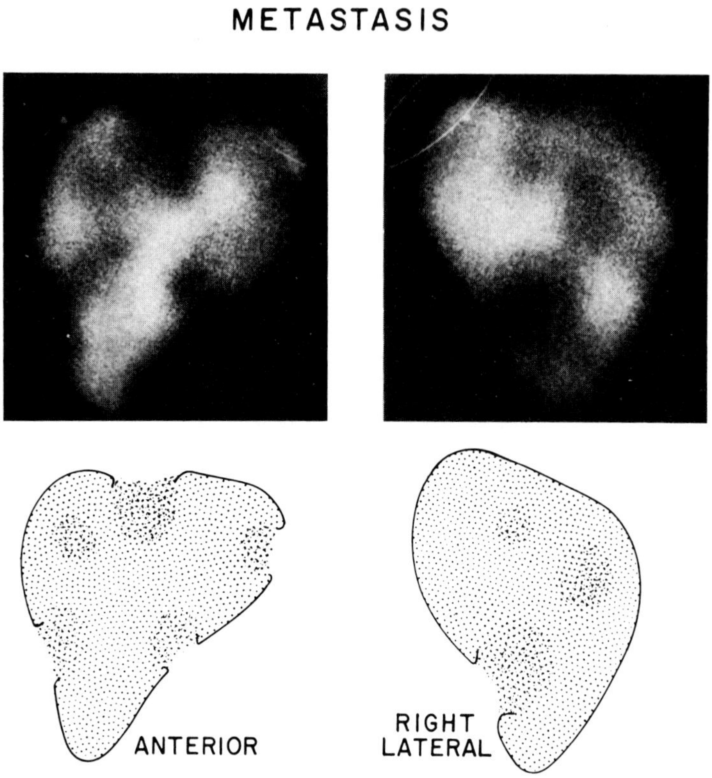

Figure 5–22. ^{99m}Tc sulfur colloid hepatic scintiscan. Hepatic metastases secondary to pancreatic cancer.

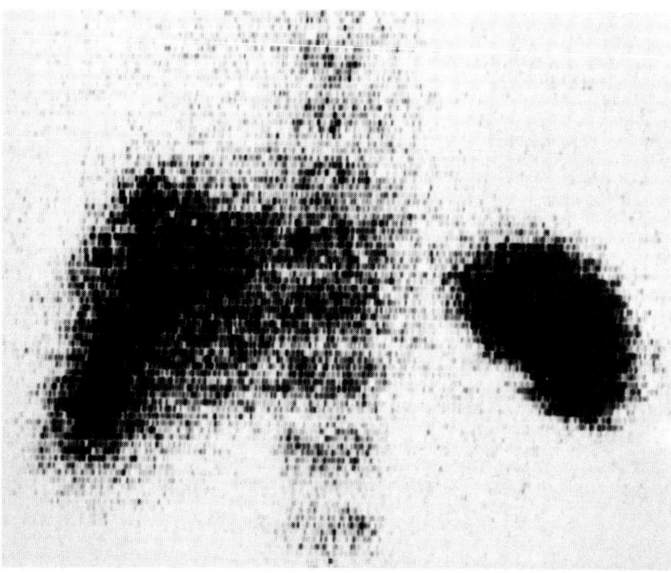

Figure 5–23. ^{99m}Tc sulfur colloid abdominal scintiscan. Nonhomogenous distribution of hepatic radioactivity, coupled with increased radioactivity in the spleen and bone marrow of the spine. This pattern is considered characteristic of hepatocellular disease.

viding significant diagnostic insight into the mechanism of jaundice in any given case. While demonstration of ductal dilatation is of more direct and specific application, these helpful, indirect signs should also be carefully sought.

PERCUTANEOUS CHOLANGIOGRAPHY

The merits and drawbacks of percutaneous cholangiography have been debated for nearly two decades. Since the chief objection to performance of this study has been fear of serious complications (of which a disturbingly large number were encountered during the early years of its employment), it is of considerable interest that an acceptably low complication rate has been reported in several recent series involving large numbers of patients (Table 5–6). (The procedural innovations presumably responsible for this improvement are discussed below.) Because of this welcome development, there has been a general trend toward increasingly widespread acceptance of the procedure in the last few years.

Successful percutaneous cholangiography can provide essential information about three related diagnostic issues which are of crucial significance in the jaundiced patient:

1. Is extrahepatic biliary obstruction present?
2. If so, where is the site of obstruction?
3. What is the nature of the obstructing process?

TABLE 5–6. Fatalities Due to Transhepatic Cholangiography in Recent Series

REFERENCE	NO. OF PATIENTS	NO. OF DEATHS
Ruzicka (1968)	66	0
Turner (1968)	115	0
Elmslie (1969)	40	0
Ritchie (1969)	54	0
Redman (1970*b*)	15	0
Weiner (1970)*	56	1
Herba (1971)	106	0
James (1971)	104	0
Machado (1971)	53	0
Ozdemir (1971)	17	0
Strack (1971)†	91	0
Greene (1972)	8	0
Teeslink (1973)	331	0
TOTAL	1,056	1

*Transjugular approach.
†"Minilaparotomy."

Is Extrahepatic Obstruction Present?

With respect to the first question, percutaneous cholangiography almost invariably provides an unequivocal answer if the biliary ducts can be opacified. In patients with hepatocellular (medical) jaundice, the intrahepatic radicals and common bile duct are of normal caliber (Fig. 5–24): common duct configuration is unremarkable – i.e., no narrowing, distortion, or cut-off is present; and contrast material passes freely into the duodenum. In patients with obstructive (surgical) jaundice, the proximal biliary tree is dilated to a point of occlusion, narrowing or other distortion, and there is little or no passage of contrast material into the duodenum (Fig. 5–25). There continues to be considerable disagreement about the significance of failure to achieve ductal opacification after four to six attempted punctures. Certain authorities (Flemma, 1963; Baum, 1971; and Teeslink, 1973) contend that this essentially excludes extrahepatic obstruction, while others (Ritchie, 1969; Turner, 1968; and Herba, 1971) maintain that unsuccessful attempts are completely inconclusive. After surveying the available literature, the authors of this monograph think that the view held by Evans (1964) is the most appropriate: failure to obtain a satisfactory cholangiogram in a jaundiced patient reduces the probability of extrahepatic obstruction, but does not exclude it and should not, of itself, preclude exploration.

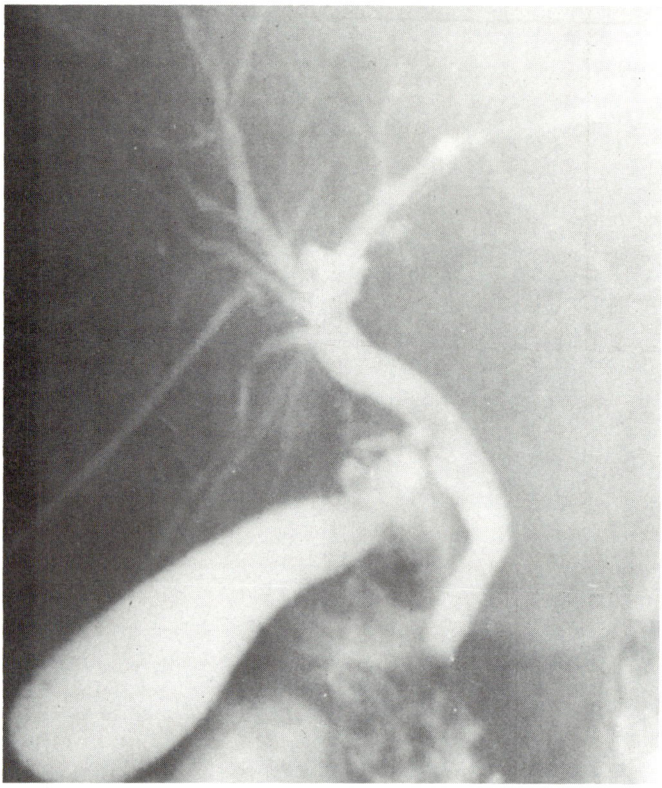

Figure 5–24. Transhepatic cholangiogram. The biliary radicals and common bile duct are nondilated; contrast passes into the duodenum. The anatomy appears normal. Cholestatic jaundice was confirmed by liver biopsy. (From Eaton, S. B., et al.: Radiologic diagnosis of extrahepatic biliary obstruction in jaundiced patients. Amer. J. Gastroent., *58*:396–405, 1972.)

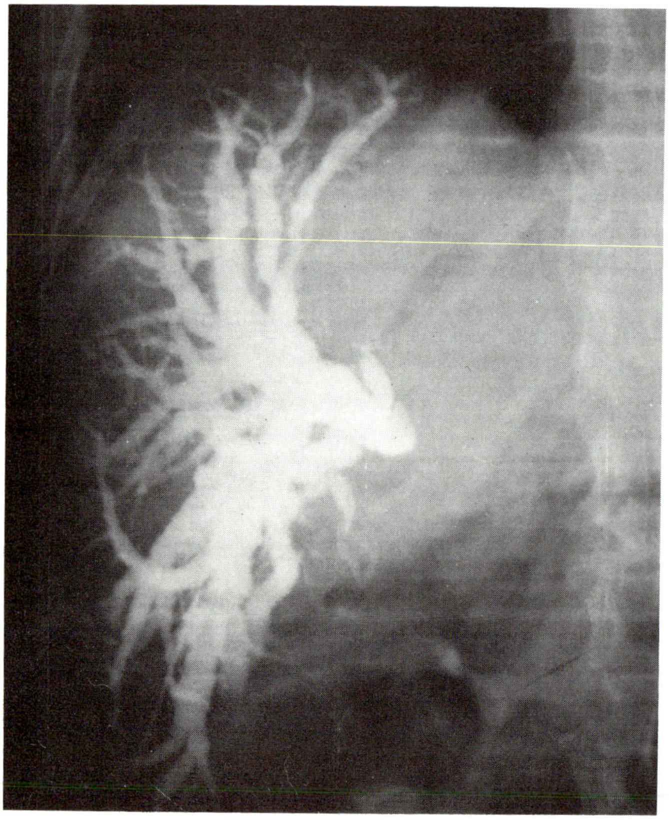

Figure 5–25. Transhepatic cholangiogram. The biliary radicals in the right lobe are dilated and the column of contrast terminates abruptly near the junction of the right and left hepatic ducts. Biliary obstruction is due to metastases in the porta hepatis from a colonic cancer.

Where is the Site of Obstruction?

With respect to the second question, successful percutaneous cholangiography nearly always demonstrates the site or level of obstruction (Fig. 5-26). This information is of major significance since it provides an opportunity for unhurried consideration of appropriate operative alternatives. Without prior knowledge, determination of the site of obstruction at celiotomy can be a difficult, lengthy task. If the point of obstruction and the type of bypass that is most likely to succeed can be determined preoperatively, literally hours of operative time can be saved. Since anesthetic morbidity and mortality are inversely related to the length of operation, preoperative determination of the site of obstruction is of significant value (Glenn, 1964; Sato, 1968).

In some circumstances, it may be desirable to leave the flexible cannula in position to allow long-term, nonsurgical decompression (Kaude, 1969). This is particularly true if blockage is demonstrated high in the porta hepatis, since attempted surgical bypass procedures under these conditions often fail.

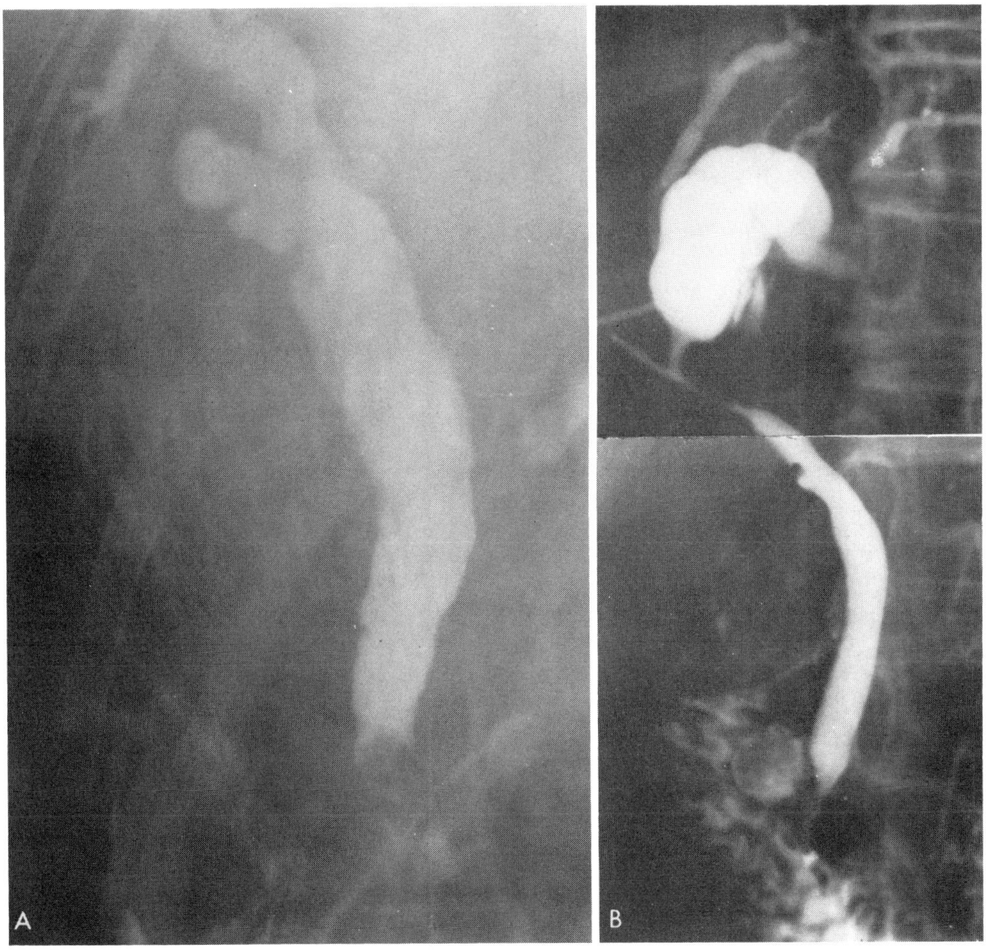

Figure 5-26. Transhepatic cholangiograms.

A, Obstruction of the distal common bile duct due to an impacted gallstone. Note the upwardly concave meniscus at the end of the contrast column. (From Eaton, S. B., et al.: Radiologic diagnosis of extrahepatic biliary obstruction in jaundiced patients. Amer. J. Gastroent., *58*:396-405, 1972.)

B, Two fluoroscopic "spot" films spliced to demonstrate the anatomy. Incompletely obstructing process at the junction of the right and left hepatic ducts. Gallbladder carcinoma.

What is Causing Obstruction?

When an obstructing process is demonstrated, the radiographic features present may or may not allow identification of its exact nature. An impacted calculus typically creates a deeply concave meniscus (Fig. 5–27) at the site of obstruction, while a funnel-like, "rat-tail," or asymmetric tapering suggests malignancy as does a raggedly irregular distal margin (Fig. 5–28). Chronic pancreatitis often produces a long, undulating, tapered narrowing of the distal common duct (Fig. 5–29), whereas complete obstruction high in the porta hepatis almost always indicates malignancy (often metastatic lymphadenopathy) (Fig. 5–30). These patterns are all highly suggestive but not completely diagnostic, and most extensive series include at least a few exceptions. Furthermore, in some instances, the appearance of the obstructing segment is quite nonspecific (Fig. 5–31). In these cases, the nature of the obstructing process cannot be determined.

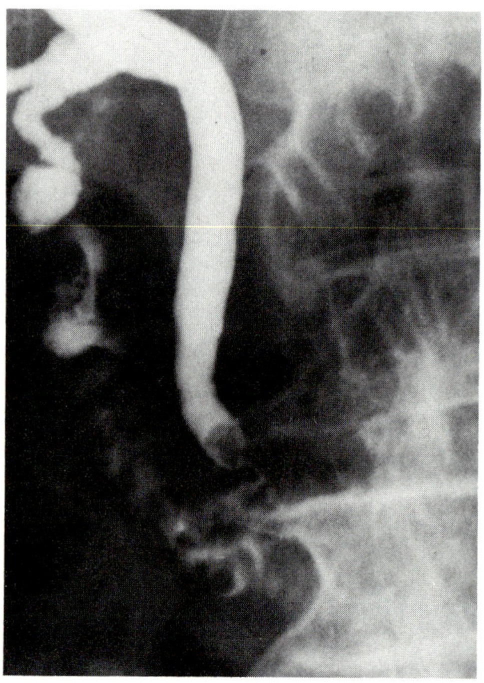

Figure 5–27. Transhepatic cholangiogram. Incompletely obstructing gallstone outlined by a contrast in the common bile duct. The upper margin of the stone produces a meniscus-like defect.

Technique

The optimal puncture site for percutaneous transhepatic cholangiography is hotly debated but, otherwise, there is fairly general consensus concerning technique. A 6- or 8-inch, 18- to 21-gauge needle assembly, with an outer teflon sleeve and a rigid inner metallic core, is employed (e.g., B-D Longdwell T^{m}). While the patient briefly suspends respiration, the needle is introduced; the inner core is then quickly withdrawn, leaving only the flexible teflon cannula in place when respiration is resumed. Position is checked fluoroscopically and the cannula is slowly withdrawn as repeated attempts are made to aspirate bile. When aspiration is successful, as much bile as possible is removed and water soluble contrast material gently introduced under fluoroscopic observation. When the biliary tree is opacified down to the level of obstruction, fluoroscopic roentgenograms are exposed. In most instances, only a predetermined number of needle passes (usually four to six) are made if aspiration is repeatedly unsuccessful. It is frequently helpful to gently inject contrast material while withdrawing the cannula during the last two or three passes. This technique often will allow identification of ducts where aspiration of bile has been unsuccessful. This has been true especially when the ducts are not dilated. When the ducts are dilated, cannulation can be achieved in approximately 80 to 90 per cent, but when ductal caliber is normal, the success rate falls to 40 to 50 per cent or less (Turner, 1968; Ritchie, 1969; Herba, 1971; and Teeslink, 1973).

Puncture sites, ranging from the posterior right axillary line all the way around the right lower rib cage near to the xiphoid, have been advocated for transhepatic cholangiography. While an inspection of available data suggests that none of these has a significantly better rate of ductal opacification or a lower incidence of complications, the authors have come to prefer a point in the right

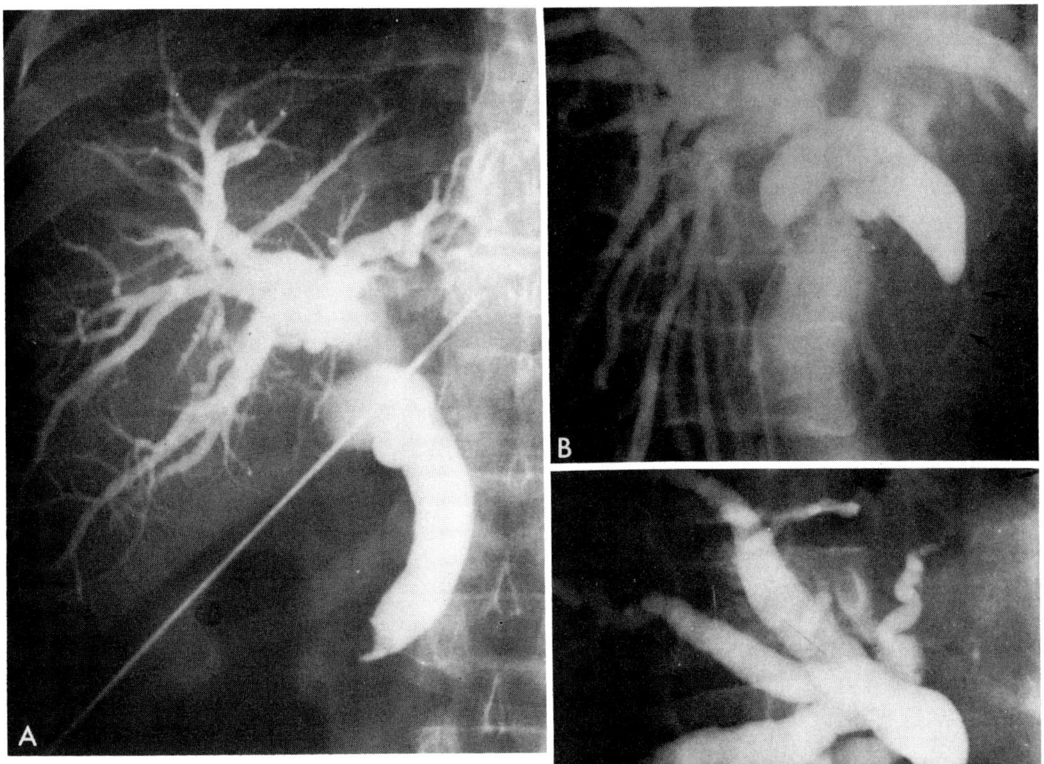

Figure 5–28. Transhepatic cholangiograms.
A, Periampullary carcinoma produces an irregular funnel-like tapered obstruction of the distal common bile duct.
B, Pancreatic cancer produces a "rat-tail" deformity of the common bile duct (*arrows*).
C, Carcinoma of the common bile duct produces a raggedly irregular obstruction of the common hepatic duct.

mid clavicular line immediately below the costal margin. Weiner and Hanafee (1970) have developed a transjugular approach for cholangiography. This method eliminates the necessity of puncturing the liver capsule, but is technically somewhat more demanding and has not, as yet, been proved to produce either a higher rate of successful biliary cannulation or a lower rate of complications. While bile leakage and intraperitoneal bleeding have been less common than with transperitoneal puncture techniques, septicemia appears to occur somewhat more often.

Strack and his co-workers (1971) have devised a still more elaborate approach. They make a 5-cm. midline subxiphoid incision (colloquially termed a "mini-laparotomy") under local anesthesia in the Radiology Department, then perform transhepatic cholangiography under direct visualization and fluoroscopic control. Successful opacification of the biliary tree has been achieved in all cases in which obstructed ducts were present and in two-thirds of those patients without obstruction. The puncture site(s) are sutured after removal of the cannula, thus diminishing the incidence of hemorrhage and bile leakage. Omentoportography and/or liver biopsy can also be performed, if desired, via the same incision.

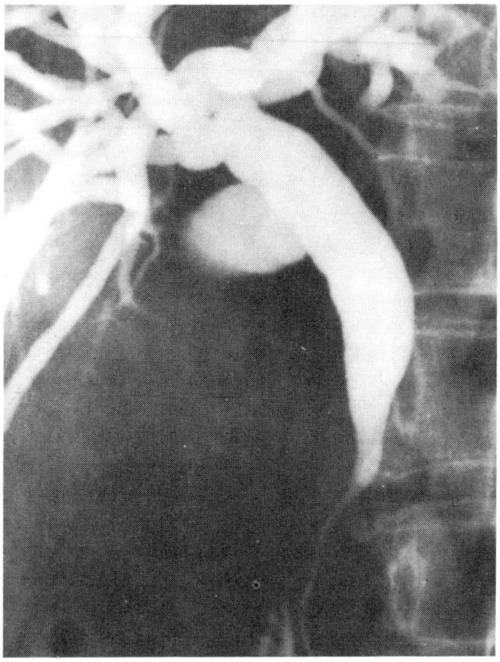

Figure 5–29. Transhepatic cholangiogram. Chronic pancreatitis produces long, tapered, undulating, incomplete narrowing of the distal common bile duct. Note the contrast material in the duodenum, which distinguishes this condition from "rat-tailing" (see Fig. 5–28,*B*) in which obstruction is nearly always complete. Chronic pancreatitis seldom produces complete obstruction.

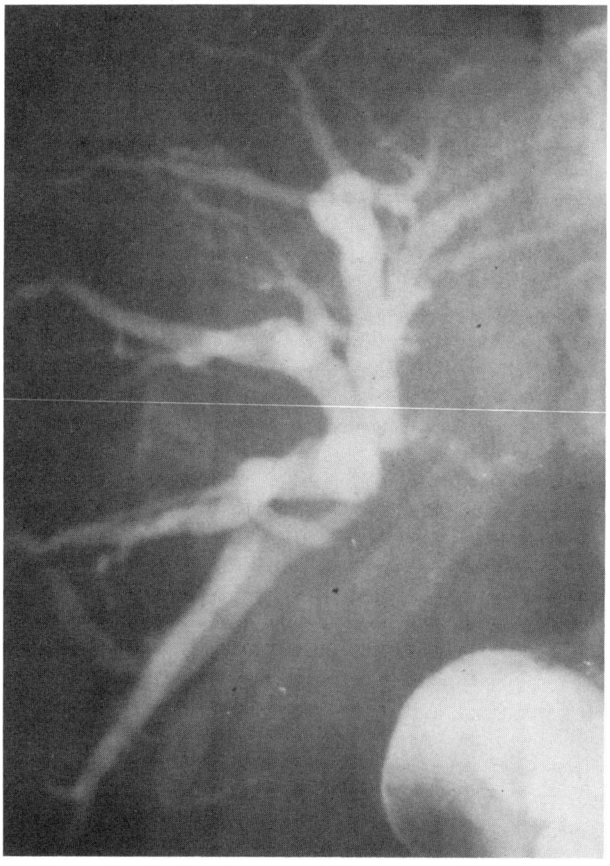

Figure 5–30. Transhepatic cholangiogram. Metastases (from pancreatic cancer) produce biliary obstruction high in the porta hepatis. A faint "rat tail" is present. The contrast in the right lower corner is residual barium. (From Eaton, S. B., et al.: Radiologic diagnosis of extrahepatic biliary obstruction in jaundiced patients. Amer. J. Gastroent., 58:396–405, 1972.)

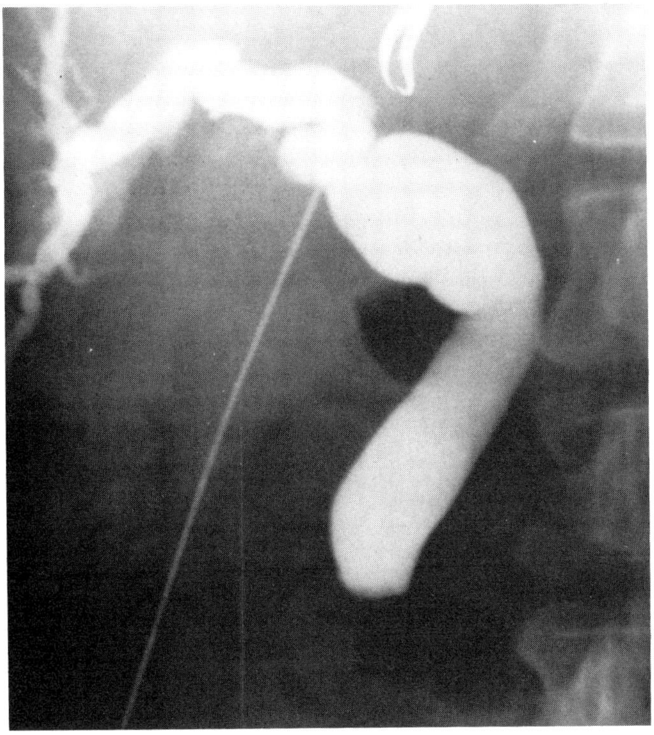

Figure 5-31. Transhepatic cholangiogram. Nonspecific complete obstruction of the distal common bile duct was found at surgery to be the result of periampullary cancer. A specific cholangiographic diagnosis is hazardous in this instance.

Complications

The most feared complications of percutaneous cholangiography include intraperitoneal hemorrhage, bile peritonitis and septicemia. Pneumothorax, inadvertent puncture of viscera adjacent to the liver, and perihepatic abscess are other occasionally encountered misadventures.

Most reported deaths have been due either to hemorrhage or septicemia. Mujahed and Evans (1966) were able to find reports of four deaths in 811 attempted studies up to that time and therefore estimated a fatality rate of 0.5 per cent. An analysis of series reported from 1968 to 1972 reveals only one death in a total of 1056 cases (0.1 per cent) (Table 5-6). Serious bleeding generally has been the result of hepatic laceration, but use of a flexible teflon cannula appears to have diminished the incidence of such injury. Of course, an incorrectably elevated prothrombin time is considered a contraindication for percutaneous cholangiography. Septicemia results chiefly from establishment of bile-blood fistulae along the puncture tract (Koch, 1969). Since intraductal pressure within an obstructed biliary tree usually exceeds hepatic venous pressure (Wiechel, 1964) flow through an iatrogenic fistula will be from the liver into the general circulation. Bile is commonly infected in patients with biliary obstruction (Flemma, 1965) and the resulting bacteremia may progress to septicemia and septic shock.

The incidence of such sequelae can be decreased by prophylactic administration of broad spectrum antibiotics (beginning 12 to 24 hours prior to the procedure), by considering fever as a contraindication, and by withdrawing as much bile as possible via the cannula to produce a relative biliary decompression. There is a tendency toward bile leakage via the puncture tract in all patients with obstruction in whom ductal cannulation is actually achieved. Progression of such leakage to actual bile peritonitis can be prevented by biliary decompression via the cannula and by prompt postprocedural surgery.

An increasing number of advocates now suggest that percutaneous cholangiography need not be confined to the immediate preoperative period (e.g., Teeslink, 1973), but the authors of this monograph still think that it should be performed only in patients scheduled for surgery immediately thereafter, since prompt surgery will ordinarily allow correction of any complications which might develop. If cholangiography reveals nondilated ducts and no evidence of obstruction, surgery is deferred and the patient is placed under close surveillance for 48 hours.

ANGIOGRAPHY AND ULTRASONOGRAPHY

Angiography

Angiographic demonstration of pancreaticoduodenal malignancy is discussed in a separate chapter but, naturally, when a tumor (or pseudocyst) is located by angiographic study in a position to produce obstruction of the common bile duct, the cause of jaundice in an icteric patient is essentially established. A less well-known application of angiography to the study of jaundiced patients lies in direct demonstration of gallbladder size. Celiac and especially hepatic arterial injections commonly produce opacification of the gallbladder wall during the parenchymal phase, and the course of the cystic artery is only slightly less helpful in identifying gallbladder enlargement (Fig. 5–32). By studying these parameters, Redman and Reuter (1970*a*) were able to prospectively identify gallbladder enlargement in nearly 90 per cent of their patients. While the angiographic limits of normal gallbladder size have not been precisely defined, these two investigators chose a width of 5 cm. as their upper normal value and, until a more extensive analysis is presented, this figure seems a reasonable one. As previously discussed, gallbladder enlargement in jaundiced patients correlates well with malignant obstruction of the distal common bile duct.

In addition to demonstrating pancreaticoduodenal malignancy, pancreatic pseudocyst, and gallbladder dilatation, angiographic studies in jaundiced patients may also demonstrate hepatic metastasis and evidence of hepatic cirrhosis. While these findings (like gallbladder enlargement) do not absolutely or precisely establish the mechanism of jaundice, they are of considerable diagnostic significance.

Ultrasonography

Ultrasonic techniques and their application to the field of pancreaticobiliary diagnosis also form the basis for a separate chapter. While this method of examination is not yet fully developed, it is clear that pseudocysts, some cancers, and inflammatory edema in the head of the pancreas are all amenable to ultrasonic demonstration (Filly, 1970; Holm, 1971). Furthermore, most normal gallbladders and nearly all those which are enlarged can be clearly represented on longitudinal and transverse ultrasonic sections of the upper abdomen (Holm, 1971) (Fig. 5–33). In some cases, dilated bile ducts at the porta hepatis can also be depicted on ultrasonic sections (Suruga, 1969). While the ultimate clinical importance of echography in jaundiced patients has not been established, the apparent potential of the technique seems impressive.

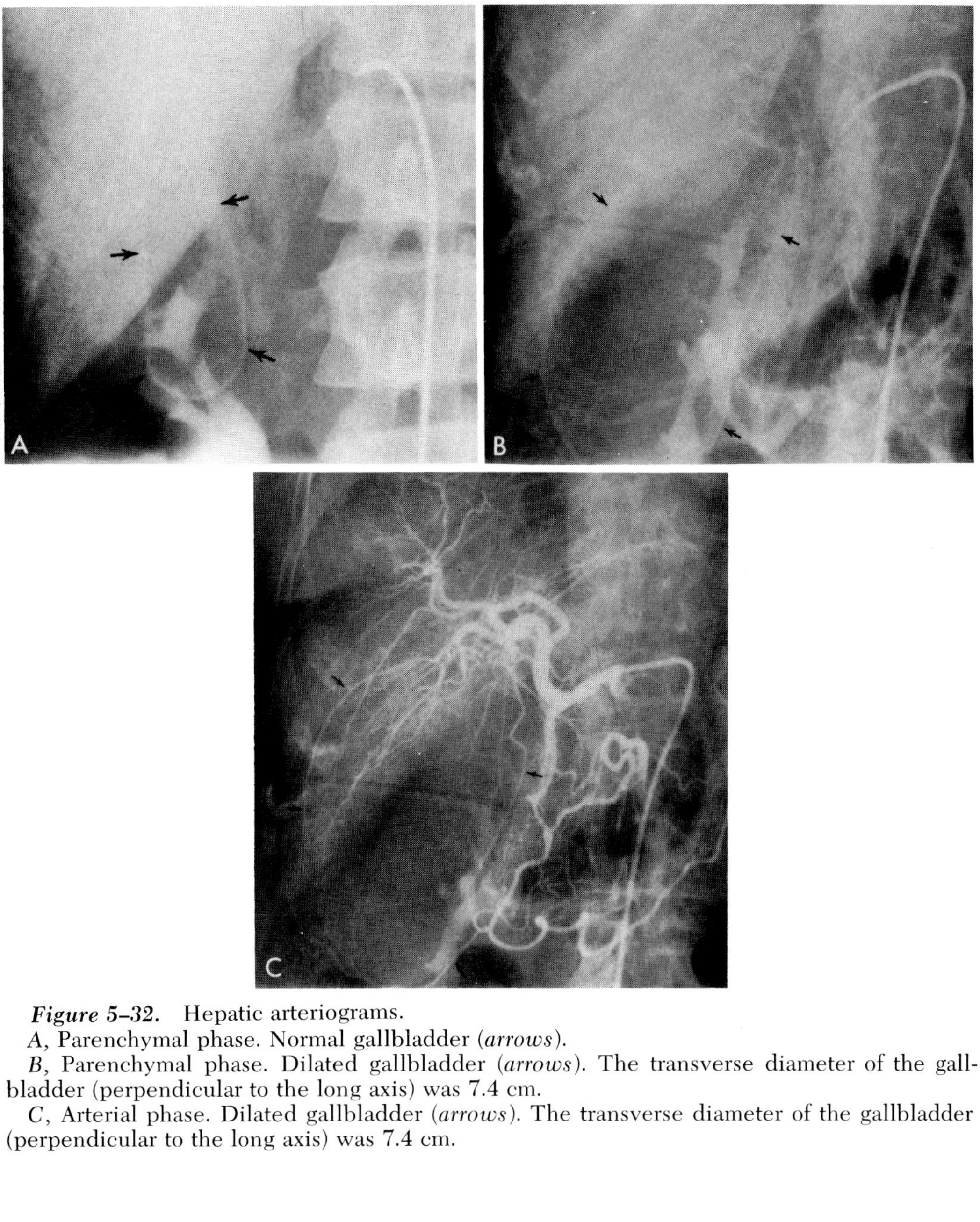

Figure 5–32. Hepatic arteriograms.

A, Parenchymal phase. Normal gallbladder (*arrows*).

B, Parenchymal phase. Dilated gallbladder (*arrows*). The transverse diameter of the gallbladder (perpendicular to the long axis) was 7.4 cm.

C, Arterial phase. Dilated gallbladder (*arrows*). The transverse diameter of the gallbladder (perpendicular to the long axis) was 7.4 cm.

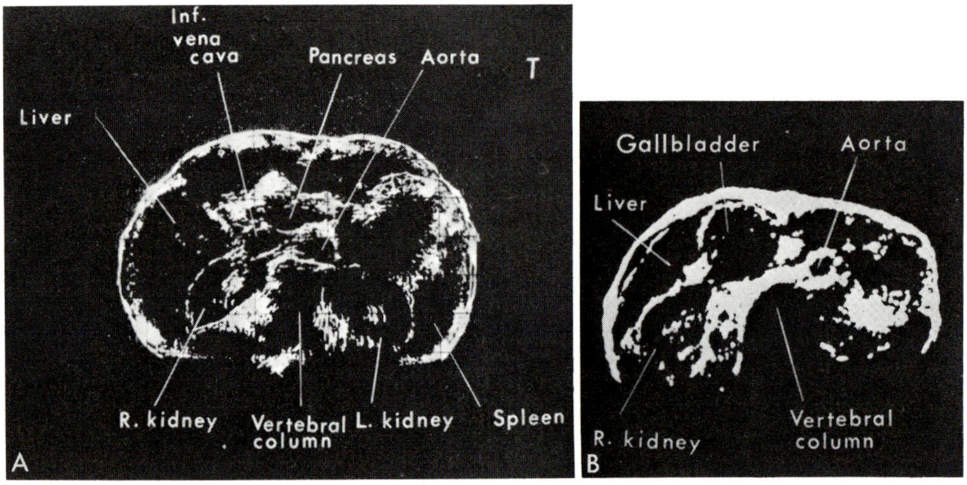

Figure 5–33. Transverse upper abdominal ultrasonic sections. *A*, Normal anatomy; *B*, dilated gallbladder. (From Holm, H. H.: Ultrasonic scanning in the diagnosis of space-occupying lesions of the upper abdomen. Brit. J. Radiol., *44*:24–36, 1971.)

STRATEGY FOR RADIOLOGIC EVALUATION OF JAUNDICE

An ideal plan for intelligent utilization of the various radiologic techniques available for evaluation of jaundiced patients must represent a compromise between three guiding principles. The first is patient *safety*. Ideally, the least dangerous procedures would be utilized first, with more hazardous studies held in reserve. The second is diagnostic *accuracy*. Those studies most likely to distinguish correctly between "surgical" and "medical" jaundice should be employed at the beginning of the work-up. Finally, the diagnostic protocol should be as *economical* as possible in terms of both cost and time. These general principles must be made to fit the clinical setting of the individual case. For example, patients with intermittent or low-grade hyperbilirubinemia are often candidates for procedures (e.g., intravenous cholangiography) not practicable in patients with persistent, severe jaundice. Another example might be the patient with severe peripheral atherosclerotic disease in whom angiographic study carries a somewhat higher risk of morbidity. Finally, the patient with incorrectable prolongation of prothrombin time belongs to a high risk category for percutaneous transhepatic cholangiography, and this study is ordinarily considered contraindicated under such circumstances.

While such considerations may influence the selection of procedures in certain individual instances, it is still possible to draw up an idealized format for radiologic evaluation of jaundice applicable in most situations. Although the recommended examinations should be employed in a specific sequence, it is not intended that each study be utilized for every patient. Once the desired information has been ascertained, the sequence is to be terminated and the appropriate therapy instituted without reference to further, superfluous examinations.

Outpatient Diagnostic Procedures

In the opinion of the authors, the initial radiologic examinations for evaluation of jaundiced patients are best performed on an outpatient basis. This approach has two economic advantages. First, a significant portion of the patient's work-up can be performed (and, in many cases, the diagnosis established) prior to hospitalization. In itself, this constitutes a significant saving. Second, barium studies (such as hypotonic duodenography) can be performed without fear of prolonging hospitalization merely to clear the bowel of barium in preparation for angiographic study.

Radioiodinated Rose Bengal Examination

The initial outpatient visit should be for administration of radioiodinated rose bengal, determination of blood clearance, and performance of early-phase abdominal imaging. If radioactivity appears in the gut, "medical" disease can be diagnosed with approximately 95 per cent confidence and further radiologic procedures canceled. If no intestinal activity is demonstrated, a second appointment is made 24 hours later. For this visit, the patient should be fasted in anticipation of possible study by hypotonic duodenography. Follow-up abdominal scintigraphy is the first item on the second day's agenda since demonstration of intestinal radioactivity may be considerably delayed in certain patients with cholestatic jaundice. If there is still no radioactivity in the intestinal tract, however, further investigation depends largely on the rose bengal blood clearance, determined during the first visit. If retention of ^{131}I rose bengal was 90 per cent or greater and the clinical course of jaundice has been brief (i.e., duration of less than ten days), "medical" disease can be diagnosed (again with approximately 95 per cent confidence) and the radiologic investigation discontinued. If jaundice has been present for longer than ten days, or if rose bengal retention is less than 90 per cent, further evaluation by means of hypotonic duodenography is recommended. If blood retention is 70 per cent or less, extrahepatic obstruction can be diagnosed with approximately 95 per cent confidence, but further radiologic investigation is recommended to better define the disease present.

Hypotonic Duodenography

The authors advocate hypotonic duodenography rather than conventional upper gastrointestinal examination for evaluation of jaundiced patients since, at the conclusion of duodenography, a reasonably satisfactory study of the stomach can be simply performed. Inhibition of gastric peristalsis seems an acceptable price to pay for optimal demonstration of the duodenum—the area of major clinical concern in such patients. This approach obviates the need for re-examination by hypotonic duodenography in circumstances in which conventional barium studies have shown questionable abnormalities. The over-all benefit is considered to outweigh the slightly increased cost and time required for hypotonic examination.

When duodenography is considered desirable, it is performed immediately after the 24-hour abdominal rose bengal image is obtained and analyzed. If the barium study is unrevealing, no diagnostic inference is justified although the likelihood of extrahepatic obstructive jaundice is somewhat reduced. On the other hand, should an anatomic lesion in the pancreaticoduodenal area be demonstrated, a potential site (and, in many instances, the pathologic nature of the obstructing process) can be established. When a mass lesion in the pancreaticoduodenal area is demonstrated in patients with jaundice, immediate progression to surgery is recommended by some authorities (Meyerowitz, 1968). An example might be the situation in which clinical and radiologic findings are entirely in accord with an impacted common duct calculus. In most circumstances, however, the authors of this monograph think that further diagnostic evaluation is of significant value, a position also adopted by Sato (1968) and Strack (1971). Additional diagnostic studies are also required when hypotonic duodenography has failed to reveal an anatomic abnormality.

Inpatient Diagnostic Procedures

Angiography

The next stages of radiologic evaluation require hospitalization which should begin several days after study by hypotonic duodenography. At this point, barium will have been cleared from the bowel and angiography can be performed on the first full hospital day. In those patients in whom hypotonic duodenography was negative, angiography sometimes reveals tumors (e.g., of the gallbladder, common bile duct or, rarely, the pancreas) located in a position to produce jaundice without causing demonstrable abnormality of the duodenum. In patients in whom hypotonic duodenography has revealed a mass lesion, angiographic study more fully defines the extent of the process and also indicates the status of adjacent vascular structures. Hepatic metastasis can also be shown in some instances. Finally, angiographic study ordinarily demonstrates gallbladder size. In most instances, the presence of an enlarged gallbladder suggests that surgical bypass procedures (either cholecystojejunostomy or choledochojejunostomy) will be reasonably simple and that the technically difficult bypass procedures necessitated by obstruction high in the porta hepatis area will probably not be required.

Transhepatic Cholangiography

When radiologic examination has been negative or indeterminate up to this point, it is logical to proceed with transhepatic cholangiography. Small choledochal tumors, choledocholithiasis, and metastatic processes in the porta hepatis may all produce obstruction and yet defy efforts at detection by barium studies and angiography. In such cases (i.e., in which biliary obstruction and ductal dilatation are actually present), transhepatic cholangiography has an excellent (80 per cent) likelihood of demonstrating the disease. In other circumstances in which a pathologic process has been clearly demonstrated by any other previously employed procedures, transhepatic cholangiography may still be of value by demonstrating a level of blockage proximal to that suggested by the less definitive studies. For example, periampullary tumors may be associated with undetected metastases to the porta hepatis area. Such metastases usually require a difficult proximal bypass procedure, the necessity for which may not have been identified by either duodenography or angiography. When jaundice results from hepatocellular disease, transhepatic cholangiography may be of aid by demonstrating nondilated bile ducts. In such instances, likelihood of ductal opacification approaches 50 per cent.

When it proves impossible to achieve biliary ductal opacification by means of transhepatic cholangiography, the authors feel no meaningful diagnostic inference can be drawn. Our recommendation under these circumstances is for either exploratory surgery or liver biopsy. Either of these procedures can be carried out on the second full hospital day immediately after attempted percutaneous cholangiography.

CONCLUSION

The sequence of examinations described in the preceding paragraphs is applicable to the great majority of patients who present with significant jaundice and in whom distinction between hepatocellular disease and extrahepatic biliary obstruction is not clinically apparent. Radiology as currently practiced can provide accurate, detailed information about the nature of nearly all obstructing processes and can definitively exclude extrahepatic obstruction in those instances in which it is absent. The sequence of examinations described is designed to provide such clear-cut diagnostic information as rapidly and economically as possible, with a minimum of patient morbidity and mortality.

REFERENCES

Baum, S.: Personal communication, 1971.

Culver, P. J.: Tests related to the liver and biliary systems. *In* A Syllabus of Laboratory Examinations in Clinical Diagnosis. Edited by L. B. Page and P. J. Culver. Cambridge, Mass., Harvard Univ. Press, 1961, pp. 406–407.

Datta, D. V., Sherlock, S., and Scheuer, P. J.: Postnecrotic cirrhosis with chronic cholestasis. Gut, *4*:223–230, 1963.

Davis, W. D.: Liver function in disease and in preoperative evaluation. *In* Current Gastro-

enterology. Edited by D. McHardy. New York, Paul B. Hoeber, Inc., 1962, pp. 418–424.
Eaton, S. B., Ferrucci, J. T., Benedict, K. T., and Margulis, A. F.: Diagnosis of choledocholithiasis by barium duodenal examination. Radiology, *102*:267–273, 1972*a*.
Eaton, S. B., Ferrucci, J. T., Margulis, A. F., and Weens, H. S.: Unfamiliar roentgen findings in pancreatic disease. Amer. J. Roentgen., *116*: 396–405, 1972*b*).
Elmslie, R. G., and Newstead, G.: The place of percutaneous cholangiography in managing the jaundiced patient. Postgrad. Med., *46*:89–94, 1969.
Evans, J. A.: Specialized technics in investigation of abdominal diseases. Radiology, *82*:578–594, 1964.
Eyler, W. R.: An evaluation of roentgen signs of pancreatic enlargement. J.A.M.A., *181*:967–971, 1962.
Filly, R. A., and Freimanis, A. K.: Echographic diagnosis of pancreatic lesions. Radiology, *96*:575–582, 1970.
Flemma, R. J., Capp, M. P., and Shingleton, W. W.: Percutaneous transhepatic cholangiography. Arch. Surg., *90*:5–10, 1965.
Flemma, R. J., Schauble, J. F., Gardner, C. E., Anlyan, W. G., and Capp, M. P.: Percutaneous transhepatic cholangiography in the differential diagnosis of jaundice. Surg. Gynec. Obstet., *116*:559–568, 1963.
Freeman, L. M., Kay, C. J.: Radioactive rose bengal abdominal scanning in jaundiced patients. New Jork J. Med., *66*:1778–1781, 1966.
Freeman, L. M., Kay, C. J., and Derman, A.: Renal excretion of radioiodinated rose bengal: a pitfall in the interpretation of rose bengal abdominal scans. J. Nucl. Med., 9:227–232, 1968.
Glenn, F., and Thorbjarnarsom, B.: Carcinoma of the pancreas. Ann. Surg., *159*:945–958, 1964.
Greene, A. G., Sadowsky, N. L.: A radiologic approach to the differential diagnosis of surgical and non-surgical jaundice. Amer. J. Roentgen., *116*:368–374, 1972.
Harville, D. D., and Summerskill, W. H. J.: Surgery in acute hepatitis. J.A.M.A., *184*:257–261, 1963.
Heck, L. L., and Gottschalk, A.: The appearance of intrahepatic biliary duct dilatation on the liver scan. Radiology, *99*:135–140, 1971.
Herba, M. J., and Kiss, J.: Percutaneous transhepatic cholangiography. Experience with 106 examinations. J. Canad. Ass. Radiol., *22*: 22–29, 1971.
Hess, W.: Surgery of the Biliary Passages and the Pancreas. Princeton, N. J., D. Van Nostrand Company, Inc., 1965, pp. 62 and 125.
Holm, H. H.: Ultrasonic scanning in the diagnosis of space-occupying lesions of the upper abdomen. Brit. J. Radiol., *44*:24–36, 1971.
Howard, J. M.: Pancreatic calcification. *In* Surgical Diseases of the Pancreas. Edited by J. M. Howard and G. L. Jordon. Philadelphia, J. B. Lippincott Company, 1960. pp. 203–222.
James, M.: Normal or "negative" percutaneous cholangiogram. Arch. Surg., *103*:31–33, 1971.
Kaude, J. V., Weidenmier, C. H., and Agee, O. F.: Decompression of bile ducts with percutaneous transhepatic technic. Radiology, *93*: 67–71, 1969.
Koch, R. L., and Borden, J. L.: Bile-blood fistula: a complication of percutaneous transhepatic cholangiography. Radiology, *93*:67–68, 1969.
Machado, A. L.: Percutaneous transhepatic cholangiography. Brit. J. Surg., *58*:616–624, 1971.
Meyerowitz, B. R.: The misuse of percutaneous transhepatic cholangiography. Surg. Gynec. Obstet., *127*:1318–1319, 1968.
Mujahed, Z., and Evans, J. A.: Percutaneous transhepatic cholangiography. Radiol. Clin. N. Amer., *4*:535–545, 1966.
Nordyke, R. A.: Surgical vs. nonsurgical jaundice: differentiation by a combination of rose bengal I^{131} and standard liver-function tests. J.A.M.A., *194*:949–953, 1965.
Ozdemir, A. I., and Lancaster, J. R.: Percutaneous transhepatic cholangiography. Arch. Surg., *103*:684–687, 1971.
Perez, C. A., Powers, W. E., Holtz, S., and Spjut, H. J.: Roentgenologic-pathologic correlation of resectable carcinoma of the pancreaticoduodenal region. Amer. J. Roentgen., *94*:438–448, 1965.
Phillips, G. B., and Davidson, C. S.: Liver disease of the chronic alcoholic simulating extrahepatic biliary obstruction. Gastroenterology, *33*:236–244, 1957.
Poppel, M. H.: Duodenocolic apposition. Amer. J. Roentgen., *83*:851–856, 1960.
Redman, H. C., and Reuter, S. R.: The angiographic evaluation of gallbladder dilatation. Radiology, *97*:367–370, 1970*a*.
Redman, H. C., Reuter, S. R., and Joseph, R. R.: Roentgenographic evaluation of patients with suspected obstructive jaundice. Surg. Gynec. Obstet., *131*:1100–1104, 1970*b*.
Ritchie, G. W., Jackson, D. C., and Eaglesham, H.: Percutaneous transhepatic cholangiography: experience with 54 cases. Canad. Med. Ass. J., *100*:110–116, 1969.
Ruzicka, F. F., and Sanchez-Ubeda, R.: Percutaneous transhepatic cholangiography. New York J. Med., *68*:3034–3039, 1968.
Sahler, O. D., and Hampton, A. O.: The roentgen appearance of common duct stone. Amer. J. Roentgen., *52*:298–302, 1944.
Salzman, E.: Opacification of bile duct calculi. Radiol. Clin. N. Amer., *4*:525–533, 1966.
Samuel, E.: The cystogastrocolic band: radiologic considerations. Brit. J. Radiol., *25*:19–21, 1952.
Sarles, H., Sarles, J. C., Camatte, R., Muratore, R., Gaini, M., Guien, C., Pastor, J., and LeRoy, F.: Observations on 205 confirmed cases of acute pancreatitis, recurring pancreatitis, and chronic pancreatitis. Gut, *6*:545–559, 1965.
Sato, T., Saitoh, Y., Koyama, K., and Watanabe, K.: Preoperative determination of operability in carcinomas of the pancreas and the periampullary region. Ann. Surg., *168*:867–886, 1968.
Shaldon, S., and Sherlock, S.: Viral hepatitis with features of prolonged bile retention. Brit. Med. J., *2*:734–738, 1957.

Sharp, H. L., Krivit, W., and Lowman, J. T.: The diagnosis of complete extrahepatic obstruction by rose bengal I^{131}. J. Pediat., *70*:46–53, 1967.

Sherlock, S.: Jaundice. Brit. Med. J., *1*:1359–1366, 1962.

Smith, R., and Sherlock, S.: Surgery of the Gallbladder and Bile Ducts. London, Butterworth & Company, 1964, p. 86.

Strack, P. R., Newman, H. K., Lerner, A. G., Green, S. H., Meng, C-H, Del Guercio, L. R. M., and State, D.: An integrated procedure for the rapid diagnosis of biliary obstruction, portal hypertension and liver disease of uncertain etiology. New Eng. J. Med., *285*:1225–1231, 1971.

Suruga, K., Kirai, Y., Nagashima, K., Wagai, T., and Inui, M.: Ultrasonic echo examinations as an aid in diagnosis of congenital bile duct lesions. J. Pediat. Surg., *4*:542, 1969.

Teeslink, R., Brown, S. W., and Pool, W. H.: Percutaneous cholangiography: a neglected diagnostic tool. Amer. J. Roentgen. (In press, 1973.)

Turner, F. E., and Costopoulous, L. B.: Percutaneous transhepatic cholangiography. A study of 115 cases. Canad. Med. Ass. J., *99*:513–521, 1968.

Weiner, M., and Hanafee, W. N.: A review of transjugular cholangiography. Radiol. Clin. N. Amer., *8*:53–68, 1970.

Weinstein, B. R., Korn, R. J., and Zimmerman, H. J.: Obstructive jaundice as a complication of pancreatitis. Ann. Intern. Med., *58*:245–258, 1963.

Whiting, E. G., and Nusynowitz, M. L.: Radioactive rose bengal testing in the differential diagnosis of jaundice. Surg. Gynec. Obstet., *127*:729–733, 1968.

Wiechel, K. L.: Percutaneous transhepatic cholangiography: technique and application. With studies of the hepatic venous and biliary duct pressure, the chemical changes in blood and bile and clinical results in a series of jaundiced patients. Acta Chir. Scand.: Suppl. 330, 1–99, 1964.

Wise, R. E.: Intravenous Cholangiography. Springfield, Ill., Charles C Thomas, Publisher, 1962.

Chapter 6

RADIONUCLIDE PANCREATOGRAPHY

Majic S. Potsaid, M.D.

The pancreas has been difficult to examine by any method and precise delineation of the organ, using a noninvasive radiologic technique, has proved to be an especially formidable task. A lead toward direct visualization of the pancreas by external means developed when Friedberg and his associates (1948) observed that amino acids concentrate rapidly in the gland after intravenous administration. Using methionine labeled with sulfur-35, they showed that the pancreas establishes a higher amino acid concentration than any other body tissue, even the liver.

Since sulfur-35 is a pure beta ray emitter, it is not suitable for clinical organ imaging. Therefore, Blau and Manske (1961) substituted gamma ray emitting selenium-75 for the sulfur atom in methionine (Fig. 6–1) and produced a radioanalog that localizes in tissues with essentially the same distribution as the naturally occurring amino acid. A comparison of the physiologic behavior of ^{75}Se-selenomethionine with the sulfur-35 labeled molecule demonstrated that the pancreas incorporates both agents at the same rate (Hansson, 1963). The compounds are biochemically similar in other ways as well (Spencer, 1962; McConnell, 1967; Awwad, 1967).

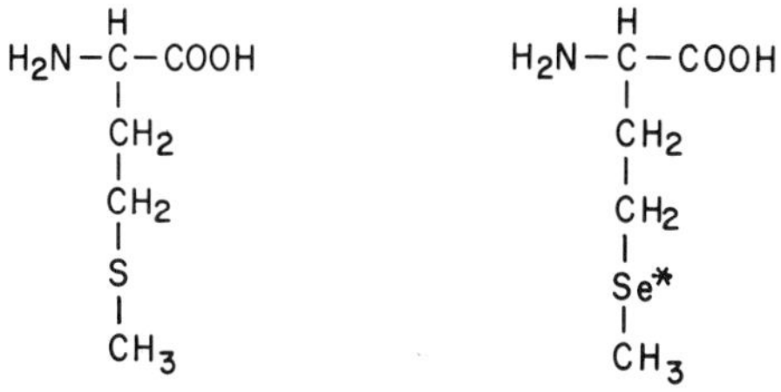

METHIONINE SELENOMETHIONINE

Figure 6–1. Selenium-75 substituted for sulfur atom in methionine.

PHYSIOLOGIC PRINCIPLES

Amino Acid Metabolism

Intravenously injected ^{75}Se-selenomethionine enters a pool of free amino acids in the blood plasma. Rapid equilibration of plasma amino acids with those of the interstitial fluid occurs by diffusion across the capillary wall: the concentration of free amino acids in interstitial fluid is almost identical to that in plasma (Guyton, 1961). Amino acids pass across cell membranes from interstitial fluid to the interior of tissue cells predominantly by active transport. The efficiency of this process is demonstrated by the concentration gradient established between interstitial fluid and the intracellular compartment; typically, tissues contain five to 15 times as much free amino acid as plasma or interstitial fluid (Friedberg, 1947; Roberts, 1962).

The time course for the entire process of amino acid transit from blood to tissue is rapid. Radioactively labeled amino acids appear in tissue cells within one minute after intravenous injection (Palade, 1961; Van Heyningen, 1965). Five minutes after administration, the radioactivity of pancreatic tissue may be five or six times that of blood, and after 15 minutes, 80 to 90 per cent of injected amino acids have been removed from the plasma (Friedberg, 1947; Hansson, 1959; Van Goidsenhoven, 1967).

Protein secretory cells (such as pancreatic acinar cells) possess an elaborate internal membranous organization and a heavy cytoplasmic concentration of ribosomes (Walker, 1966) (Fig. 6–2). The membranes (the endoplasmic reticulum) enclose a complex intracellular space (the cisternae) and separate it from the residual cytoplasmic matrix. Most membranes, particularly those in the basal portion of the cell, are studded with ribosomes on their external surface (i.e., facing the cytoplasmic matrix). Membranes without associated ribosomes are located in the Golgi region.

That protein synthesis occurs in the ribosomes has been abundantly demonstrated by ultracentrifugal cell fractionation and by radioautography (Palade, 1961; Morris, 1960; Warshawsky, 1963; and Caro, 1964). Newly synthesized pro-

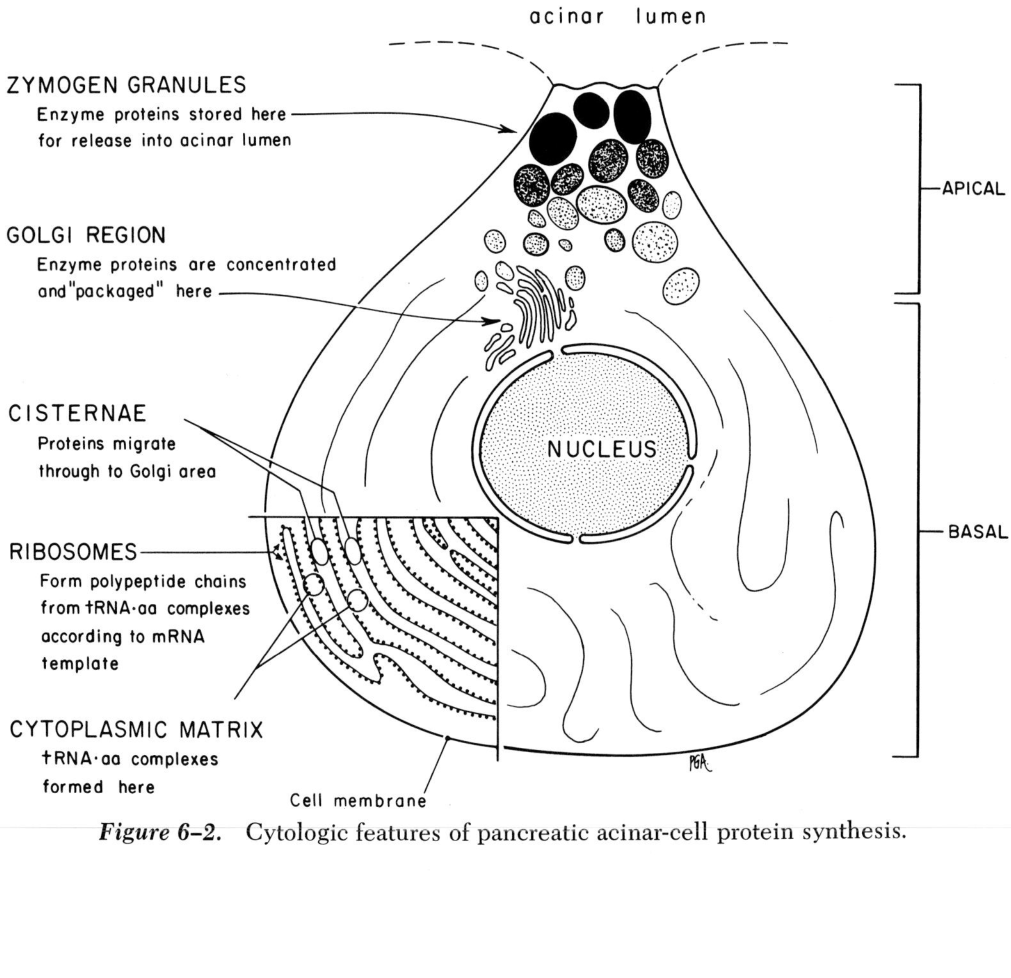

Figure 6–2. Cytologic features of pancreatic acinar-cell protein synthesis.

teins are released from the ribosomes into the cisternae of the endoplasmic reticulum (Palade, 1961; Caro, 1964). Through the cisternae, proteins migrate to the Golgi region, a portion of the cell where numerous smooth-surfaced membranes enclose irregularly shaped vacuoles. The Golgi apparatus appears to be engaged in concentration and "packaging" of newly synthesized "exportable" proteins (Caro, 1961). Golgi vacuoles progressively enlarge, then migrate to the apical region of the cell adjacent to the acinar lumen; in this position, they are known as zymogen (secretory) granules. There is a close parallel between the enzyme content of pancreatic juice and that of the zymogen granules (Keller, 1971). Zymogen granules are ultimately discharged into the acinar lumen; the discharge process involves coalescence of the zymogen granule-limiting membrane with the plasma membrane of the luminal aspect of the cell (Palade, 1961).

Function of the Exocrine Pancreas

The rate of penetration of labeled amino acids from plasma into cells varies directly with the protein synthetic activity of the tissue being studied (Neuberger, 1964). The pancreas (which in man weighs about 90 gm. and can secrete as much as 6 gm. of protein per 24 hours) is especially active in protein synthesis and has been shown to possess a higher rate of amino acid accumulation than any other tissue in all the mammalian species examined (Hansson, 1959; Van Goidsenhoven, 1967; Cardell, 1966; Haverback, 1965; Awwad, 1966; and Zuidema, 1963).

The time course of pancreatic protein synthesis has been well documented by both ultracentrifugal cell fractionation and radioautographic studies (Palade, 1961; Warshawsky, 1963; and Nadler, 1963). Only one minute after intravenous injection, at least some labeled amino acids have been incorporated into protein by pancreatic ribosomes (Palade, 1961). Turnover time in the ribosomes is short (three to six minutes), indicating that migration of proteins toward the Golgi region begins very soon after their formation (Palade, 1961; Nadler, 1963). Twenty minutes after injection, most radioactively labeled proteins are in the Golgi region (Caro, 1964). Turnover time in this portion of the cell is eight to 15 minutes and, by 60 minutes, labeled proteins are predominantly in the zymogen granules (Palade, 1961; Nadler, 1963; and Junqueira, 1956). Turnover time for zymogen granule protein is about 36 minutes (Nadler, 1963). Different authorities have calculated the over-all mean life span for newly formed exportable proteins in pancreatic acinar cells to be 52.4 minutes (Nadler, 1963) and from three to six hours (Van Heyningen, 1965).

Proteins released from zymogen granules into the acinar lumen proceed distally through the pancreatic ductal system. The time necessary for secreted protein to traverse the whole length of the pancreatic ductal system has been estimated to be about three minutes (Junqueira, 1956). Multiple studies in numerous mammalian species have demonstrated that radioactive proteins begin to appear in pancreatic juice about 45 minutes after intravenous injection of labeled amino acids (Hansson, 1963; Van Goidsenhoven, 1967; Rotschild, 1957). Radioactivity is maximal between 90 and 180 minutes, and gradually diminishes over the next several hours. All these studies have utilized secretin to stimulate the flow of pancreatic juice.

At any given time, over-all pancreatic radioactivity after intravenous administration of labeled amino acids is the result of amino acid uptake, protein synthesis and protein secretion. The pancreas accumulates amino acids so avidly that its peak level of radioactivity occurs at about 30 minutes (at which time it achieves greater radioactivity per gram of tissue than any other organ) (Awwad, 1966). Radioactivity then decreases relatively rapidly; six hours after injection, its level approaches that of other organs (Hansson, 1959). The concomitant radioactivities of free amino acids, pro-

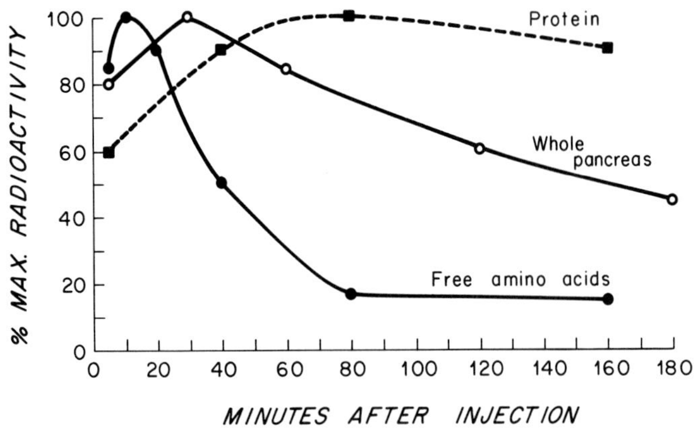

Figure 6–3. Relationship between time and pancreatic radioactivity after intravenous radiomethionine injection in normally fed mice. (Adapted from Hansson, E.: The formation of pancreatic juice proteins studied with labeled amino acids. Acta Physiol. Scand., *46*:Suppl. 161, 1959.)

tein and whole pancreas, following intravenous injection of ^{35}S methionine, have been studied in mice by Hansson (1959) (Fig. 6–3). Labeled free amino acids attain peak concentration about ten minutes after injection and, thereafter, rapidly decline. Total glandular radioactivity is maximal at 30 minutes and is only 45 per cent of maximal at three hours. Radioactively labeled pancreatic protein attains its highest concentration about 80 minutes after injection and decreases relatively slowly. Turnover time for nonexportable protein has been calculated to be 62.5 hours as opposed to estimates of 52.4 minutes (Nadler, 1963) and three to six hours (Van Heyningen, 1965) for exportable digestive enzyme protein. Accordingly, the over-all accumulation of radioactivity by pancreatic acinar cells after administration of labeled amino acids reflects primarily the labeling of digestive enzymes (Hansson, 1959).

Regulation of Pancreatic Secretion

It is generally accepted that, in controlling pancreatic secretions, hormones from the stomach and the proximal small intestine work in concert with the autonomic nervous system. In particular, actions of the vagus nerve complement the effects of the hormones, pancreozymin and secretin. Recent evidence, however, has shown that hormonal influences are considerably more important than are those of the vagus (Dupre, 1970).

Pancreozymin, vagal stimulation and *cholinergic drugs* (e.g., pilocarpine) produce essentially similar effects on pancreatic acinar cells: the number of visible zymogen granules decreases, the enzyme content of pancreatic juice increases and that of pancreatic tissue decreases (Daley, 1952; Laird, 1958; Gregory, 1962; Ichikawa, 1965; Rothman, 1966). When labeled amino acids are administered under such conditions, they are more rapidly incorporated into pancreatic enzyme protein than they are in the control state, and the resulting labeled proteins are more rapidly secreted (Farber, 1956; Hansson, 1959; Webster, 1966). Little or no increase in the volume of pancreatic secretion occurs (Nardi, 1963). *Anticholinergic drugs* (e.g., atropine) inhibit enzyme secretion in response to vagal stimulation and cholinergic drugs, but have no effect upon the action of pancreozymin (Davies, 1949; Junqueira, 1958). Anticholinergics do not suppress pancreatic uptake of labeled amino acids (Junqueira, 1958). *Secretin* markedly increases the volume and bicarbonate content of pancreatic juice (Janowitz, 1961). No detectable cytologic alterations are produced and there is no significant change in protein secretion (Nardi, 1963; Ichikawa, 1965). It is thought that secretin acts on the centroacinar and/or the intralobular duct epithelial cells (where carbonic anhydrase is localized) to regulate secretion of fluid and electrolytes by the pancreas (Becker, 1961; Dreiling, 1964). Intravenous administration of secretin also causes a significant temporary increase in pancreatic blood flow and, more importantly, increases the proportion of total cardiac output reaching the pancreas (Delaney, 1966).

On entering the stomach, *food* stimulates acid production and also triggers release of gastrin from the gastric antrum. Gastrin has been shown to produce effects very much like those of pancreozymin and, to a lesser extent, like those of secretin (Preshaw, 1965*a*; 1965*b*). To what extent these actions are due to a direct effect on the pancreas or to the release of pancreozymin and secretin from the duodenal mucosa has not been clearly established.

Although, in man, there is probably a basal level of continuous pancreatic secretion, ingestion and subsequent digestion of food produce an increase in both the volume and enzyme content of pancreatic juice (Dreiling, 1964). The early phase of the pancreatic response to eating appears to depend upon vagal pancreatic stimulation, but when the gastric contents empty into the duodenum, secretin and pancreozymin are liberated (into the blood stream) from the duodenal mucosa (Gregory, 1962). Most foodstuffs, to some degree, cause the release of both hormones; peptones and amino acids, however, are most effective in causing pancreozymin release, whereas acid most effectively triggers secretin release. These hormones act on the pancreas to produce the major portion of the pancreatic secretory response to a meal (Gregory, 1962).

The effects of eating on pancreatic enzyme secretion and synthesis are comparable in magnitude to those of a single intravenous injection of pancreozymin or pilocarpine, but are less reproducible and of longer duration. The continuous entry of gastric contents into the duodenum sustains the release of secretin and pancreozymin over a fairly long period. In particular, a longer period of time is required for restitution of full pancreatic activity after feeding (Daley, 1952).

The enzyme content of pancreatic tissue is lower in fasted animals than in those stimulated to secrete, then allowed to recover. When fasting is continued for a relatively long period (e.g., 48 hours), pancreatic enzyme activity falls significantly (Daley, 1952). These observations are partially explained by slow, but continuous, pancreatic enzyme secretion during fasting (Daley, 1952; Morris, 1960). In addition, secretion exceeds enzyme synthesis during this period; it has been demonstrated that pancreas slices from fasted pigeons incorporate amino acids into protein less rapidly than do pancreas slices from fed birds (Webster, 1966). Despite this, fasted animals have been reported to accumulate labeled amino acids (in the pancreas) at the same rate as do normally fed animals (Hansson, 1959).

RADIOPHARMACEUTICAL

Production Methods

^{75}Se-L-selenomethionine can be synthesized either biologically or chemically; the radiopharmaceuticals produced have comparable physiologic activity. Biosynthesis was the original technique. Blau and Bender (1962) grew yeast on a low-sulfur medium which contained selenium-75 as selenite. The yeast accommodatingly synthesized ^{75}Se-L-selenomethionine which was thereafter isolated using a cation exchange resin technique. A purely chemical method of synthesizing ^{75}Se-L-selenomethionine has also been developed. Proponents of this technique claim that it provides a radiopharmaceutical with greater chemical and radiochemical purity (Amersham, 1968).

Pharmacologic Considerations

Because methionine is an essential amino acid, its analog, selenomethionine, could be considered an antimetabolite. Actually, some investigators (Schwarz, 1957; Schwarz, 1961; Rosenfeld, 1964) feel that stable selenium is probably an essential trace element in man and that it almost certainly enters the body in the form of seleno-amino acids. Male adults in the United States have been found to have a mean whole blood selenium concentration of about 20 μgm. per 100 ml. (Allaway, 1968). Since, for radioisotopic pancreatic imaging, only a fraction of a milligram of selenium (including both radioactive and stable forms) is administered (Squibb, 1970), there is little risk of significant antimetabolic effect and currently accepted dosages are considered safe. Chemically produced selenomethionine does contain some ^{75}Se-D-selenomethionine (the dextrorotatory form), but the amount present is below any known chemotoxic levels.

Radiation Risk

The average adult patient receives about 250 μCi. of selenium-75 as selenomethionine for pancreas visualization. Dose limitations are imposed primarily by the 120-day physical half-life of selenium-75. It has been estimated that 13 per cent of intravenously administered ^{75}Se-L-selenomethionine has a biologic half-life of 0.55 days; 44 per cent, a biologic half-life of 46 days; and 42 per cent, a biologic half-life of 220 days, with an over-all biologic half-life of about 70 days (Lathrop, 1972). When physical decay is taken into account, the effective half-life has been calculated to be 47 days. An average pancreatic examination, in which an adult patient receives 250 μCi. of ^{75}Se-L-selenomethionine, exposes various organs to the following estimated absorbed doses of radiation: (a) ovaries, 1.3 rad.; (b) whole body, 2.0 rad.; (c) blood, 2.2 rad.; (d) testes, 2.8 rad.; (e) pancreas, 3.0 rad.; (f) spleen, 4.6 rad.; (g) kidneys, 5.5 rad.; and (h) liver, 5.8 rad. (Lathrop, 1972). Since the radiation is delivered over an extended period, the potential damaging effects are probably reduced significantly. It should be pointed out that selenium-75 has small internal conversion coefficients which result in a low dose from nonpenetrating radiation. Since ^{75}Se-selenomethionine is widely distributed in the tissues and will cross the placental barrier, pancreatic studies in pregnant women should be avoided, especially in the first trimester.

PHYSIOLOGIC ENHANCEMENT

The counting statistics (i.e., signal photons) available for ^{75}Se-selenomethionine pancreatography are significantly less than the number of gamma rays per unit time desirable for image formation. Since the maximum amount of radiopharmaceutical which can be given for a single examination has been rather firmly fixed, other methods of increasing the information content of pancreatic imaging have been sought. These enhancement attempts have centered on physiologic means of increasing the concentration of selenomethionine in the pancreas or of delaying the secretion of labeled enzymes into the duodenum. Dietary, hormonal, and pharmacologic approaches have all been tried.

Numerous dietary modifications have been proposed (Blau, 1962; Rodriguez-Antunez, 1964; Sodee, 1964; Bender, 1965; Tabern, 1965; Sodee, 1966), but none have been proven to influence accumulation of radioactivity by the human pancreas. Rodriguez-Antunez (1964) advocated morphine and Bender (1965) tried propantheline bromide in efforts to delay pancreatic secretion of radiolabeled enzymes, again without noticeable success. At the Massachusetts General Hospital, it has been our impression that pancreatic images made in the morning after the patient has had a protein-rich breakfast are of generally better quality than those made under other circumstances. This observation has not been rigorously substantiated, but has the virtues of simplicity and good patient acceptance.

IMAGE FORMATION AND DISPLAY

Selenium-75 Nuclear Data

Selenium-75 disintegrates at a rate that results in a physical half-life of 120 days.

Decay is by electron capture so that the gamma rays emitted have a wide spectrum of energies. In addition to K and L x-rays, 10 separate gamma emissions contribute to the radiation dose. Only those photons with energies of 121, 136, 265, 280, and 400 keV. are important for image formation (Lathrop, 1972). About 85 per cent of all selenium-75 nuclear disintegrations result in emission of either 280 or 265 keV. photons. Therefore, for clinical pancreatic imaging, the detector is set to encompass these energy levels. The 400 keV. photons are emitted by only just over 10 per cent of selenium-75 disintegrations and the photons with lower energies are less desirable for image formation (see Table 6–1).

TABLE 6–1. Selenium-75 Nuclear and Radiation Dose Data

MEAN ENERGY (KEV.)	MEAN NUMBER PER DISINTEGRATION	G-RAD. μCI.-HR.
121	0.16	0.04
136	0.56	0.16
265	0.59	0.33
280	0.25	0.15
400	0.13	0.11

Imaging Procedures

Initially, a rectilinear scanner (with a 3- or 5-inch scintillation crystal) was used for almost all radionuclide pancreatograms (Fig. 6–4), but more recently, the stationary scintillation camera has been advocated for this purpose (Fig. 6–5). After analyzing large numbers of images made by each type of equipment, the authors have come to prefer the scintillation camera. This instrument can be oriented in various angulations so that oblique images can be obtained while the patient lies in a comfortable supine position. In addition, serial images can be made more easily than with a rectilinear scanner.

If a scanner is to be employed for pancreatic imaging, an 80 to 90 hole focusing collimator should be used and the spectrum window set to fully encompass the 265 and 280 keV. photopeaks. Gamma rays have been recorded at a rate of 1500 to 3000 per minute from the pancreatic region (Agnew, 1969). It has been necessary to run the detector at a speed of 20 to 40 cm. per minute. As a rule, the line spacing has been around 0.25 cm. To project the pancreas away from the liver as much as possible, the patient can be placed in an oblique position by putting a pillow or wedge under his left side.

When the scintillation camera or the

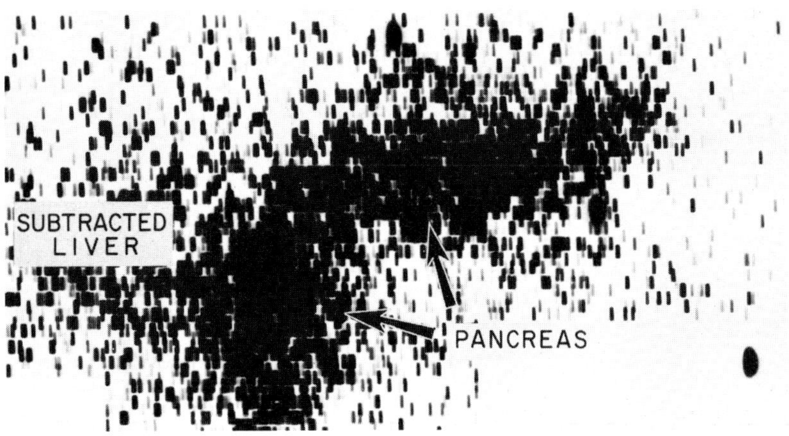

Figure 6–4. Normal pancreas obtained with a rectilinear scanner.

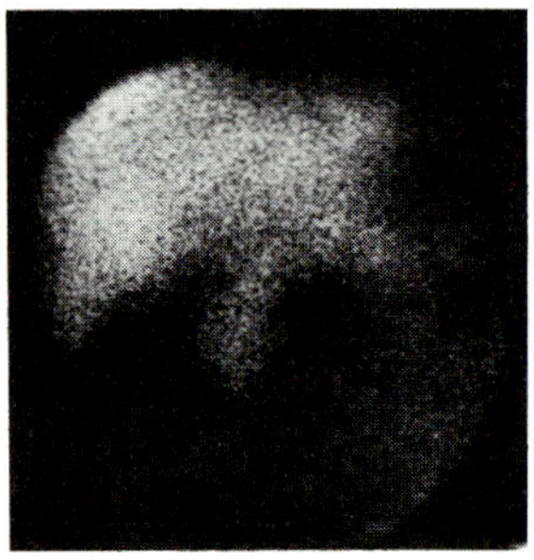

Figure 6–5. Normal pancreas obtained with a scintillation camera.

autofluoroscope is used, the patient need not move from the supine position. The camera detector is angled about 10° cephalad and about 10° toward the right in order to "peek" under the liver (Fig. 6–6). The geometry is so arranged that the center of the crystal is aimed at the mid portion of the pancreas which is in the general region marked by a point 2 inches caudad to the xiphoid and 2 inches to the left of the midline. Positioning can be corrected easily after an initial, briefly exposed image outlines the liver edge. The two photon peaks (265 and 280 keV.) used for imaging are bracketed by a 15 to 20 per cent window. A collimator suitable for gamma rays up to at least 300 keV. must be used. Serial studies are obtained, each view being timed from 10 to 30 minutes. Single exposures of up to three-quarters of an hour or even a full hour have been tried to improve the quality of the image by increasing the number of counts outlining the pancreas.

The following is the Massachusetts General Hospital protocol:

1. The patient is fasted overnight.
2. Early in the morning, he has a high-protein breakfast.
3. About one-half hour later, he is given an intravenous injection of ^{75}Se-selenomethionine (250 μCi. for an adult).
4. An immediate scan, taking three to five minutes, is carried out to determine the liver edge.
5. With a scintillation camera angled 5° to 10° cephalad and 12° to the right, the first 20-minute view of the pancreatic region is obtained.

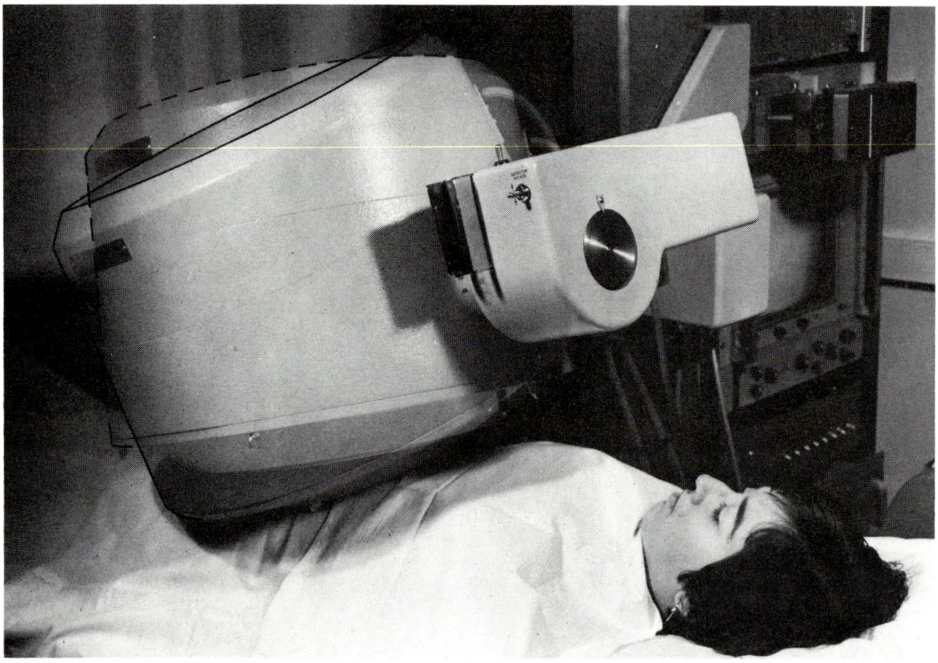

Figure 6–6. Pancreas study (patient-detector relationships) double-exposure photograph showing changes in the position of the detector to obtain a stereoscopic pair of images.

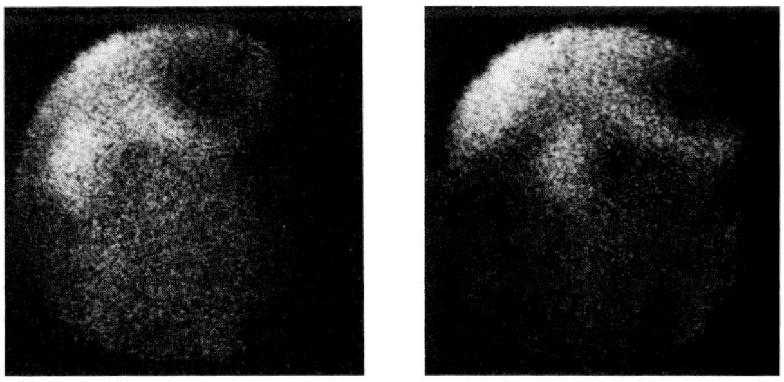

Figure 6–7. Stereoscopic radionuclide pancreatogram (normal study). *A*, Oblique view; *B*, anterior view.

6. The head of the scintillation camera is then placed in a directly anterior position with only the cephalad angulation, and another 20-minute view is recorded.
7. The scintillation camera is then placed in the same position as in step 5, and another 20-minute view is obtained.
8. If the liver is hiding a significant part of the pancreas, the patient is kept in the position described in step 5, and 2 to 3 mCi. of ^{99m}Tc sulfur/sulfide colloid is administered intravenously.
9. After a suitable waiting period, images of the liver are recorded on film for "eyeball" subtraction, and are also stored in a computer for electronic subtraction.

The timing of pancreatic imaging can provide an additional index of the gland's ability to accumulate ^{75}Se-selenomethionine. Serial views more precisely indicate the time course of pancreatic radioactivity during the hour after injection. Furthermore, the second and third images can be used for stereoscopic viewing (Fig. 6–7). (If a stereoscopic pair of images is considered unnecessary, the position described in step 5 can be used for all the views.) In any event, 20-minute images are recommended as they provide a better statistical representation of the pancreas than is possible with 10-minute exposures. When, in the judgment of the examiner, a poorly visualizing pancreas needs to be scanned for longer than one hour, the study may be extended, but images made after two or three hours seldom yield any additional information.

Viewing Techniques

Images obtained with older rectilinear scanners portray the pancreas on a one to one basis, recording the actual size and configuration of the gland. The newer scanners can reduce image size if desired, and images made by the scintillation camera or autofluoroscope are routinely minified. Minification does not reduce information content in the image, however, because of the resolution limitations of the system as a whole. Blending can produce an image that is more esthetically pleasing and sometimes easier to interpret, even though the total amount of information has been compromised because each bit of information (dot) has been degraded by the defocusing process (Fig. 6–8).

Radionuclide stereoscopy, accomplished by a simple movement of angulation of the scintillation camera head, has been found to be a worthwhile modification for ^{75}Se-selenomethionine pancreatic imaging (Potsaid, 1973). The stereoscopic approach facilitates distinction between overlapping structures (e.g., the liver and pancreas) and also doubles image information content since two distinct images are visually fused by the observer during inspection.

Many radionuclide pancreatograms clearly delineate the gland but, in some instances, the liver's concentration of

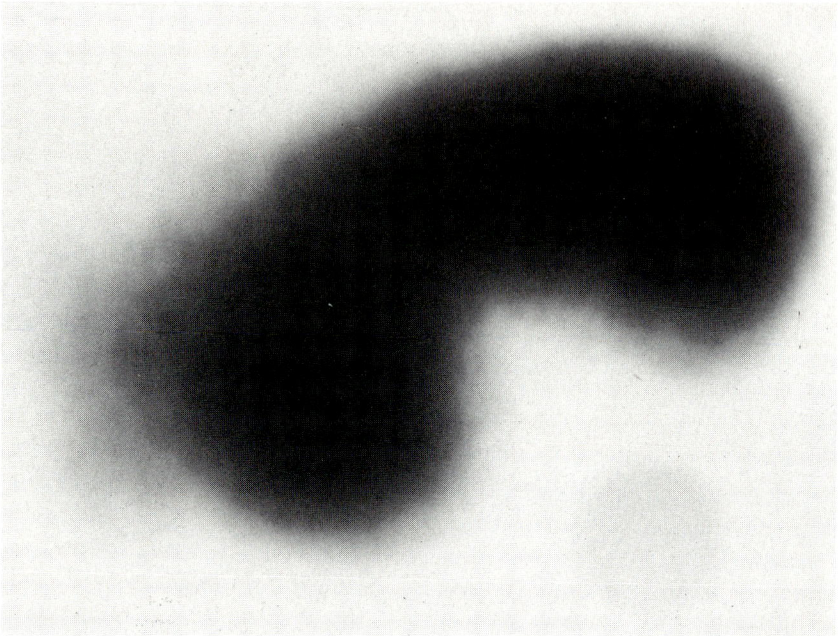

Figure 6–8. Blended or defocused pancreas scan (normal study).

^{75}Se-selenomethionine interferes with pancreatic detection and visualization. For this reason, several techniques for "subtracting" the hepatic image have been developed. Most employ an additional radiopharmaceutical (e.g., colloidal ^{198}Au; ^{99m}Tc sulfur colloid) which localizes in the liver, but not in the pancreas. Dual isotope methods for pancreatic imaging have taken several forms. The simplest requires that the patient maintain exactly the same position for an initial ^{75}Se-selenomethionine pancreas-liver image and, after injection of the second radiopharmaceutical, a subsequent colloidal liver-spleen image. By comparing the position of the inferior hepatic margin in the two studies, ^{75}Se-selenomethionine radioactivity in the liver can be relatively effectively differentiated from that in the pancreas. Electronic means of subtracting have been reported by a number of investigators (Kaplan, 1966; Eaton, 1967*a*; Blanquet, 1968; Fink, 1969; Charlesworth, 1970; Bergeron, 1970; Heslip, 1971; Staab, 1971; Landman, 1971; and Overton, 1971). Two major methods of electronic subtraction have been employed. In the initial scanner procedures, the signals emitted by radioselenomethionine and the radiocolloid used were electronically channelled so as to produce an image in which the liver was cancelled out (Fig. 6–9). Too often, this analogue approach left no room for data manipulation. Later, as multichannel analyzers and computers became available for storage, retrieval and processing, digital handling of radionuclide pancreatographic data and computerized subtraction became more popular than the earlier electronic analogue techniques. Despite the claims made for various types of subtraction pancreatic radioimaging, however, other authors (e.g., Landman, 1971) have concluded that subtraction is only rarely necessary for clinically adequate radionuclide pancreatography. Even though we were initially enthusiastic about subtraction pancreatic scanning (Eaton, 1967*a*), the authors of this monograph have come to believe that conventional (unsubtracted) ^{75}Se-selenomethionine pancreatic images are seldom substantially improved by application of subtraction techniques.

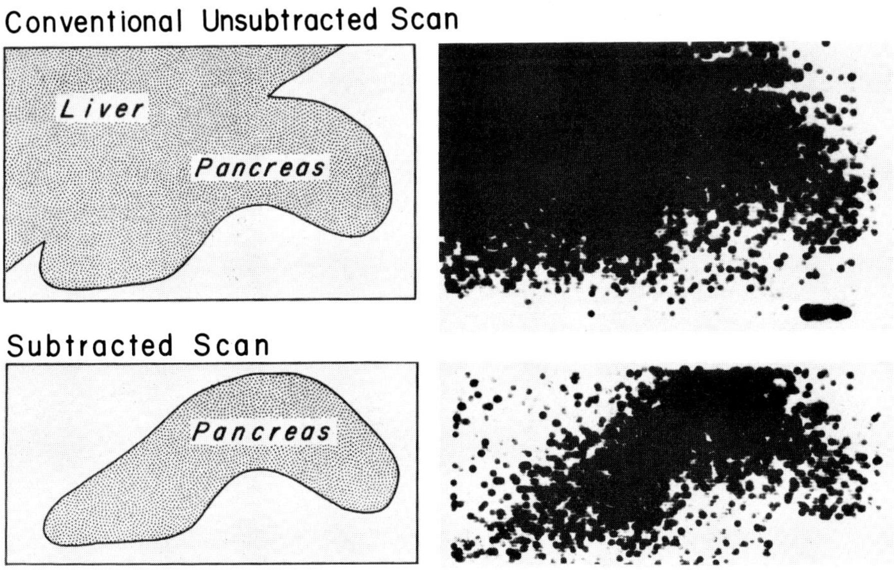

Figure 6–9. Subtraction study, eliminating liver interference and showing a normal pancreas. (From Eaton, S. B., et al.: Radioisotope "subtraction" scanning for pancreatic lesions. Radiology, 89:1033–1039, 1967a.)

IMAGE INTERPRETATION

Normal Patterns

In most patients, the pancreas lies just below the porta hepatis in an essentially horizontal plane at the level of the first and second lumbar vertebral bodies. Classically, it is described as having a somewhat globular head which fits snugly into the duodenal loop. The body, smaller in width than the head, gradually tapers to form a short tail which ends in the region of the splenic hilum. There may be some thinning of the organ in the midline in the region of the aorta, inferior vena cava, and the spine. The superior mesenteric artery and vein are probably the two principal structures adjacent to the thinned portion of the gland. The superior aspect of the pancreatic head and body usually lies partly behind the left lobe of the liver; accordingly, when this portion of the liver enlarges, bothersome interference with direct pancreatic visualization can result, especially on images made in a direct anterior projection (Fig. 6–10). Scan measurements in one series of cases revealed the average length of the pancreas to be 15.5 cm. and the average width, 4.1 cm. (Riccobono, 1968).

In the normal pancreatic scan, there is usually a fairly even distribution of radioactivity throughout the organ (Fig. 6–11). The outline should not be distorted and there should be no missing

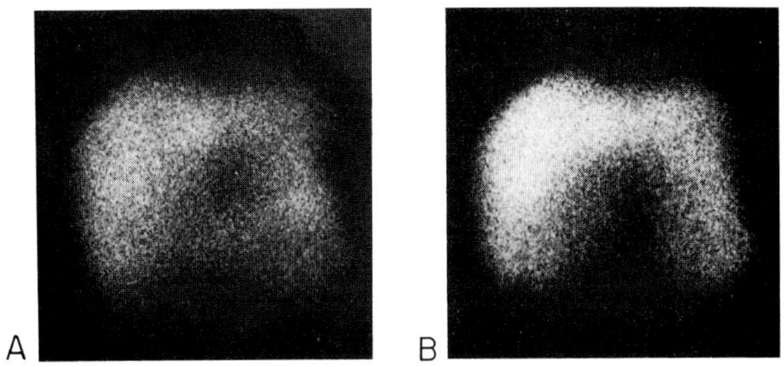

Figure 6–10. Pancreas beneath the left lobe of the liver in a patient with an unusually large left lobe. *A*, ^{75}Se-selenomethionine study; *B*, ^{99m}Tc colloid study.

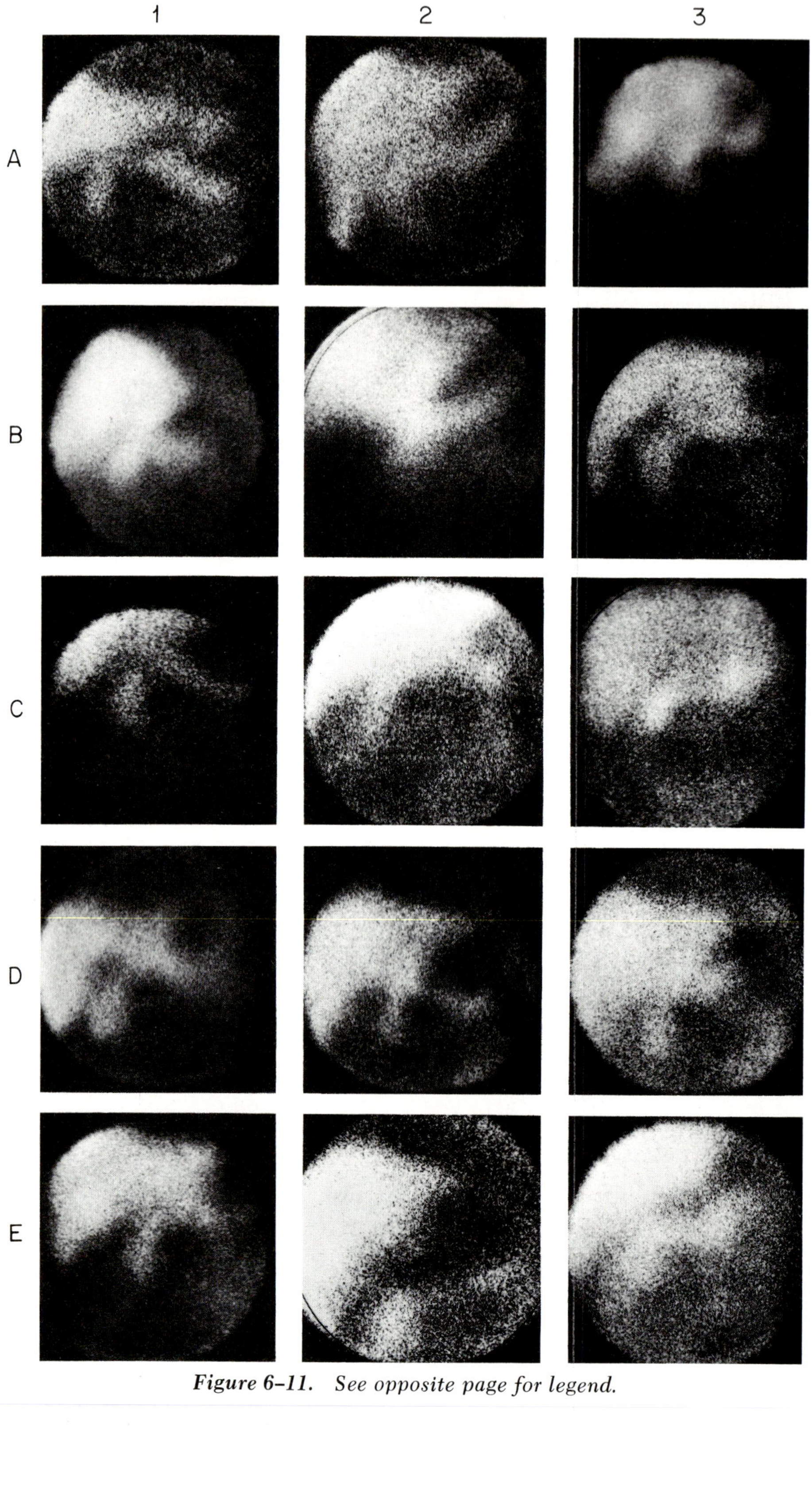

Figure 6–11. *See opposite page for legend.*

segments (e.g., the body or tail). Slight variations in radionuclide concentration throughout the gland can be seen in normal individuals (Agnew, 1969). One commonly encountered, but confusing, normal subpattern occurs when radioactivity in the head and tail of the pancreas is considerably more prominent than that in the thinner "neck" area where the gland is compressed by midline vascular structures (Fig. 6–12). Numerous false-positive misinterpretations have understandably resulted when this configuration has been demonstrated. In some cases, serial views show a "filling-in" of the questionable area, possibly as radioactively labeled digestive enzymes from the distal pancreas pass through. Landman (1971) has advocated a bolus injection of ^{99m}Tc pertechnetate so that the position of the defect with relation to the aorta and superior mesenteric artery can be ascertained. If the defect and the vessels can be superimposed, it may be assumed with some (but not complete) assurance that the study is normal. Images made more than an hour after administration of ^{75}Se-selenomethionine may reveal a mottled pattern of radioactivity as the pancreas begins to secrete its labeled enzyme protein.

A number of authors have described the varying shapes which can be identified on pancreatic images made in normal patients (King, 1966; Colella, 1967; Riccobono, 1968; Rodriguez-Antunez, 1970, etc.). In the classic pattern, the head

---

Figure 6–11. Normal pancreas scans showing a fairly even distribution of radioactivity throughout the delineated organ.

A-1, This 51-year-old man was admitted because of recurrent pancreatitis and an abdominal mass. He had been a heavy beer drinker for many years. After a thorough work-up, he underwent surgery. A pseudocyst with bloody fluid was found and a cystgastrostomy was performed. The scan was performed three years after surgery.

A-2, A pancreas scan was done on this middle-aged man because of some vague abdominal pains.

A-3, This 56-year-old woman, a diabetic patient, was admitted because of epigastric distress. A questionable rise in serum amylase was noted.

B-1, This 81-year-old woman was admitted to the hospital because of weight loss and many digestive symptoms.

B-2, This 80-year-old woman was admitted because of thrombophlebitis.

B-3, This is a 58-year-old woman with multiple sclerosis.

C-1, This 55-year-old woman was admitted because of an abdominal mass. The pancreas scan showed a perfectly normal gland. At surgery, a retroperitoneal lymphoma was found to be of lymphocytic type.

C-2, This 62-year-old woman was admitted because of chronic duodenal ulcer disease.

C-3, Eight years before this study, this 67-year-old woman had a cholecystectomy and a sphincterotomy for supposed chronic pancreatitis. Many abdominal explorations followed because of abdominal pain for which no cause could be found.

D-1, This 53-year-old man was admitted because of recurrent pancreatitis or duodenal ulcer. At the age of 15, he had a cholecystectomy because of chronic cholecystitis. At 46, he developed persistent abdominal pains. At 47, he had a sphincterotomy of the papilla of Vater which was fibrotic and stenotic.

D-2, This 36-year-old woman gave a history of chronic midabdominal pains of 7 years' duration.

D-3, This 31-year-old woman was examined as an outpatient because of recurrent abdominal pains following an automobile accident that occurred three weeks earlier.

E-1, This 55-year-old woman had a subtotal gastrectomy and a vagotomy for duodenal ulcer disease three years earlier. She had the dumping syndrome and a reaction hypoglycemia.

E-2, This 69-year-old man has diabetes mellitus controlled by oral medication. He also had a subacute hepatitis proven by a needle biopsy of the liver.

E-3, This 64-year-old woman was admitted to the hospital for recurrent abdominal pains suspected to be of pancreatic origin. No pancreatic pathology was demonstrated.

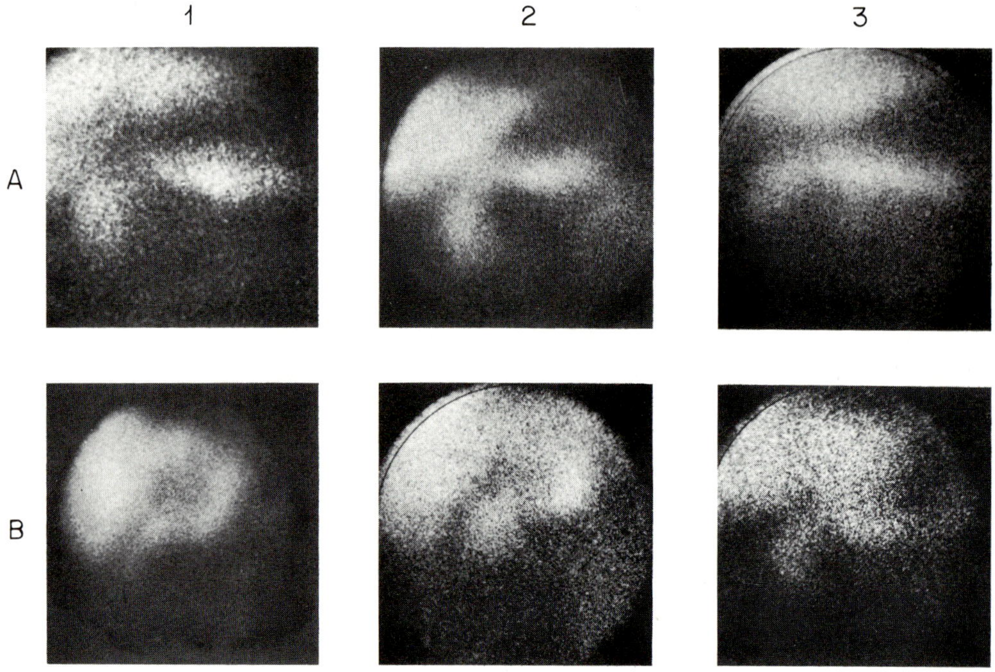

Figure 6–12. Normal pancreas showing the thinned-out portion of the body as well as better uptake in the tail than in the head of the gland.

A-1, This 35-year-old woman is a chronic alcoholic who was admitted with a diagnosis of chronic relapsing pancreatitis. Several months before the scan, the patient had an acute episode of pancreatitis, with an extremely high serum amylase level.

A-2, This 54-year-old man was an outpatient who complained of upper gastrointestinal distress.

A-3, This is a 46-year-old male diabetic patient who had abdominal pains of uncertain etiology. He probably had an acute gastritis.

B-1, This 56-year-old woman, a patient with Parkinson's disease on L-Dopa therapy, is suspected of having peptic ulcer disease.

B-2, This 54-year-old woman has diabetes which is controlled by diet.

B-3, This 36-year-old man gave a history of pancreatitis five years earlier. He was admitted because of numbness and tingling of the hands and feet, and was considered to have a neuritis of unknown etiology.

is clearly the largest part of the gland, while the body and tail can vary somewhat in size and orientation. The axis of the organ can be horizontal or angled cephalad (as much as 45°). The commonest normal variants have been described as pistol-shaped, horseshoe-shaped, and sigmoid-shaped. The patient's position in relation to the detector (Fig. 6–7) and the type of imaging system employed can alter the apparent configuration produced.

Abdominal scintigrams made after administration of ^{75}Se-selenomethionine demonstrate several extrapancreatic structures (Fig. 6–13). The most prominent is the liver, but the spleen and proximal small bowel are also routinely shown. Small intestinal activity appears to result partially from direct mucosal accumulation and partially from the presence of intraluminal digestive enzymes secreted by the pancreas. Rodriguez-Antunez (1970) feels that the latter component is more significant and that if there is a good deal of small bowel radioactivity, this indicates satisfactory pancreatic secretory function. He suggests that, in instances where the pancreatic image itself appears equivocal,

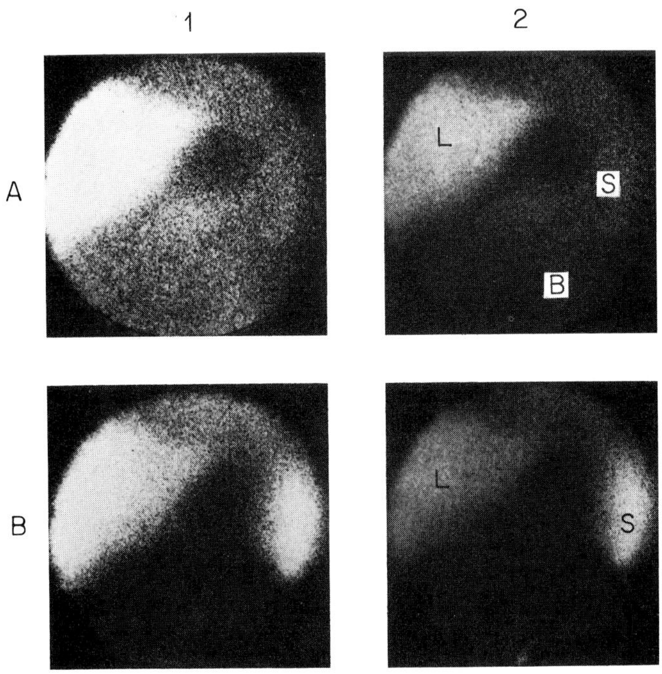

Figure 6–13. Pancreas scan in a patient with pancreatitis, showing poor delineation of the gland, as well as some activity in the spleen *(S)* and proximal small bowel *(B)* and obvious activity in the liver *(L)*. *A*, ^{75}Se-selenomethionine studies; *B*, ^{99m}Tc colloid studies.

the presence of normal intestinal radioactivity can be used as the basis for a normal interpretation.

Abnormal Patterns

The abnormal patterns demonstrable by radionuclide pancreatography are limited in their range. As a result, pancreatic imaging with ^{75}Se-selenomethionine is useful chiefly for demonstrating the presence or absence of abnormality and not for indicating the specific nature of the disease process present. The two principal scintigraphic manifestations of pancreatic abnormality are generalized dysfunction and the presence of a focal defect.

Generalized dysfunction can vary in appearance from complete absence of any identifiable pancreatic radioactivity (Fig. 6–14) through degrees of definite but uniform diminution in radioactivity to a generally mottled or patchy appearance. Pancreatitis is a common cause of generalized dysfunction. *Acute pancreatitis* usually produces total nonvisualization whereas patients with resolving or subacute pancreatitis often have a mottled or spotty-appearing pancreas, frequently with some delay in accumulation (Fig. 6–15). In *chronic pancreatitis*, a generalized dysfunction pattern is often present. This may take the form of complete nonvisualization (usually in cases where there has been a recent acute

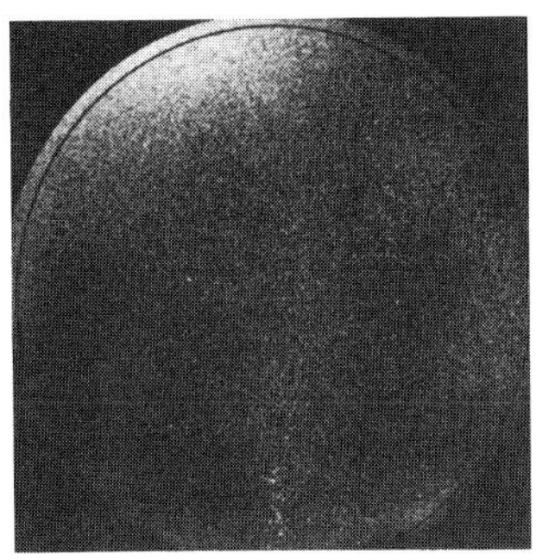

Figure 6–14. Pancreas scan showing no visualization of the organ in a 53-year-old man admitted because of abdominal pains and findings of pancreatic insufficiency. At surgery, the pancreas was found to be completely replaced by tumor, with metastases to omental lymph nodes. Histologic examination indicated adenocarcinoma.

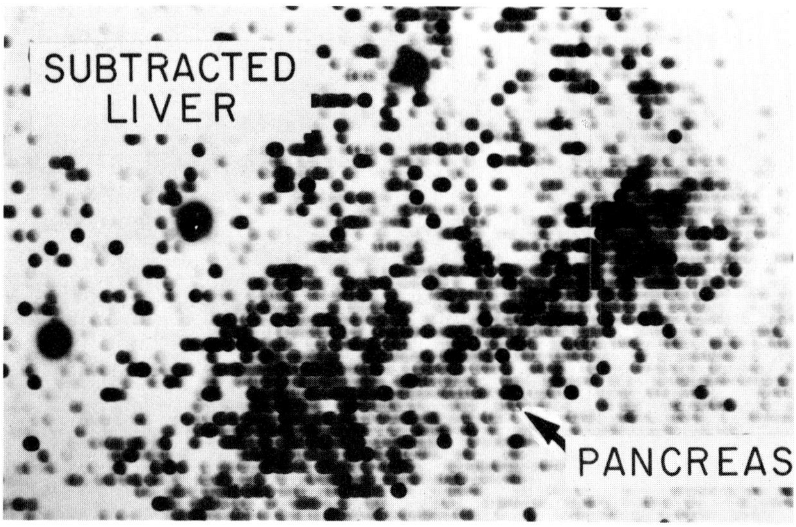

Figure 6–15. Subacute or chronic pancreatitis. In this instance, the gland has a mottled appearance and is not well delineated.

exacerbation) or of patchy mottling (this is especially common in quiescent chronic alcoholic pancreatitis). In certain patients with chronic relapsing gallstone pancreatitis where there has been no irreversible pancreatic damage (see Chapter 11), ^{75}Se-selenomethionine scintigraphic images made during symptom-free periods may be entirely normal. In some instances, *pancreatic pseudocysts* produce generalized dysfunction. This is most frequent when the cyst is large or when there is considerable associated inflammation in the pancreas itself. Generalized dysfunction can also result from *pancreatic neoplasms* arising in the *head* of the gland. Malignant tumors in this location are especially prone to occlude the pancreatic duct. Such ductal obstruction produces a profound diminution in protein synthesis by pancreatic acinar cells "upstream" from the point of blockage. Thus tumors located in the head can produce a generalized decrease in pancreatic radioactivity and poor visualization of the entire organ. About two-thirds of all patients with carcinomas arising in the head of the pancreas have this sort of scintigraphic pattern (McCarthy, 1972). In some series, nearly half of all patients with carcinoma arising in the *body* of the pancreas have had generalized reduction in uptake involving the whole gland (McCarthy, 1972). The mechanism for decreased radionuclide accumulation in the seemingly uninvolved portion of the pancreas (i.e., the head) has not been explained.

Other types of pancreatic disorders which have been associated with a generalized dysfunction pattern include total pancreatectomy, recent sphincterotomy (Eaton, 1971), infiltrative pancreatic diseases such as amyloidosis (Melmed, 1968; Hatchette, 1972), and invasion of the pancreas by malignancies arising in adjacent viscera (e.g., the stomach). In the latter instance, the degree of scan abnormality varies markedly with the amount of pancreatic involvement present (Fig. 6–14). Many patients with diabetes mellitus have generally decreased pancreatic ^{75}Se-selenomethionine uptake (Miale, 1965; Melmed, 1968; Landman, 1971). In some instances, this probably results from associated, but clinically occult chronic pancreatitis. Whether such a relationship explains all such cases remains to be determined.

Extrapancreatic disorders such as hepatocellular disease (especially cirrhosis), uremia, and generalized carcinomatosis with debilitation are all capable of producing a generalized dysfunction pattern on radionuclide pancreatic imaging. The common feature in many of these patients appears to be the presence of a systemic derangement of protein metabolism. Animal studies have shown that protein metabolism and exocrine pancreatic function are closely interrelated and that severe limitation of food intake can provide abnormal histologic changes in the pancreas.

Focal defects can be either easier or more difficult to identify on ^{75}Se-selenomethionine pancreatic images than the generalized dysfunction pattern. The straightforward focal defects occur when either the entire head or the entire body-tail segments are missing in patients where the remainder of the gland is well visualized. False-positive diagnoses are made least often in circumstances of this type. As previously discussed, an apparent focal defect in the neck of the pancreas is usually due to pancreatic thinning produced by adjacent vascular and body structures. Since the shape of the pancreas as shown by ^{75}Se-selenomethionine imaging can be so variable, interpretation of apparent defects involving the periphery of the head or body is fraught with hazard. Similarly, determining whether or not the distal pancreatic tail is intact is quite difficult.

Focal defects can result from many of the same forms of pancreatic disease which can also produce a generalized dysfunction pattern. *Acute pancreatitis* may be restricted to a limited portion of the organ (especially in gallstone pancreatitis where the head may be involved with relative sparing of the body and tail [Howard, 1960]). In quiescent *chronic pancreatitis*, one portion of the gland may have considerably more irreversible acinar destruction and fibrotic scarring than the remainder of the organ. In these instances, a focal defect may be demonstrated. Smaller *pseudocysts* (especially those with a sizeable intrapancreatic component) and occasional larger ones may also produce only focal abnormality on radionuclide pancreatic images (Fig. 6–16).

Exocrine *pancreatic malignancies* produce discrete defects fairly often. About one-third of tumors arising in the head and a little over one-half of those arising in the body are demonstrated as localized reductions of radioactivity (McCarthy, 1972) (Fig. 6–17). Most *islet-cell neoplasms* are too small to be detected by ^{75}Se-selenomethionine pancreatography; however, relatively large lesions of this sort may produce definite focal defects. Highly differentiated peptide-secreting islet-cell tumors may rarely appear as areas of focally increased ^{75}Se-selenomethionine uptake. This phenomenon

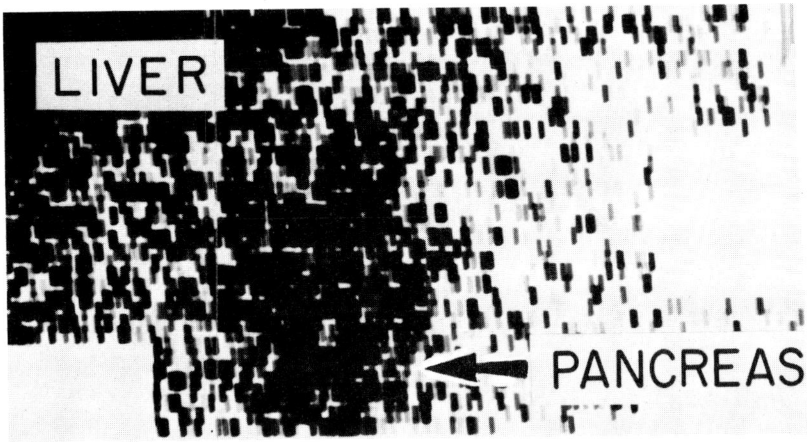

Figure 6–16. Large pseudocyst of the pancreas causing interference of uptake in the body and tail, with only the head of the gland visualized. (From Eaton, S. B., et al.: Comparison of current radiologic approaches to the diagnosis of pancreatic disease. N. E. J. Med., 279:389–396, 1968.)

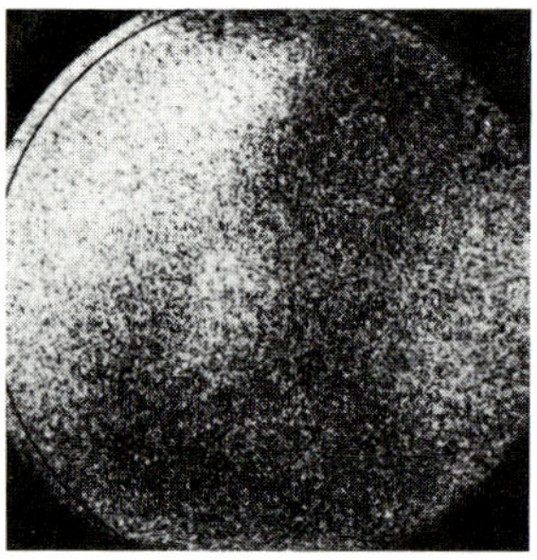

Figure 6–17. Carcinoma of the body of the pancreas. This 60-year-old man had diarrhea, fatty, foul-smelling, and frothy stools as well as persistent weight loss. At surgery, a hard mass, 6 cm. in diameter, was found in the midpancreas, with metastases to the liver and lymph nodes. Only the head of the gland is visualized on the radionuclide pancreatogram.

has been reported by several authors (Melmed, 1968; Brown, 1968; Thomas, 1968) and, in some instances, even metastases from such tumors may demonstrate significant accumulation of ^{75}Se-selenomethionine (Staab, 1971).

Reliability

If ever an imaging study in nuclear medicine has met with mixed acceptance, it has been radionuclide pancreatography. For a decade, its merits have been supported by a persistent band of advocates, its limitations have been stressed by a well-meaning group of doubters, and most nonpartisans have been confused by the polarity. As experience with the procedure has increased, a considerable body of data concerning its value and limitations has been accumulated (Table 6–2). Published reports of series involving use of ^{75}Se-selenomethionine pancreatic imaging now exceed 2000 cases, a number considered sufficient to allow meaningful evaluation of its place in clinical medicine.

An inspection of Table 6–2 indicates that the technique has considerable sensitivity (that is, it seldom fails to detect pancreatic abnormality when present) but limited specificity (that is, it is incapable, by itself, of identifying the etiologic factors involved). The over-all incidence of false-negative results (which can be taken as a measure of sensitivity) is less than 10 per cent. This figure, while not optimal, establishes that radionuclide imaging is the most reliable screening test for pancreatic disorders currently available. The technique will fail to identify pancreatic disease less often than any method now in use. On the other hand, nearly a third of all abnormal pancreatic scans are false-positives (at least in the sense that no anatomic pancreatic abnormality is present). Furthermore, the examination cannot identify the type of disease present. These considerations dictate that a positive pancreatic scan should be taken as an indication for further, more specific, radiologic investigation and not as an indication for immediate surgical exploration.

POTENTIAL METHODS OF IMPROVING RADIONUCLIDE PANCREATOGRAPHY

Even though pancreatic visualization with ^{75}Se-selenomethionine has been found to be of considerable value, the technique is distinctly limited in comparison with what radioisotope organ imaging can accomplish in other viscera (e.g., brain, liver, thyroid, etc.). In general, two approaches for improving radionuclide pancreatography are available: one attempts to increase the percentage of a given administered dose of ^{75}Se-selenomethionine which localizes in the pancreas. The other focuses on developing an improved radiopharmaceutical for pancreatic visualization.

As previously discussed, attempts to increase the amount of ^{75}Se-selenomethionine accumulated by the pancreas by dietary or pharmacologic means lack a scientifically documented theoretical basis. In addition, there has been little or no effort to rigorously demonstrate, either in a series of human patients or in animal experiments, that any of the numerous protocols which have been espoused by various authors has any

TABLE 6–2. Accuracy of Pancreatic Imaging in Published Clinical Series

AUTHOR	YEAR	TOTAL NO. OF CASES	NORMAL DIAGNOSIS *Correct*	NORMAL DIAGNOSIS *Incorrect*	PERCENTAGE OF FALSE NEGATIVES	ABNORMAL DIAGNOSIS *Correct*	ABNORMAL DIAGNOSIS *Incorrect*	PERCENTAGE OF FALSE POSITIVES	COMMENTS
Sodee	1966	218	146	5	3	58	9	13	
Melmed	1968	170	95	9	9	46	20	30	Emphasized that extrapancreatic disorders (e.g., liver disease) and diabetes mellitus can adversely affect pancreatic uptake of ^{75}Se-selenomethionine.
Riccobono	1968	211	153	7	4	42	9	18	
Brown	1968	72	33	3	8	30	6	17	
Fink	1969	82	38	8	17	21	15	42	Stressed that cirrhosis can be associated with abnormal pancreatic scintigrams.
Rodriguez-Antunez	1970	439	281	23	8	69	66	49	
Landman	1971	94	42	6	13	37	9	20	
Heslip	1971	23	6	0	0	16	1	6	Data restricted to 23 patients with obstructive jaundice or other symptoms suggesting pancreatic malignancy; proven final diagnoses available for all.
Staab	1971	61	42	3	7	9	7	44	
McCarthy	1972	387	101	26	20	177	83	32	Of the false-negative diagnoses, 21 were in patients with pancreatitis, often when the process was in clinical remission. Authors also stress tendency for extrapancreatic disorders to adversely affect pancreatic accumulation of ^{75}Se-selenomethionine.
Espiritu	1972	178	77	10	11	55	36	40	
Hatchette	1972	125	78	5	6	34	8	19	
Miale	1972	339	221	11	5	77	30	28	Also note that systemic disorders (e.g., uremia, carcinomatosis, etc.) can produce abnormal pancreatic scans.
TOTALS		2399	1313	116	8	671	299	31	

TABLE 6–3. Pancreatic ^{75}Se-selenomethionine Accumulation in Animals

EXPERIMENTAL CONDITION	NO. OF ANIMALS	ADMINISTERED DOSE (%) PER GRAM OF PANCREATIC TISSUE (MEAN ± S.D.)
The Rabbit		
Controls: allowed to feed ad lib. (~ 2.5 kg. males)	4	3.92 ± 0.75
Pancreozymin: 12.5 units, IV, 3 hr. before ^{75}Se-selenomethionine (see Blau, 1962)	4	3.94 ± 0.65
Secretin: 12.5 units, IV, simultaneously with ^{75}Se-selenomethionine (see Delaney, 1966)	4	4.46 ± 1.59
The Rat		
Controls: allowed to feed ad lib. (~ 400 gm. males)	10	3.15 ± 0.28
Fasted (allowed water ad lib.) 24 hr. before ^{75}Se-selenomethionine (see Hansson, 1959; Webster, 1966)	6	3.18 ± 0.75
Pro-Banthine: 0.5 mg., IP, simultaneously with ^{75}Se-selenomethionine (see Bender, 1965)	4	3.38 ± 0.59
Pilocarpine: 20 mg., IP, 3 hr. before ^{75}Se-selenomethionine (see Farber, 1956)	4	2.93 ± .09
Pilocarpine: 2 mg., IP, 3 hr. before ^{75}Se-selenomethionine	3	2.83 ± 0.14
Pilocarpine: 2 mg., IP, 3 hr. before and Pro-Banthine, 0.5 mg., IP, simultaneously with ^{75}Se-selenomethionine	4	2.91 ± 0.40
Solu-Cortef: 5 mg., IP, 2 hr. before ^{75}Se-selenomethionine (see Kaplan, 1961)	4	1.80 ± 0.46*
Raw soybean flour: 1 gm., PO, 2 hr. before ^{75}Se-selenomethionine (see Guggenheim, 1964; Rothman, 1967)	4	3.65 ± 0.87
Soybean tryptic inhibitor: 50 mg., PO, 2 hr. before ^{75}Se-selenomethionine (see Lyman, 1957)	3	3.26 ± 0.07
CZI insulin: 1 unit, IP, simultaneously with ^{75}Se-selenomethionine (see Ben Abdeljil, 1965; Wool, 1965)	4	3.14 ± 0.62
Glucose: 80 mg., IP, 30 min. before ^{75}Se-selenomethionine (see Sodee, 1966)	4	3.21 ± 0.14
Ethionine: 0.5 mg., IP, 30 min. before ^{75}Se-selenomethionine (see Eaton, 1967*b*)	6	4.84 ± 0.53*

*Statistically different from controls; $p < 0.001$ (t test).

actual beneficial effect. The authors of this monograph have conducted a series of modest experimental studies in animals in an effort to find means of improving pancreatic ^{75}Se-selenomethionine uptake (Table 6–3). Our data suggest that pancreatic amino acid accumulation is a relatively autonomous function. Among the numerous protocols analyzed, only pretreatment with ethionine produced a statistically significant increment (Eaton, 1967*b*). This agent, which is the ethyl analogue of methionine, appears to affect pancreatic amino acid accumulation by suppressing acinar cell enzyme release rather than by increasing amino acid uptake or protein synthesis per se (Lin, 1954; Kahn, 1959; Ekholm, 1962). Unfortunately, ethionine causes pancreatitis when given in large doses (Farber, 1950; Ekholm, 1962) and is carcinogenic when given in small daily doses over a prolonged period (Farber, 1963). Since the dose of ethionine required to increase pancreatic ^{75}Se-selenomethionine accumulation is only one-thousandth that used to produce pancreatitis, it might be possible to employ this agent as an adjunct to pancreatic scanning in humans, but the requisite clinical trials have not been performed.

An improved radiopharmaceutical for pancreatic imaging would be more desirable than any of the physiologic alterations so far advanced. Since the avidity of normal pancreatic acinar cells for amino acids is the most distinctive biochemical function amenable to use for radionuclide imaging of the pancreas, it seems reasonable to seek a radioactively labeled amino acid which can be safely administered in greater doses than can ^{75}Se-selenomethionine. Amino acids "tagged" with radioactive halogens (e.g., tryptophan and phenylalanine labeled with ^{123}I [Lambrecht, 1972] and phenylalanine labeled with ^{18}F [Hoyte, 1971]) have been developed, but the addition of a relatively large halogen atom to an amino acid tends to decrease the affinity of the combined molecule for the enzyme systems which transport amino acids across the pancreatic cell membrane.

A more promising possibility has been advanced by Miale (1972) who suggests development of ^{73}Se-selenomethionine. Selenium-73 has a physical half-life of 7.1 hours and decays by positron emission (which, in turn, results in 511 keV. positron annihilation radiation) and electron capture (with emission of 359 keV. gamma rays). A suitably rapid technique for incorporating Selenium-73 into selenomethionine remains to be devised and, at present, the high production cost of the isotope itself is a limiting factor. Nevertheless, if these problems could be overcome, a dose of ^{73}Se-selenomethionine which would result in a tenfold increase in peak pancreatic radioactivity could be given as safely as the currently accepted dose of ^{75}Se-selenomethionine.

REFERENCES

Agnew, B. A., McCarthy, D. M., Melmed, R. N., and Bouchier, A. D.: Count rate analysis as an adjunct to the ^{75}Se-selenomethionine pancreas scan. Brit. J. Radiol., *42*:762–769, 1969.

Allaway, W. H., Kubota, J., Losee, F., et al: Selenium molybdenum and vanadium in human blood. Arch. Environ. Health, *16*:342–348, 1968.

Amersham/Searle Radiopharmaceuticals RP-1, Des Plaines, Ill., November, 1968.

Awwad, H. K., Adelstein, S. J., Potchen, E. J., et al: The interconversion and reutilization of injected 75-Se-selenomethionine in the rat. J. Biol. Chem., *242*:492–500, 1967.

Awwad, H. K., Potchen, E. J., Adelstein, S. J., et al: The regional distribution of Se-75-selenomethionine in the rat. Metabolism, *15*: 370–378, 1966.

Becker, V.: Histochemistry of the exocrine pancreas. *In* The Exocrine Pancreas. Edited by A. V. S. deReuck and M. P. Cameron. Boston, Little, Brown and Company, 1961, pp. 56–66.

Ben Abdeljil, A., et al: Effect of insulin on pancreatic amylase and chymotrypsinogen. Biochem. Biophys. Res. Commun., *18*:71–75, 1965.

Bender, M. A.: Pancreas photoscanning. *In* Nuclear Medicine. Edited by W. H. Blahd. New York, McGraw-Hill, 1965, pp. 298–302.

Bergeron, D. A., and Veogel, J. M.: Dual isotope pancreatic imaging utilizing the Anger camera and Tc-99m sulfur colloid. Amer. J. Roentgen., *109*:764–768, 1970.

Blanquet, P. C., Beck, C. R., Fleury, J., and Polais, C. J.: Pancreas scanning ^{75}Se-selenomethionine and ^{198}Au using digital-data-processing techniques. J. Nucl. Med., 9:486–488, 1968.

Blau, M.: Biosynthesis of ^{75}Se-selenomethionine

and ^{75}Se-selenocystine. Biochim. Biophys. Acta, *49*:389–390, 1961.

Blau, M., and Bender, M. A.: ^{75}Se-selenomethionine for visualization of the pancreas by isotope scanning. Radiology, *78*:974, 1962.

Blau, M., and Manske, R. F.: The pancreas specificity of Se^{75}-selenomethionine. J. Nucl. Med., *2*:102–105, 1961.

Bonte, R. J., and Curry, T. S.: Radionuclide cineangiography of the pancreas in dogs. J. Nucl. Med., *10*:389, 1969.

Brown, P. W., Sircus, W., Smith, A. N., Donaldson, A. A., Dymock, I. W., Falconer, C. W. A., and Small, W. P.: Scintillography in the diagnosis of pancreatic disease. Lancet, *1*:160–163, 1968.

Cardell, B. S.: The pancreas. *In* Systemic Pathology. Edited by G. P. Wright and W. St. C. Symmers. London, Longmans, 1966, pp. 688–707.

Caro, L. G.: Electronic microscopic radioautography of thin sections: the Golgi zone as a site of protein concentration in pancreatic acinar cells. J. Biophys. Biochem. Cytol., *10*:37–45, 1961.

Caro, L. G., and Palade, G. E.: Protein synthesis, storage and discharge in the pancreatic exocrine cell: an autoradiographic study. J. Cell. Biol., *20*:473–495, 1964.

Charlesworth, D., Testa, H. J., Pullan, B. R., and Torrance, H. B.: Experiences with data processing to separate the images in pancreatic scanning. Gut, *11*:261–267, 1970.

Colella, A. C., and Pigorini, F.: Experiences in pancreas scanning using ^{75}Se-selenomethionine. Brit. J. Radiol., *40*:662–669, 1967.

Daley, M. M., and Mirsky, A. E.: Formation of protein in the pancreas. J. Gen. Physiol., *36*: 243, 1952.

Davies, R. E., et al.: A comparison of the respiratory activity and histological changes in isolated pancreatic tissue. Amer. J. Physiol., *157*:278–282, 1949.

Delaney, J. P., and Grim, E.: Influence of hormones and drugs on canine pancreatic blood flow. Amer. J. Physiol., *211*:1398, 1966.

Dreiling, D. A., et al: Pancreatic Inflammatory Disease. New York, Hoeber, 1964.

Dupre, J.: Regulation of the secretions of the pancreas. Ann. Rev. Med., *21*:299–316, 1970.

Eaton, S. B., Potsaid, M. S., Lo, H. H., and Beaulieu, E.: Radioisotope "subtraction" scanning for pancreatic lesions. Radiology, *89*:1033–1039, 1967*a*.

Eaton, S. B., Potsaid, M. S., Lo, H. H., et al.: A potential method for increasing pancreatic accumulation of Se-75-selenomethionine. Radiology, *89*:933, 1967*b*.

Eaton, S. B., James, A. E., Potsaid, M. S., and Nardi, G. L.: Evaluation of Corrective Surgery for Pancreatitis by Se^{75}-selenomethionine pancreatic imaging. Amer. J. Roentgen., *112*: 678–681, 1971.

Ekholm, R., Zelander, T., and Edlund, Y.: The ultrastructure of the rat exocrine pancreas after brief ethionine exposure. J. Ultrastruct. Res., *7*:102–120, 1962.

Espiritu, C. R., and Rolfs, H. E.: Diagnostic accuracy of pancreatic scanning. Amer. J. Dig. Dis., *17*:539–543, 1972.

Farber, E.: Ethionine carcinogenesis. Advances Cancer Res., *7*:383–474, 1963.

Farber, E., and Popper, H.: Production of acute pancreatitis with ethionine and its prevention with methionine. Proc. Soc. Exp. Biol. Med., *74*:838, 1950.

Farber, E., and Sidransky, H.: Changes in protein metabolism in the rat pancreas on stimulation. J. Biol. Chem., *222*:237–248, 1956.

Fink, S., Ben-Porath, M., Jacobson, B., Clayton, G. B., and Kaplan, E.: Current status of dual channel pancreas scanning. J. Nucl. Med., *10*:78–82, 1969.

Friedberg, F., and Greenberg, D. M.: Partition of intravenously administered amino acids in blood and tissues. J. Biol. Chem., *168*:411, 1947.

Friedberg, F., Tarver, H., and Greenberg, D. M.: The distribution pattern of sulfur-labeled methionine in the protein and the free amino acid fraction of tissues after intravenous administration. J. Biol. Chem., *173*:355–361, 1948.

Gregory, R. A.: The pancreas. *In* Secretory Mechanisms of the Gastrointestinal Tract. London, Edward Arnold Publishers, 1962, pp. 134–191.

Guggenheim, K., and Goldberg, A.: Endogenous loss of nitrogen originating in the pancreas. *In* The Role of the Gastrointestinal Tract in Protein Metabolism. Edited by H. N. Monro. Philadelphia, F. A. Davis Co., 1964, pp. 63–82.

Guyton, A. C.: Osmotic equilibria and fluid shifts between the extracellular and intracellular fluids. Medical Physiology. Philadelphia, W. B. Saunders Company, 1961, pp. 42–51.

Hansson, E.: The formation of pancreatic juice proteins studied with labeled amino acids. Acta. Physiol. Scand., *46*:Suppl. 161, 1959.

Hansson, E., and Blau, M.: Incorporation of Se^{75} selenomethionine into pancreatic juice proteins in vivo. Biochem. Biophys. Res. Commun., *13*:71–74, 1968.

Hatchette, J. B., Shuler, S. E., and Murison, P. J.: Scintiphotos of the pancreas: analysis of 134 studies. J. Nucl. Med., *13*:51–57, 1972.

Haverback, B. J.: Exocrine function of the pancreas. J.A.M.A., *193*:279–283, 1965.

Heslip, P. G., and Overton, T. R.: The value of radioisotope scanning in the investigation of suspected carcinoma of the pancreas. Amer. J. Roentgen., *112*:667–677, 1971.

Howard, J. M.: Pancreatitis associated with gallstones. *In* Surgical Diseases of the Pancreas. Edited by J. M. Howard and G. L. Jordan. Philadelphia, J. B. Lippincott Company, 1960.

Hoyte, R. M., Lin, S. S., Christman, D. R., Atkins, H. L., Hauser, W., and Wolf, A. P.: Organic radiopharmaceuticals labeled with short-lived nuclides. III. ^{18}F labeled phenylalanines. J. Nucl. Med., *12*:280–286, 1971.

Ichikawa, A.: Fine structural changes in response to hormonal stimulation of the perfused canine pancreas. J. Cell. Biol., *24*:369, 1965.

Janowitz, H. D., and Dreiling, D. A.: Secretion of

fluid and electrolytes. *In* The Exocrine Pancreas. Edited by A. V. S. deReuck and M. P. Cameron. Boston, Little, Brown and Company, 1961, pp. 115–137.
Junqueira, L. C. U., and Hirsch, G. C.: Cell secretion: a study of pancreas and salivary glands. Int. Rev. Cytol., *V*:323–364, 1956.
Junqueira, L. C. U., et al.: The action of atropine on pancreatic secretion. Brit. J. Pharmacol., *13*:71, 1958.
Kahn, D. B., and Carlson, A. B.: On the mechanism of experimentally induced ethionine pancreatitis. Ann. Surg., *150*:42–48, 1959.
Kaplan, E., Ben-Porath, M., Fink, S., Clayton, G. D., and Jacobson, B.: Elimination of liver interference from the selenomethionine pancreas scan. J. Nucl. Med., *7*:807–816, 1966.
Kaplan, S. A., and Nagareda, C. S.: Effects of hydrocortisone and adrenalectomy on uptake of X-Amino-Isobutryic acid. Amer. J. Physiol., *200*:1035, 1961.
Keller, P. J., and Cohen, E.: Enzymatic composition of some cell fractions of bovine pancreas. J. Biol. Chem., *236*:1407–1413, 1971.
King, E. R., Sharpe, A., Grubb, W., Brock, J. S., and Greenberg, L.: A study of the morphology of the normal pancreas using Se^{75} methionine photoscanning. Amer. J. Roentgen., *96*:657–663, 1966.
Laird, A. K., and Barton, A. D.: Protein synthesis in the rat pancreas. II. Changes in the intracellular distribution of pancreatic amylase during the secretory cycle. Biochim. Biophys. Acta, *27*:12, 1958.
Lambrecht, R. M., Mantescu, C., Atkins, H. L., and Wolf, A. P.: Development of New ^{123}I Radiopharmaceuticals. American Nuclear Society Transactions, Vol. 15. 1972.
Landman, S., Polcyn, R. E., and Gottschalk, A.: Pancreatic imaging: is it worth it? Radiology, *100*:631–636, 1971.
Lathrop, K. A., Johnston, R. E., Blau, M., and Rothschild, E. O.: Radiation dose to humans from ^{75}Se-L-selenomethionine. J. Nucl. Med., *13*:Suppl., 1972.
Lin, T. M., and Grossman, M. I.: Reversal by dl-methionine of acute effect of dl-ethionine on pancreatic enzyme output in dogs. Amer. J. Physiol., *176*:377, 1954.
Lyman, R. L., and Lepkovsky, S.: The effect of raw soy bean meal and trypsin inhibitor diets on pancreatic enzyme secretion in the rat. J. Nutr., *62*:269–284, 1957.
McCarthy, D. M., Brown, P., Melmed, R. N., Agnew, J. E., and Bouchier, I. A. D.: ^{75}Se-selenomethionine scanning in the diagnosis of tumours of the pancreas and adjacent viscera: the use of the test and its impact on survival. Gut, *13*:75–87, 1972.
McCarthy, D. M., Kreel, L., Agnew, J. E., and Bouchier, I. A. D.: Value of hypotonic duodenography as an adjunct to pancreatic scanning. Gut, *10*:665–673, 1969.
McConnell, K. P., and Cho, G. J.: Active transport of L-selenomethionine in the intestine. Amer. J. Physiol., *213*:150–156, 1967.
Melmed, R. N., Agnew, J. E., and Bouchier, I. A. D.: The normal and abnormal pancreatic scan. Quart. J. Med., *37*:607–624, 1968.
Miale, A.: Personal communication, 1972.
Miale, A., Rodriguez-Antunez, A., and Gill, W. M.: Pancreatic scanning after ten years. Seminars Nucl. Med., *2*:201–219, 1965.
Morris, A. J., and Dickman, S. R.: Biosynthesis of ribonuclease in mouse pancreas. J. Biol. Chem., *235*:1404–1408, 1960.
Nadler, N. J.: Calculations of the turnover times of proteins in each region of the acinar cells of the pancreas. J. Cell. Biol., *16*:24, 1963.
Nardi, G. L.: Physiologic peregrinations in pancreatic perfusion. Ann. Surg., *158*:830, 1963.
Neuberger, A., and Richards, F. F.: Protein biosynthesis in mammalian tissues. *In* Mammalian Protein Metabolism. Edited by H. N. Munro and J. B. Allison. New York, Academic Press, 1964, pp. 243–296.
Overton, T. R., Heslip, P. G., Barrow, P. A., and Jelinek, J.: Dual radioisotope techniques and digital image subtraction methods in pancreatic visualization. J. Nucl. Med., *12*:493–498, 1971.
Palade, G. E., et al.: Structure, chemistry, and function of the pancreatic exocrine cell. *In* The Exocrine Pancreas. Edited by A. V. S. deReuck and M. P. Cameron. Boston, Little Brown and Company, 1961, pp. 23–55.
Potsaid, M. S.: Stereoscopic radionuclide pancreatography. (In preparation.)
Preshaw, R. M., Cooke, A. R., and Grossman, M. I.: Pancreatic secretion induced by stimulation of the pyloric gland area of the stomach. Science, *148*:1347–1348, 1965*a*.
Preshaw, R. M., Cooke, A. R., and Grossman, M. I.: Stimulation of pancreatic secretion by a humoral agent from the pyloric gland area of the stomach. Gastroenterology, *49*:617–622, 1965*b*.
Riccobono, X. J.: Pancreatic scanning. Seminars Roentgen., *3*:310–317, 1968.
Roberts, H., and Simonsen, D. G.: Free amino acids in animal tissue. *In* Amino Acid Pools. Edited by J. T. Holden. Amsterdam, Elsevier Publishing Company, 1962, pp. 284–349.
Rodriguez-Antunez, A.: Pancreatic scanning with selenium-75 methionine utilizing morphine to enhance contrast. Cleveland Clin. Quart., *31*:213–218, 1964.
Rodriguez-Antunez, A., Alfidi, R. J., and Gill, W. M.: Pancreas scanning. CRC Critical Reviews in Radiological Sciences, *1*:26–46, 1970.
Rothman, S. S.: Trypsin and chymotrypsin secretion from rabbit pancreas in vitro. Amer. J. Physiol., *211*:777–780, 1966.
Rothman, S. S., and Wells, H.: Enhancement of pancreatic enzyme synthesis by pancreozymin. Amer. J. Physiol., *213*:215–218, 1967.
Rosenfeld, I., and Beath, O. A.: Selenium. New York, Academic Press, 1964.
Rotschild, H. A., et al.: Radioactive amino acid incorporation into the rat pancreatic juice proteins. Experimentia, *13*:158, 1957.
Schwarz, K.: Development and status of experimental work on factor 3 selenium. Fed. Proc., *20* (Part 1):663–673, 1961.
Schwarz, K., and Foltz, C. M.: Selenium as an

integral part of factor 3 against dietary necrotic liver degeneration. J. Amer. Chem. Soc., *79*:3292–3293, 1957.

Sodee, D. B.: Pancreatic scanning. Radiology, *87*:641–645, 1966.

Sodee, D. B.: Radioisotope scanning of the pancreas with selenomethionine (Se^{75}). Radiology, *83*:910–916, 1964.

Spencer, R. P., and Blau, M.: Intestinal transport of Selenium-75 selenomethionine. Science, *136*:155, 1962.

Squibb Technical Data Sheet "Sethotope" Division of Nuclear Medicine, New Brunswick, N. J., April, 1970.

Staab, E. V., Babb, O. A., Klatte, E. C., and Brill, A. B.: Pancreatic radionuclide imaging using electronic subtraction technique. Radiology, *99*:633–640, 1971.

Tabern, D. L., Kearney, M. D., and Dolbow, A.: The use of intravenous amino acids in the visualization of the pancreas with Seleno-75-methionine. J. Nucl. Med., *6*:762–766, 1965.

Thomas, R. L., Robinson, A. E., Johnsrude, I. S., Goodrich, J. K., and Lester, R. G.: The demonstration of an insulin and gastrin producing pancreatic tumor by angiography and pancreatic scanning. Amer. J. Roentgen., *104*: 646–651, 1968.

Van Goidsenhoven, G. E., et al: Pancreatic metabolism of Se-75-selenomethionine in dogs. Gastroenterology, *53*:403–411, 1967.

Van Heyningen, H. E.: Secretion of protein enzymes by the acinar cells of the rat pancreas. *In* The Use of Radioautography in Investigating Protein Synthesis. Edited by C. P. LeBland. New York, Academic Press, 1965, pp. 261–272.

Walker, D. G.: Cytoarchitecture of protein secretory and active transport cells. *In* The Physiological Basis of Medical Practice. Edited by C. H. Best and N. B. Taylor. Baltimore, Williams & Wilkins Co., 1966, pp. 1055–1058.

Warshawsky, H., Leblond, C. P., Droz, B., et al.: Synthesis and migration of proteins in the cells of the exocrine pancreas as revealed by specific activity determination from radioautography. J. Cell. Biol., *16*:1–27, 1963.

Webster, P. D., and Tyor, M. P.: Effect of intravenous pancreozymin on amino acid incorporation in vitro by pancreatic tissue. Amer. J. Physiol., *211*:157–160, 1966.

Wool, I. G.: Relation of effects of insulin on amino acid transport and on protein synthesis. Fed. Proc., *24*:1060–1070, 1965.

Zuidema, G. D., et al: Pancreatic uptake of Se^{75}-selenomethionine. Ann. Surg., *158*:894–897, 1963.

Chapter 7

ANGIOGRAPHY

Stanley Baum, M.D. and Christos A. Athanasoulis, M.D.

ANATOMY AND TECHNIQUE

The arterial and venous anatomy of the pancreas and duodenum are outlined in detail in Chapter 1. As is seen in Figures 1–5 and 1–6, the origins of the arterial branches to the pancreas are multiple and varied. Approximately 50 per cent of patients have some form of anatomic variation other than the classic three-vessel celiac axis (Fig. 7–1).

Satisfactory pancreatic arteriography is technically much more difficult to perform than other selective angiographic examinations. Boijsen (1966*a*) approached the problem of the dual blood supply to the pancreas by injecting simultaneously into the celiac and superior mesenteric arteries, utilizing two catheters passed retrograde from each femoral artery (Fig. 7–1, *A*). Because of the potential increase in morbidity involved with double catheterization techniques, and the superimposition of the many injected vessels, alternative methods were devised. These involve separate injections into the celiac and superior mesenteric arteries as well as superselective techniques with injections into the hepatic, gastroduodenal and splenic arteries (Figs. 7–2 and 7–3). Superselective injection of relatively large volumes of contrast material (30 to 40 cc.) into intrapancreatic branches such as the dorsal pancreatic artery is a technique that has recently been introduced in an attempt to define greater detail in this otherwise elusive organ (Eisenberg, 1973) (Fig. 7–4).

Description of the techniques and operative details involved in performing safe and technically diagnostic studies is beyond the scope of this chapter. Many excellent articles have been written on the choice of catheter material, catheter shapes, as well as catheter manipulators (Boijsen, 1961; Baum, 1964; Judkins, 1967; Reuter, 1969*a*; and Rösch, 1969). In addition, direct serial magnification as well as pharmacoangiographic studies are now frequently employed in an attempt to increase the diagnostic yield of the examination (Figs. 7–3 and 7–5).

Duodenum

Tumors

Selective angiography has been of very limited value in the diagnosis of gastrointestinal tumors. Adenocarcinoma, the most common malignant duodenal tumor, is not a particularly vascular lesion, and therefore the angiographic findings are usually not very remarkable. Some authors have described hypervascularity, luminal irregularity and occasional staining of the area of the tumor (Boijsen, 1966*b*), but these findings are in most cases very difficult to evaluate. More often than not, the angiographer is em-

(Text continued on page 233)

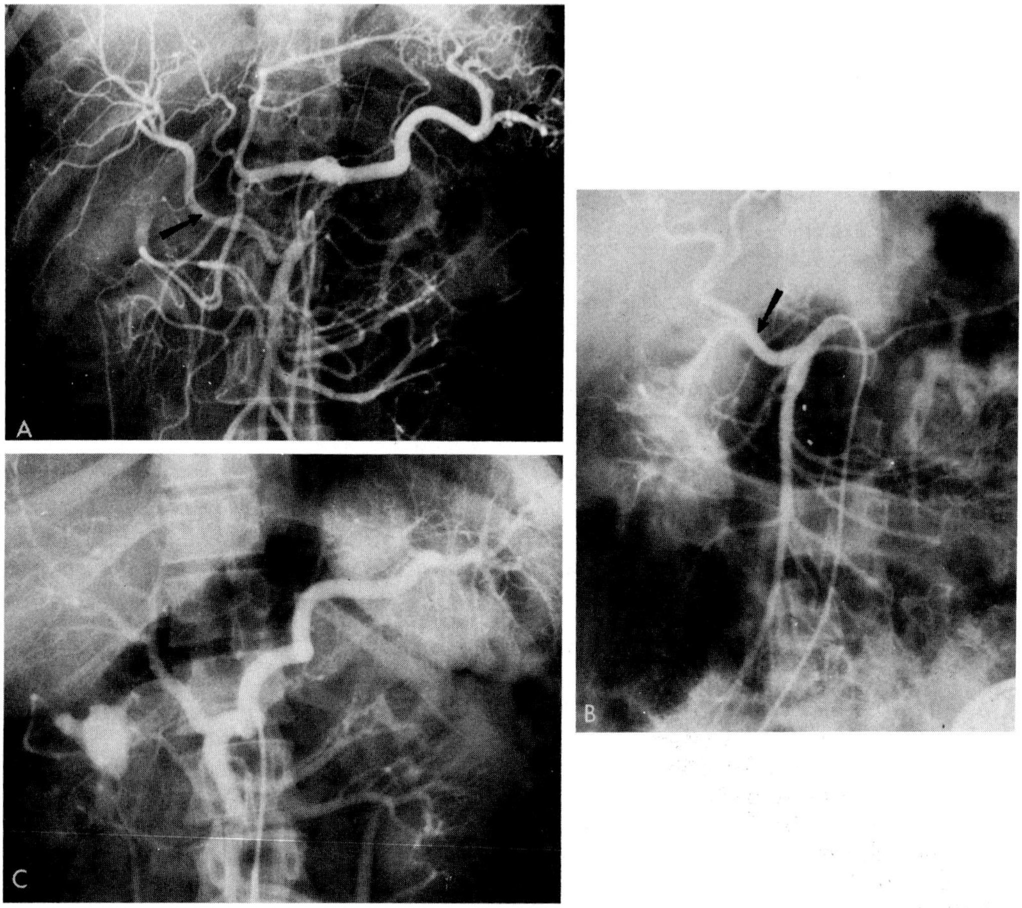

Figure 7–1. Variations of normal celiac and superior mesenteric anatomy.

A, Contrast injected simultaneously into two catheters: one positioned in the celiac axis, and the other in the superior mesenteric artery.

The right hepatic artery takes origin from the superior mesenteric artery (*arrow*). The celiac axis gives origin to the left and middle hepatic arteries. The gastroduodenal artery takes origin from the left hepatic artery.

B, Superior mesenteric arteriography shows the entire hepatic artery originating from the superior mesenteric artery. The splenic and the left gastric arteries have a common, separate origin from the aorta.

C, The superior mesenteric, hepatic and splenic arteries originate from the aorta as a common celiacomesenteric trunk. The left gastric artery in the same patient came directly from the aorta.

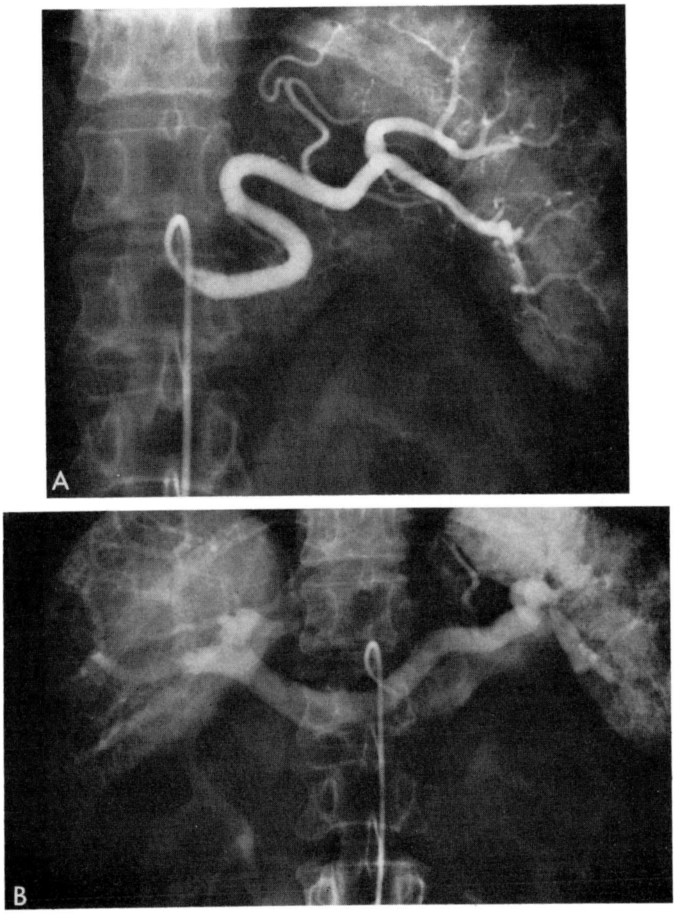

Figure 7–2. Normal splenic arteriogram in the evaluation of the pancreatic body and tail.

A, Arterial phase of a selective splenic arteriogram demonstrates the pancreatica magna and short pancreatic arteries supplying the body and tail of the pancreas.

B, During the venous phase of the same injection, the splenic vein and portal vein are optimally visualized. The close association of the splenic vein with the opacified normal pancreatic body and tail is apparent.

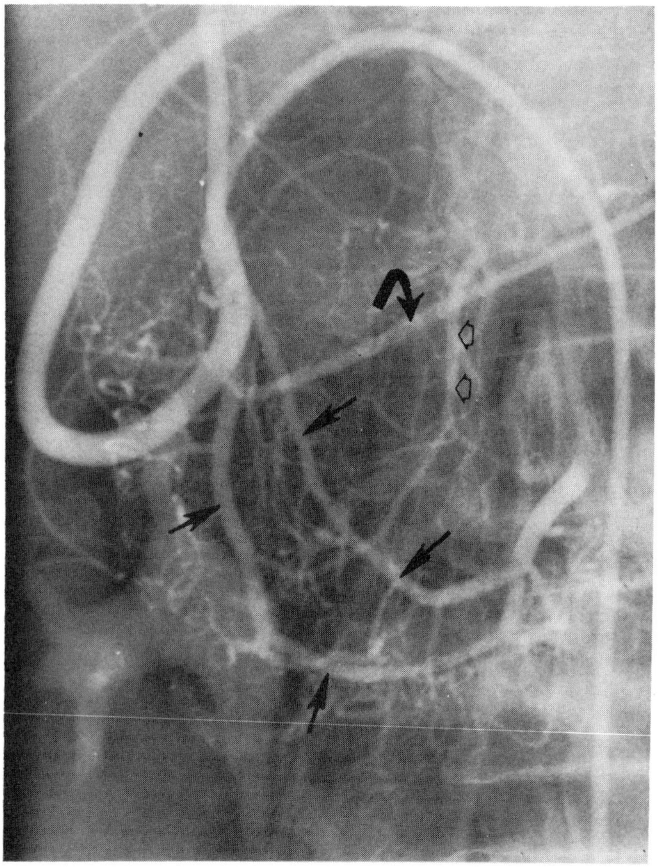

Figure 7–3. Normal pancreatic arcades. Direct serial magnification angiography during a gastroduodenal artery injection clearly demonstrates the pancreatic arcades (*straight arrows*), the transverse pancreatic artery (*curved arrow*) and the dorsal pancreatic artery (*open arrow*).

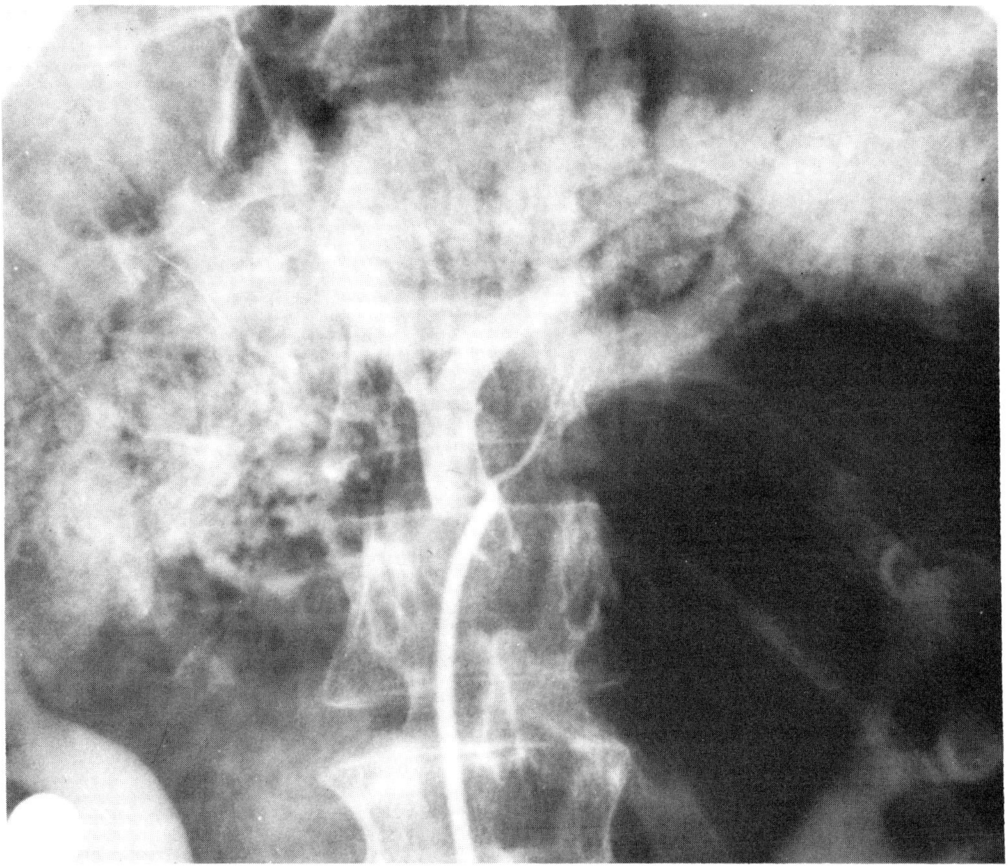

Figure 7–4. Total opacification of the pancreatic head, body and tail. Direct magnification (3 ×) arteriography shows intense opacification of the entire organ following the injection of 40 cc. of contrast injected selectively into the dorsal pancreatic artery after stimulation with intravenous secretin. (Courtesy of Dr. Harvey Eisenberg, Boston, Mass.)

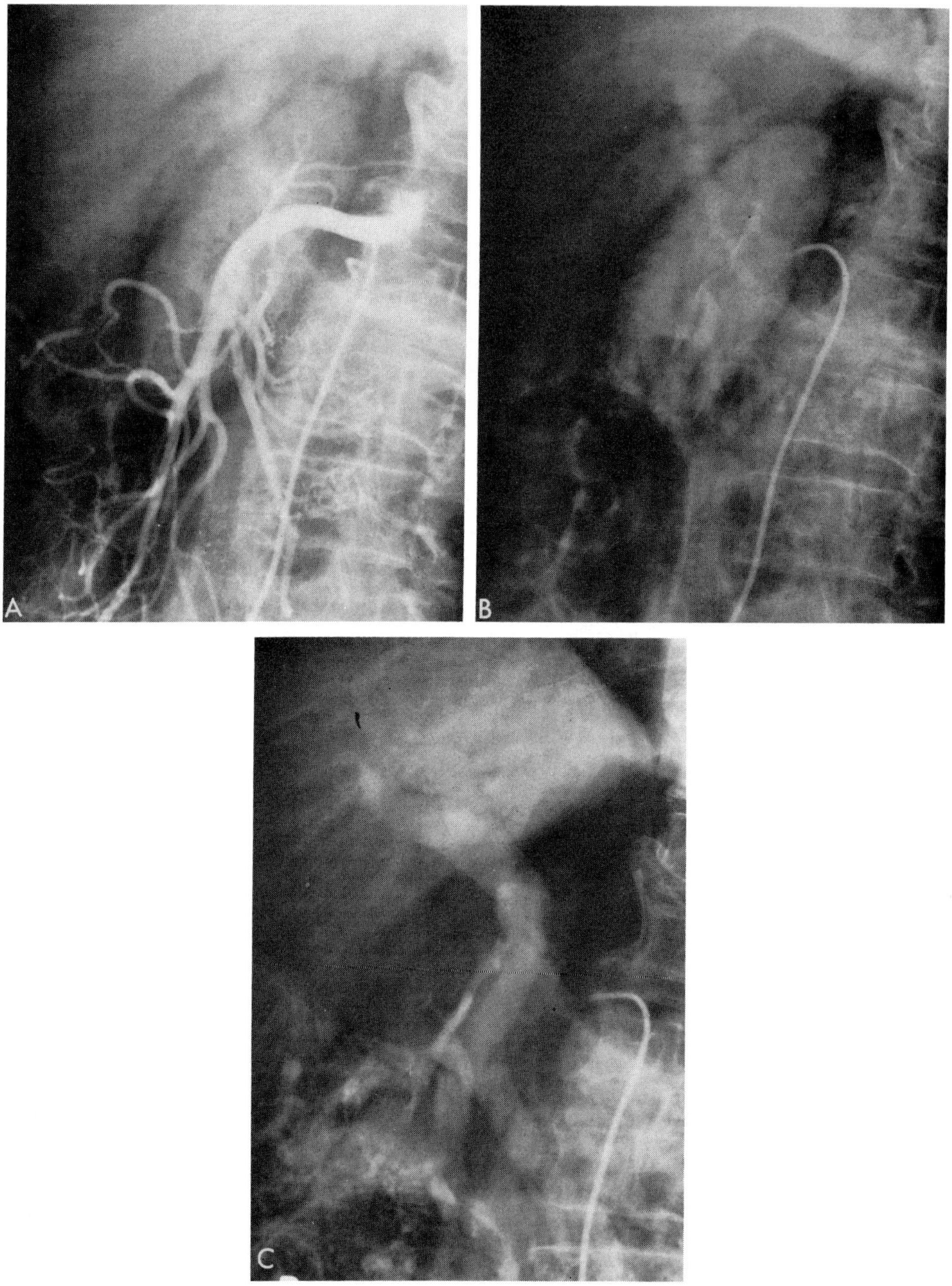

Figure 7–5. Improved opacification of the portal venous system with pharmacological means.
A, Superior mesenteric arteriogram, arterial phase.
B, During the venous phase of the superior mesenteric arteriogram, there is inadequate opacification of the mesenteric and portal veins because of contrast dilution.
C, In the same patient, the opacification of the superior mesenteric and portal veins was markedly improved when the superior mesenteric arteriogram was repeated after the injection of 25 mg. of tolazoline into the superior mesenteric artery.

barrassed by the very meager findings on selective angiography of the duodenum when compared with the gross changes of malignancy in the conventional barium examination (Baum, 1971*a*). It is probably fair to state that present angiographic techniques will probably never replace barium studies for the detection of early gastrointestinal cancer. Angiography can, however, evaluate the extent of the cancer and detect metastatic disease in the area of the head of the pancreas and porta hepatis. An additional benefit derived from selective angiography in patients with adenocarcinoma of the gastrointestinal tract is the delineation of a preoperative arterial road map, since it is obviously important for the surgeon to know anatomic variations prior to any attempt at radical surgery.

Strictures in the duodenum can, on occasion, be confused with primary adenocarcinoma, and angiography can be very helpful in separating out those patients who have strictures secondary to ischemic changes, or direct extension by adjacent tumors such as pancreatic carcinoma (Figs. 7–6 and 7–7).

Tumors that are characteristically vascular, such as leiomyomas, angiomatous

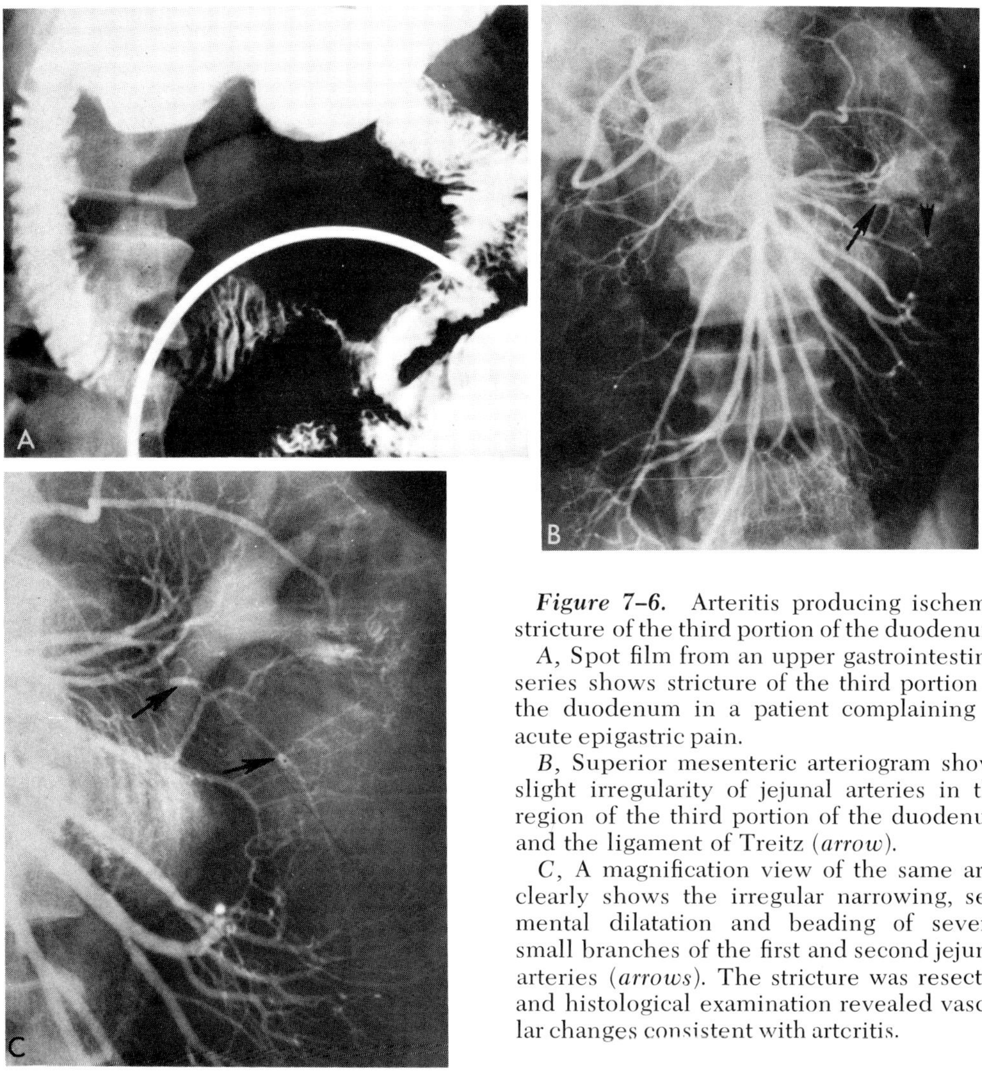

Figure 7–6. Arteritis producing ischemic stricture of the third portion of the duodenum.

A, Spot film from an upper gastrointestinal series shows stricture of the third portion of the duodenum in a patient complaining of acute epigastric pain.

B, Superior mesenteric arteriogram shows slight irregularity of jejunal arteries in the region of the third portion of the duodenum and the ligament of Treitz (*arrow*).

C, A magnification view of the same area clearly shows the irregular narrowing, segmental dilatation and beading of several small branches of the first and second jejunal arteries (*arrows*). The stricture was resected and histological examination revealed vascular changes consistent with arteritis.

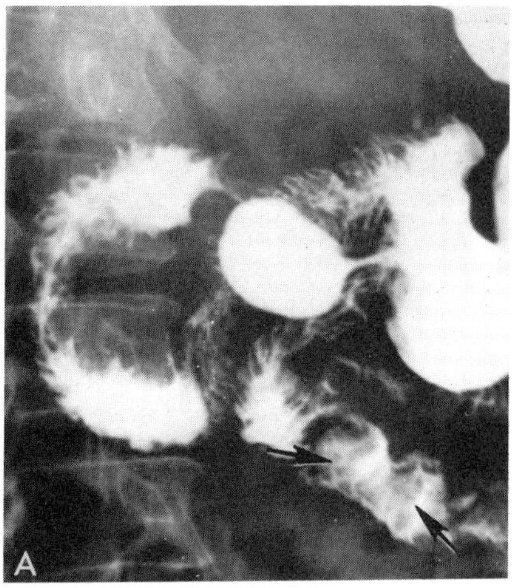

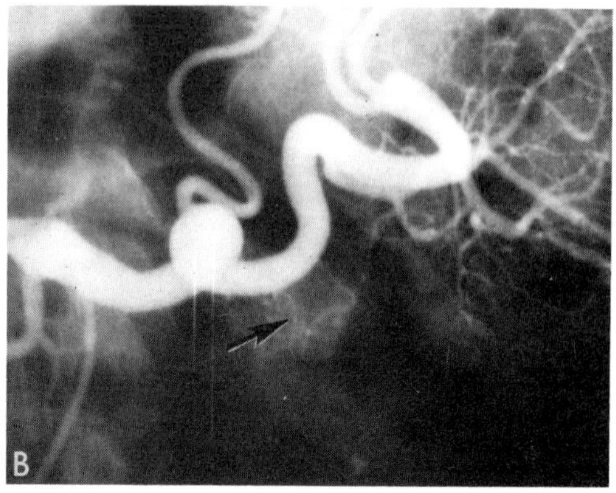

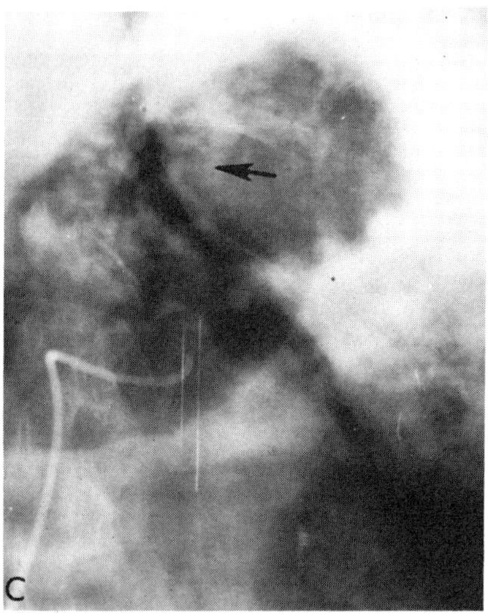

***Figure* 7–7.** Extension of pancreatic carcinoma into the adjacent jejunum.

A, A radiograph from an upper gastrointestinal series shows deformity of the inner aspect of the duodenal sweep from a pancreatic mass lesion. A segment of the proximal jejunum is constricted and the pattern of normal folds has been disrupted in an adjacent loop of small bowel (*arrows*).

B, Selective celiac arteriogram shows irregularity of arterial branches to the body of the pancreas (*arrow*). The splenic artery is normal.

C, The venous phase of a selective splenic arteriogram shows complete occlusion of the splenic vein with opacification of gastric varices (*arrow*). At surgery, carcinoma of the body and tail of the pancreas was found that had involved the ligament of Treitz and proximal jejunum.

malformations or carcinoids, exhibit the same hypervascular appearance when they involve the duodenum as well as other areas of the gastrointestinal tract. These lesions are "hypervascular," with an increase in the apparent number and size of the vessels within the tumor, prominent early filling veins and an intense parenchymal blush (the so-called tumor stain) seen best during the capillary phase of the examination (Figs. 7–8 and 7–9).

Bleeding Duodenal Ulcers

Active bleeding in the gastrointestinal tract, regardless of its location, can be detected angiographically as extravasation of contrast material into the lumen of the gut if the bleeding rate is in excess of 0.5 cc./minute (Nusbaum, 1963). A bleeding duodenal ulcer due to acid peptic disease is best seen when the contrast is injected directly into this gastroduodenal artery, although celiac and superior mesenteric arteriography are also capable of demonstrating the bleeding site. Ulcers in the first portion of the duodenum bleed most often from a branch of either the anterior or posterior pancreaticoduodenal artery and, fortunately for the patient, less often from direct erosion into the gastroduodenal artery.

The angiographic demonstration of bleeding ulcers has assumed even greater

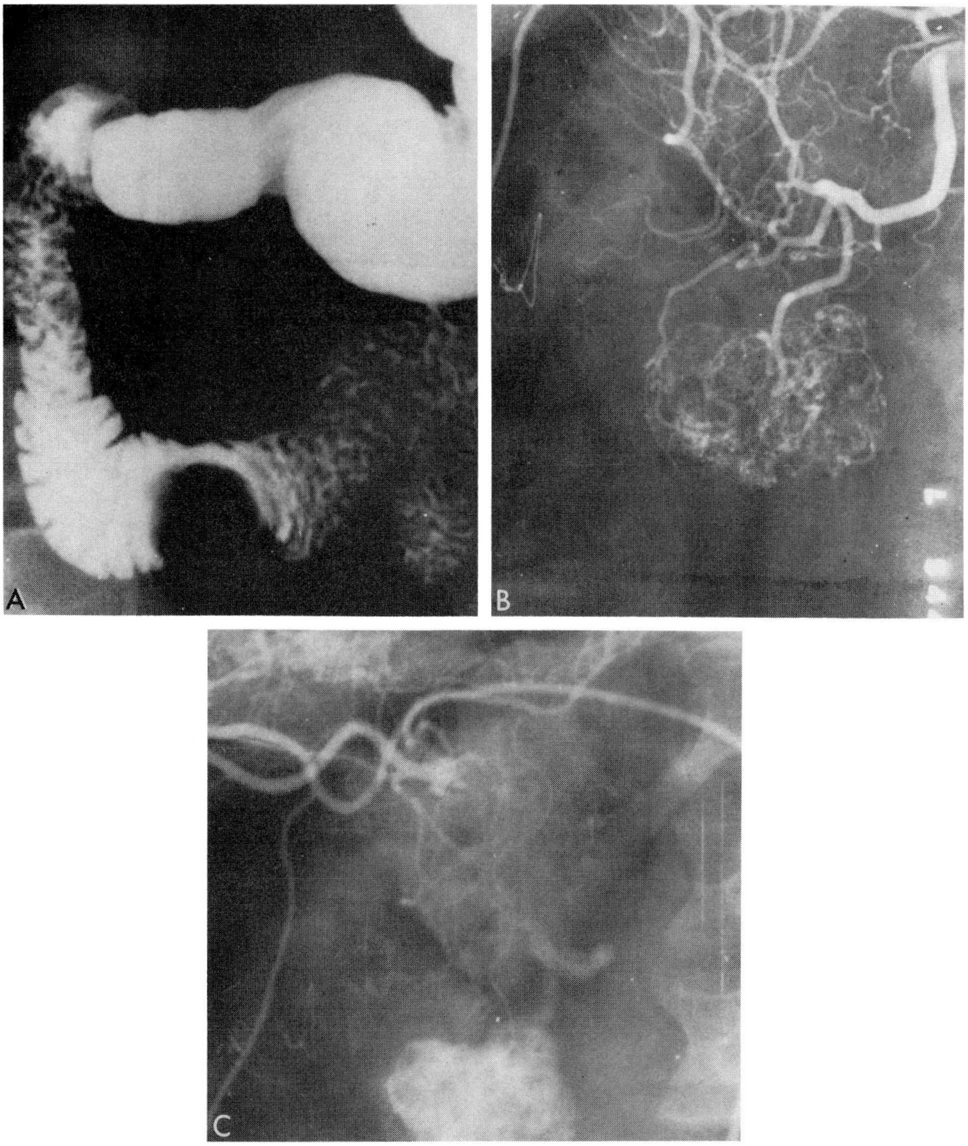

Figure 7–8. Leiomyoma of the third portion of the duodenum.

A, A spot film of an upper gastrointestinal series shows a submucosal mass in the third portion of the duodenum. The patient presented with low-grade gastrointestinal bleeding.

B, Selective magnification gastroduodenal arteriography shows abundant tumor vessels arising from the inferior pancreaticoduodenal artery supplying a mass corresponding to the defect noted in the barium study.

C, During the late phase of the same injection there is an intense blush in the same area.

At surgery this was a duodenal leiomyoma.

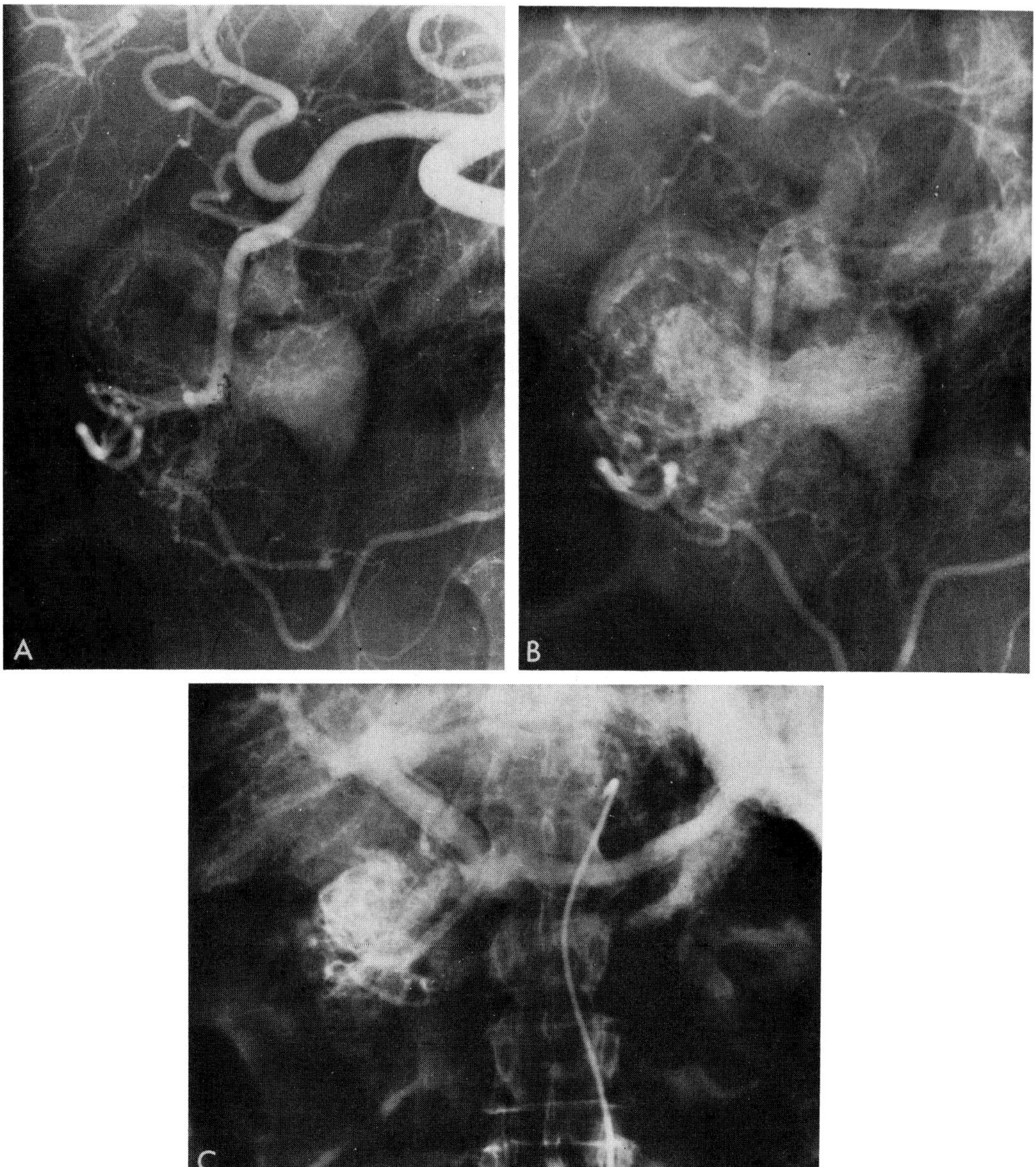

Figure 7–9. Duodenal arteriovenous malformation. A 70-year-old woman with gastrointestinal bleeding, normal gastrointestinal barium studies and a negative exploratory laparotomy.

A, Arterial phase of a selective celiac arteriogram shows an increase in the number of vessels in the distal portion of the gastric antrum and the first portion of the duodenum.

B, The capillary phase of the injection shows an intense blush in the same area.

C, During the venous phase of the celiac arteriogram, the intense blush in the distal antrum and proximal duodenum persists and there is opacification of markedly dilated veins.

The patient was re-explored and biopsy confirmed the presence of an arteriovenous malformation.

importance since the introduction of catheter techniques to control gastrointestinal bleeding. The selective infusion of vasoconstricting agents such as surgical pituitrin (Pituitrin-S) is capable of decreasing arterial flow for long enough periods of time so as to allow stable clot formation in the bleeding vessel (Baum, 1971*b*; Rösch, 1971; Conn, 1972; and Baum, 1973) (Fig. 7–10). In addition to the infusion of vasoconstricting agents, several case reports have described the use of autologous clots (Rösch, 1972), injected through the catheter, as a means of achieving hemostasis (Fig. 7–11). Although all of these techniques are new, preliminary experience suggests that they will become increasingly important in the management of patients hemorrhaging from the gastrointestinal tract.

Stress ulcers frequently involve the stomach and duodenum. These lesions are particularly suitable for arteriography because (a) the ulcers are usually shallow and generally not visualized by barium contrast studies; (b) the ulcers are not surrounded by an indurated inflammatory mass, making them very difficult to detect by surgical palpation (Freeark, 1967); and (c) most stress ulcer bleeding is massive, facilitating arteriographic localization.

Bleeding duodenal stress ulcers occur very often in the descending duodenum (Fig. 7–12) and, in one study, five of eight patients with duodenal stress bleeding had the ulceration at the junction of the second and third portions of the duodenum (Baum, 1971*c*). This is at variance with the previously reported incidence of postbulbar ulceration which runs from 2 per cent in a barium series of peptic ulcers (Salter, 1968) to 8 per cent in an autopsy-diagnosed series of patients with Curling's ulcers (Sevitt, 1967). It has been suggested that the reason acute ulcers occur in this location is that the junction of the second and third portions of the duodenum is at the periphery of the celiac and superior mesenteric

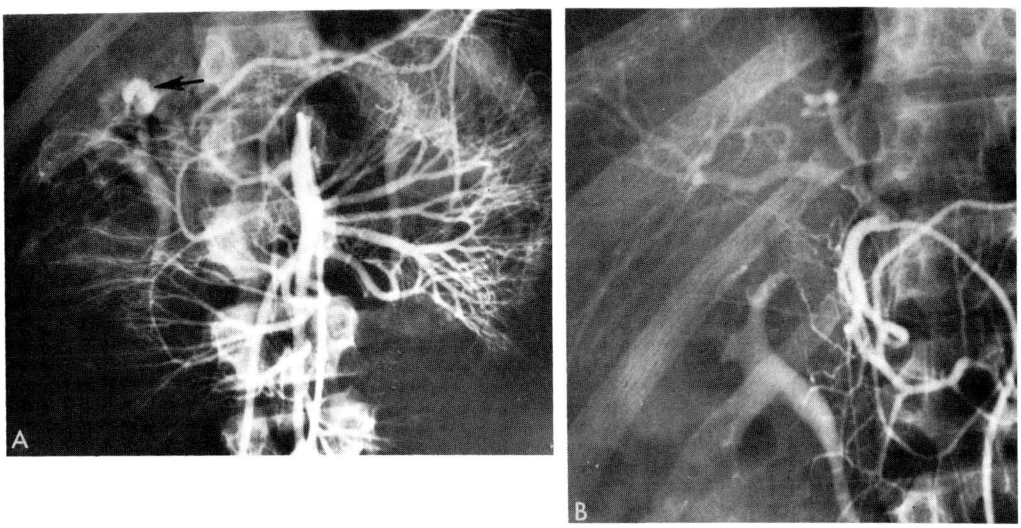

Figure 7–10. Bleeding duodenal ulcer in a twelve-year-old boy controlled with the intra-arterial infusion of pituitrin (Pituitrin-S).

A, Superior mesenteric arteriogram shows a bleeding duodenal ulcer with extravasation from a branch of the superior pancreaticoduodenal artery (*arrow*).

B, The gastroduodenal artery was selectively catheterized and Pituitrin infused at a rate of 0.2 units/minute for 15 minutes. Repeat arteriography no longer shows extravasation. The infusion was continued for 24 hours and the bleeding did not recur.

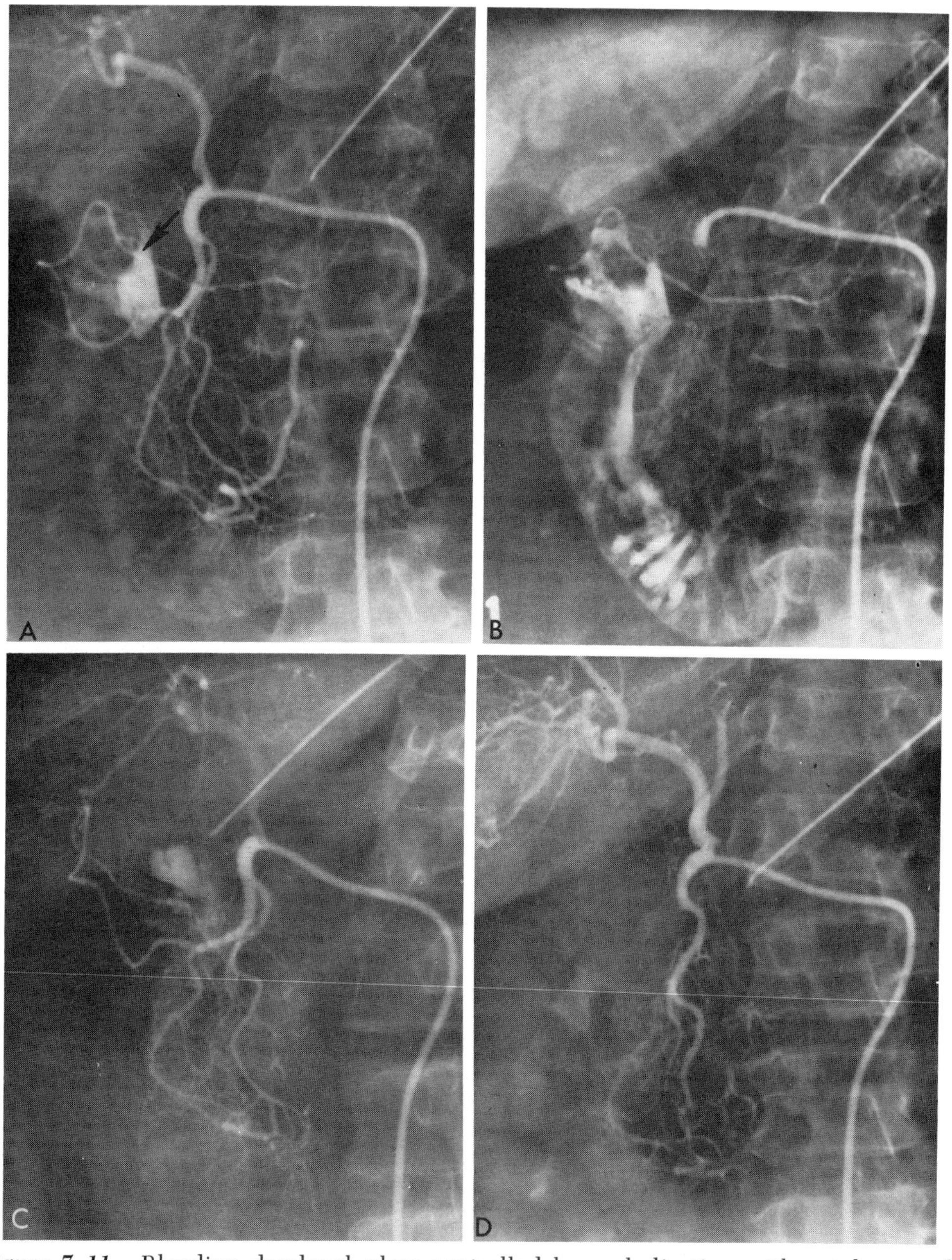

Figure 7–11. Bleeding duodenal ulcer controlled by embolization with autologous clot.

A, Selective gastroduodenal artery injection shows gross extravasation from a branch of the superior pancreaticoduodenal artery into a bleeding duodenal ulcer (*arrow*).

B, Later, during the same injection, the extravasated contrast opacifies the second and third portions of the duodenum.

C, Fifteen minutes after the intraarterial infusion of Pituitrin, at a rate of 0.2 units/minute, a repeat gastroduodenal arteriogram shows persistent bleeding.

D, The branch of the bleeding superior pancreaticoduodenal artery was embolized with autologous clot. Repeat arteriogram after embolization shows no extravasation.

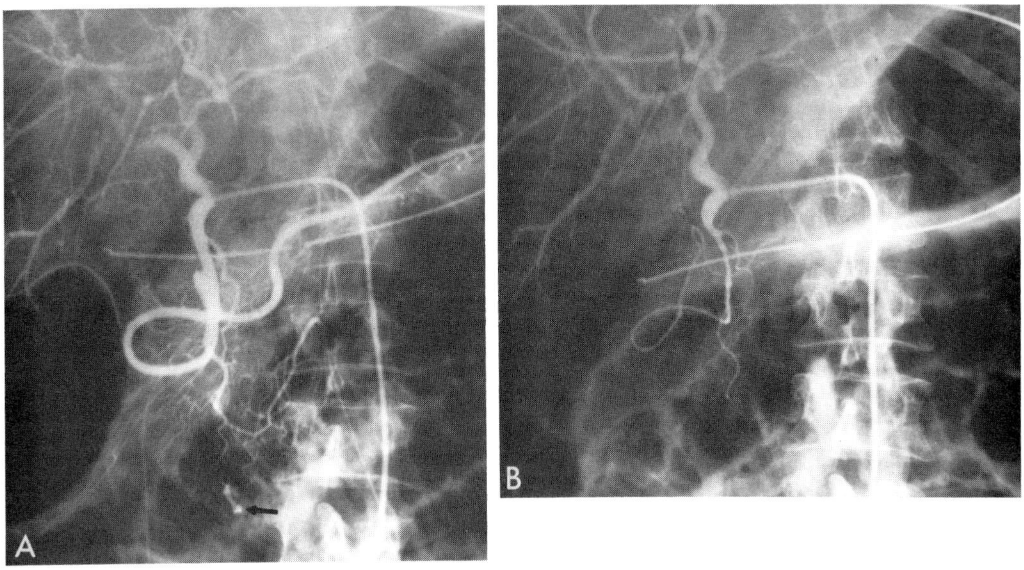

Figure 7–12. Bleeding stress ulcer in the descending duodenum.

A, Selective gastroduodenal arteriogram shows extravasation of contrast from a branch of the inferior pancreaticoduodenal artery (*arrow*) corresponding to an ulceration at the junction of the second and third portion of the duodenum.

B, The arteriogram was repeated during the intraarterial infusion of Pituitrin, at a rate of 0.2 units/minute, for 15 minutes. There is constriction of the gastroduodenal and pancreaticoduodenal arteries with control of the bleeding.

arterial systems. The splenic flexure of the colon, also at the periphery of two arterial systems, is particularly prone to ischemia (Marston, 1966), and the same may therefore be true of the mid-duodenum. All of the patients with ulcers at the junction of the second and third portions of the duodenum had been or were receiving digitalis. This gives further support to the ischemic theory of the origin of these ulcers, since digitalis is a very potent splanchnic arterial vasoconstrictor (Ferrer, 1965) and may further promote ischemia at the junction of the celiac and superior mesenteric arterial systems.

Since emergency arteriography is not performed in many hospitals, these massively bleeding ulcerations are sometimes never detected. It is suggested, therefore, that when confronted with massively bleeding stress ulcers and no other source can be located for the bleeding, an enterostomy should be done at the junction of the second and third portions of the duodenum and a careful search made for a bleeding ulceration.

Extrinsic Pressure Defects of the Duodenal Loop in Mesenteric Occlusive Disease

A major link in the collateral chain between the superior mesenteric artery and celiac axis is by way of pancreaticoduodenal arterial arcades (Fig. 7–13). When either the celiac or superior mesenteric artery is occluded, these arcades enlarge and appear, on angiography, as a vascular loop extending from the superior mesenteric artery around the head of the pancreas to the gastroduodenal and hepatic arteries. In this event, a large arterial channel is formed, coursing between the pancreas and duodenum (Baum, 1965). Such vessel enlargement can produce deformity and expansion of the duodenal loop, mimicking enlargement of the head of the pancreas (Fig. 7–14). It is obviously important to recog-

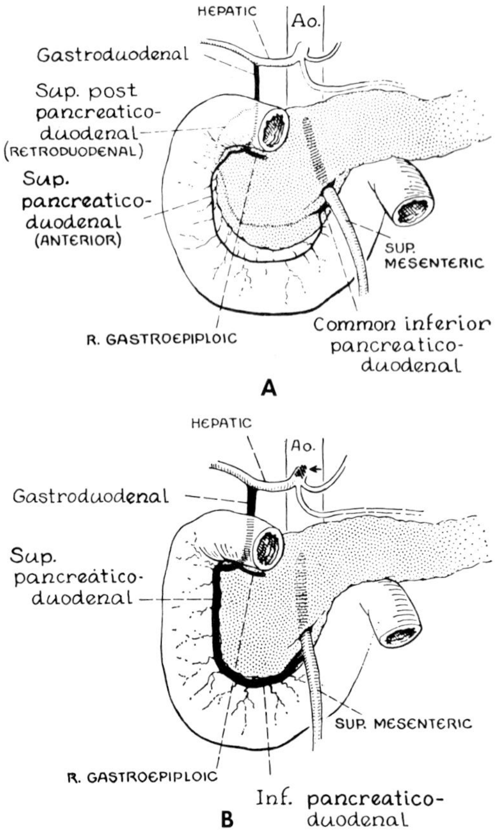

Figure 7–13. Normal anastomosis between the celiac and superior mesenteric arteries.

A, The inferior pancreaticoduodenal artery communicates with the gastroduodenal artery via the pancreaticoduodenal arcades.

B, When the celiac axis is occluded at its origin, the anastomosis between the celiac and superior mesenteric arteries becomes very large because of collateral flow. The arcades, which course along the medial aspect of the descending limb of the duodenum, become enlarged and tortuous. (Reproduced by permission of *Radiology*.)

(From Baum, S., Stein, G. N., and Baue, A.: Extrinsic pressure defects on the duodenal loop in mesenteric occlusive disease. Radiology 85:866–874, 1965.)

nize that these medial wall defects in the descending duodenum can be caused by collateral vessels associated with mesenteric vascular occlusive disease. The symptoms of this latter condition are similar to those of pancreatic cancer—namely, mid epigastric pain, anorexia, weight loss and cachexia.

Congenital Anomalies

Congenital anomalies of fixation and rotation of the intestinal tract are uncommon and generally not symptomatic (Wang, 1963). Malrotation of the gut may be discovered unexpectedly during laparotomy or as an incidental finding at a barium examination performed for other reasons. When symptoms do exist, they are generally those of partial, recurrent obstruction due to midgut volvulus with or without vascular occlusion. The physical findings during the attacks are nonspecific, and the diagnosis is usually not made. The correct diagnosis of malrotation can be established only by complete barium examination including evaluation of the stomach and small and large bowel. It is possible to miss gross abnormalities if only the stomach and duodenum are examined.

Angiography can play an important role in demonstrating the presence of volvulus with coexisting blood vessel traction. In chronic reversible midgut volvulus, the conventional radiographic examination may not demonstrate any abnormal findings other than malrotation. The indications for early elective surgery, therefore, are difficult to establish when the patient has only minimal symptoms. Once hemorrhagic infarction occurs, resection of the small bowel is usually fatal (Amend, 1968). The angiographic diagnosis can be made and, in at least one case (Buranasiri, 1973), the superior mesenteric artery and vein looked very much like a "barber pole" because of the rotation of the small intestines around the root of the mesentery (Fig. 7–15).

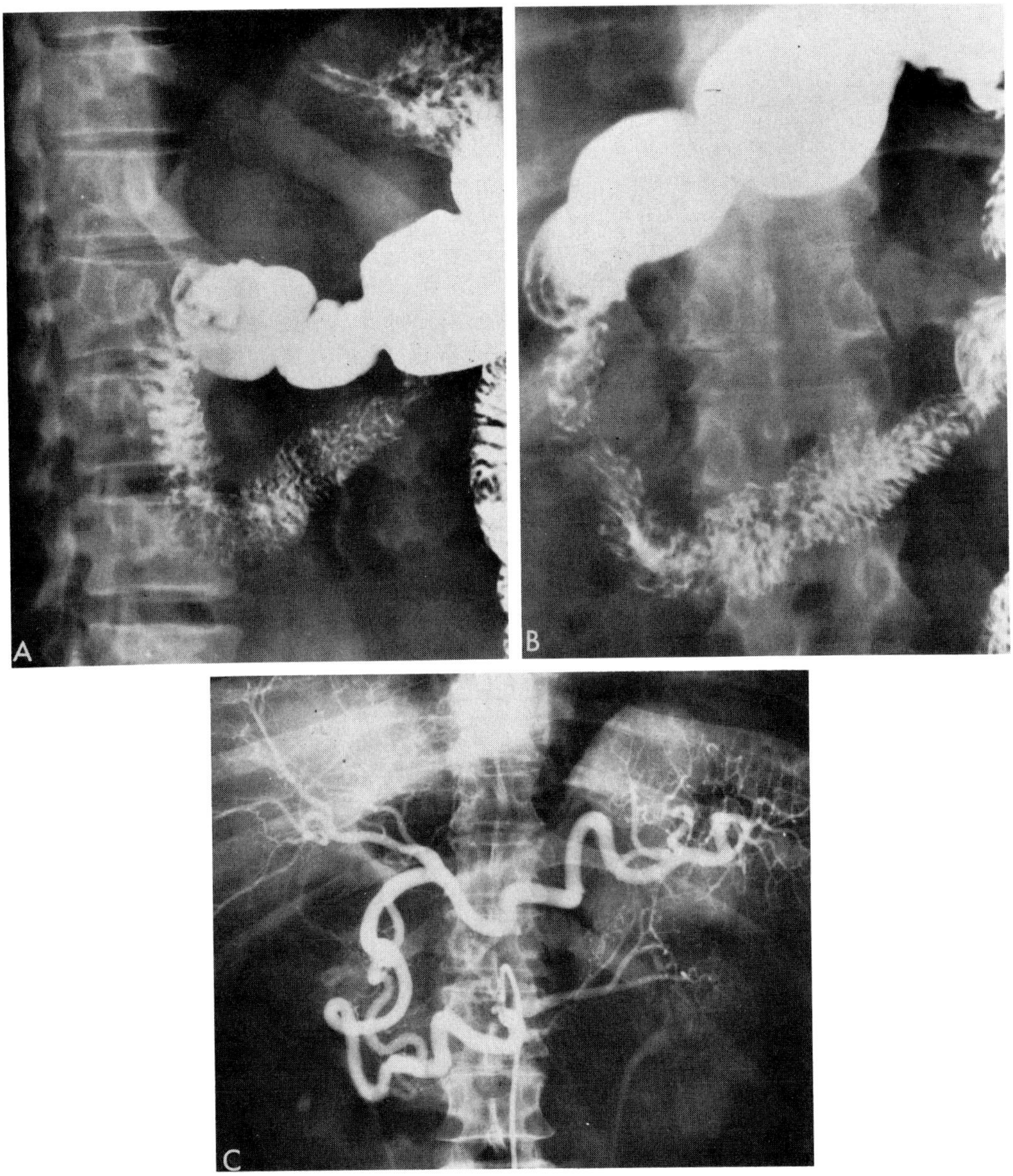

Figure 7–14. Large pancreatic arcades producing defects on the barium-filled duodenal sweep. This 64-year-old man was evaluated by angiography for recurrent epigastric pain.

A, A radiograph from an upper gastrointestinal series performed five years prior to the angiographic examination shows the duodenal sweep to be normal.

B, Upper gastrointestinal series performed five days prior to the angiographic examination shows extrinsic defects and a double contour along the inner aspect of the duodenal sweep.

C, Selective inferior pancreaticoduodenal artery injection shows enlarged tortuous pancreatic arcades which serve as collateral pathways for the retrograde opacification of the hepatic artery and splenic artery. The celiac axis is occluded at its origin from the aorta. The tortuous course of the enlarged pancreatic arcades corresponds to the pressure defects noted during the barium examination.

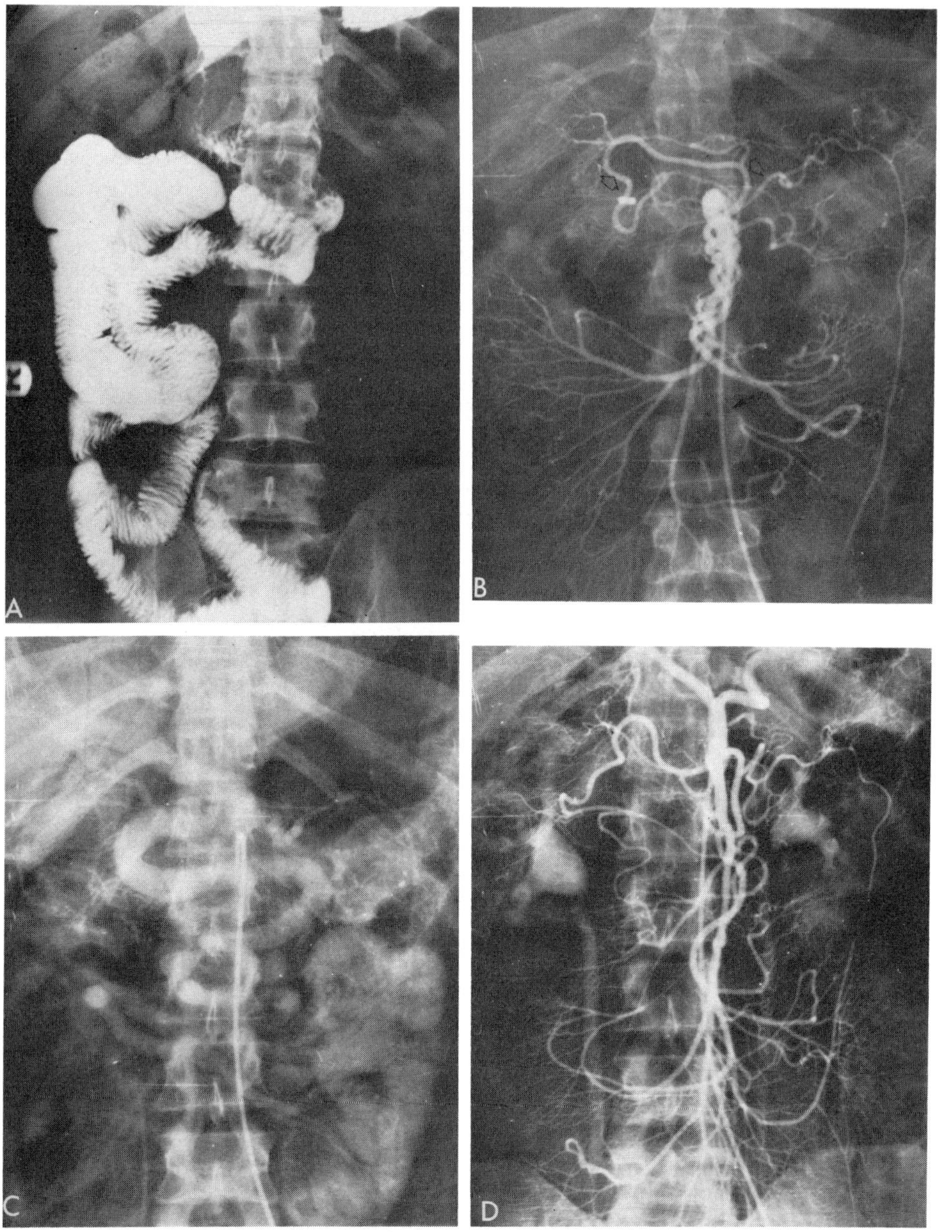

Figure 7–15. Mid gut malrotation with volvulus of the small bowel. A 26-year-old woman with abdominal pain since childhood.

A, Upper gastrointestinal series shows malrotation of the small bowel with the ligament of Treitz and the jejunum occupying the right side of the abdomen.

B, Superior mesenteric arteriogram, arterial phase, demonstrates marked twisting of the jejunal and ileal branches upon the ileocolic branch, giving the appearance of a "barber pole." There is narrowing of the proximal portion of a mid jejunal artery (*black arrow*) that is probably caused by the mid gut volvulus. Also note the abnormal position of the middle and right colic arteries (*open arrows*) which are in the upper and left portions of the abdomen.

C, The venous phase of the superior mesenteric arteriogram demonstrates dilatation of the jejunal, ileal and superior mesenteric veins. The veins are being twisted around the root of the mesentery, presumably as a result of the volvulus.

Upon exploration, a congenital band was found attaching the cecum to the left upper quadrant with rotation of the mesentery. This was released and the jejunum and ileum returned to their normal positions.

D, Superior mesenteric arteriogram postoperatively shows that the jejunal and ileal arteries have returned to normal position. (From Buranasiri, S., Baum, S., Nusbaum, M., and Tumen, H.: The angiographic diagnosis of mid-gut malrotation with volvulus in adults. Radiology. [In press.])

The severity of the mesenteric vascular occlusion varies with the number of rotations and the degree of tightness of the mesenteric pedicle.

Surgical correction requires accurate reduction of the volvulus, with restoration of mesenteric attachments, severance of congenital bands and closure of internal hernias.

Superior Mesenteric Artery Syndrome

Another disorder that can be documented angiographically is the superior mesenteric artery syndrome. This will be discussed in detail in Chapter 10, but it should be emphasized that, in order to appreciate the relationship of the superior mesenteric artery to the aorta, it is important to film the abdominal aortogram in a lateral position.

Pancreas

Since its introduction by Per Odman in 1958, selective pancreatic arteriography has become established as a safe, accurate method for evaluating the presence and extent of pancreatic disease. Direct pancreatography, echography, isotopic scanning and angiography are at present the only four radiographic techniques that attempt to establish a diagnosis of pancreatic disease on the basis of direct pancreatic visualization. All other radiographic studies rely on the changes the pancreas produces on adjacent structures such as the stomach, duodenum and small bowel.

Carcinoma

Adenocarcinoma of the pancreas, similar to other infiltrating malignancies of the gastrointestinal tract, is poorly vascularized. The most common arterial abnormality in pancreatic cancer is encasement of the intrapancreatic and adjacent larger arteries (Lunderquist, 1965; Boijsen, 1969*a*; and Bookstein, 1969). Displacement, evidence of tumor vessels, and early venous filling are changes that are only occasionally seen. The appearance of arterial invasion may range from an almost pathognomonic serrated or serpiginous encasement to much less specific forms of smooth narrowing (Figs. 7–16, 7–17 and 7–18).

With the increasing popularity of angiographic studies, it was hoped that early diagnosis could be made by this direct approach to pancreatic visualization. Even though many of these pancreatic tumors are relatively large in size, the angiographic findings may be very subtle. The very fine tumor vessels and tumor stains that some investigators have described are frequently seen only when superselective examinations are performed, and these sometimes require direct serial magnification (Fig. 7–19). Since many laboratories do not have the catheter expertise for routine superselective studies, or the special equipment required for direct serial magnification angiography, many angiographers have become discouraged in attempting to make the diagnosis of pancreatic carcinoma. In 1972, Buranasiri and Baum emphasized the importance of the venous phase of the pancreatic arteriogram in diagnosing pancreatic cancer. Forty-six of 47 patients with adequate portal system visualization demonstrated venous involvement. This would suggest, therefore, that venous involvement is perhaps the single most important criterion for the diagnosis of pancreatic carcinoma. This finding is also much easier to evaluate than minimal arterial irregularity, displacement or tumor vessels described by others. These findings are in agreement with reports by earlier authors (Rösch, 1964) who reported venous involvement as seen by splenoportography in 92 per cent of their patients with pancreatic neoplasms.

Because the venous phase of the examination is obviously so important in the evaluation of pancreatic disease, particular care must be taken to inject adequate volumes of contrast material as well as to carry out the filming for 30 seconds after the injections. Better venous visualization is accomplished when the rate of injection is kept below

(Text continued on page 247)

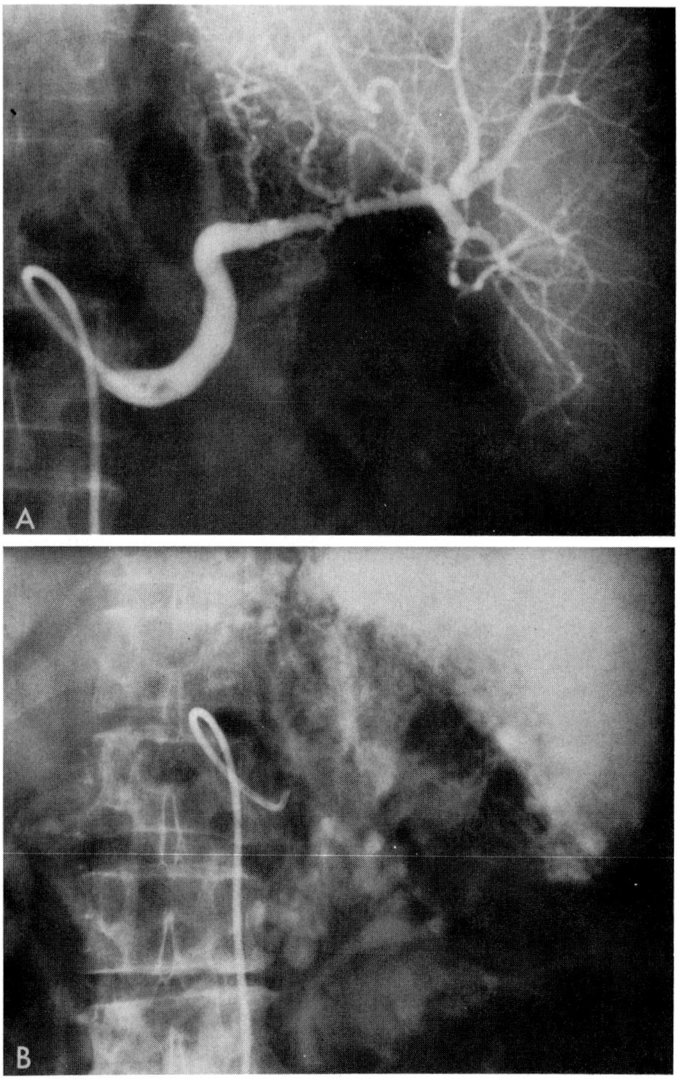

Figure 7–16. Carcinoma of the tail of the pancreas.

A, Selective splenic arteriogram shows tumor encasement of the distal end of the splenic artery as well as several of its branches in the region of the splenic hilum.

B, The venous phase of the selective splenic arteriogram shows complete occlusion of the splenic vein. There is collateral drainage via the gastroepiploic and short gastric veins.

At surgery, this was a carcinoma of the pancreatic body and tail.

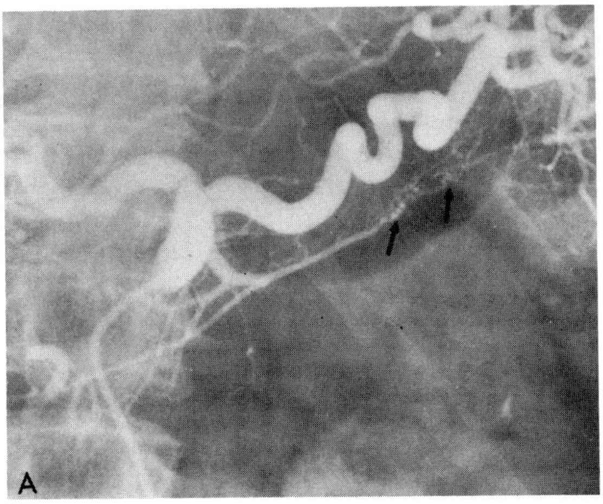

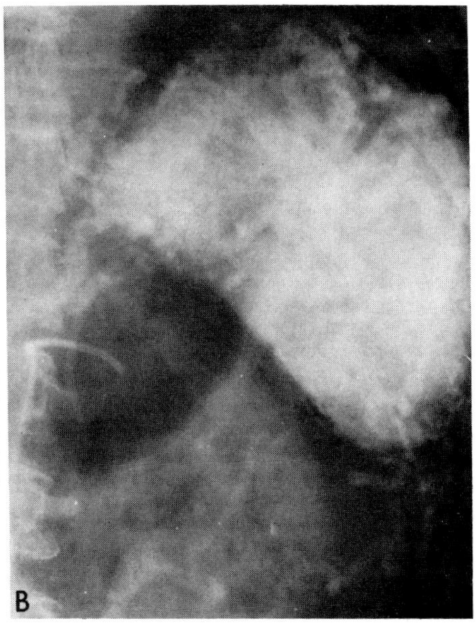

Figure 7–17. Carcinoma of the body of the pancreas.

A, Selective celiac axis arteriogram demonstrates tumor encasement of the transverse pancreatic artery (*arrows*).

B, During the venous phase of the examination, there is complete occlusion of the splenic vein with collateral drainage via the epiploic veins. (From Buranasiri, S., and Baum, S.: The significance of the venous phase of celiac and superior mesenteric arteriography in evaluating pancreatic carcinoma. Radiology, *102*:11–20, 1972.)

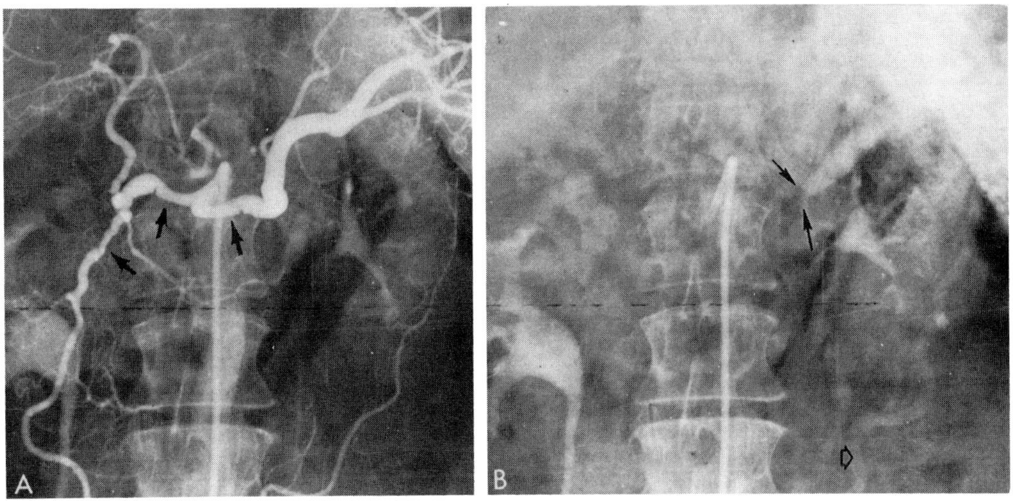

Figure 7–18. Carcinoma of the head and body of the pancreas.

A, Selective celiac arteriogram shows encasement of the hepatic, gastroduodenal and splenic arteries (*arrows*).

B, During the venous phase of the celiac arteriogram, there is complete occlusion of the splenic vein (*straight arrows*), and collateral drainage via a dilated gastroepiploic vein (*open arrow*). (From Buranasiri, S., and Baum, S.: The significance of the venous phase of celiac and superior mesenteric arteriography in evaluating pancreatic carcinoma. Radiology, *102*:11–20, 1972.)

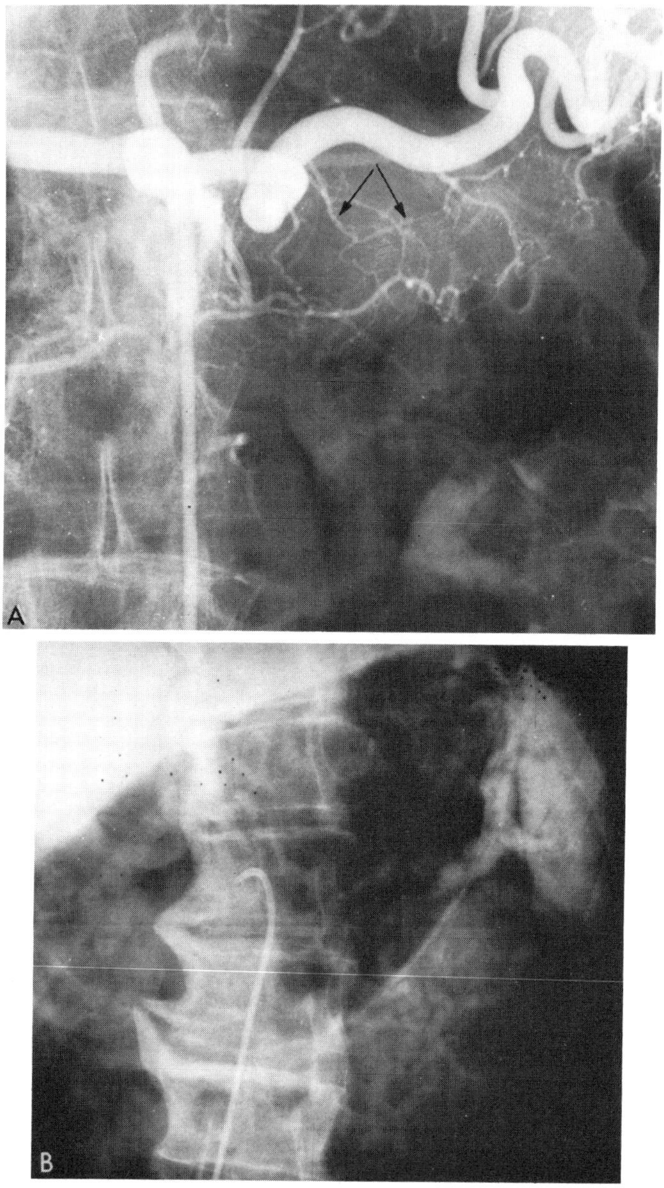

Figure 7–19. Carcinoma of the body of the pancreas.

A, Selective direct magnification celiac arteriogram shows minimal irregularity of the transverse pancreatic and short pancreatic arteries (*arrows*). This type of irregularity can be produced by arteriosclerotic changes as well.

B, During the venous phase of the examination, the splenic vein is completely occluded and there is filling of collateral epiploic and retroperitoneal veins.

On the basis of the venous occlusion, the minimal arterial changes seen in *A* assume more importance in establishing the correct preoperative diagnosis of a pancreatic carcinoma. (From Buranasiri, S., and Baum, S.: The significance of the venous phase of celiac and superior mesenteric arteriography in evaluating pancreatic carcinoma. Radiology, *102*:11–20, 1972.)

8 ml./second (Fig. 7–20). If the veins are not adequately visualized using this technique, pharmacoangiographic manipulation of blood flow may be employed with 25 mg. of tolazoline (Priscoline) injected directly into the superior mesenteric artery immediately prior to the arteriogram (Redman, 1969) (Fig. 7–21).

The evaluation of minimal marginal arterial irregularities can be difficult and easily confused with atheromatous disease, especially in the older age group. For this reason, the status of adjacent veins assumes even greater importance (Figs. 7–22 and 7–23). The problem of false-positive examination occasionally arises in patients who have venous occlusions on the basis of chronic pancreatitis. In this group, however, arterial changes will also be frequent (Moskowitz, 1968), so that the incidence of false-positive studies in chronic pancreatitis will probably not be higher than if the diagnosis relied only on the arterial or capillary phase of the study.

Eisenberg (1973) has pointed out that the over-all arteriographic picture of pancreatic carcinoma is that of an arterial "wipe out" or sparse filling in the arterial and capillary phases of the study as contrasted with pancreatitis where one has a normal or slightly increased capillary stain.

Carefully performed selective pancreatic arteriography that includes satisfactory detail of pancreatic vessels as well as visualization of the portal venous system should yield a diagnostic accuracy of approximately 95 per cent in patients with pancreatic carcinoma.

In addition to being able to make the diagnosis of pancreatic carcinoma, the

(Text continued on page 251)

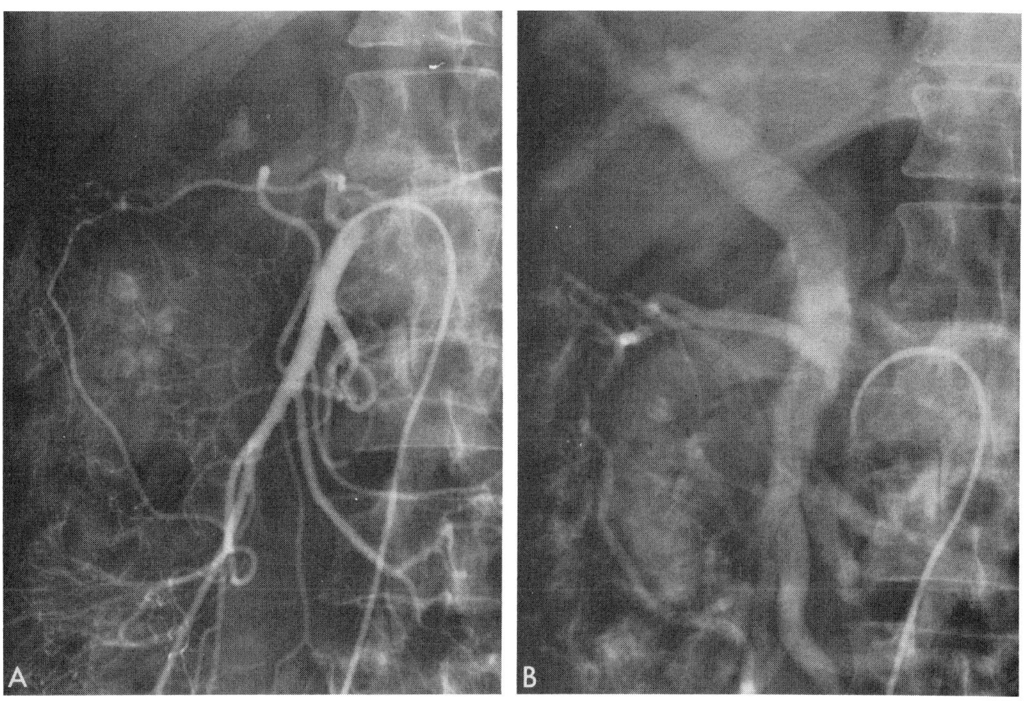

Figure 7–20. Normal superior mesenteric and portal veins.

A, Superior mesenteric arteriogram, arterial phase.

B, During the venous phase of the superior mesenteric arteriogram, there is excellent opacification of jejunal, superior mesenteric and portal veins. The patient is in a 15 degree right posterior oblique position so that the mesenteric vein is not superimposed on the spine.

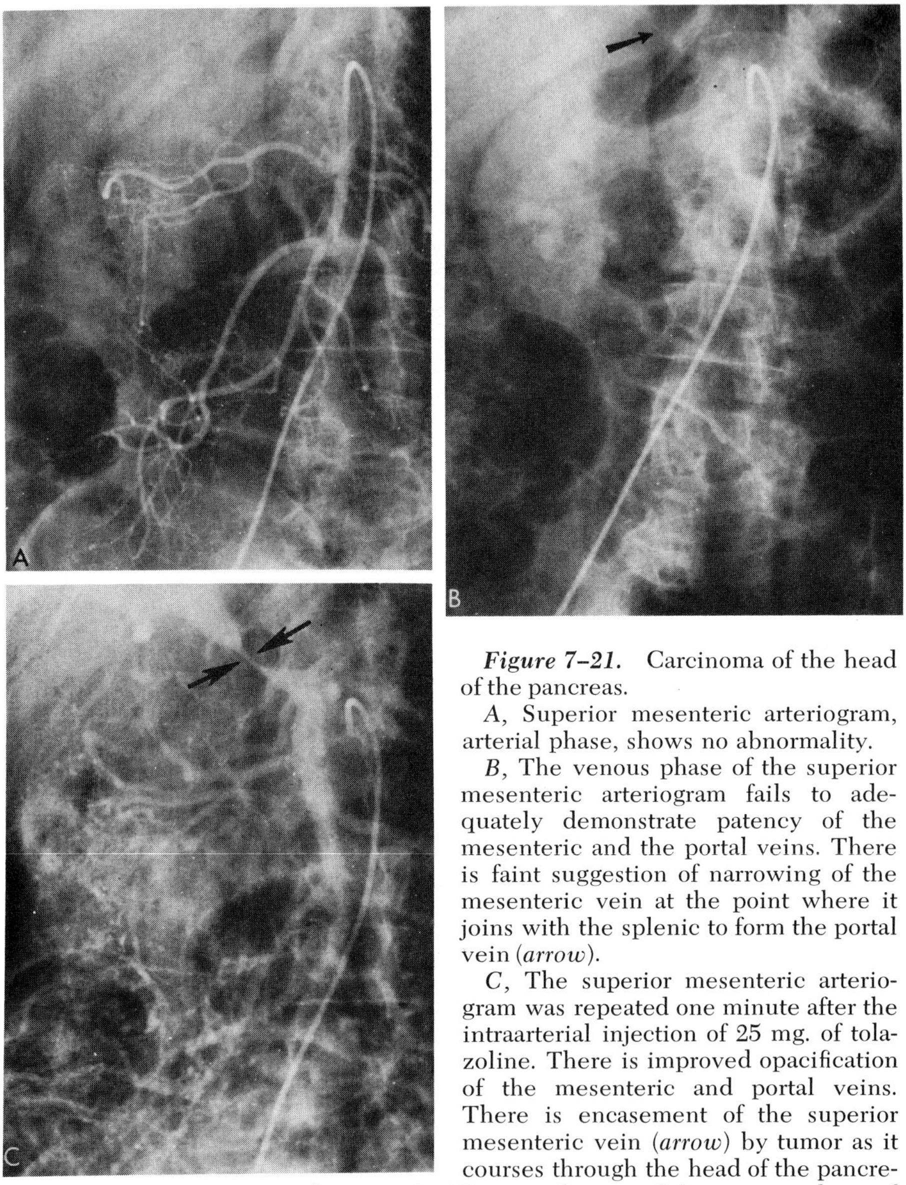

Figure 7–21. Carcinoma of the head of the pancreas.

A, Superior mesenteric arteriogram, arterial phase, shows no abnormality.

B, The venous phase of the superior mesenteric arteriogram fails to adequately demonstrate patency of the mesenteric and the portal veins. There is faint suggestion of narrowing of the mesenteric vein at the point where it joins with the splenic to form the portal vein (*arrow*).

C, The superior mesenteric arteriogram was repeated one minute after the intraarterial injection of 25 mg. of tolazoline. There is improved opacification of the mesenteric and portal veins. There is encasement of the superior mesenteric vein (*arrow*) by tumor as it courses through the head of the pancreas. (From Buranasiri, S., and Baum, S.: The significance of the venous phase of celiac and superior mesenteric arteriography in evaluating pancreatic carcinoma. Radiology, *102*:11–20, 1972.)

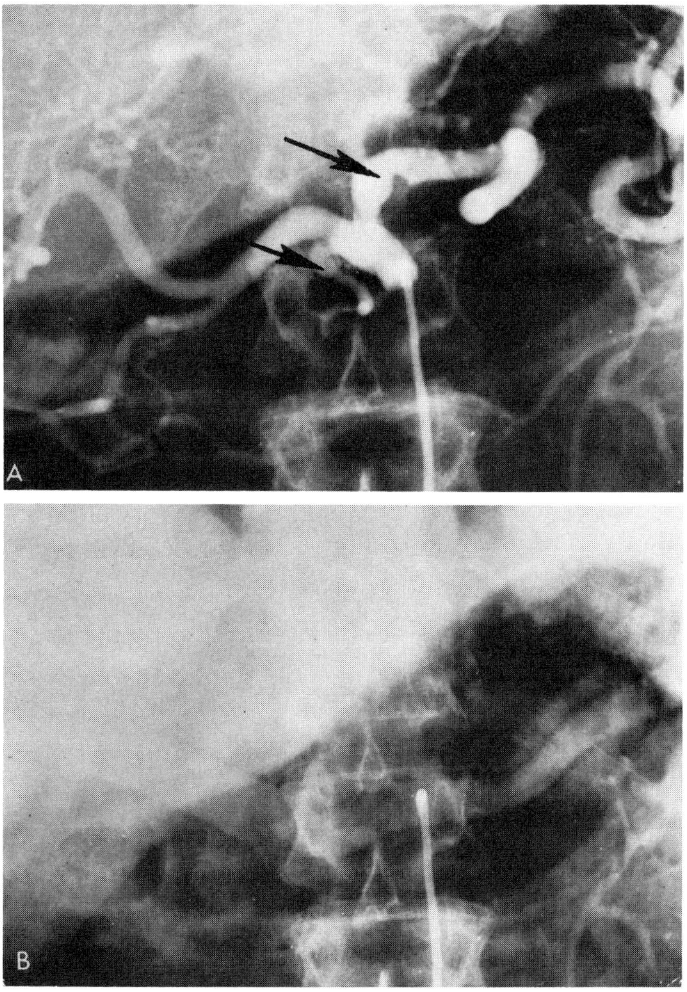

Figure 7–22. The significance of the venous appearance in the differentiation between arteriosclerotic and neoplastic arterial involvement.

A, Selective celiac arteriogram in this 60-year-old man who presented with epigastric pain shows narrowing of the splenic and the dorsal pancreatic arteries (*arrows*).

B, During the venous phase of the same injection, the splenic and portal veins are normal. This finding helps to distinguish arteriosclerotic from neoplastic arterial involvement. This patient has been followed for seven years since the examination was performed, and there has been no clinical evidence of pancreatic malignancy. (From Buranasiri, S., and Baum, S.: The significance of the venous phase of celiac and superior mesenteric arteriography in evaluating pancreatic carcinoma. Radiology, *102*:11–20, 1972.)

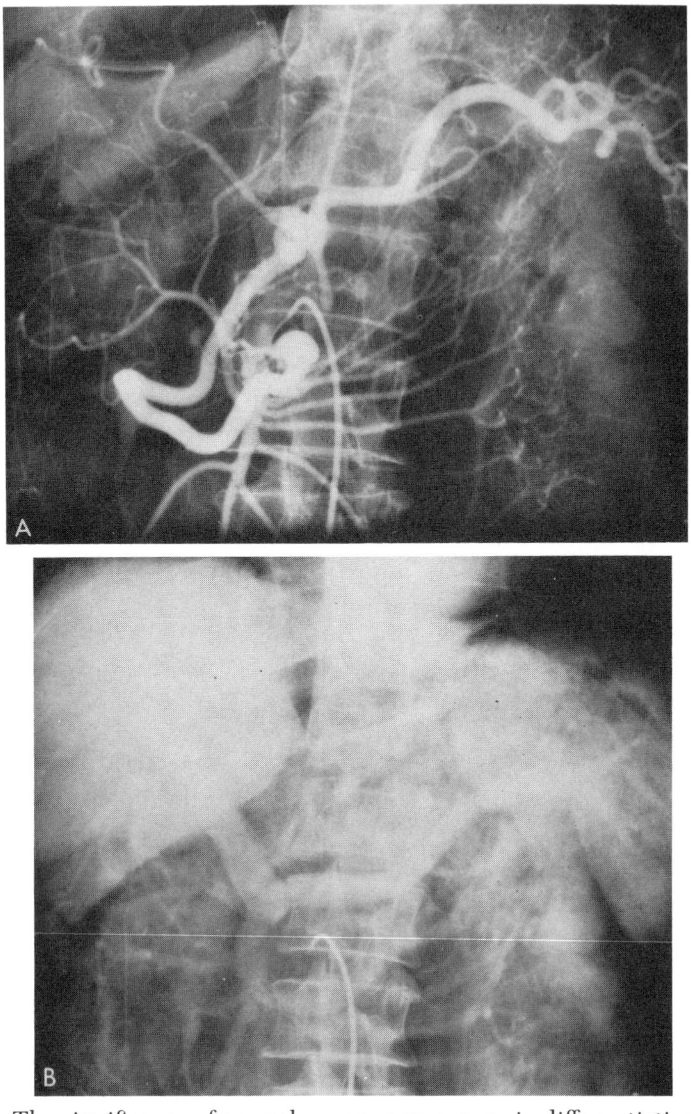

Figure 7–23. The significance of normal venous appearance in differentiating arteriosclerotic from neoplastic arterial changes.

A, Selective superior mesenteric arteriogram in this 60-year-old man with epigastric pain shows retrograde opacification via the pancreatic arcades of the entire celiac axis and its branches. On the basis of the arterial phase alone, it would be difficult to attribute the celiac axis occlusion to arteriosclerosis or involvement by neoplastic process.

B, During the venous phase of the same injection, the superior mesenteric, splenic and portal veins are all patent and normal. This normal appearance of the venous structures surrounding the body and the head of the pancreas makes the presence of neoplastic disease unlikely. This patient has been followed for eighteen months since the examination was performed, and there has been no clinical evidence of pancreatic malignancy.

preoperative arteriogram gives the surgeon an opportunity to evaluate the arterial anatomy prior to any attempt at radical surgery. The preoperative knowledge of superior mesenteric or portal venous occlusion, encasement of hepatic or jejunal arterial branches, or the presence of anatomic variations such as a replaced right hepatic artery which courses from the superior mesenteric artery to the liver through the head of the pancreas is obviously of great preoperative interest to the surgeon.

Secondary Malignancy of the Pancreas

When the pancreas is secondarily involved with malignancy, it is most often due to direct extension of a cancer that arises in an adjacent organ such as the stomach or colon. True hematogenous metastasis to the pancreas is rare (Robbins, 1967); however, it has been seen angiographically in patients with carcinoid tumors as well as hypernephromas (Fig. 7–24).

Pancreatitis

There are marked discrepancies in the angiographic literature concerning the findings in pancreatitis (Rösch, 1963; Hepp, 1968; Reuter, 1969*b*; and Boijsen, 1972). An entire spectrum of changes has been seen, and one can find descriptions of marked pancreatic hypervascularity

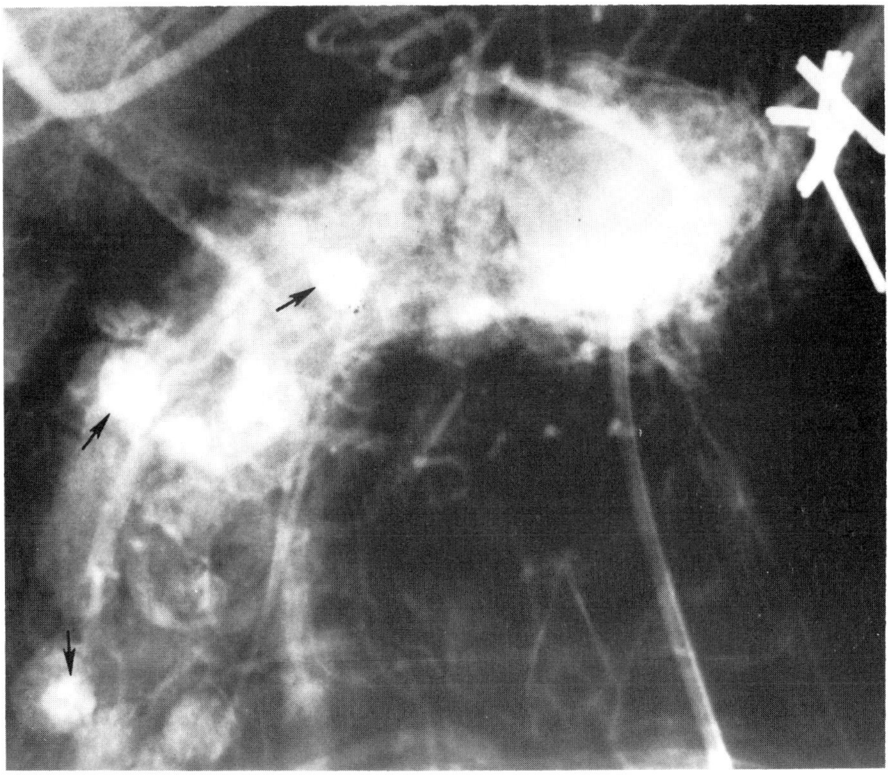

Figure 7–24. Metastatic disease to the pancreas demonstrated by angiography. This 60-year-old male patient had his right kidney removed because of a hypernephroma. Five months following nephrectomy, the patient was readmitted to the hospital because of persistent back and right flank pain. During an angiographic evaluation, a selective dorsal pancreatic arteriogram was performed showing hypervascular metastatic deposits scattered throughout the entire pancreas (*arrows*). (Courtesy of Dr. Harvey Eisenberg, Boston, Mass.)

as well as hypovascularity. This apparent contradiction in findings is probably due to various authors studying different phases of the same disease.

The arteriogram in acute pancreatitis may be perfectly normal (Reuter, 1972). If, however, the pancreas is enlarged, the angiographic picture is one of increased size of the intrapancreatic arteries and an increase in the parenchymal staining during the capillary phase. The differential diagnosis between pancreatic cancer and pancreatitis is at this stage of the disease quite simple, since cancer tends to have very sparse filling of the small intrapancreatic vessels.

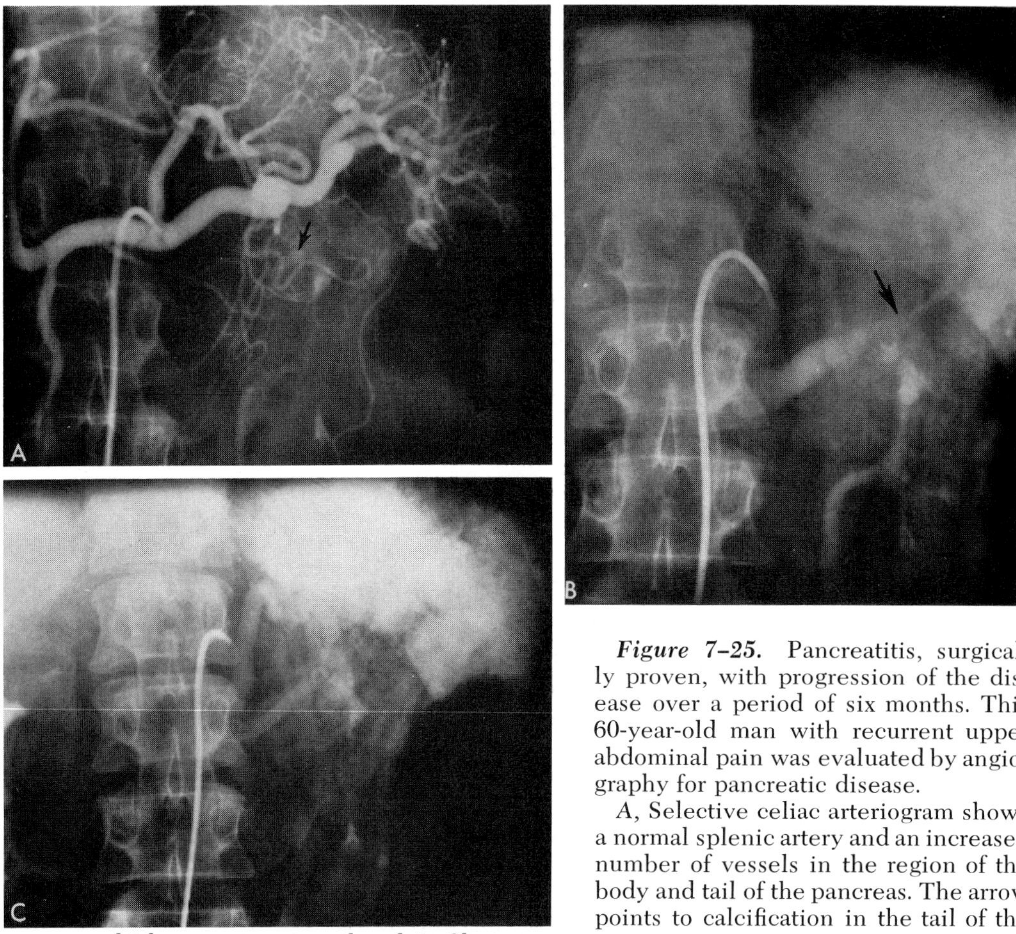

Figure 7–25. Pancreatitis, surgically proven, with progression of the disease over a period of six months. This 60-year-old man with recurrent upper abdominal pain was evaluated by angiography for pancreatic disease.

A, Selective celiac arteriogram shows a normal splenic artery and an increased number of vessels in the region of the body and tail of the pancreas. The arrow points to calcification in the tail of the pancreas which was present on the plain films.

B, During the venous phase of the celiac arteriogram, there is narrowing of the splenic vein (*arrow*) adjacent to the pancreatic calcification.

The patient was treated medically and six months later, because of continued abdominal pain, he was re-evaluated by angiography.

C, The venous phase of the celiac arteriogram six months later shows progression of the disease with complete occlusion of the splenic vein and collateral flow via a dilated coronary vein and epiploic veins.

At surgery, the diagnosis of pancreatitis was confirmed and a distal pancreatectomy performed. The patient is asymptomatic 18 months later.

As the disease enters the relapsing recurrent phase, there is progressive fibrosis and destruction of the gland. It is this phase of the disease that presents difficulties in differential diagnosis. As fibrosis occurs, the smaller pancreatic arteries frequently have a characteristic "beaded" segmental narrowing that is quite different from the serpiginous encasement seen in carcinoma. Other arteriographic changes include straightening of the intrapancreatic vessels and tapered narrowing of the adjacent splenic and hepatic arteries and veins (Fig. 7–25).

A fairly specific arteriographic finding in pancreatitis is the presence of aneurysms within the intrapancreatic or adjacent arteries (Boijsen, 1969*b*) (Figs. 7–26 and 7–27). This is presumably due to digestion of the vessel wall by pancreatic enzymes, and has not been described in carcinoma. Both the splenic and superior mesenteric veins may be either narrowed or occluded as a result of the intense fibrotic reaction occurring within the pancreas.

Cysts and Pseudocysts

True epithelium-lined cysts of the pancreas are rare. With the exception of the neoplastic cystadenoma (Bieber, 1963; and Abrams, 1967), true cysts are thin-walled and very difficult to diagnose angiographically. If the cysts are confined to the pancreas itself, a diagnosis may be established by intrapancreatic arterial displacement and filling defects during the capillary and parenchymal phase of the study. If the cysts become exophytic and leave the substance of the pancreas, they may be impossible to diagnose angiographically since they generally do not have surrounding vessels.

Pseudocysts are by far the most common form of pancreatic cystic disease. The wall of a pseudocyst tends to be thick and fibrous, and the contents of the cyst may include pancreatic secretions, blood, and necrotic or suppurative pancreatic tissue. It is at times impossible to differentiate between a pancreatic pseudocyst and a pancreatic abscess. Pancreatitis is the etiologic fac-

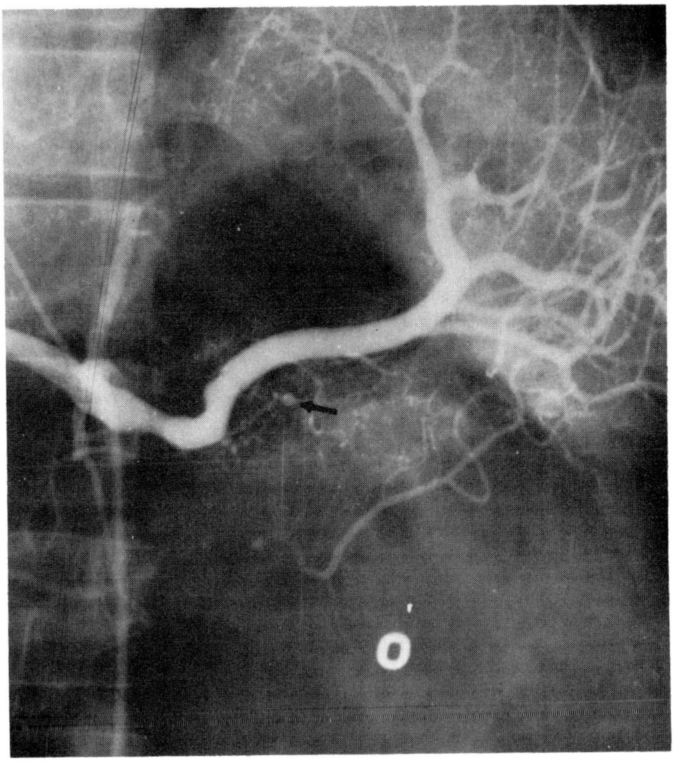

Figure 7–26. Pancreatitis with microaneurysm formation. Selective celiac arteriogram shows irregularity of several pancreatic arteries in the region of the body and tail with a small aneurysm of the transverse pancreatic artery (*arrow*). The splenic artery is normal. Due to persistent symptomatology, the patient was operated upon and the diagnosis of pancreatitis was confirmed.

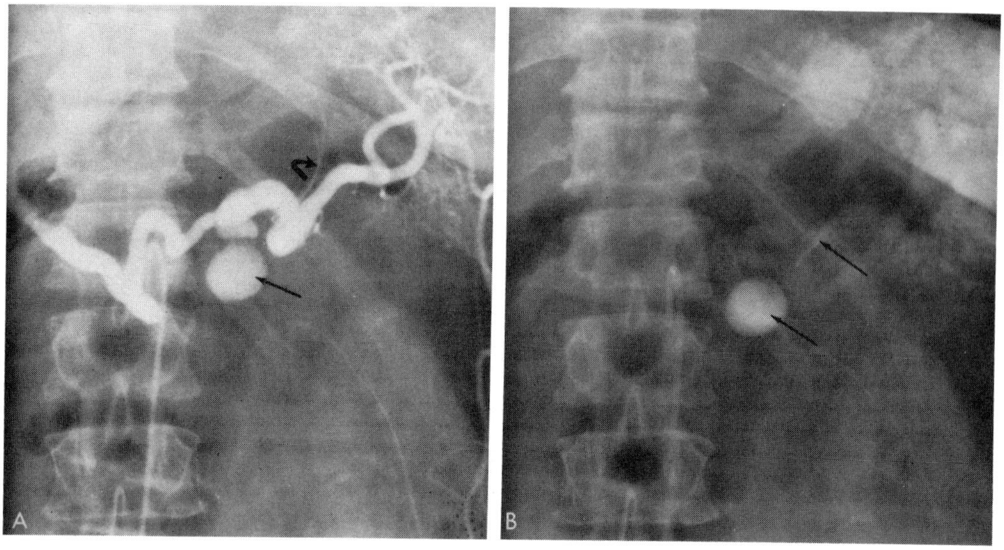

Figure 7–27. Rupture of a noncalcified splenic artery aneurysm secondary to pancreatitis.

A, Selective celiac arteriogram demonstrates a splenic artery aneurysm with opacification of a false sac (*arrow*). There is displacement of pancreatic branches (*curved arrow*) apparently due to the presence of a large hematoma around the aneurysm.

B, During the venous phase of the celiac arteriogram, there is persistent opacification of the false sac with a rim of contrast outlining a wall of a hematoma (*arrows*).

These findings were confirmed at surgery, at which time a successful distal pancreatectomy was performed.

tor in approximately 75 per cent, and trauma in the remaining 25 per cent of pancreatic pseudocysts. The angiographic findings depend on the thickness of the fibrous wall as well as the size of the mass (Kadell, 1967; and Fu, 1969). In large masses, the splenic, hepatic and even superior mesenteric artery may be displaced (Figs. 7–28 and 7–29). If the fibrous wall of the pseudocyst is very thick, it is occasionally possible to see mural staining. Pseudocysts are capable of eroding blood vessels and, therefore, may be responsible for massive gastrointestinal bleeding (Fig. 7–30). Large pseudocysts also can compress or obstruct the adjacent splenic or superior mesenteric veins, with resulting gastric or duodenal varices.

Islet Cell Tumors

Several distinct clinical syndromes are associated with hyperfunction of the islets of Langerhans; namely, hyperinsulinism, multiple endocrine adenomatosis and the Zollinger-Ellison syndrome. Each of these clinical entities can be caused by diffuse hyperplasia of islet cells, single or multiple adenomas or malignant tumors.

Three distinctive cells have been identified in the islets of Langerhans in man. The beta-cells produce insulin; hence, tumors involving this cell result in hyperinsulinism. The alpha-cells secrete glucagon, which induces glycogenolytic activity in the liver and results in hyperglycemia. Glucagon-secreting tumors of

(Text continued on page 257)

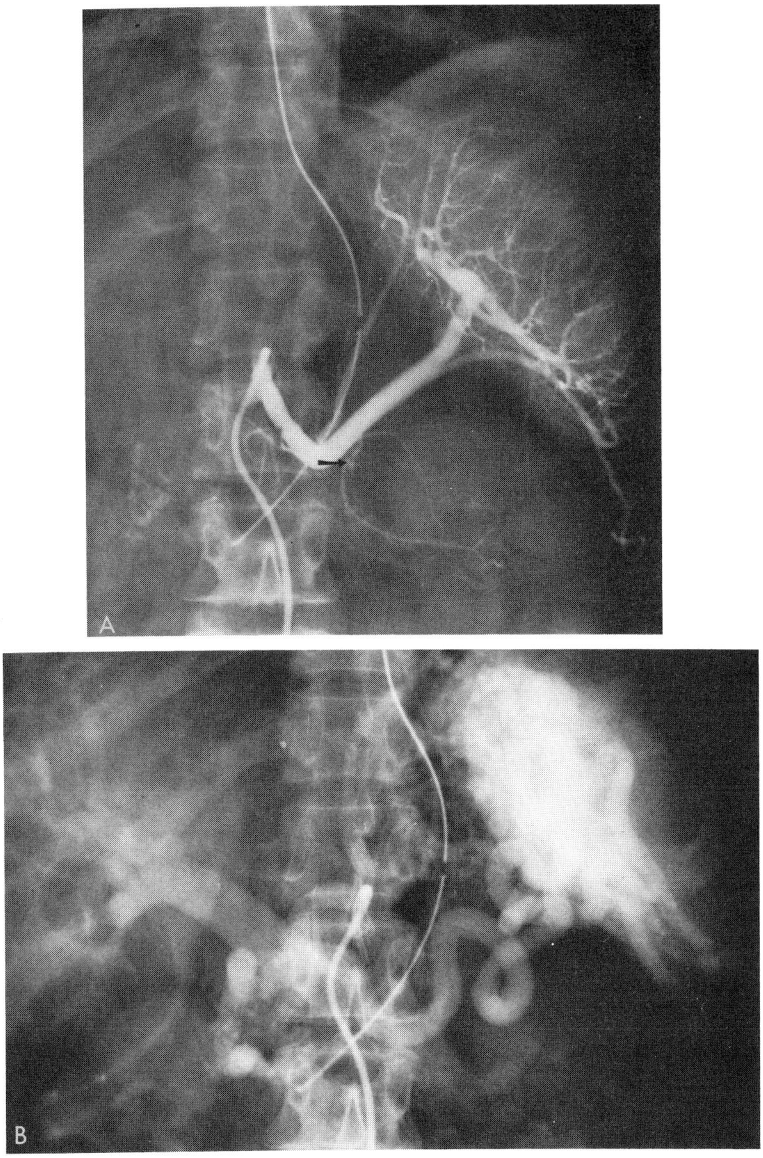

Figure 7–28. Pancreatitis with pancreatic pseudocyst.

A, Selective splenic arteriogram shows stretching and splaying of branches of the splenic artery by a mass lesion in the region of the pancreatic body and tail. The arrow points to a small aneurysm of the pancreatica magna artery.

B, During the venous phase of the selective splenic arteriogram, there is complete occlusion of the splenic vein and collateral drainage via dilated gastroepiploic, short gastric and coronary veins.

At surgery, a pseudocyst of the pancreatic body and tail was found and internally drained.

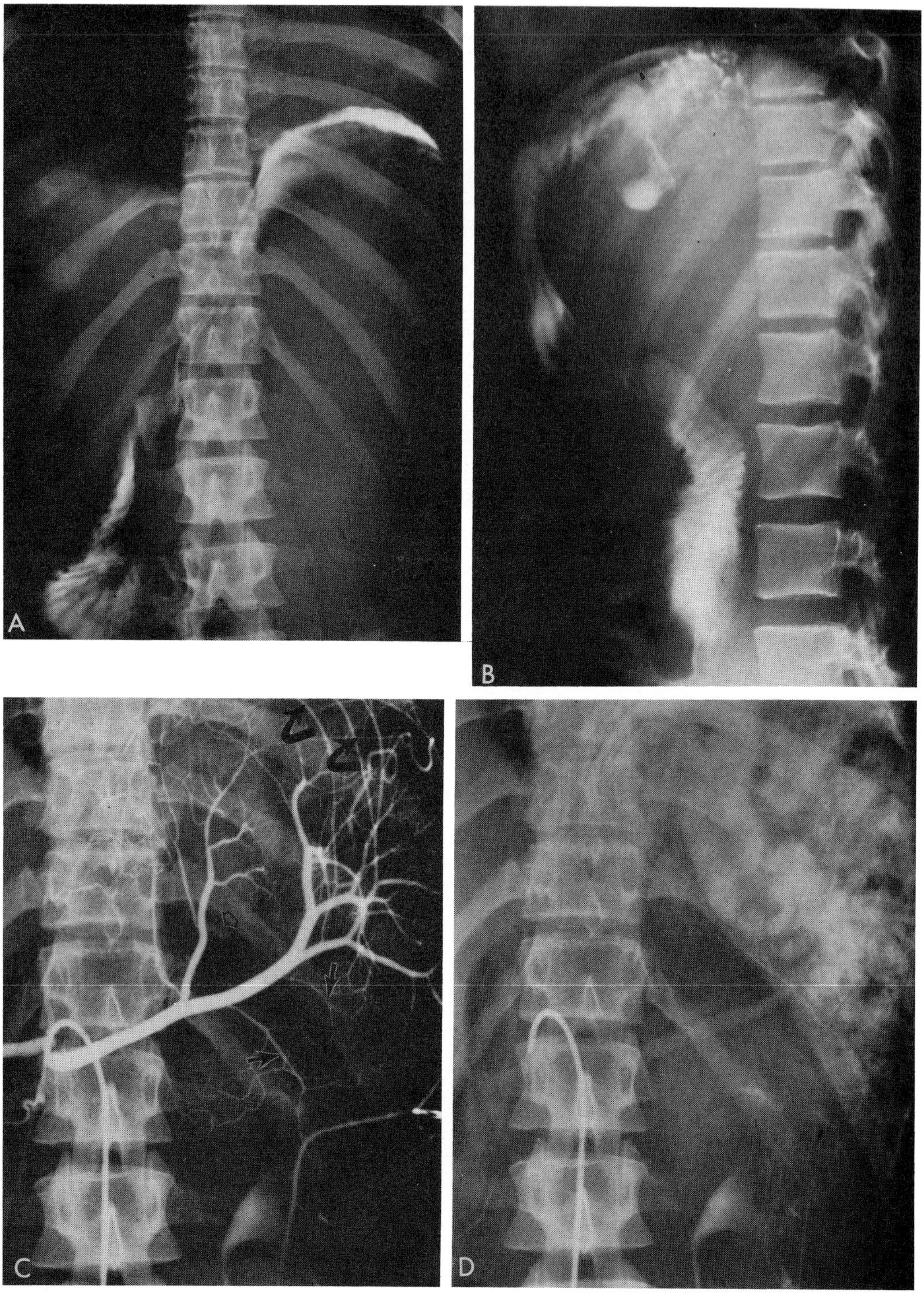

Figure 7–29. Traumatic pancreatic pseudocyst. One week after blunt trauma to the upper abdomen, this 20-year-old woman was admitted to the hospital with fullness in the epigastrium and a dropping hematocrit. Abdominal exploration at the time of the initial injury had shown no abnormality.

A, A radiograph from an upper gastrointestinal series shows displacement of the fundus and body of the stomach superiorly and to the right.

B, A lateral radiograph shows displacement of the barium-filled stomach anteriorly by a retrogastric mass lesion.

C, Selective splenic arteriogram shows stretching and attenuation of splenic artery branches to

 (*Legend continued on next page*)

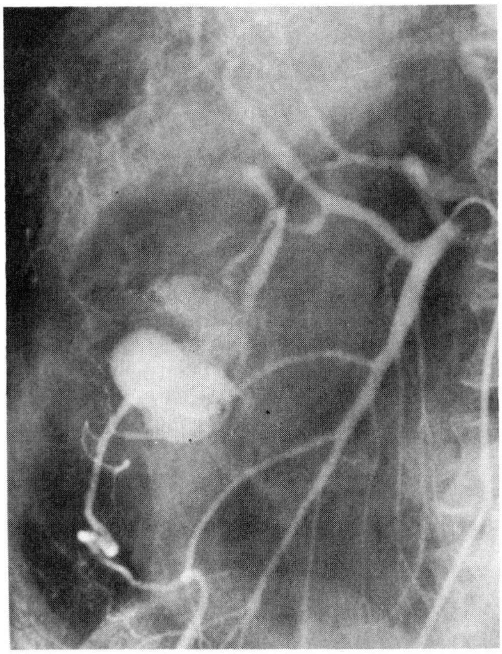

Figure 7–30. Pancreatic abscess eroding into the duodenum, causing massive gastrointestinal hemorrhage. Selective superior mesenteric arteriogram shows massive extravasation originating from a branch of the retroduodenal artery. The right hepatic artery originates from the superior mesenteric artery. On exploration, a pancreatic abscess was found eroding into the second portion of the duodenum. The bleeding resulted from erosion into a branch of the gastroduodenal artery.

the alpha-cells are very rare. The delta-cells are nonscreting, and their function is poorly understood. It is thought that perhaps the delta-cell is the origin of nonfunctioning adenomas and carcinomas of the pancreas.

The Zollinger-Ellison syndrome (see also Chapters 10 and 11) consists of the association of islet cell tumors with overproduction of gastrin, gastric hypersecretion and peptic ulceration. The underlying lesion in these patients is neoplasia or hyperplasia of a nonbeta islet cell. The exact origin of the cell type is not known, although it is clear that it is neither a beta- nor an alpha-cell tumor.

Although the presence of insulin-producing tumors can generally be detected clinically, detection of their exact location within the pancreas is a matter of considerable importance. Eighty-five per cent of insulinomas are single and, of these, approximately three-quarters are between 1 and 3 cm. in diameter. Although surgical removal of the insulinoma affords a cure, their small size frequently makes surgical identification exceedingly difficult. However, by virtue of the abundant blood supply of the cells of Langerhans, islet cell tumors tend to be very vascular (Fig. 7–31). Angiographically, small islet cell tumors exhibit very well circumscribed tumor blushes that can be seen during the parenchymal phase of the arteriogram. In larger lesions, tumor vessels as well as tumor staining are seen. Most reports describe an 80 to 90 per cent accuracy in diagnosis (Madsen, 1966; Rösch, 1968; Epstein, 1969; and Boijsen, 1970), although Bookstein (1966) reports a considerably lower success rate. All reports

---

Figure 7–29. Continued.
the pancreatic body and tail (*arrow*), as well as draping of the short gastric arteries (*curved arrow*) around a mass lesion in the region of the pancreas. A small amount of extravasation (*open arrow*) is noted originating from a polar branch of the splenic artery.

D, The venous phase of the selective splenic arteriogram demonstrates the splenic vein to be narrowed but patent.

At surgery, a bleeding pancreatic pseudocyst was found.

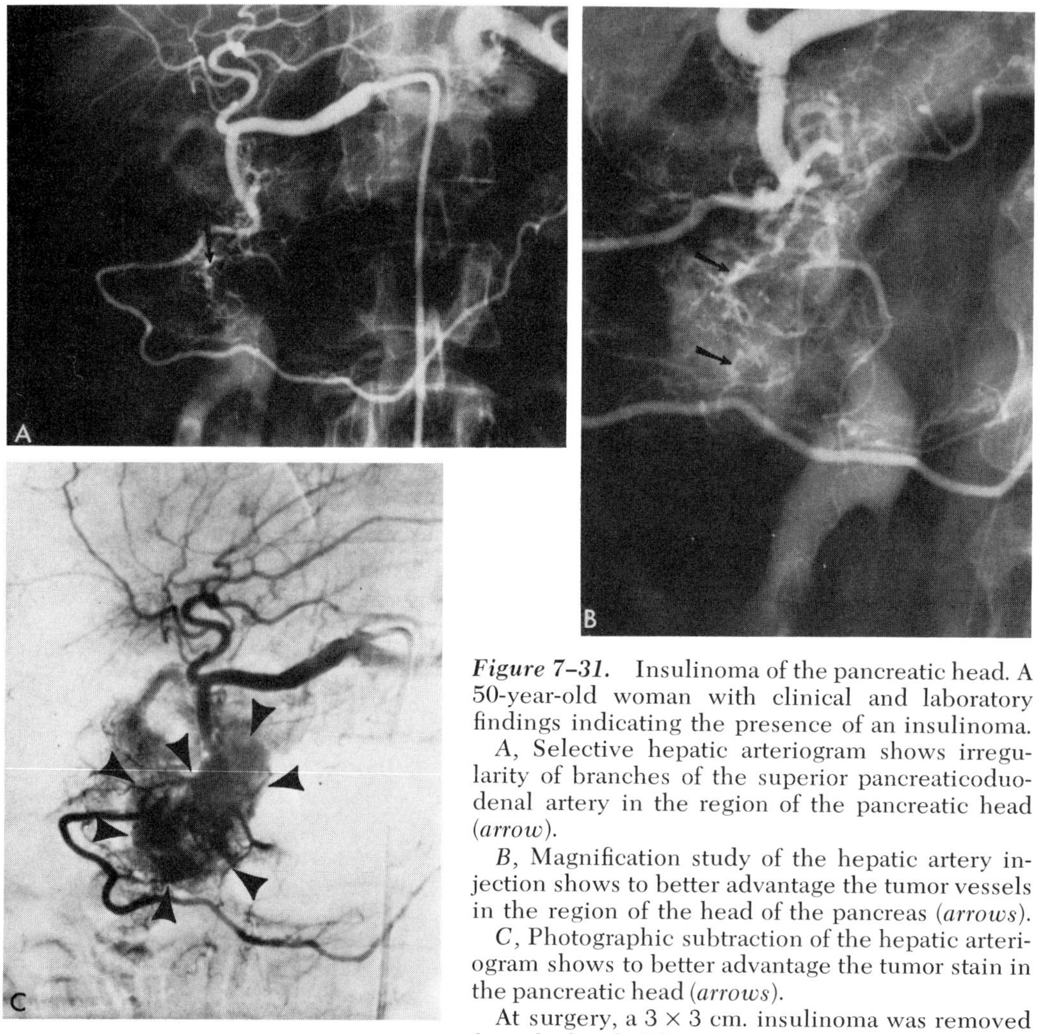

Figure 7–31. Insulinoma of the pancreatic head. A 50-year-old woman with clinical and laboratory findings indicating the presence of an insulinoma.

A, Selective hepatic arteriogram shows irregularity of branches of the superior pancreaticoduodenal artery in the region of the pancreatic head (*arrow*).

B, Magnification study of the hepatic artery injection shows to better advantage the tumor vessels in the region of the head of the pancreas (*arrows*).

C, Photographic subtraction of the hepatic arteriogram shows to better advantage the tumor stain in the pancreatic head (*arrows*).

At surgery, a 3 × 3 cm. insulinoma was removed from the head of the pancreas.

agree that angiography cannot distinguish between benign and malignant tumors except when metastatic lesions are identified. It is also generally agreed that the Zollinger-Ellison tumor tends to be less vascular than the insulinoma (Clemett, 1967).

REFERENCES

Abrams, R. M., Beranbaum, E. R., Beranbaum, S. L., and Ngo, N. L.: Angiographic studies of benign and malignant cystadenoma of the pancreas. Radiology, *89*:1028, 1967.

Amend, F.: The importance of x-ray diagnosis in the determination of congenital torsion and fixation disorders of the intestinal tract. (Thereto a clinical case of fatal small intestine volvulus in connection with a rare congenital anomalous position of the colon). Radiology, *8*:43–48, 1968.

Baum, S.: Angiography of localized gastric lesion. Seminars Roentgen., *6*:207–219, 1971*a*.

Baum, S., and Abrams, H. L.: A J-shaped catheter for retrograde catheterization of tortuous vessels. Radiology, *83*:436, 1964.

Baum, S., and Nusbaum, M.: Control of gastrointestinal hemorrhage by selective mesenteric arterial infusion of vasopressin. Radiology, *98*:497–505, 1971*b*.

Baum, S., Rösch, J., Dotter, C. T., Ring, E. J., Athanasoulis, C. A., Waltman, A. C., and Courey, R.: The role of angiography and selective mesenteric arterial infusions in the management of massive diverticular hemorrhage. New Eng. J. Med., *288*:1269–1272, 1973.

Baum, S., Stein, G. N., and Baue, A.: Extrinsic pressure defects on the duodenal loop in mesenteric occlusive disease. Radiology, *85*:866–874, 1965.

Baum, S., Ward, S., Nusbaum, M., and Tumen, H.: Stress bleeding from the mid-duodenum: an often unrecognized source of gastrointestinal hemorrhage. Radiology, *95*:595–602, 1971*c*.

Bieber, W. P., and Albo, R. J.: Cystadenoma of the pancreas: its arteriographic diagnosis. Radiology, *80*:766, 1963.

Boijsen, E.: Angiographic diagnosis of pancreatic disease. T. Gastroent., *12*:219, 1969*a*.

Boijsen, E.: Selective pancreatic angiography. Brit. J. Radiol., *39*:481, 1966*a*.

Boijsen, E., and Feinstein, G. L.: Arteriographic catheterization techniques. Amer. J. Roentgen. Radium Ther. Nucl. Med., *85*:1037, 1961.

Boijsen, E., and Samuelsson, L.: Angiographic diagnosis of tumors arising from the pancreatic islets. Acta Radiol. (Diagn.) (Stockh.), *10*:161, 1970.

Boijsen, E., and Tylen, U.: Vascular changes in chronic pancreatitis. Acta Radiol., *12*:34, 1972.

Boijsen, E., Göthlin, J., Hallbook, T., and Sandblom, P.: Preoperative angiographic diagnosis of bleeding aneurysms of abdominal visceral arteries. Radiology, *93*:781, 1969*b*.

Boijsen, E., Wallace, S., and Kanter, I. E.: Angiography in tumors of the stomach. Acta Radiol. (Diagn.), *4*:306, 1966*b*.

Bookstein, J. J., and Oberman, H. A.: Appraisal of selective angiography in localizing islet-cell tumors of the pancreas. Radiology, *86*:682, 1966.

Bookstein, J. J., Reuter, S. R., and Martel, W.: Angiographic evaluation of pancreatic carcinoma. Radiology, *93*:757, 1969.

Buranasiri, S., and Baum, S.: The significance of the venous phase of celiac and superior mesenteric arteriography in evaluating pancreatic carcinoma. Radiology, *102*:11–20, 1972.

Buranasiri, S., Baum, S., Nusbaum, M., and Tumen, H.: The angiographic diagnosis of mid-gut malrotation with volvulus in adults. Radiology, 1973. (In press.)

Clemett, A. R., and Park, W. M.: Arteriographic demonstration of pancreatic tumor in the Zollinger-Ellison syndrome. Radiology, *88*: 32, 1967.

Conn, H. O., Ramsy, G. R., and Storer, E. K.: Selective intra-arterial vasopressin in the treatment of upper gastrointestinal hemorrhage. Gastroenterology, *63*:634, 1972.

Eisenberg, H.: Pancreatic angiography. *In* Small Vessel Angiography. Edited by S. Hilal. St. Louis, Mo., C. V. Mosby Co., 1973. (In press.)

Epstein, H. Y., Abrams, R. M., Beranbaum, E. R., and Localio, S. A.: Angiographic localization of insulinomas: high reported success rate and two additional cases. Ann. Surg., *169*:349, 1969.

Ferrer, M. I., Bradley, S. E., Wheeler, H. O., et al: The effect of digoxin in the splanchnic circulation in ventricular failure. Circulation, *32*: 524–537, 1965.

Freeark, R. J., Norcross, W. J., and Baker, R. J.: Exploratory gastrostomy in management of massive upper gastrointestinal hemorrhage. Arch. Surg., *94*:684–695, 1967.

Fu, W. R., and Stanton, L. W.: Angiographic study of pseudocysts of the pancreas. J. Canad. Ass. Radiol., *20*:176, 1969.

Hepp, J., Hernandez, C., Moreaux, J., and Bismuth, H.: L'Arteriographie dans les affections chirurgicales du foie, du pancreas et de la rate. Paris, Masson, 1968.

Judkins, M. P., Kidd, H. J., Frische, L. H., and Dotter, C. T.: Lumen-following safety J-guide for catheterization of tortuous vessels. Radiology, *88*:1127, 1967.

Kadell, B. M., and Riley, J. M.: Major arterial involvement by pancreatic pseudocysts. Amer. J. Roentgen., *99*:632, 1967.

Lunderquist, A.: Angiography in carcinoma of the pancreas. Acta Radiol.: Suppl. 235, 1965.

Madsen, B.: Demonstration of pancreatic insulinomas by angiography. Brit. J. Radiol., *39*: 488, 1966.

Marston, A., Pheils, M. T., Thomas, M. L., et al: Ischaemic colitis. Gut, *7*:1–15, 1966.

Moskowitz, H., Chait, A., and Mellins, H. Z.: "Tumor encasement" of the celiac axis due to chronic pancreatitis. Amer. J. Roentgen., *104*: 641–645, 1968.

Nusbaum, M., and Baum, S.: Radiographic demonstration of unknown sites of gastrointestinal bleeding. Surg. Forum, *14*:374–375, 1963.

Odman, P.: Percutaneous selective angiography of the coeliac artery. Acta Radiol.: Suppl. 159, 1958.

Redman, H. C., Reuter, S. R., and Miller, W. J.: Improvement of superior mesenteric and portal vein visualization with tolazoline. Invest. Radiol., *4*:24–27, 1969.

Reuter, S. R.: Superselective pancreatic angiography. Radiology, *92*:74, 1969*a*.

Reuter, S. R., and Redman, H. C.: Gastrointestinal Angiography. Philadelphia, W. B. Saunders Company, 1972.

Reuter, S. R., Redman, H. C., and Joseph, R. R.: Angiographic findings in pancreatitis. Amer. J. Roentgen., *107*:56, 1969*b*.

Robbins, S. L.: Pathology. 3rd ed. Philadelphia, W. B. Saunders Company, 1967.

Rösch, J., and Bret, J.: Arteriografie pankreatu. Cesk. Roentgen., *17*:192, 1963.

Rösch, J., and Grollman, J. H., Jr.: Superselective arteriography in the diagnosis of abdominal pathology. Technical considerations. Radiology, *92*:1008, 1969.

Rösch, J., and Herfort, K.: Splenoportographic diagnosis of pancreatic disease. Geriatrics, *19*:725–734, 1964.

Rösch, J., and Judkins, M. P.: Angiography in the diagnosis of pancreatic disease. Seminars Roentgen., *3*:296, 1968.

Rösch, J., Dotter, C. T., and Brown, M. J.: Selective arterial embolization: a new method for control of acute gastrointestinal bleeding. Radiology, *102*:303, 1972.

Rösch, J., Dotter, C. T., and Rose, R. W.: Selective arterial infusions of vasoconstrictors in acute gastrointestinal bleeding. Radiology, 99:27–36, 1971.

Salter, R. H.: Aspirin and gastrointestinal bleeding. Amer. J. Dig. Dis., *13*:38–58, 1968.

Sevitt, S.: Duodenal and gastric ulceration after burning. Brit. J. Surg., *4*:32–41, 1967.

Wang, C. A., and Welch, C. E.: Anomalies of intestinal rotation in adolescents and adults. Surgery, *54*:839–855, 1963.

Chapter 8

PANCREATOGRAPHY

Welland F. Short, M.D.

Pancreatography, the radiographic delineation of pancreatic ducts, was first performed in 1919 by Pallin, who used it for the study of postmortem specimens (Millbourn, 1950). Except for occasional visualization by fistulography or cholangiography, however, no method for clinical evaluation of the ducts was available until 1951 when operative pancreatography was introduced by Doubilet and Mulholland. Since then, the examination has been used almost exclusively by surgeons primarily as a guide to the treatment of pancreatitis. However, with the recent introduction of a peroral fiberoptic technique, pancreatography promises to become one of the most important methods of pancreatic diagnosis. For this reason, there is an increasing interest both in its techniques and in its interpretation by clinicians and radiologists alike.

METHODS OF EXAMINATION

Pancreatic Reflux

Pancreatic duct opacification most often is secondary to reflux from the common duct during cholangiography. This reflux is usually incidental although it is sometimes deliberately attempted (Hayes, 1960; Thal, 1959). It occurs in as many as half of all T-Tube cholangiograms and is more apt to be seen with increased resistance or obstruction at the papilla and with high injection pressure (Hess, 1965; Yvergneaux, 1969) (Fig. 8–1). In most instances, it is probably of no clinical significance.

Duodenal-pancreatic reflux has been attempted in humans but, to date, has been unsuccessful except in the presence of duodenal diverticula involving the major papilla (Waldron, 1972). In the absence of diverticula or prior sphincteromy, its occurrence should be considered abnormal (Fig. 8–2). Biliary or pancreatic reflux has been described in carcinomas of the papillary region (Eaton, 1970) as well as in Crohn's disease (Legge, 1970) and strongyloidiasis (Berkman, 1972) of the duodenum.

Operative Techniques

Retrograde catheterization of the papilla, as described by Leger (1952, 1953), is the most frequently used approach to operative pancreatography (Fig. 8–3). It entails duodenotomy and passage of a small catheter through the intact papilla. In 80 to 90 per cent of cases, the pancreatic duct is entered preferentially (Nardi, 1966). Occasionally, intravenous secretin is helpful in locating the papilla and in opening the pancreatic duct to cannulation (Howard, 1969). After the position of the catheter is checked, 1 to 2 cc. of contrast material (preferably meglumine diatrizoate, 60 per cent) (Kasugai, 1972*a*) is injected and films are exposed immediately and at one minute.

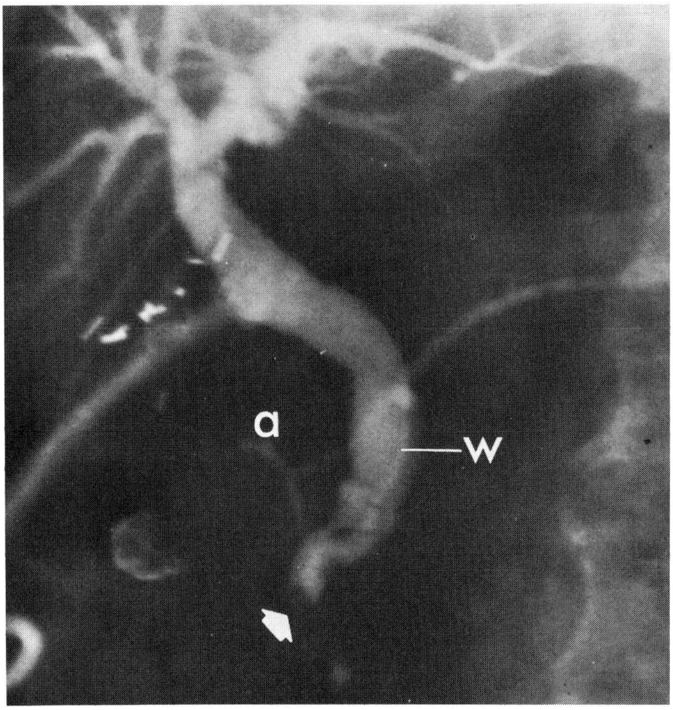

Figure 8–1. Marked pancreatic reflux during T-tube cholangiography in a patient with a retained common duct stone (*arrow*). A large accessory pancreatic duct (*a*) is filling from the duct of Wirsung (*w*), which is partially superimposed upon the dilated common duct.

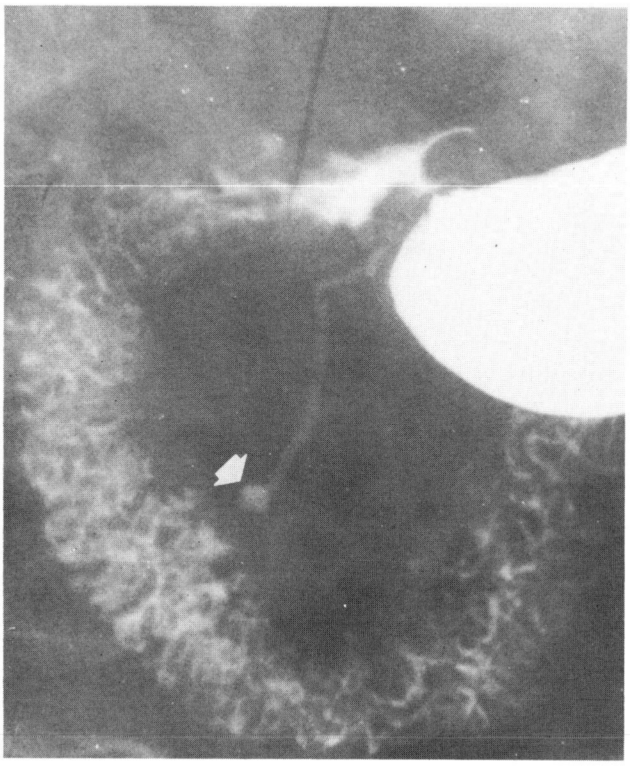

Figure 8–2. Spontaneous duodenal-pancreatic reflux during routine barium meal in a patient without evidence of duodenal or pancreatic disease. This rare occurrence should be considered abnormal until proved otherwise. What appears to be an ampulla of the duct of Wirsung (*arrow*) may represent a duodenal diverticulum and may be the cause of reflux. (Courtesy of Dr. Max W. Safely.)

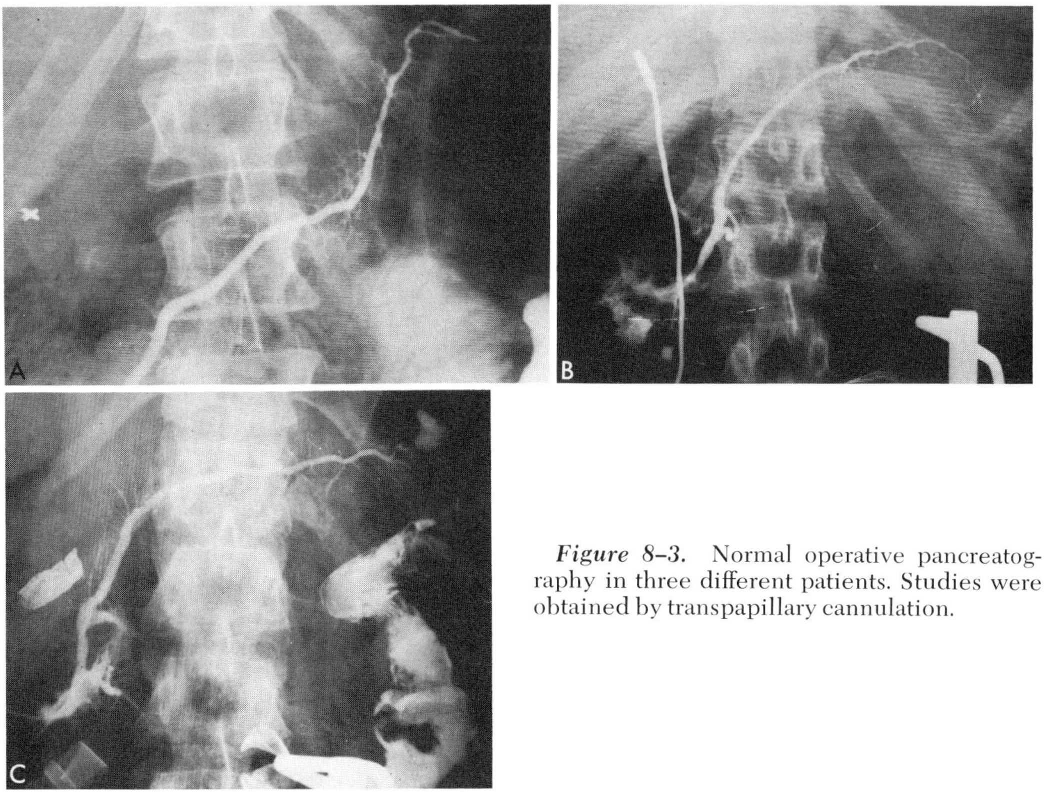

Figure 8–3. Normal operative pancreatography in three different patients. Studies were obtained by transpapillary cannulation.

When filling of the main duct is incomplete, reinjection with a larger volume is necessary.

The preferred approach in the presence of marked ductal dilatation or a pseudocyst is by direct needle puncture. This technique involves aspiration of fluid from the duct or cyst and its replacement with dilute contrast material (Trapnell, 1967). When this and the transpapillary methods fail and when retrograde drainage is anticipated, the main duct can be cannulated after amputation of the tail of the pancreas.

Although a valuable tool, operative pancreatography has been used relatively seldom. Perhaps the main reason has been the fear that it may cause acute pancreatitis. The association of this complication with pancreatography dates from early reports in which sphincterotomy preceded cannulation (Pollock, 1958) or in which large volumes of contrast material were injected, sometimes with excessive force (Hess, 1965). Sphincterotomy which, by itself, is complicated by pancreatitis in up to 14 per cent of the cases was undoubtedly responsible for some of these complications (Hess, 1965). Great emphasis has been placed on the danger of injecting a volume of more than 2 cc. or of filling more than the main duct and a few collecting ducts (Hess, 1965; Trapnell, 1966). However, the remarkable safety of pancreatography without sphincterotomy suggests that this view may need modification.

Work with experimental animals has shown that modern water-soluble contrast material (50 per cent sodium diatrizoate) is safe when infused in relatively large amounts and at pressures of 65 to 70 cm. of water (Waldron, 1968). Even infusions at greater than 100 cm. of water, the accepted pressure necessary to cause ductule rupture, resulted in no more than a mild pancreatitis. As is true in clinical studies (Cotton, 1972;

Howard, 1969; Kasugai, 1972*a*), marked elevations in serum amylase were seen in the absence of pancreatitis. Radiographic evidence of acinar filling may be seen in such cases (Birnstingl, 1959) (Fig. 8–4). From this experiment and others, it would appear that the opening of potential ductule-interstitial-capillary pathways allows absorption of water-soluble contrast agents with little damage to acinar cells (Bockman, 1971; Waldron, 1971). On the other hand, insoluble substances such as Ethiodol and barium, which cannot follow this pathway and are poorly cleared from the ducts, may cause severe pancreatitis (Waldron, 1968).

Fiberoptic Pancreatocholangiography

Peroral pancreatography was first performed in 1965 by two radiologists, Rabinov and Simon, using a modified intestinal tube and fluoroscopic guidance. At that time, they suggested the use of fiberendoscopy as a guide to cannulation. The latter technique was successfully demonstrated by McCune in 1968. One year later, Oi (1969) reported success with a new fiberduodenoscope designed specifically for pancreatocholangiography. Since then, a number of reports have attested to the feasibility, value and safety of this technique (Classen, 1971; Cotton, 1972; Kasugai, 1972*a*; Kasugai, 1972*b*).

This procedure may be indicated when, following routine radiologic workup, additional study of the pancreas is needed (Fig. 8–5). In theory, at least, it should precede angiography or transhepatic cholangiography. Its contraindications include the acute phase of pancreatitis and septic conditions such as cholangitis or suspected infectious hepatitis in which inability to sterilize the instrument may lead to cross-infection (Cotton, 1972). Because large doses of anticholinergic drugs are required to produce duodenal atony, glaucoma is also a contraindication, and the procedure must be cautiously employed in patients

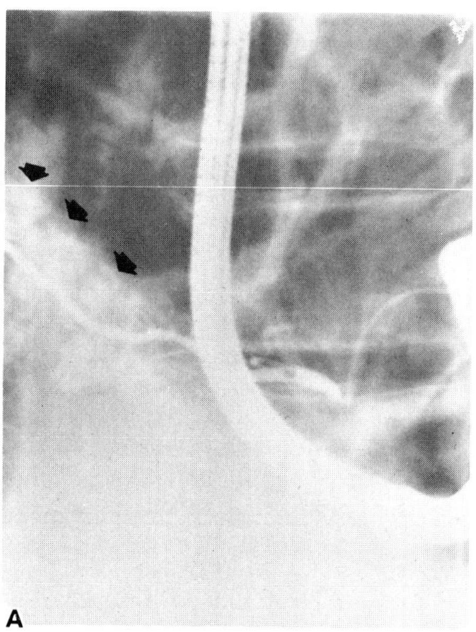

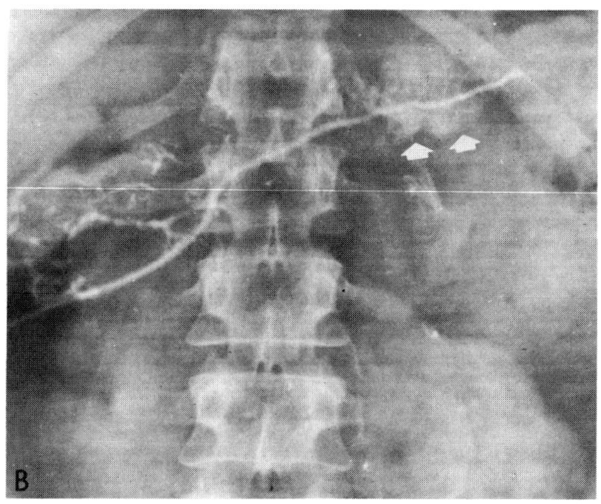

Figure 8–4. Acinar opacification. Possible overfilling versus pancreatitis.

A, Normal endoscopic pancreatogram demonstrating so-called acinar filling (*arrows*) due to a large injection of contrast material. The caudocranial course of the right half of the duct is a normal variation. Radiolucencies in the main duct are due to injected air. (Courtesy of Dr. George J. Brodmerkel, Jr.)

B, Operative transpapillary pancreatogram in known chronic pancreatitis. Acinar filling is localized to the affected area (*arrows*). The appearance is indistinguishable.

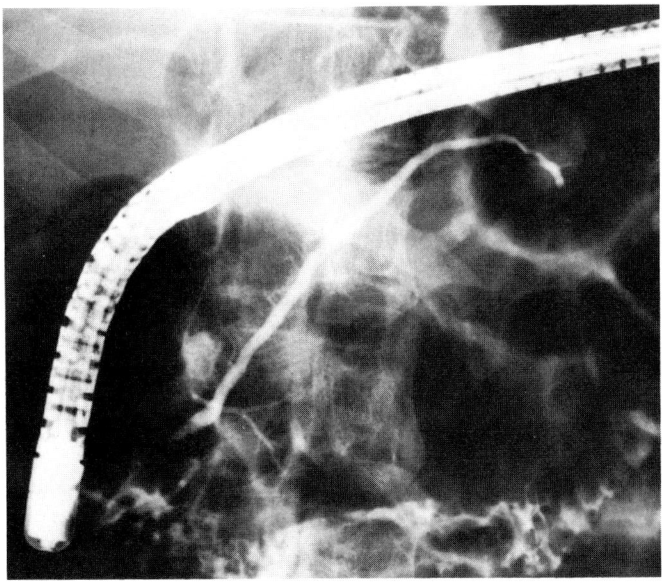

Figure 8–5. Normal endoscopic pancreatogram. (Reproduced by courtesy of the *New England Journal of Medicine.*)

with urinary retention or severe cardiac disease. In the first four years since its introduction, only two (both nonfatal) complications were reported—one was an instance of acute pancreatitis (Galvan, 1972) and the other, of bile peritonitis (Cotton, 1972). More recently, a single case of fatal necrotizing pancreatitis has been recorded (Amman, 1973).

NORMAL ANATOMY

Terminology

The following are definitions of key anatomic terms as they are used here. The *duct of Wirsung* (also referred to by many investigators as *the main pancreatic duct*) is that duct emptying at the major papilla whether or not it is the major excretory pathway or communicates with the duct of Santorini. The *duct of Santorini* is that duct which ends at the minor papilla whether or not it is the main or accessory route of excretion. Note that the entire central duct is named according to its dominant excretory pathway. The *accessory pancreatic duct* is synonymous with the duct of Santorini but only when the duct of Wirsung is dominant. The *ventral pancreatic duct* is that of the ventral pancreatic anlage. The *dorsal pancreatic duct* is that of the dorsal pancreatic anlage. The adjectives "ventral" and "dorsal" incorrectly describe the positions of the adult ducts to which they are sometimes applied and are best limited to describe the embryo (Millbourn, 1950).

Embryology

The pancreatic ducts, including their drainage patterns and biliary and duodenal relationships, are easily understood after their embryologic development is studied (Millbourn, 1950). The pancreas originates from two primordia on the dorsal and ventral aspects of the gut, the latter in turn being part of the more distally located hepatobiliary anlage (Callender, 1934) (Fig. 8–6, *A*). Rotation of the duodenum and of the ventral pancreas brings the primordia to a left lateral position, and the major and minor papillas to their respective adult dorsolateral and ventrolateral positions (Fig. 8–6, *B*, *C*). During fusion of the two glands, the duct systems usually anastomose and the cephalic portion of the dorsal duct tends to diminish in

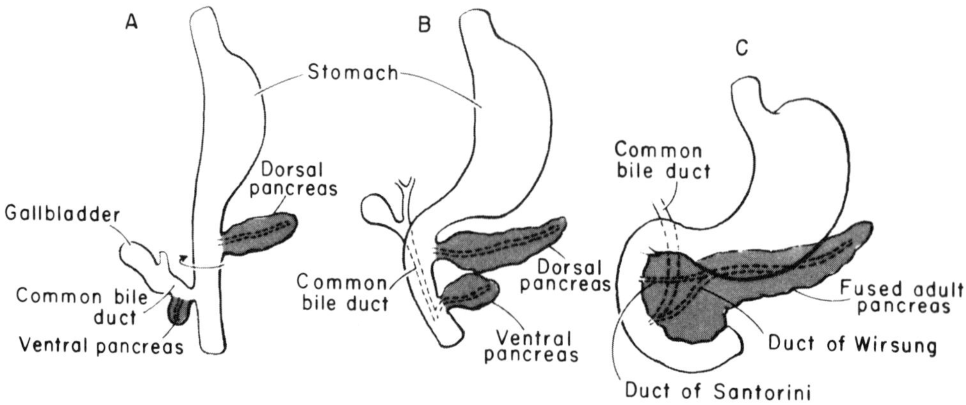

Figure 8–6. Embryologic development of the pancreas.
A, Left lateral view. The arrow indicates the future direction of rotation.
B and *C*, Frontal views during and after rotation, respectively. (Modified from Callender, C. L.: Surgical Anatomy. Philadelphia, W. B. Saunders Company, 1934, p. 440.)

size, giving way to a dominant duct of Wirsung. Almost all duct patterns in the adult can be explained on the basis of variations in the presence and site of anastomosis and the degree of atrophy of the dorsal duct. The adult form of annular pancreas is thought to be due to adherence, during rotation, of the tip of the ventral pancreas to the anterior aspect of the duodenum. Therefore, the duct of the annulus is always the duct of Wirsung or one of its branches (Doubilet, 1965; McNaught, 1935; Millbourn, 1950) (see also Fig. 4–85, Chapter 4).

Adult Duct System

Of the anatomic studies of the major pancreatic ducts which are in good agreement (Berman, 1960; Hjorth, 1947; Millbourn, 1950, 1959), those of Millbourn are the best documented and most detailed. Figure 8–7, which draws heavily upon the latter work, illustrates the main patterns of pancreatic drainage. Notice that the duct of Wirsung is the main excretory pathway in approximately 91 per cent of the adults, and communicates through an accessory duct with the minor papilla in 39 per cent of these. (One study has shown that in infants and small children, patency of the accessory duct is much more common [Dawson, 1961].) However, in only about half of the latter group is this second pathway large enough to act as a functional substitute for the main duct. It is also noteworthy that when the duct of Santorini is dominant, the duct of Wirsung is separate in approximately 61 per cent, whereas an isolated accessory duct is quite rare (Millbourn, 1950). Duplication of the ducts is occasionally seen and is most common in the tail of the pancreas (Howard, 1969).

The pancreatic and common bile ducts, according to a recent authoritative study by Barraya and his colleagues (1971), form a common channel in approximately 90 per cent of the cases. The common channel is usually a direct extension of the pancreatic duct, whereas the common bile duct enters the superior surface of the common channel at a more acute angle (Fig. 8–8). This probably explains why the pancreatic duct is entered first in the majority of transpapillary cannulations (Nardi, 1966).

As noted in Chapter 4, the term "ampulla of Vater" refers to a dilatation of the ductal system immediately below the papillary orifice. This dilatation is commonly present during fetal development, but is seldom present as a noticeable dilatation during adult life. The reported incidence of an ampulla of the duct of Wirsung (i.e., the ampulla of Vater) varies from 1 to 8.8 per cent (Kasugai, 1972*a*; Millbourn, 1959) and is occasionally demonstrable radiographically during hypotonic duodenography or postoperative

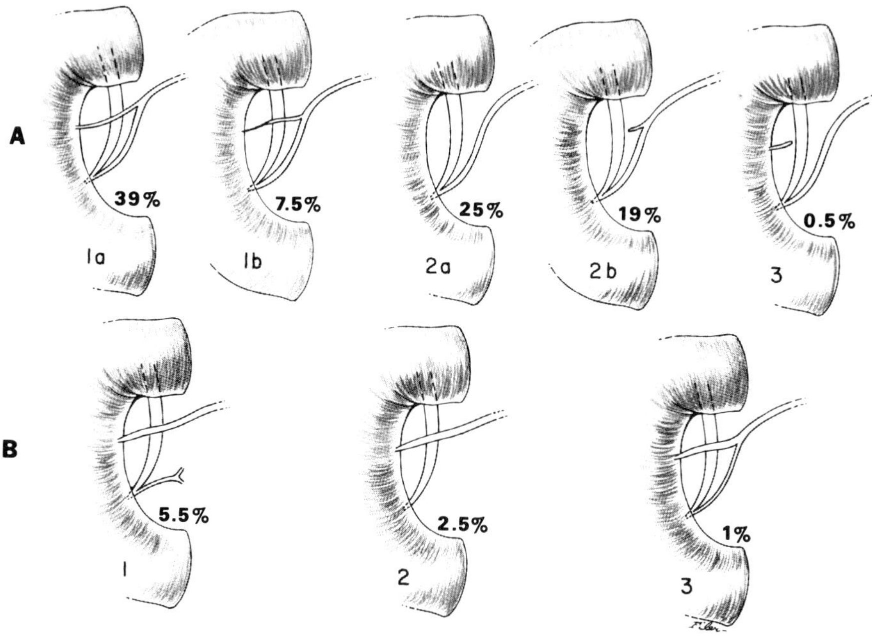

Figure 8–7. Patterns of the pancreatic ducts.
A, Duct of Wirsung predominates. *1a*, Patent duct of Santorini. *1b*, Duct of Santorini ending blindly at the lesser papilla. *2a* and *b*, Duct of Wirsung, the only effluent, the latter showing a small accessory duct remnant. *3*, Small isolated duct of Santorini.
B, Duct of Santorini predominates. *1*, Small isolated duct of Wirsung. *2*, Absent duct of Wirsung. *3*, Small duct of Wirsung communicating with duct of Santorini. (Percentages are based on the work of Millbourn in 1950.)

cholangiography (see also Fig. 4–55, Chapter 4). In contrast, an ampullary dilatation occurs at the orifice of the duct of Santorini in about 20 per cent of these instances in which it acts as an accessory duct, and in nearly 50 per cent, in which the duct of Santorini is dominant (Millbourn, 1959) (Fig. 8–9).

The main pancreatic duct is centrally located in the body and tail of the pancreas (Hayasaka, 1970) and courses in a variable direction from the region of the spleen. In approximately half of the cases, its initial course is cephalocaudad, whereas in about a quarter, it is horizontal and in the remainder, either sigmoid or ascending (Kasugai, 1972*a*). Upon reaching the neck or isthmus of the gland, it usually either angles inferiorly, paralleling the common duct in a slightly ventral plane or, when the duct of Santorini is dominant, follows a fairly straight but dorsal pathway towards the minor papilla.

Measurements of the width of the normal pancreatic duct depend upon a number of variables, including the site being measured, the patient's age, the degree of ductal distention, and the amount of x-ray magnification. The maximum diameter of the main duct is usually found in the head of the pancreas, but its caliber varies little except for slight tapering in the tail (Millbourn, 1959; Trapnell, 1967). There is a progressive increase in the diameter of the average duct as the patient advances in age (Table 8–1). Interestingly, the common duct shows a similar trend although there is no useful correlation between its diameter and that of the pancreatic duct in the same individual (Millbourn, 1959). Comparison of in vivo cholangiographic examinations with autopsy examinations requires correction for injection pressure (higher in the autopsy series) and magnification (greater in the cholangiographic series). When both

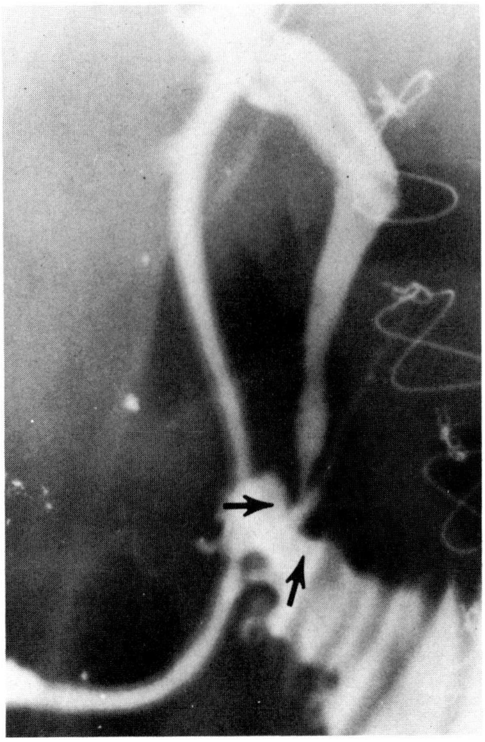

Figure 8–8. Oblique entrance of the common duct into the superior aspect of the main pancreatic duct forming a common channel. This arrangement accounts for the greater ease in entering the pancreatic duct than the bile duct during perendoscopic or transpapillary cannulation of the papilla.

factors are taken into account, it becomes apparent that figures based on postmortem examination require subtraction of approximately 1 mm. before they can be applied to the evaluation of living patients. Autopsy studies in which small injections were made confirm that the differences result chiefly from the effects of injection pressure rather than from postmortem changes (Trapnell, 1966). The differentiation of unusually large, but otherwise normal, pancreatic ducts (greater than 3 mm. in diameter in persons under the age of 30, and six mm. in those over the age of 30 on standard radiograms) from those with obstructive dilatation should be based on a consideration of all clinical and radiologic evidence.

The duct of Wirsung may show localized narrowing in two areas—namely, at its orifice and, when dominant, in the neck of the gland where fusion of the pancreatic primordia took place (Fig. 8–10). Narrowing at its orifice is usually limited to tapering of the sphincteric segment but may be nontapered and extend for about 1.5 cm. (Millbourn, 1950). Narrowing at the isthmus is seen in approximately 4 per cent of the individuals and may be striking in degree (Birnstingl, 1959; Howard, 1969; Leger, 1952). Pathologic strictures may occur in these same areas but usually should be obvious because of resulting presentotic ductal dilatation (Thal, 1959).

Collecting ducts enter the main pancreatic duct in radial and evenly spaced fashion, except in the head where they tend to be larger and less numerous (Hayasaka, 1970). The one closest to the major papilla usually drains the uncinate process and may, through a looping course, anastomose with a branch of the accessory duct. This communication is not uncommon and has been named the *ansa pancreatica* (Dawson, 1961). Drain-

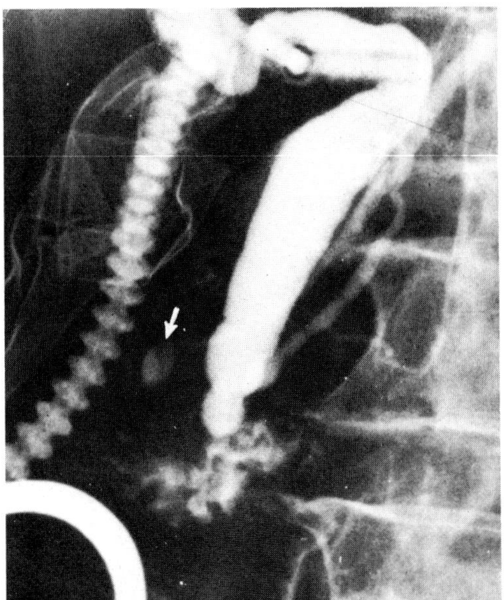

Figure 8–9. Ampulla of the duct of Santorini (*arrow*). A visible ampulla of Santorini is more common than is an ampulla of Wirsung.

TABLE 8–1. Pancreatic Duct Diameters*

AUTOPSY SERIES (150 CASES)			CHOLANGIOGRAPHY SERIES (81 CASES)	
Age Group (years)	*Maximum Diameter (mm.)*† *Average*	*Range*	*Maximum Diameter (mm.) Average*	*Range*
	DUCT OF WIRSUNG (PRINCIPAL DUCT)			
16–20	3.3	3.0–4.0	–	–
21–30	3.5	2.5–4.5	2.2	1–3
31–40	3.9	3.0–6.0	3.0	1–5
41–50	4.2	2.5–5.0	3.2	1–5
51–60	4.3	2.0–7.0	3.6	1–7
61–70	4.5	3.0–10.0	3.4	2–4
71–80	5.0	2.5–11.0	–	–
81–92	6.0	3.5–10.0	–	–
	DUCT OF SANTORINI (PRINCIPAL DUCT)			
20–50 (4 cases)	2.9	2.5–3.0		
50–90 (13 cases)	3.5	2.0–6.0		

*See Millbourn, E.: Calibre and appearance of the pancreatic ducts and relevant clinical problems. A roentgenographic and anatomical study. Acta Chir. Scand., *118*:286–303, 1959–60.

†Before clinical use, 1 mm. should be subtracted to correct for the effects of magnification and injection pressure (see page 268).

ing into the collecting ducts are the intermediate ducts which, in turn, receive the terminal ductules and acini (Callender, 1934).

With advancing age, in the majority of individuals there is a tendency for more and more collecting ducts to be obstructed and thus nonvisualized (Berman, 1960). This finding has been noted in association with a variety of histologic pictures including inspissated ductal secretions, hyperplasia and metaplasia of ductal epithelium, and chronic inflammation, fibrosis and fatty atrophy of the

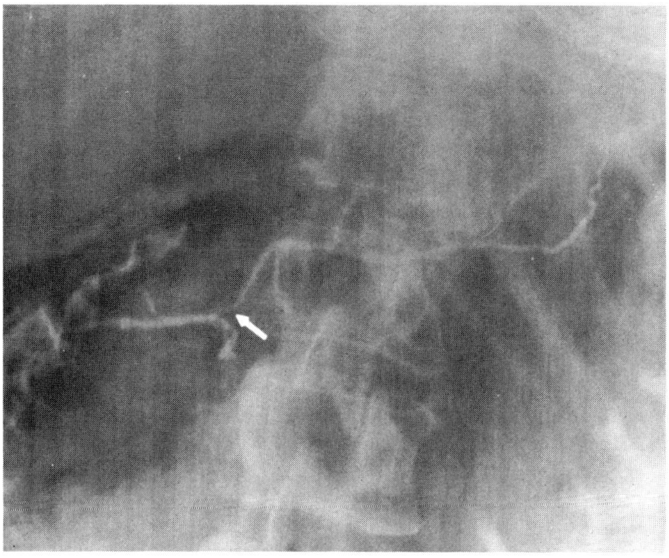

Figure 8–10. Operative pancreatogram in a 41-year-old female with mild chronic pancreatitis. The main pancreatic duct is of normal caliber except for an area of tapered narrowing in the head (*arrow*). The latter does not cause obstruction and is thought to represent a normal variant of the type which is occasionally seen at or near the neck of the gland. Another variant is seen to the left of the arrow where the duct of Wirsung follows a figure-eight course.

gland (Berman, 1960; Birnstingl, 1959; Warter, 1965). In addition, Berman's work (1960) suggests that it occurs more frequently in the presence of cholelithiasis. It is important to recognize that this change is not always the result of chronic inflammation and that it should be evaluated in light of the patient's age and other clinical and radiologic evidence.

DIAGNOSTIC CRITERIA

Acute Pancreatitis

Injection of the ducts during an acute episode of pancreatitis is contraindicated since it does not give immediately useful information and may further damage the gland. Moreover, acute and acute relapsing pancreatitis are seldom associated with pancreatographic abnormalities. Occasionally, however, an inciting stricture or a pancreatic abscess is discovered. In addition, during the acute or subacute phases of an attack, pancreatography may result in a hazy type of parenchymal staining presumably due to increased permeability of the ductal epithelium (Doubilet, 1955; Elmslie, 1963; Leger, 1952). Such opacification is nonspecific and is similar to the appearance of acinar filling which may be seen in normal glands with large injections of contrast material (Birnstingl, 1959) (Fig. 8–4, *A*).

Chronic Pancreatitis

Pancreatography is a valuable supplement to inspection and palpation of the gland in the surgical management of chronic relapsing pancreatitis. When obstruction of the main pancreatic duct is not present, treatment of related diseases such as alcoholism, cholelithiasis or hyperparathyroidism is often sufficient. However, once obstruction has occurred, pancreatic drainage or resection is frequently indicated (Warren, 1971).

In early or mild cases of chronic pancreatitis, the main pancreatic duct is, as a rule, normal (Fig. 8–11) although irregular filling and small cystic dilatations of its branches may be seen (Howard, 1971; Kasugai, 1972*b*). Later, however, the central duct usually dilates while the secondary ducts decrease in number and become more deformed (Fig. 8–12). The enlarged duct may be smooth but is more often similar in appearance to a string of sausages or beads (Hepp, 1959). In most instances, the entire duct is involved, but occasionally

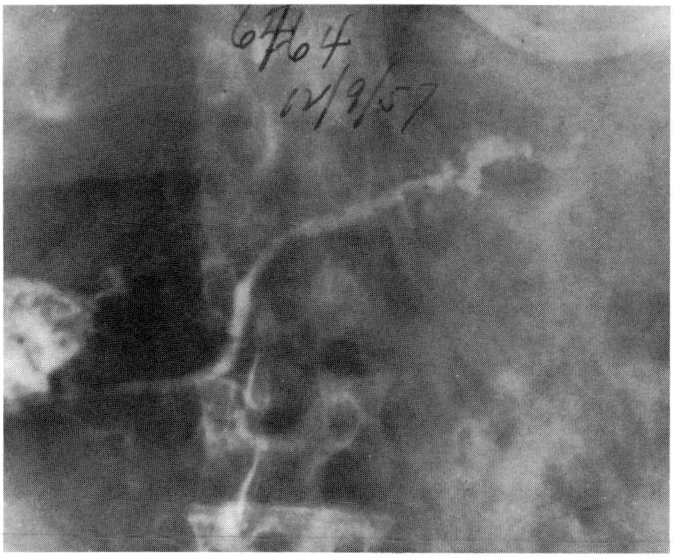

Figure 8–11. Operative transpapillary pancreatogram in chronic calcific pancreatitis. The duct of Wirsung shows only slight dilatation and irregularity in outline, whereas the secondary ducts in the tail of the gland exhibit typical changes of chronic inflammatory disease—stenoses and dilatation.

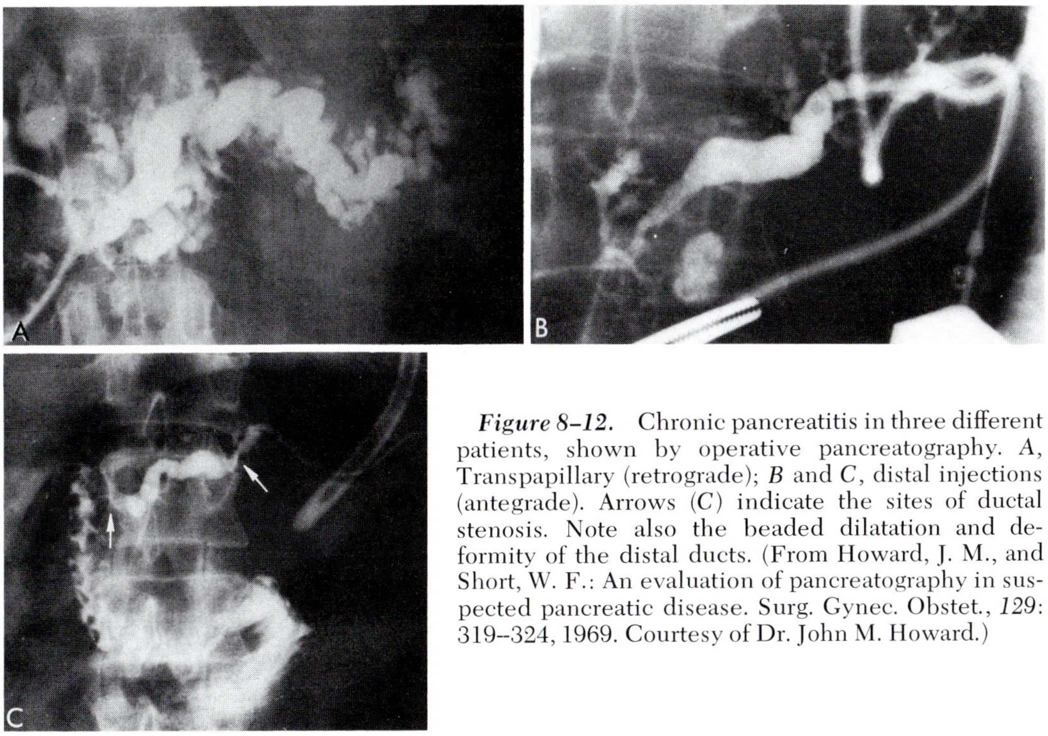

Figure 8–12. Chronic pancreatitis in three different patients, shown by operative pancreatography. *A*, Transpapillary (retrograde); *B* and *C*, distal injections (antegrade). Arrows (*C*) indicate the sites of ductal stenosis. Note also the beaded dilatation and deformity of the distal ducts. (From Howard, J. M., and Short, W. F.: An evaluation of pancreatography in suspected pancreatic disease. Surg. Gynec. Obstet., *129*: 319–324, 1969. Courtesy of Dr. John M. Howard.)

with peripheral obstruction those portions in the head and body are spared. Obstruction is seldom complete and is primarily due to stricture, with calculi playing a secondary role. When advanced disease is not accompanied by obstruction, the main pancreatic duct is normal in caliber but is more tortuous and receives only scattered, deformed collection ducts (Hepp, 1959; Sarles, 1965). Presumably due to increased ductal rigidity and decreased capacity, there tends to be better filling of the remaining peripheral branches by the usual 2 cc. injection of contrast material (Nardi, 1966). However, this is not a reliable criterion for the diagnosis of chronic pancreatitis.

Pseudocyst

Pseudocysts, which may accompany acute or chronic pancreatitis, can be studied by radiopaque contrast material. The small intrapancreatic variety which is fairly common in chronic disease may be detected only by pancreatography (Nardi, 1969; Sarles, 1965) (Fig. 8–13, *A*). Injection of large pseudocysts can be helpful in outlining them and in tracing suspected extensions such as those into the mediastinum (McClintock, 1965). Complete obstruction of the main pancreatic duct is sometimes found in the presence of large pseudocysts (Howard, 1969). In this instance, the duct may be visualized either by direct needle puncture or, not uncommonly, through a communication with the opacified pseudocyst (Fig. 8–13, *B*).

Tumor

Pancreatography has played a relatively minor role in the diagnosis of pancreatic carcinoma. However, the advent of peroral studies has led to greater interest in its use for this purpose. Early reports by endoscopists are encouraging, although much more experience will have to be accumulated before its place in our diagnostic armamentarium is clear.

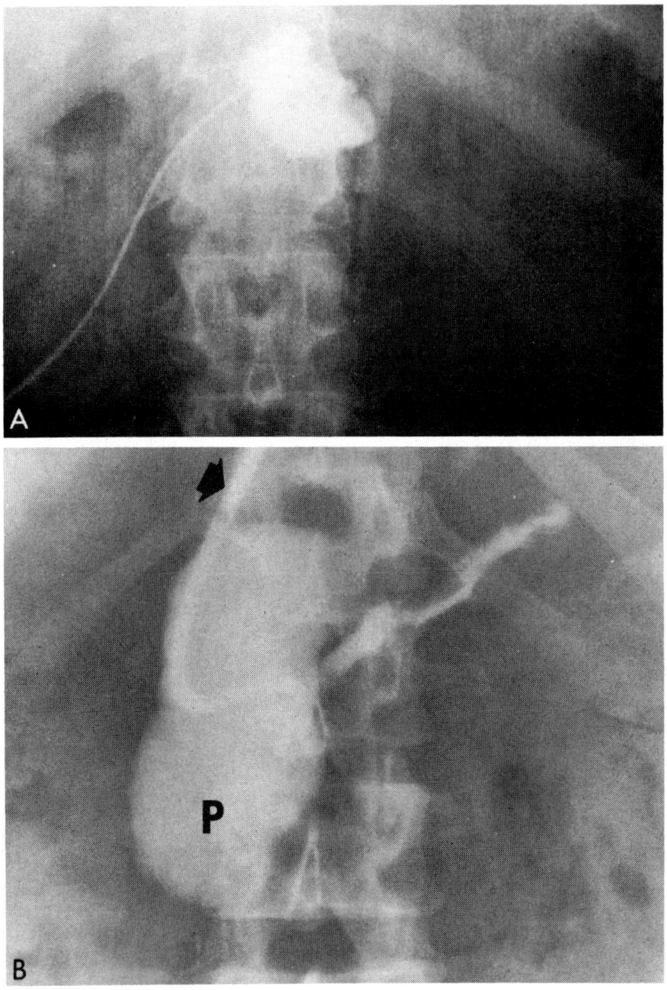

Figure 8–13. Pseudocysts. *A*, Intrapancreatic pseudocyst. (From Nardi, G. L.: Solitary occult retention cyst of the pancreas. New Eng. J. Med., *280*:11–15, 1969. Courtesy of the *New England Journal of Medicine* and of Dr. George L. Nardi.)

B, Fistulography in a patient who had acute pancreatic necrosis six months earlier reveals a pseudocyst (*P*) which is communicating with an obstructed, dilated pancreatic duct. Contrast material outlines the tube through which the injection was made (*arrow*). (From Howard, J. M., and Short, W. F.: An evaluation of pancreatography in suspected pancreatic disease. Surg. Gynec. Obstet., *129*:319–324, 1969. Courtesy of Dr. John M. Howard.)

Specific unanswered questions include the frequency with which the main pancreatic duct is involved, the accuracy of differentiation between benign and malignant disease, this accuracy relative to other diagnostic techniques, and the effectiveness of this tool in the early diagnosis of carcinoma.

Pancreatographic findings suggestive of carcinoma include complete obstruction as well as tapered, concentric ductal stenosis (Fig. 8–14), especially when the secondary radicals in the vicinity of the stenosis fail to fill. When a transpancreatic injection is given, smooth, uniform dilatation of the distal duct is typical of tumor in the pancreatic head (Anacker, 1962; Artigas, 1965; Hess, 1965; and Warter, 1965) (Fig. 8–15). While smoothly uniform dilatation is common in carcinoma, some patients with such lesions develop secondary pancreatitis (Castleman, 1972; Hayes, 1960), while in other cases chronic pancreatitis precedes the development of carcinoma (Johnson, 1963; Sarles, 1965). Accordingly, the presence of an inflammatory type of change cannot exclude malignancy (Fig. 8–16).

Carcinoma of the papilla of Vater is usually suspected preoperatively by means of a barium study or fiberoptic duodenoscopy. Operative pancreatography, when performed, can be expected

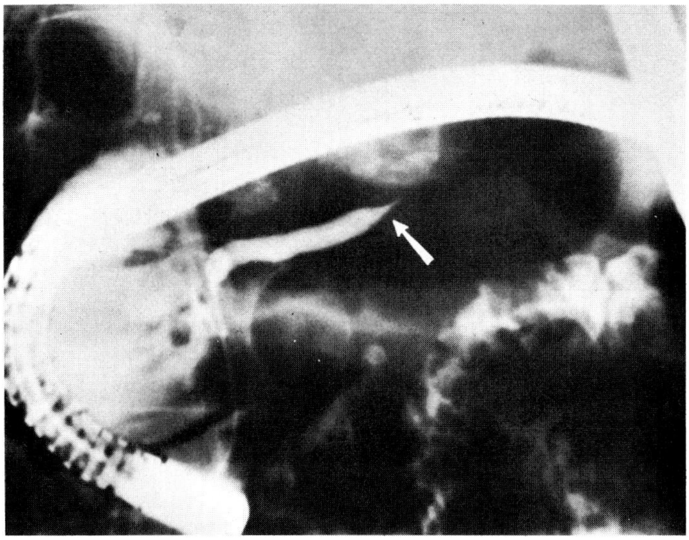

Figure 8–14. Endoscopic pancreatography in carcinoma of the body of the pancreas demonstrates a cone shaped stricture (*arrow*) characteristic of malignancy. The true diameter of the duct is obtained by comparison with that of the tip of the fiberscope (actual diameter, 10 mm.). (From Short, W. F., Bron, K. M., Eaton, S. B., Jr., and Leopold, G. R.: Pancreatic evaluation by roentgenography, ultrasound and radioisotopes. *In* Diseases of the Pancreas. Edited by L. C. Carey. St. Louis, Mo., C. V. Mosby Company, 1973. Courtesy of C. V. Mosby Company and Dr. George J. Brodmerkel, Jr.)

to show partial or complete obstruction of the Vaterian canal and of the adjoining portion of the pancreatic duct (Howard, 1969). However, cholangiography is more easily performed and is, as a rule, more useful in evaluating this lesion.

To the author's knowledge, pancreatography has not been used successfully in the diagnosis of other pancreatic tumors. It has been suggested that small lesions such as islet cell tumors might be detectable in glands which were completely opacified by the injection of relatively large amounts of contrast material (Doubilet, 1955). However, potential difficulties with this method include the low percentage of cases in which acinar filling occurs, the patchy type of opacification frequently obtained, and the added risk of producing pancreatitis (Birnstingl, 1959; Kasugai, 1972*a*).

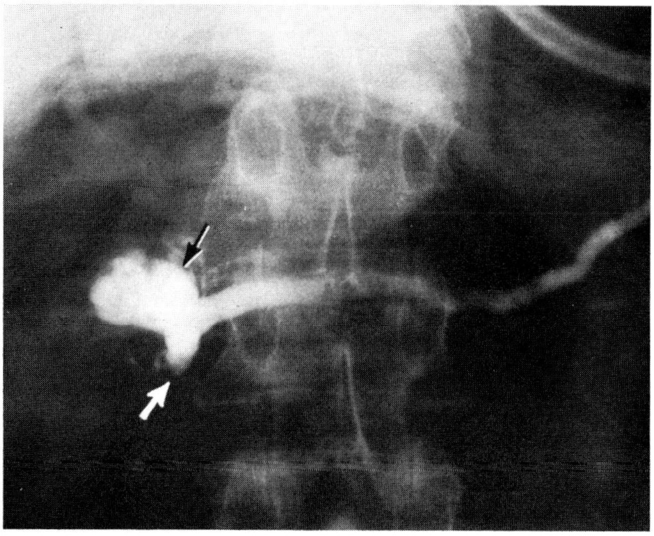

Figure 8–15. Complete obstruction of the pancreatic duct due to carcinoma of the head of the pancreas is demonstrated by intraoperative transparenchymal injection. Concentric narrowing, smooth dilatation and complete obstruction of the duct favor a malignant rather than an inflammatory stricture (*lower white arrow*). The cyst-like structure in the head of the pancreas is thought to be an area of tumor necrosis (*upper black arrow*). (From Howard, J. M., and Short, W. F.: An evaluation of pancreatography in suspected pancreatic disease. Surg. Gynec. Obstet., *129*:319–324, 1969. Reproduced by permission of the authors and publisher.)

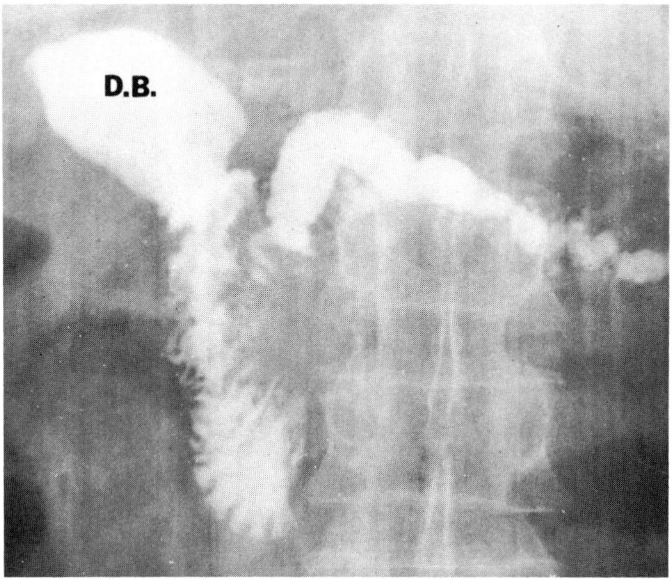

Figure 8–16. Operative pancreatogram performed by transparenchymal injection in a patient with carcinoma of the common bile duct. Stenosis just proximal to its orifice has resulted in incomplete obstruction of the duct of Wirsung. The beaded type of dilatation of the main and secondary pancreatic ducts is characteristic of chronic pancreatitis. Contrast material fills the duodenal bulb (*D.B.*) and loop. (From Howard, J. M., and Short, W. F.: An evaluation of pancreatography in suspected pancreatic disease. Surg. Gynec. Obstet., *129*:319–324, 1969. Reproduced by permission of the authors and publisher.)

REFERENCES

Amman, R. W., Deyhle, P., and Butikofer, E.: Fatal necrotizing pancreatitis after peroral cholangiopancreatography. Gastroenterology, *64*: 320–323, 1973.

Anacker, H.: Die Pathologischen Veränderungen des Pankreasgangsystems im Röntgenbild. Fortschr. Roentgenstr., *96*:455–470, 1962.

Artigas, D. V., and LaCalle, J.: Pancreatografía—técnica, indicaciones y resultados. Prensa Med. Argent., *52*:1713–1719, 1965.

Barraya, L., Pujol Soler, R., and Yvergneaux, J.-P.: La region Oddienne. Anatomie millimetrique. Presse Med., *79*:2527–2534, 1971.

Berkman, Y. M., and Rabinowitz, J.: Gastrointestinal manifestations of the strongyloidiasis. Amer. J. Roentgen., *115*:306–311, 1972.

Berman, L. G., Prior, J. T., Abramow, S. M., and Ziegler, D. D.: A study of the pancreatic duct system in man by the use of vinyl acetate casts of postmortem preparations. Surg. Gynec. Obstet., *110*:391–403, 1960.

Birnstingl, M.: A study of pancreatography. Brit. J. Surg., *47*:128–139, 1959–60.

Bockman, D. E., Schiller, W. R., and Anderson, M. C.: Route of retrograde flow in the exocrine pancreas during ductal hypertension. Arch. Surg., *103*:321–329, 1971.

Callender, C. L.: Surgical Anatomy. Philadelphia, W. B. Saunders Company, 1934, p. 440.

Castleman, B., Scully, R. E., and McNeely, B. U.: Case records of the Massachusetts General Hospital: Case 25–1972. New Eng. J. Med., *286*:1353–1359, 1972.

Classen, M.: Progress report. Fibroendoscopy of the intestines. Gut, *12*:330–338, 1971.

Cotton, P. B., Blumgart, L. H., Davies, G. T., Pierce, J. W., Salmon, P. R., Burwood, R. J., Lawrie, B. W., and Read, A. E.: Cannulation of papilla of Vater via fiber-duodenoscope. Lancet, *1*:53–58, 1972.

Dawson, W., and Langman J.: An anatomical-radiological study on the pancreatic duct pattern in man. Anat. Rec., *139*:59–68, 1961.

Doubilet, H., and Mulholland, J. H.: Intubation of the pancreatic duct in the human. Proc. Soc. Exp. Biol. Med., *76*:113–144, 1951.

Doubilet, H., and Worth, M. H.: Pseudocyst of annular pancreas demonstrated by operative pancreatography. Surgery, *58*:824–827, 1965.

Doubilet, H., Poppel, M. H., and Mulholland, J. H.: Pancreatography. Radiology, *64*:325–339, 1955.

Eaton, S. B., Benedict, K. T., Ferrucci, J. T., and Fleischli, D. J.: Hypotonic duodenography. Radiol. Clin. N. Amer., *8*:125–137, 1970.

Elmslie, R. G., White, T. T., and Magee, D. F.: Pancreatography with particular reference to activation of pancreatic enzymes. Surg. Gynec. Obstet., *117*:405–410, 1963.

Galvan, A., and Klotz, A. P.: Is transduodenal pancreatography ever contraindicated? Abstr. Gastroent., *62*:888, 1972.

Hayasaka, N., and Sasano, N.: Vascular and ductal patterns of pancreas by microradiology and their relation to lesions of pancreatitis. Tohoku J. Exp. Med., *100*:327–347, 1970.

Hayes, M. A.: Operative pancreatography. Surg. Gynec. Obstet., *110*:404–408, 1960.

Hepp, J., Tourneur, R., and Moreaux, J.: Les lésions anatomiques du pancréas confrontées avec les données de la pancréatographie dans les pancréatitis chroniques calcifiantes. Presse Med., *67*:1275–1278, 1959.

Hess, W.: Surgery of the Biliary Passages and the Pancreas. Princeton, N.J., D. Van Nostrand Company, Inc., 1965, p. 298.

Ibid., pp. 302–308.
Ibid., p. 458.
Hjorth, E.: Contributions to the knowledge of pancreatic reflux as an etiologic factor in chronic affections of the gall bladder. Acta Chir. Scand., *96*:Suppl. 134, 1947.
Howard, J. M., and Nedwich, A.: Correlation of the histologic observations and operative findings in patients with chronic pancreatitis. Surg. Gynec. Obstet., *132*:387–395, 1971.
Howard, J. M., and Short, W. F.: An evaluation of pancreatography in suspected pancreatic disease. Surg. Gynec. Obstet., *129*:319–324, 1969.
Johnson, J. R., and Zintel, H. A.: Pancreatic calcification and cancer of the pancreas. Surg. Gynec. Obstet., *117*:585–588, 1963.
Kasugai, T., Kuno, N., Kobayashi, S., and Hattori, K.: Endoscopic pancreatocholangiography. I. The normal endoscopic pancreatocholangiogram. Gastroenterology, *63*:217–226, 1972*a*.
Kasugai, T., Kuno, N., Kizu, M., Kobayashi, S., and Hattori, K.: Endoscopic pancreatocholangiography. II. The pathological endoscopic pancreatocholangiogram. Gastroenterology, *63*: 227–234, 1972*b*.
Leger, L.: L'exploration radio-chirurgicale du pancréas et le drainage trans-papillaire du canal de Wirsung. J. Chir., *68*:518–536, 1952.
Leger, L.: Surgical contrast visualization of the pancreatic ducts with a study of pancreatic external secretion. Amer. J. Dig. Dis., *20*: 8–12, 1953.
Legge, D. A., Carlson, H. C., and Judd, E. S.: Roentgenologic features of regional enteritis of the upper gastrointestinal tract. Amer. J. Roentgen., *110*:355–360, 1970.
McClintock, J. T., McFee, J. L., and Quimby, R. L.: Pancreatic pseudocyst presenting as a mediastinal tumor. J.A.M.A., *192*:573–574, 1965.
McCune, W. S., Shorb, P. E., and Moscovitz, H.: Endoscopic cannulation of the ampulla of Vater: a preliminary report. Ann. Surg., *167*: 752–756, 1968.
McNaught, J. B., and Cox, A. J.: Annular pancreas. Amer. J. Path., *11*:179–184, 1935.
Millbourn, E.: Calibre and appearance of the pancreatic ducts and relevant clinical problems. A roentgenographic and anatomical study. Acta Chir. Scand., *118*:286–303, 1959–60.
Millbourn, E.: On the excretory ducts of the pancreas in man, with special reference to their relations to each other, to the common bile duct and to the duodenum. Acta Anat., *9*: 1–34, 1950.
Nardi, G. L., and Acosta, J. M.: Papillitis as a cause of pancreatitis and abdominal pain: role of evocative test, operative pancreatography and histologic evaluation. Ann. Surg., *164*:611–621, 1966.
Nardi, G. L., Lyon, D. C., Sheiner, H. J., and Bartlett, A.K.: Solitary occult retention cysts of the pancreas. New Eng. J. Med., *280*:11–15, 1969.
Oi, I., Takemoto, T., and Kondo, T.: Fiberduodenoscope: direct observation of the papilla of Vater. Endoscopy, *3*:101–103, 1969.
Pollock, A. V.: Pancreatography in the diagnosis of chronic relapsing pancreatitis. Surg. Gynec. Obstet., *107*:765–770, 1958.
Rabinov, K. R., and Simon, M.: Peroral cannulation of the ampulla of Vater for direct cholangiography and pancreatography. Radiology, *85*:693–697, 1965.
Sarles, H., Sarles, J. C., Camatte, R., Muratore, R., Gaini, M., Guien, C., Pastor, J., and LeRoy, F.: Observations on 205 confirmed cases of acute pancreatitis, recurring pancreatitis and chronic pancreatitis. Gut, *6*:545–559, 1965.
Thal, A. P., Goott, B., Margulis, A. R.: Sites of pancreatic duct obstruction in chronic pancreatitis. Ann. Surg., *150*:49–56, 1959.
Trapnell, J. E.: Pancreatography: a reassessment. Brit. J. Surg., *54*:934–939, 1967.
Trapnell, J. E., Howard, J. M., and Brester, J.: Transduodenal Pancreatography: an improved technique. Surgery, *60*:1112–1119, 1966.
Waldron, R. L.: Reflux pancreatography: an evaluation of contrast agents for studying the pancreas. Amer. J. Roentgen., *104*:632–640, 1968.
Waldron, R. L., Seaman, W. B., and Foster, S.: Reflux pancreatography and distension duodenography in humans. Radiology, *104*:295–300, 1972.
Waldron, R. L., Luse, S. A., Wollowick, H. E., and Seaman, W. B.: Demonstration of a retrograde pancreatic pathway: correlation of roentgenographic and electron microscopic studies. Amer. J. Roentgen., *111*:695–699, 1971.
Warren, K. W., and Mountain, J. C.: Comprehensive management of chronic relapsing pancreatitis. Surg. Clin. N. Amer., *51*:693–710, 1971.
Warter, M. M. J., Weill, J.-P., Buchser, P., and Weill-Bousson, M. M.: Contribution à l'étude de la pancréatographie post mortem. Arch. Mal. App. Dig. Nutr., *54*:1219–1239, 1965.
Yvergneaux, J. P.: Le reflux wirsungien à la lumière du cliché dentaire intra-abdominal, complément de la radiomanométrie. Acta Gastroent. Belg., *32*:225–264, 1969.

Chapter 9

PANCREATIC ECHOGRAPHY

Paul C. Kahn, M.D.

Unlike the instantaneous development of the x-ray from discovery to medical use, exploitation of the ultrasound beam was slow. A quarter century elapsed between the first patent of an ultrasonic transducer by Langevin in 1917 (Howry, 1965) and its initial application in medicine by Dussik (1942). A decade went by before devices for cross-sectional display of ultrasonic echoes were developed (Howry, 1952; Wild, 1952), another passed before the first tentative reports of the clinical application of abdominal echography were published (Holmes, 1963), and the better part of a third elapsed before the first analyses of pancreatic examination by ultrasound appeared (Engelhart, 1970; Filly, 1970).

The long delay was undoubtedly the result of the technical problems and cost of the equipment required to produce and display echo maps. It was prolonged by the controversy over the choice between water path and contact scanners for mass production. The former tend to be clumsy, expensive, immobile, and unsuited to sick patients but produce clean, reliable and rapid echograms. The latter are usually light in weight, cheaper, and can be brought to the bedside of the most critically ill patient but require manual operation, and produce scans slowly, with considerably more artifacts. It was the commercial production of contact scanners in the late 1960's that finally brought diagnostic ultrasound into hospital practice.

Medical ultrasound owes much of its technology to spin-off from military programs. Nonetheless, we feel that the field is sufficiently remote from sound navigation and ranging that the acronym "sonar" is an unnecessary affectation, and that "echography" or "echoscopy" sufficiently differentiates the recording or viewing of ultrasound echoes from other ultrasonic techniques such as detection of motion by the Doppler principle.

Reflections of ultrasound (echoes) occur whenever a sound wave encounters a structure of different acoustical impedance. Density, elasticity, and architecture at the magnitude of the length of the sound waves (roughly 0.1–1 mm.) determine the strength of echoes in a manner which is difficult to predict mathematically. Clear fluids are usually free of echoes, homogenous organs (e.g., liver, spleen, and kidneys) have a few echoes (anechoic), and less uniform structures (fascia, muscle bundles, and bone) reflect much sound. Since most of the unidentifiable structures in the abdomen tend to produce numerous echoes, the basis of echographic interpretation is the recognition of relatively echo-free organs.

This physical principle clearly explains one of the difficulties encountered in pancreatic echography. The pancreas, probably because of its numerous ducts and blood vessels and its lobular structure, belongs to the category of heavily echo-producing organs. This has been shown clearly in vitro by Filly and

Freimanis (1970). The relative thinness and irregularity of the organ, as well as its lack of a dense capsule, further encourage its disappearance into the indefinable echoes of the retroperitoneum. Thus, the normal pancreatic echogram is one in which the pancreas is not demonstrated! Although it is theoretically possible that the thicker portions of the head of the pancreas might produce a small relatively echo-free area behind the liver, this has never been convincingly differentiated from a fluid-containing duodenal loop.

The transmission of ultrasound in a semifluid medium is inversely related to the production of echoes. Thus, regions which are anechoic also transmit sound well (transonic, sonolucent). In order to obtain a useful echo, the region between the transducer and the structure being studied must be relatively transsonic. Thus, deep organs such as the pancreas must be viewed through an "access window." This presents the second major problem in pancreatic echography, since bone (lower ribs and spine) and air (stomach, bowel, and lung bases) present essentially absolute impediments to sound transmission. Therefore, great care must be taken in selecting planes for pancreatic ultrasonic studies, and even greater caution must be used in the interpretation of echograms to make certain that "through transmission" has been achieved (Freimanis, 1970).

A third problem is presented by the fact that scans are most easily performed in planes perpendicular or parallel to the major body axes. The oblique orientation of the pancreas assures that any one standard cross-section will include only a small part of the organ.

In view of this bleak assessment, the reader may wonder why pancreatic echography is to be considered at all. The answer is that while the normal pancreas is essentially invisible by present ultrasonic scanning techniques, the edematous organ of pancreatitis, the tumor within the pancreas, and especially the fluid containing pancreatic cyst and pseudocyst often are clearly apparent. Furthermore, the echogram permits simultaneous study of associated disease in the liver, gallbladder, spleen, retroperitoneal lymph nodes, and peritoneal cavity.

TECHNIQUE

The patient ordinarily requires no special preparation. If he is severely ill, he should be well hydrated and made as comfortable as possible with appropriate medication, since he must be able to lie still in order that the examination have a reasonable chance of success. Barium in the stomach or bowel absorbs a great deal of sound and is a serious barrier to the examination (Leopold, 1971). Water-soluble contrast media, on the other hand, have only a minimal effect. Bowel gas also presents a serious impediment and, in the less seriously ill patient, premedication with vasopressin may be considered (Göthlin, 1972). Filling the stomach with water has been utilized as a method of displacing gas-containing structures (Holmes, 1967; Holm, 1971), but in our hands it has not been too helpful, perhaps because of the air inevitably swallowed at the same time.

A contact scanner with a 2-MHz transducer is generally employed (a 5-MHz transducer may be used in infants or small children). The patient is marked with a crayon so that scans can be identified in the coordinate grid (discussed below; see Fig. 9–1), and his abdomen is covered with a thin layer of glycerine or mineral oil to assure proper sonic contact. Transverse and vertical scans are then performed both with the patient supine and prone, as well as special views of the gallbladder, spleen, and any recognized abnormalities in various oblique planes.

Discipline in the use of scanning equipment is essential to success in pancreatic echography. There are four important principles: (1) A sufficient number of sections must be obtained. These should include scans on either side of the area of interest, as well as several sections through the area. "Spot filming" of lesions is hazardous to accuracy. (2) Scans of the same plane must be obtained at

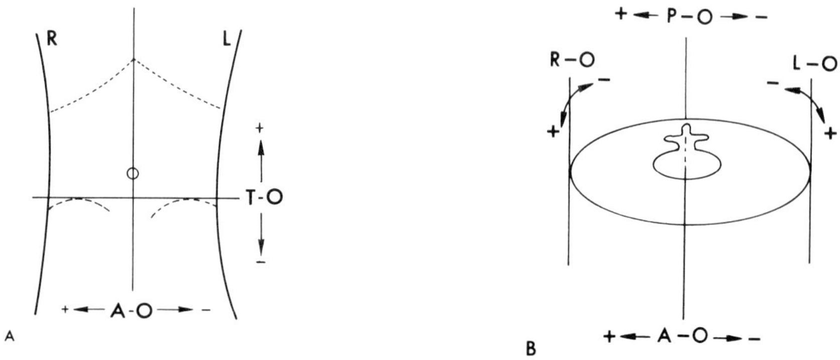

Figure 9–1. Basic orientation to the abdominal echogram.

A, Transverse planes are measured in centimeters above or below the iliac crest (*T*), and sagittal planes, in centimeters to the right or left of the midline (*A*). Plus (+) signifies upward or to the right, and minus (−), downward or to the left. Reference planes are indicated as A−O and T−O.

B, Other vertical sections are related to the posterior axis (*P*) or to the right or left midaxillary lines (*R* or *L*). Plus (+) is to the right or anteriorly, and minus (−) is to the left or posteriorly.

different, but standardized, sensitivity settings (Lehman, 1966; Holm, 1968). Since the recording of echoes tends to be an all-or-none affair, demonstration of lesions at various gain settings is necessary for a confident diagnosis. (3) All areas should be demonstrated in two intersecting (preferably perpendicular) planes (Freimanis, 1970). This helps to eliminate some of the many artifacts of contact scanning, and permits better analysis of the shape of organs and lesions. (4) All echograms should be clearly marked and identified on a coordinate grid so that they can be related easily to each other, to the patient's topographic anatomy, and to his radiographs or nuclide scans.

Figure 9–2 illustrates typical cross-sections that might be obtained in a pancreatic study. Figure 9–3 shows a representative panel of Polaroid films from a typical examination. The usual complete study consists of about three

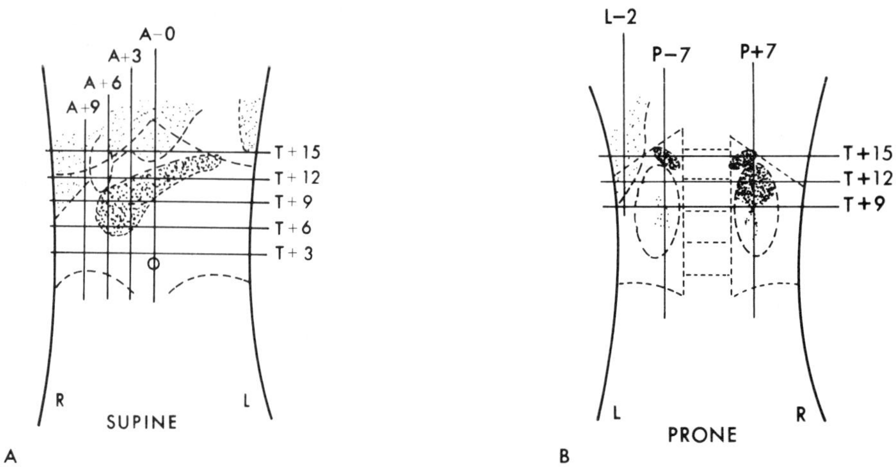

Figure 9–2. Typical basic sections in a pancreatic echogram.

A, Supine sections extend from just above the crest to just below the xiphoid. Vertical sections are primarily to the right of the midline.

B, Prone sections. Transverse sections are taken through the upper portions of both kidneys. Vertical sections also extend through both kidneys, and a left lateral section passes through the spleen.

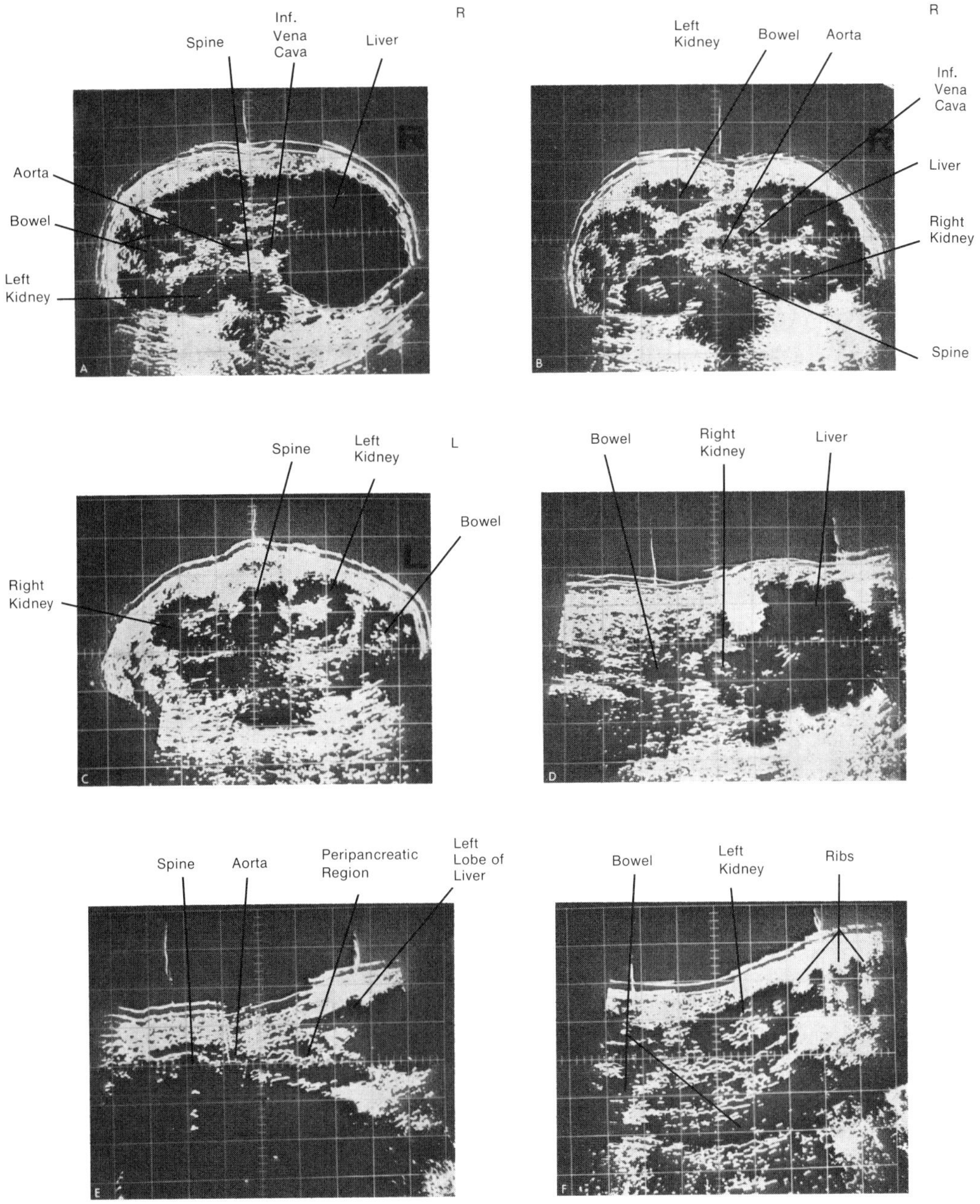

Figure 9–3. Six representative frames from a normal pancreatic echogram. *A*, Supine transverse ($T + 15$); *B*, supine transverse ($T + 9$); *C*, prone transverse ($T + 7$); *D*, supine vertical ($A + 6$); *E*, supine vertical ($A - 1$); and *F*, prone vertical ($P - 7$). Outlines of the liver, kidneys, spine, aorta, and vena cava are readily recognizable. No pancreatic tissue can be identified. In the vertical sections, the cephalic end is to the right. Each vertical mark equals 3 cm. unless otherwise specified.

such panels. We image the head and body of the pancreas with a series of supine horizontal sections from just below the xiphoid to above the iliac crest, and with a series of supine vertical sections from the right midclavicular line to the midline. We obtain spot views of the gallbladder and turn the patient on his right side to obtain vertical sections of the splenic area. The patient is then asked to lie in the prone position, and horizontal and vertical sections are taken with special attention to the left upper quadrant.

The marking method we employ (Fig. 9–1) is a simplification of the elegant system devised by Holm and his coworkers (1971). The transverse plane through the crests of the ilium is the "zero plane," all transverse sections above being defined as positive. Thus (T + 8) is a transverse section 8 cm. above the iliac crest. Vertical sections are related to the anterior (A) or posterior (P) midline, with + to the right. Vertical echograms taken far laterally are related to the right or left midaxillary lines (R or L), with + anterior. Thus (L–2) is a vertical section 2 cm. posterior to the left midaxillary line. Angulation of the probe is indicated in degrees (+ is toward the zero plane). Oblique views are identified by marking the coordinates of two points. Thus, a typical oblique subcostal section of the liver might be indicated as (A 0, T + 15; A + 10, T + 6; – 15°). Complicated identifications like this are very rarely needed.

INTERPRETATION

The person interpreting the scan must first assure himself that an adequate number of sections have been obtained, and must then orient himself, one by one, to the plane of each section. Training oneself to read only the labels for a minute or two requires discipline but saves time in the long run. The next step is to judge the information content of each film. The key to this evaluation is the "through transmission sign" (Freimanis, 1970). Each picture is an incomplete map, with areas obscured by bone, gas, or poor transducer-skin contact. Transmitted echoes appear as short lines perpendicular to the axis of the beam, while electronic artifacts form irregular dots.

The third step is to identify those organs which are normally seen – the liver, gallbladder, spleen, aorta, inferior vena cava, kidneys, and spine. Each structure should be identified in as many sections as possible, with frequent cross-reference between horizontal and vertical planes.

Now the time has come to begin looking for abnormalities – displacement, abnormal size or distortion of the normal organs, transonic areas other than those usually seen, or increased echoes in normally sonolucent structures. Freimanis (1970) has described several useful signs to assist in this phase of the analysis. A mass lesion will frequently obliterate the borders of adjacent organs (echo silhouette sign), particularly if it is infiltrative in type. A physically well-defined mass will tend to be marginated more sharply (mass outline sign). Part of this definition may be due to the increased echoes produced by compression of the adjacent tissues by expanding lesions (compressed tissue sign).

PANCREATIC TUMORS

Pancreatic tumors may be visualized as relatively echo-free zones in the retroperitoneum (Figs. 9–4 and 9–5). Engelhart and Blauenstein (1970) identified tumors in 12 patients seen because of jaundice. In ten of these, the diagnosis was unknown prior to the scan. In a subsequent study, Engelhart (1971) was able to diagnose correctly 38 of 41 patients with suspected carcinoma of the pancreas, missing only two of 30 tumors, and one false positive in nine patients free of tumor. Filly and Freimanis (1970) identified four of five pancreatic tumors. Templeton and Stuber (1971) found six tumors in patients with normal or equivocal barium or nuclide studies.

Although the tumor is initially detected as a sonolucency, unlike a cyst, it fills in as the gain setting is increased (Fig. 9–6). It may have an irregular, lumpy

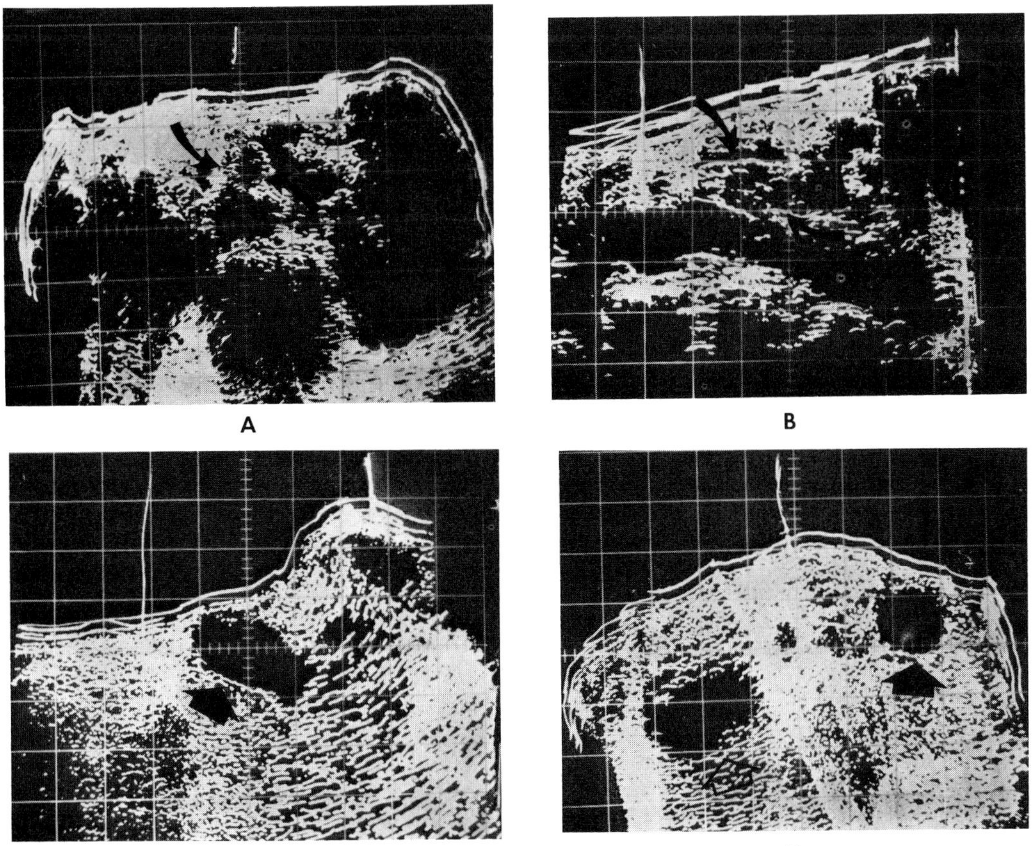

A B C D

Figure 9–4. Pancreatic echogram in 79-year-old man with jaundice.

A, A supine transverse section ($T + 10$) reveals a 3–4 cm. midepigastric mass (*arrows*) anterior to the dilated abdominal aorta.

B, A vertical section ($A - 0$) confirms the presence of this mass.

C, A vertical section at high gain ($A + 7$) shows the enlarged gallbladder (*arrow*) approximately 8×4 cm. in size.

D, A horizontal section at high gain ($T + 7$) again shows the enlarged gallbladder (*black arrow*) as well as another lucent mass on the left side (*white arrow*). The epigastric mass was confirmed at surgery to represent a carcinoma of the body of the pancreas, extending into the head to produce biliary obstruction. The transsonic mass on the left was an incidental renal cyst.

appearance. A compressed tissue sign may be present (Filly, 1970). It may not be possible to differentiate between a pancreatic tumor and other retroperitoneal lesions (Fig. 9–7). The smallest tumors that can be demonstrated by the present technique are probably about 3 cm. in diameter (Filly, 1970).

Several associated signs of pancreatic disease may be demonstrated. One of these is the presence of an enlarged gallbladder, found by Engelhart and Blauenstein (1970) in all of their jaundiced patients. The contractility of a questionably abnormal gallbladder may be challenged with a fatty meal (Hublitz, 1972) (Fig. 9–8). The presence of retroperitoneal lymph nodes (Asher, 1969), hematomas, or abscesses (Leopold, 1972) may also be shown. Ascites is sometimes seen in the B-scan or can be shown by an A-mode technique developed by Goldberg and his co-workers (1970). Enlargement of the spleen can also be evaluated (Lehman, 1966).

The value of echography in diagnosing

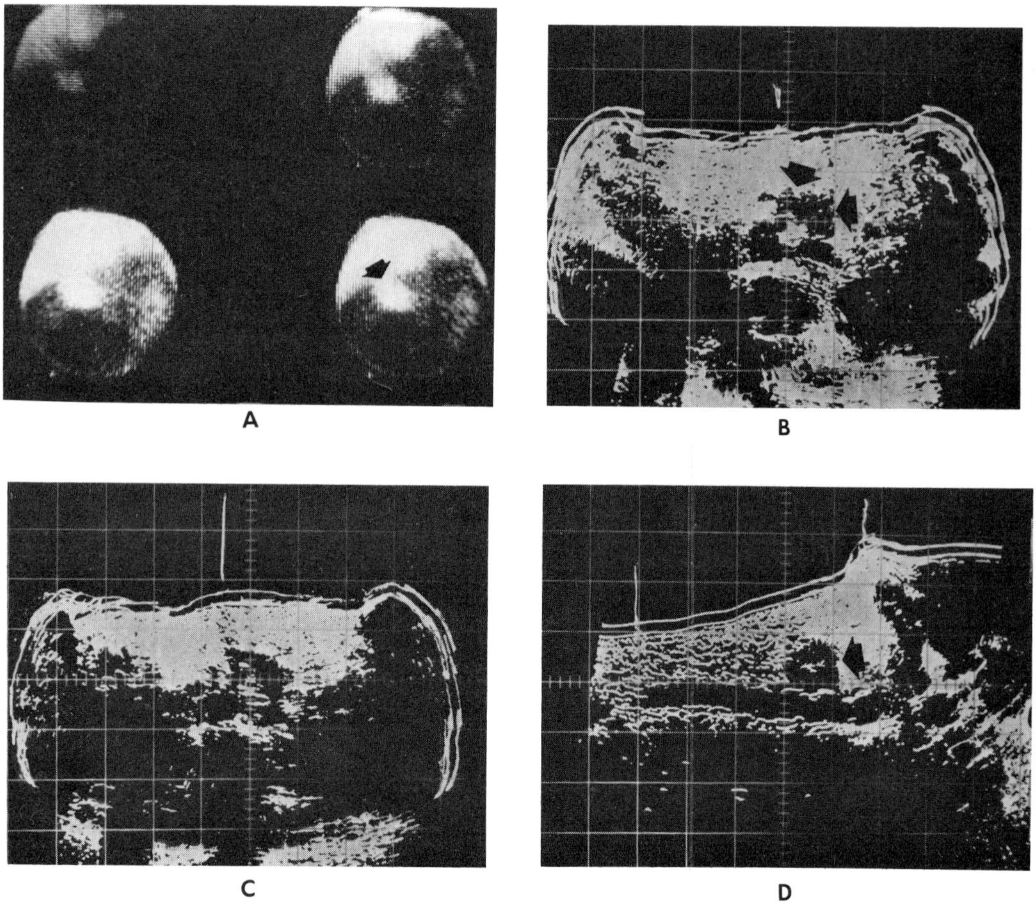

Figure 9–5. A 64-year-old man with unexplained back pain and weight loss.

A, A pancreatic Se-75 selenomethionine scan shows visualization of only the head of the pancreas (*arrow* in lower right hand frame). On this basis, carcinoma of the body of the pancreas was suspected.

B, A supine transverse scan ($T + 11$) shows a mass anterior to the aorta and the inferior vena cava (*arrows*).

C, A supine transverse scan ($T + 10$) again reveals the mass.

D, A supine vertical scan (A − 0) clearly delimits the mass lesion (*arrow*) with the aorta well seen beneath it. Carcinoma of the pancreas was confirmed at surgery.

liver metastases is still a somewhat controversial issue. McCarthy and his colleagues (1970) found the ultrasonic scan inferior to the radionuclide scan for the diagnosis of metastases, an observation with which we agree. Earlier studies which attributed up to 90 per cent accuracy to the echogram (Holmes, 1966; Holmes, 1967) were probably unduly optimistic. Nevertheless, the liver is clearly seen as a relatively lucent region in the pancreatic echogram, and metastases may sometimes be shown as ring-like echoes, whose centers may have more, less, or the same echo density as the liver parenchyma. Care must be taken not to confuse them with the flake-like echoes of cirrhosis and other liver

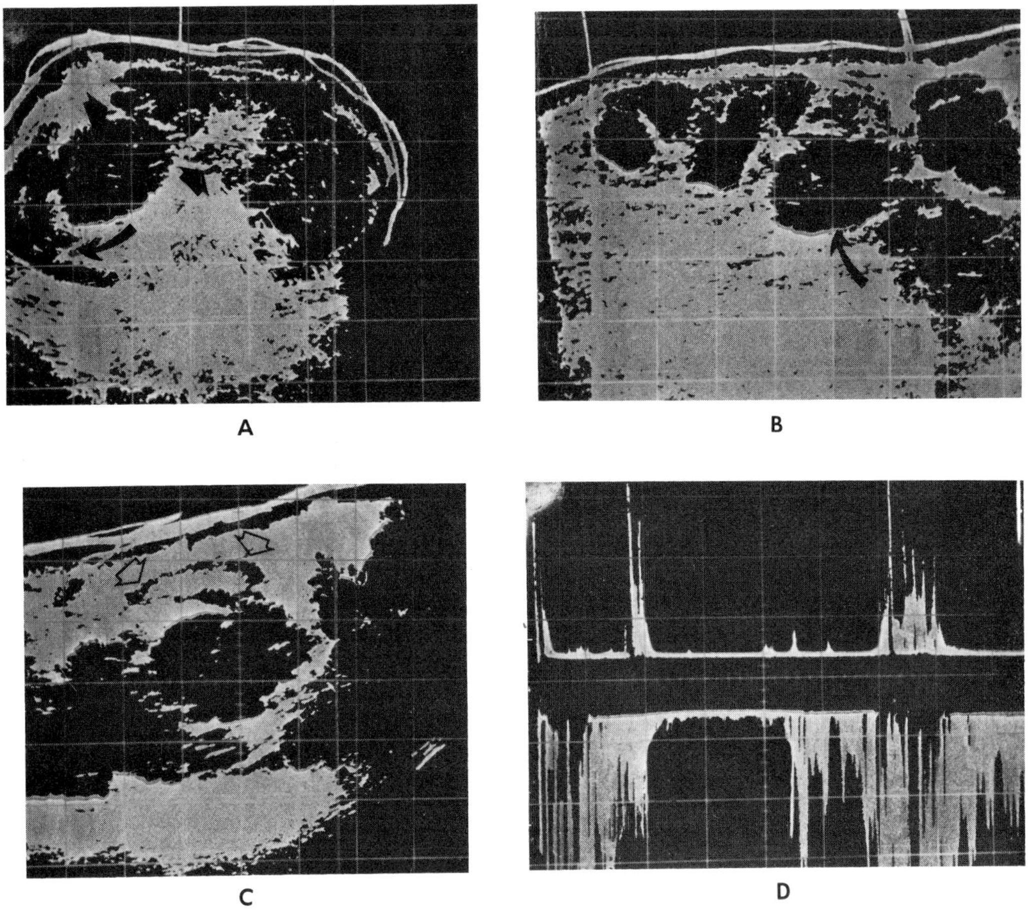

Figure 9–6. Pancreatic echogram of a 35-year-old woman with a left upper quadrant mass which was revealed in barium studies.

A, A supine transverse section (*T* + 10) shows a large, mainly transonic mass extending from the left lobe of the liver (*short arrows*) to the spleen (*long arrow*).

B, A supine vertical section (*A* − 4) again reveals the mass. Fluid-filled bowel loops interfere with visualization of the lower abdomen.

C, A prone vertical section (*P* − 7) once more reveals the mass, this time through a compressed left kidney (*white arrow*).

D, An A-scan (scale × 2) shows the mass to be fairly transonic at low gain (upper half), but to have a few echoes within it at high gain (lower half), suggesting a partly solid lesion. At surgery, a large cystadenocarcinoma of the pancreas was found.

parenchymal diseases (Lehman, 1966), or the sound reflections from dilated bile ducts.

The main role of echography in the diagnosis of pancreatic tumor appears to be to expedite the identification of a pancreatic mass. The method is not sufficiently reliable to be used as a definitive screening technique, and not sufficiently specific to make a final diagnosis possible. However, it may lead the clinician to turn more quickly to specific diagnostic techniques such as arteriography, pancreatography, or laparotomy. Another use of echography is that of following patients who are undergoing radiation or chemotherapy for known tumors (Cohen, 1969).

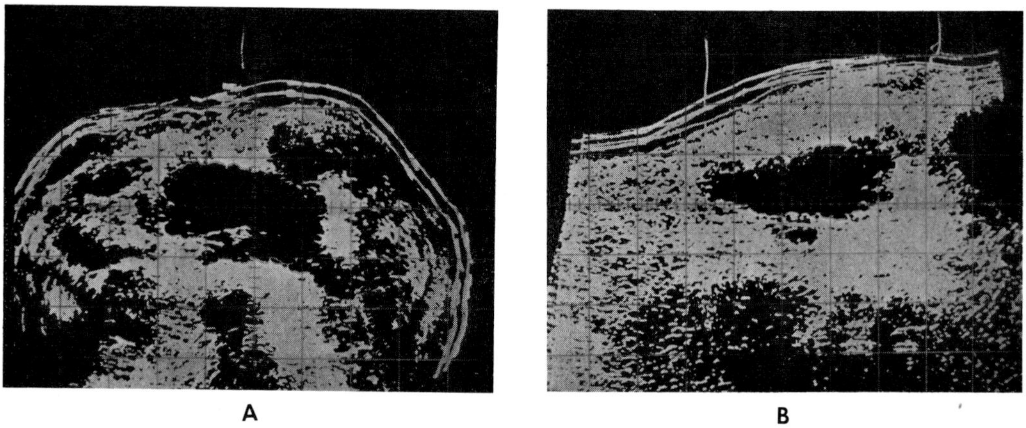

Figure 9–7. Pancreatic echogram in a 54-year-old man with a retroperitoneal mass following treatment of lymphoma.

A, A supine transverse scan ($T + 5$) shows a large transonic area in the anterior retroperitoneum obscuring the great vessels.

B, A supine vertical section at high gain ($A - 0$) shows partial filling in of the mass, but a persistently transonic center. The echogram was considered unable to differentiate between a cystic pancreatic lesion and a cystic degeneration of retroperitoneal lymph nodes.

PANCREATITIS AND PSEUDOCYST

Unlike the normal, the inflamed pancreas can often be separated from the other structures of the retroperitoneum. Filly and Freimanis (1970) suggest that this may be due to the sonolucency of edema fluid. They do not consider it possible to distinguish acute from chronic pancreatitis with acute exacerbation, but can follow progressive resolution as the disease responds to treatment. Templeton and Stuber (1971) also believe that they are able to show an enlarged pancreas in pancreatitis. Filly and Freimanis (1970) caution that bizarre peripancreatic echoes may be seen occasionally in patients with cirrhosis.

Our impressions are more like those of Leopold (1972) who has found the echogram frequently inconclusive in

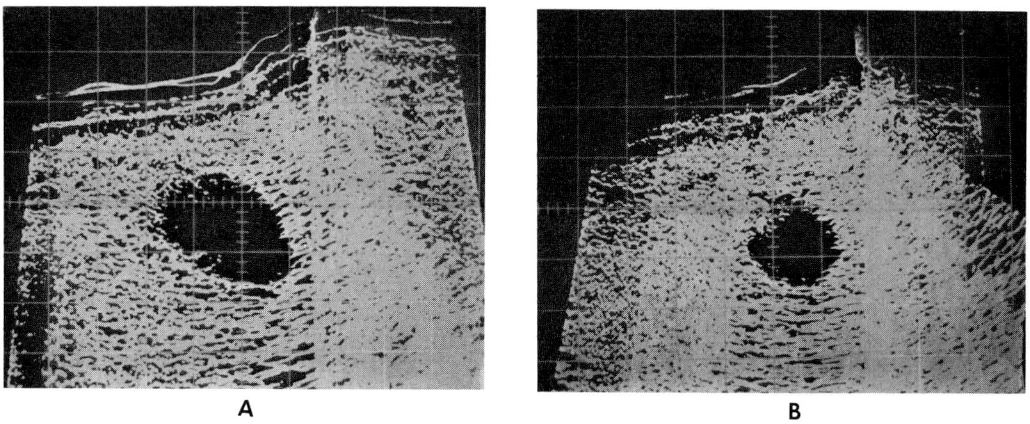

Figure 9–8. Supine vertical sections ($A + 7$) through a normal gallbladder (scale × 2).
A, An initial echo reveals a normal, transsonic gallbladder.
B, Following a fatty meal, the gallbladder is reduced in size.

pancreatitis (Fig. 9–9). These patients are often very ill and difficult to study because of the severe ileus that is usually present. While occasionally we suggest pancreatitis in studies that are done for other reasons, we do not at present think that we have enough to contribute to justify transporting patients with a primary diagnosis of pancreatitis to the Ultrasound Department.

We have an entirely different attitude when a pancreatic pseudocyst is suspected. Filly and Freimanis (1970), Holm (1971), Weill and his co-workers (1971), Templeton and Stuber (1971) and, most recently, Leopold (1972) have all mentioned the feasibility of diagnosing pseudocysts with echography. They usually present as rounded, transsonic zones with a strong posterior wall echo, but may be irregular after they have been drained (Filly, 1970). Pseudocysts occasionally are lobulated (Leopold, 1972). An A-scan should be used to prove their total sonolucency, and to differentiate them from tumor (Holm, 1971). Distention of the gallbladder may occur in pancreatitis, and must not be confused with pseudocyst, nor should a fluid-filled stomach be so misinterpreted. A naso-

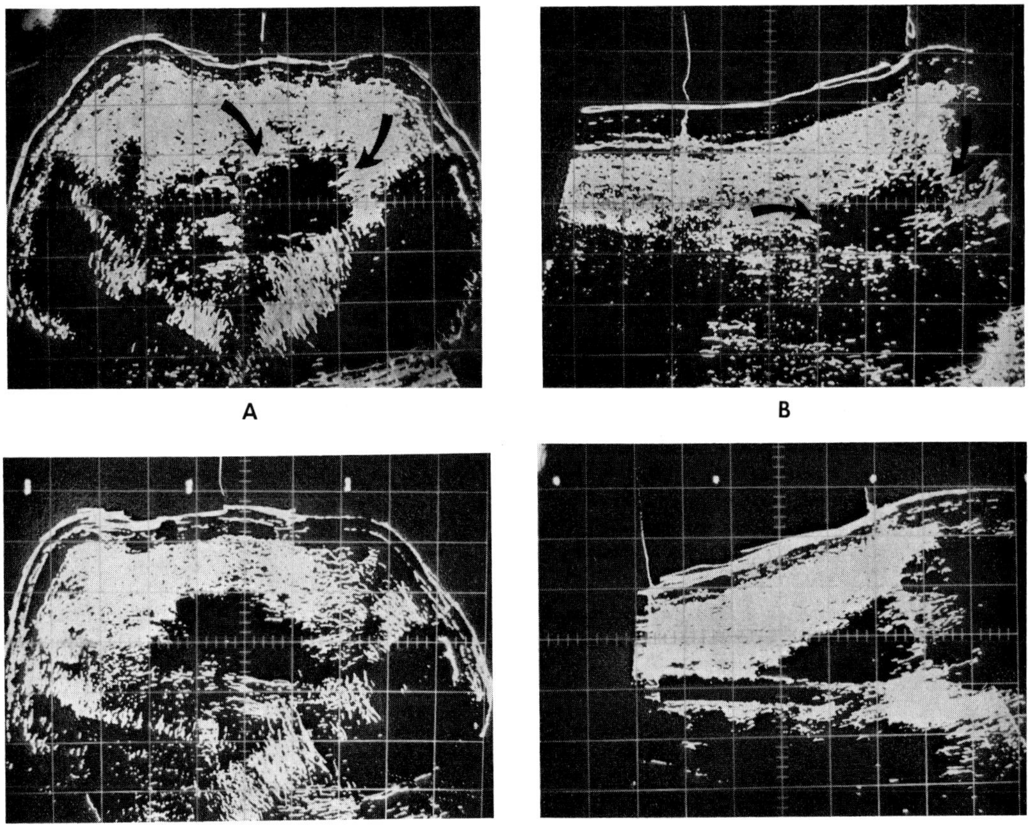

A B C D

Figure 9–9. Pancreatic echogram of a 42-year-old man with acute pancreatitis and a suspected pseudocyst.

A, A supine transverse section (*T* + 13) shows a poorly defined lucent mass in the region of the head of the pancreas (*arrows*).

B, A supine vertical section (*A* + 3) confirms this mass (*arrows*) which was thought to represent either an edematous pancreatic head or an early pseudocyst formation. A repeat echogram was suggested.

C and *D*, Corresponding views four days later show that the mass is larger, more sharply demarcated and extends across the midline. It is now easily defined as a pancreatic pseudocyst.

gastric tube must be passed when there is doubt (Leopold, 1972). The evolution of pseudocysts can be followed with echography. Recently, Leopold and his co-workers (1972) documented the spontaneous rupture of a pseudocyst into the duodenum both by ultrasound and barium.

We consider echography to be the method of choice for the imaging of pseudocysts; in accuracy, it is superior to plain films, barium studies, selenomethionine scans, and even arteriography. The main role of the other radiologic studies is to exclude other causes of cystic masses in the upper abdomen since the echogram is low in specificity. The absence of morbidity and significant discomfort also makes ultrasound the ideal method of following the course of pseudocysts during observation or after surgery (Fig. 9–10).

CONCLUSIONS

Less than ten years ago, Holmes and Howry (1963), in their comments on ultrasonic diagnosis of abdominal disease, wrote: "Visualization of the pancreas is the ultimate goal but this will require further improvement in technique and equipment." There has been little improvement in both technique and

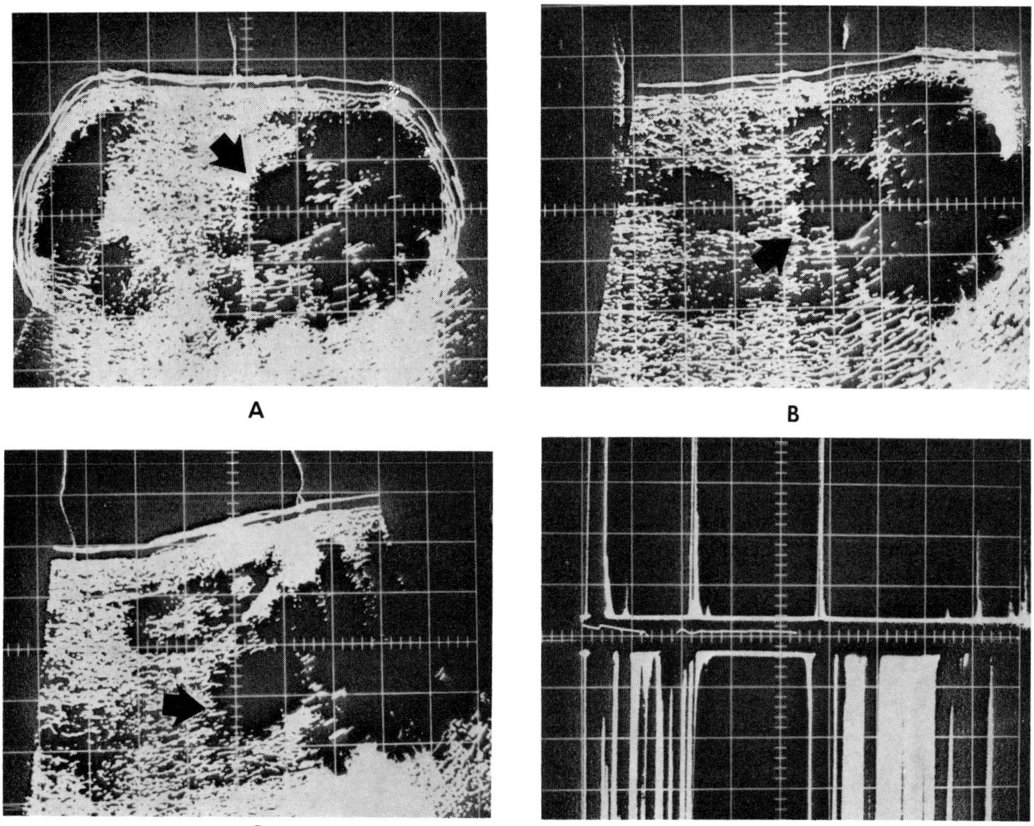

A B C D

Figure 9–10. Pancreatic echogram of a 56-year-old woman with known chronic pancreatitis.

A, A supine transverse section (*T* + 15) shows a round, lucent 5 cm. area in the region of the liver hilus (*arrow*).

B, A supine vertical scan (*A* + 5) confirms this finding (*arrow*).

C, A prone vertical scan (*P* + 5) also shows the lucent mass through the right kidney.

D, An A-scan (scale × 2) reveals the mass to be totally lucent at both high and low gains. The mass was considered to be a pseudocyst.

equipment, but a great deal of experience has been gathered because B-scanning has become commercially available. As a result, it has been shown that the normal pancreas still cannot be visualized. Tumors 3 cm. in diameter or larger can often be recognized, but their diagnosis by ultrasound has not made a major impact on the problem of pancreatic malignancy. Changes may be seen in pancreatitis, but the examination is usually more trouble than it is worth. On the other hand, echography should be considered the method of choice for diagnosing and following pseudocysts and other cystic lesions of the pancreas.

Repeated studies demonstrating the great safety margins in echography (Woodward, 1970) encourage the wider application of this technique. Greater automation of scanning equipment and, particularly, better methods of data display are expensive but, when adequately developed for widespread use, will undoubtedly increase the value of echography in treating pancreatic disease in the future.

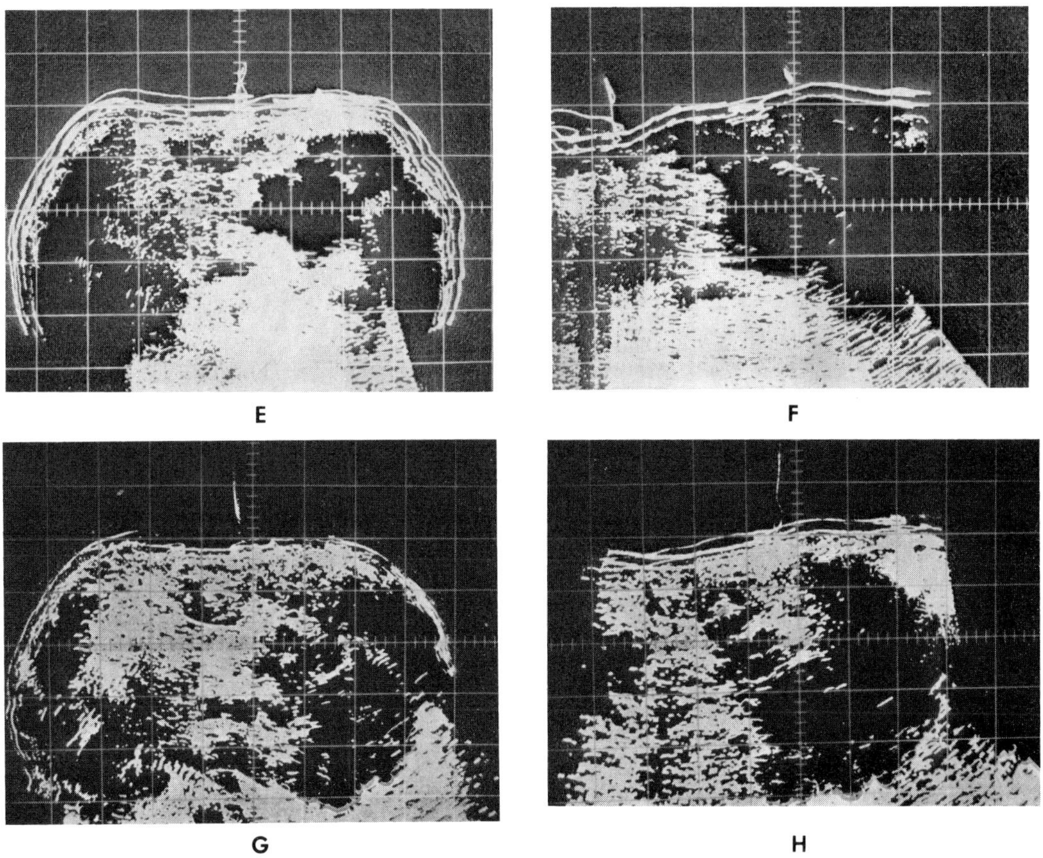

Figure 9–10 Continued. The patient was observed during medical therapy, and repeat corresponding scans two months later.

E, A supine transverse section revealed enlargement of the mass. Surgery was undertaken at this time.

F, A supine vertical section also showed enlargement of the mass.

G and *H*, Matching postoperative scans four months later show no evidence of recurrence.

REFERENCES

Asher, W. M., and Freimanis, A. K.: Echographic diagnosis of retroperitoneal lymph node enlargement. Amer. J. Roentgen., *105*:438–445, 1969.

Cohen, W. N.: B-scan ultrasonography of abdominal mass lesions. Radiology, *93*:589–591, 1969.

Dussik, K. T.: Ueber die Moeglichkeit Hochfrequente Mechanische Schwingungen als Diagnostisches Hilfsmittel zu verwenden. Z. Neurol., *174*:153, 1942.

Engelhart, G. J.: Ultraschalldiagnostik retroperitonaaler Prozess. Schweiz. Med. Wschr., *101*: 745–747, 1971.

Engelhart, G., and Blauenstein, V. W.: Ultrasound in the diagnosis of malignant pancreatic tumors. Gut, *11*:443–449, 1970.

Filly, R. A., and Freimanis, A. K.: Echographic diagnosis of pancreatic lesions. Radiology, *96*:575–582, 1970.

Freimanis, A. K., and Asher, W. M.: Development of diagnostic criteria in echographic study of abdominal lesions. Amer. J. Roentgen., *108*: 747–755, 1970.

Goldberg, B. B., Goodman, G. A., and Clearfield, H. R.: Evaluation of ascites by ultrasound. Radiology, *96*:15–22, 1970.

Göthlin, J.: Vasopressin in the elimination of intestinal gas. Acta Radiol. [Diagn] (Stockholm), *12*:100–112, 1972.

Holm, H. H.: Ultrasonic scanning in the diagnosis of space-occupying lesions of the upper abdomen. Brit. J. Radiol., *44*:24–36, 1971.

Holm, H. H., and Mortensen, T.: Ultrasonic scanning in diagnosis of abdominal disease. Acta. Chir. Scand., *134*:333–341, 1968.

Holm, H. H., Rasmussen, S. N., and Kristensen, J. K.: Identification of ultrasonic scanning pictures of the abdomen. Ultrasonics, *9*:49–53, 1971.

Holmes, J. H.: Diagnosis of tumor by ultrasound. Progr. Clin. Cancer, *3*:135–150, 1967.

Holmes, J. H.: Ultrasonic diagnosis of liver disease. *In* Diagnostic Ultrasound: Proceedings of First International Conference, University of Pittsburgh, 1965. Edited by C. C. Grossman, J. H. Holmes, C. Joyner, and E. W. Purnell. New York, Plenum Press, 1966, pp. 249–263.

Holmes, J. H., and Howry, D. H.: Ultrasonic diagnosis of abdominal disease. Amer. J. Dig. Dis., *8*:12–32, 1963.

Howry, D. H.: A brief atlas of diagnostic ultrasonic radiologic results. Radiol. Clin. N. Amer., *3*:433–452, 1965.

Howry, D. H., and Bliss, W. R.: Ultrasonic visualization of soft tissue structures of the body. J. Lab. Clin. Med., *40*:579–592, 1952.

Hublitz, U. F., Kahn, P. C., and Sell, L. A.: Cholecystosonography: An approach to the nonvisualized gallbladder. Radiology, *103*:645–649, 1972.

Lehman, J. S.: Ultrasound in the diagnosis of hepatobiliary disease. Radiol. Clin. N. Amer., *4*:605–623, 1966.

Lehman, J. S., Evans, G. C., and Brady, L. W., Jr.: Ultrasound exploration of the spleen. *In* Diagnostic Ultrasound: Proceedings of First International Conference, University of Pittsburgh, 1965. Edited by C. C. Grossman, J. H. Holmes, C. Joyner, and E. W. Purnell. New York, Plenum Press, 1966, pp. 264–295.

Leopold, G. R.: Pancreatic echography: A new dimension in the diagnosis of pseudocyst. Radiology, *104*:365–369, 1972.

Leopold, G. R., and Asher, W. M.: Deleterious effects of gastrointestinal contrast material on abdominal echography. Radiology, *98*:637–640, 1971.

Leopold, G. R., and Asher, W. M.: Diagnosis of extraorgan retroperitoneal space lesions by B-scan ultrasonography Radiology, *103*:133–138, 1972.

Leopold, G. R., Berk, R. N., and Reinke, R. T.: Echographic-radiological documentation of spontaneous rupture of a pancreatic pseudocyst into the duodenum. Radiology, *120*:699–700, 1972.

McCarthy, C. F., Davies, E. R., Wells, P. N. T., Ross, F. G. M., Follett, D. H., Muir, K. M., and Read, M. D.: A comparison of ultrasonic and isotope scanning in the diagnosis of liver disease. Brit. J. Radiol., *43*:100–109, 1970.

Templeton, A. W., and Stuber, J. L.: Abdominal and retroperitoneal sonography. Amer. J. Roentgen., *11*:741–748, 1971.

Weill, F., Kraehenbuhl, J., Ricatte, J. P., Gillet, M., and Becker, J.: L'exploration tomoechographique du pancreas. Presse Med., *79*:1641–1644, 1971.

Wild, J. J., and Reid, J. M.: Application of echoranging techniques to the determination of structure of biological tissues. Science, *115*: 226–230, 1952.

Woodward, B., Pond, J. B., and Warwick, R.: How safe is diagnostic sonar? Brit. J. Radiol., *43*: 719–725, 1970.

Chapter 10

RADIOLOGY OF SELECTED DUODENAL DISORDERS

TUMORS OF THE DUODENUM

Although tumors of the duodenum account for a minute fraction of alimentary tract neoplasms, they pose an interesting diagnostic problem. Clinicians rarely, if ever, suspect the presence of a duodenal tumor since symptoms and signs referable to the epigastrium are usually attributed to ulcer, cancer, or gallbladder disease. Hence, duodenal neoplasms are generally discovered unexpectedly by the radiologist, surgeon, or pathologist.

Commonly occurring types of duodenal tumors are listed in Table 10–1. Histologically, a wide variety of neoplasms is encountered in the duodenal area, and some of those occurring most frequently are quite specific for the duodenum—e.g., Brunner's gland adenoma and carcinoid-islet cell tumors. There is a wide variation in the gross morphology of duodenal tumors and the radiographic

TABLE 10–1. Duodenal Tumors*

Benign Tumors
Common
Adenomatous polyp
Brunner's gland adenoma
Leiomyoma
R/O ectopic pancreas, retention cyst
Uncommon
Lipoma
Fibroma
Carotid body tumor
Tumors of Variable Malignant Potential
Villous adenoma
Carcinoid-islet cell tumor
Malignant Tumors
Common
Adenocarcinoma
Carcinoma of the ampulla of Vater
Metastases
Uncommon
Lymphosarcoma
Other sarcomas

*See also Table 4–6.

differential diagnosis includes a host of inflammatory, traumatic, and neoplastic disorders arising within the duodenum itself or in surrounding structures. Table 10–2 indicates salient clinical and radiographic features of duodenal neoplasms.

Benign and Malignant Neoplasms: Distinguishing Features

Incidence and Distribution

Benign and malignant tumors occur with approximately equal frequency if the duodenum is considered as a whole. However, considering the four portions of the duodenum separately, benign tumors are far more common than malignant ones in the duodenal cap, in a ratio of approximately 5:1. In the second and third portions of the duodenum, benign and malignant tumors occur with equal frequency, while in the fourth portion of the duodenum, malignant tumors predominate in a ratio of 6:1 (Stassa, 1969). It has been observed frequently in the literature that "inch per inch the duodenum is the most frequent site of malignancy in the small bowel" (Bruno, 1970) and approximately 45 per cent of all small-bowel malignancies affect the duodenum (Bosse, 1969). As one traverses the intestinal tract from the duodenum to the ileocecal valve, the incidence of carcinoma decreases and that of sarcoma increases. Histologically, the commonest benign duodenal tumors are leiomyomas, adenomatous polyps, and carcinoid-islet cell tumors. Less common are Brunner's gland adenomas, lipomas, fibromas, hamartomas, angiomas, and carotid body tumors (Freedman, 1955; Stassa, 1969; and Bruno, 1970). Among the malignant tumors of the duodenum, adenocarcinoma is the most common, leiomyosarcoma and lymphosarcoma together comprising only 10 per cent (Bruno, 1970). Malignant carcinoid and other sarcomatous lesions are occasionally encountered.

Symptomatology

Benign duodenal tumors are often asymptomatic. They may be merely an incidental finding on upper gastrointestinal series or at surgical or pathologic examination. Occasionally, however, benign tumors can produce symptoms, particularly acute and chronic gastrointestinal hemorrhage. Constitutional symptoms in benign duodenal tumors are absent and objective findings are infrequent. Rarely is anemia present. On the other hand, patients with malignant duodenal neoplasms may have ominous constitutional symptoms such as weight loss, anorexia, pain, upper gastrointestinal bleeding, and jaundice. Development of jaundice may occur, with highly invasive malignancy of the second portion of the duodenum as the result of metastases to regional lymph nodes in the porta hepatis (Freedman, 1955; Bosse, 1969; Stassa, 1969; and Bruno, 1970).

Radiographic Appearance

BENIGN TUMORS. These usually present as discrete filling defects. As noted

TABLE 10–2. Primary Duodenal Mass Lesions

	BENIGN	MALIGNANT
Site	Lesions in the bulb; more often benign	Elsewhere; more often malignant
Symptoms	Often asymptomatic; may be an incidental finding	Symptoms may be ominous; jaundice, pain, bleeding
Radiographic appearance	Discrete, smooth, or lobulated; occasional central ulcer; malignancy usually not excluded	Polypoid; ulceration; infiltrating; often obvious malignancy

in Chapter 4, differential diagnosis includes a variety of pseudotumoral appearances, including foreign bodies and swelling of the papilla of Vater. True tumors often have a smooth or slightly lobulated surface. However, often it is difficult to distinguish whether such lesions are mucosal or submucosal in origin. They may be single or multiple, occasionally may demonstrate a pedicle, and may intussuscept. Discrete central ulceration is not infrequent. Unfortunately, there are few distinguishing radiographic features among the benign neoplasms, and one frequently has to rely on statistical frequency of occurrence for differential diagnosis. A few points of characterization can, however, be made. In the following section, specific tumors are listed in approximate order of statistical occurrence.

Adenomatous Polyps. These are usually small, measuring 1 to 2 cm. in diameter, and may present as smooth or lobulated intraluminal filling defects (Fig. 10–1). A stalk is occasionally demonstrable. Bleeding is common but usually occurs as a blood loss anemia rather than macroscopic hemorrhage. Roentgenographically, these polyps are indistinguishable from small polypoid adenocarcinomas (Fig. 10–2).

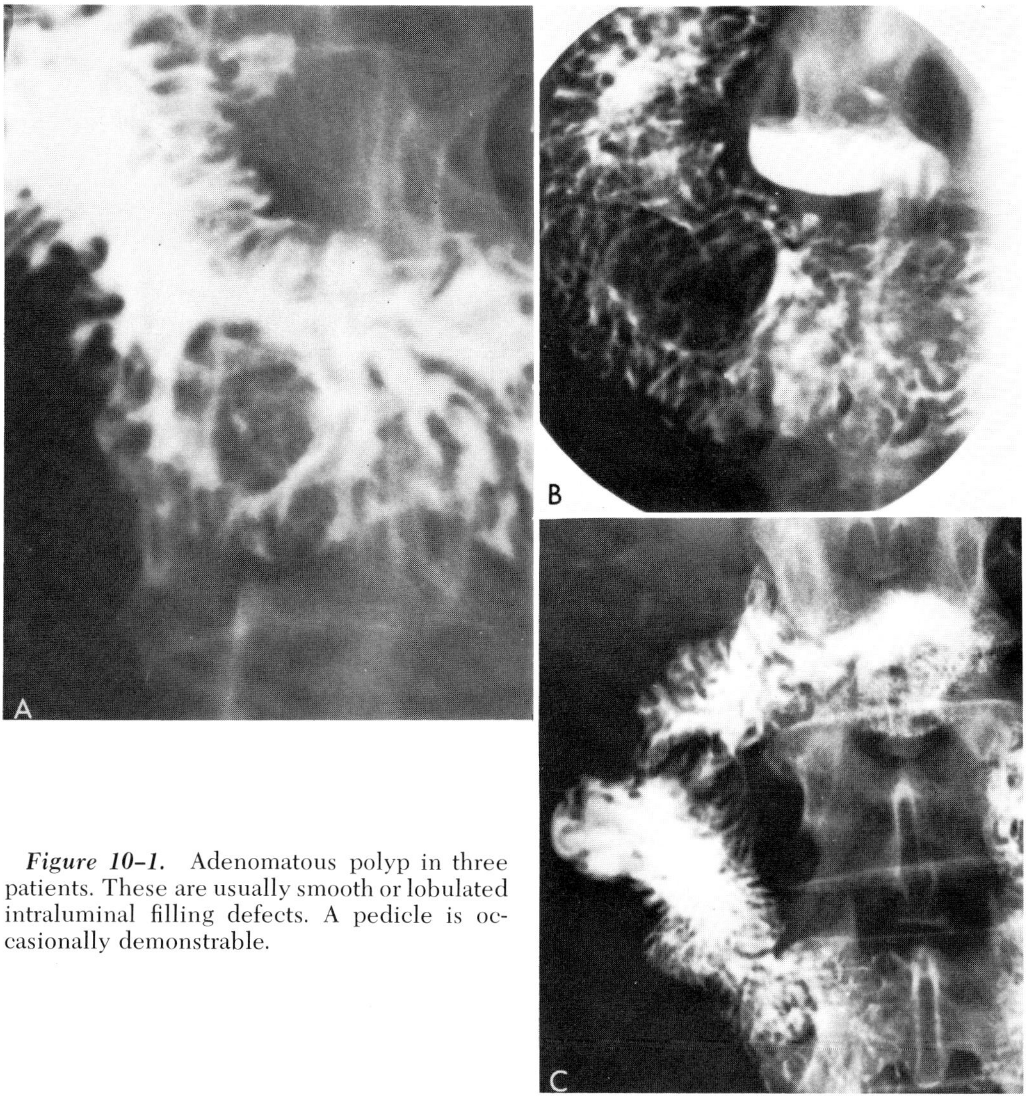

Figure 10–1. Adenomatous polyp in three patients. These are usually smooth or lobulated intraluminal filling defects. A pedicle is occasionally demonstrable.

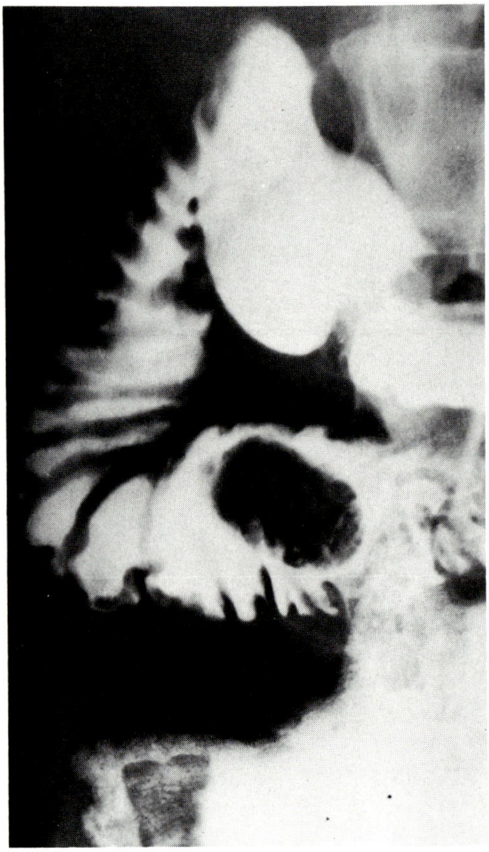

Figure 10–2. Small sessile polypoid adenocarcinoma. This is indistinguishable from a benign adenomatous polyp.

Leiomyomas. These usually have a typical intramural configuration but may present as an intraluminal or primarily extrinsic mass. A characteristic central punched-out ulceration is common (Fig. 10–3). Hence, gastrointestinal bleeding may be severe. These are often vascular neoplasms and may be discovered during angiographic investigation for gastrointestinal bleeding (Meyers, 1968) (Fig. 10–4). As in the case of adenomatous polyps, the gross appearance of smooth-muscle tumors is not reliable in distinguishing between benign and malignant growths since discrete smooth-surfaced tumors may be histologically malignant (Fig. 10–5).

Carcinoid-Islet Cell Tumor. This is a term used to describe a fascinating group of duodenal neoplasms which morphologically and functionally have features of both foregut carcinoids and islet cell tumors of the pancreas. They are believed to arise from the argentaffin cells situated in the base of the crypts of Leiberkuhn. The usual location is the first or second portions of the duodenum, and the radiographic appearance is that of a smooth, intramural filling defect (Fig. 10–6). More than half of these tumors are ulcerogenic and are associated with the Zollinger-Ellison syndrome (Oberhelman, 1972). As in the case of islet cell tumors of the pancreas, malignancy is frequent although it has been difficult to predict the biologic behavior of the lesion from histologic examination. In a recent report of 21 carcinoid-islet cell tumors (Weichart, 1971), their remarkable endocrine activity was noted; serotonin, insulin, and gastrin-like substances have all been extracted from tumor tissue. A frequent association with multiple endocrine adenomatosis (Wermer's syndrome) also has been noted (Weichart, 1971).

Brunner's Gland Adenoma. This may present as a single discrete filling defect, usually in the duodenal cap or loop (Fig. 10–7). Diffuse or circumscribed nodular hyperplasia of Brunner's glands may also occur, appearing as multiple, small, circumscribed nodules in the first and second portions of the duodenum. Brunner's glands are situated in the mucosa and submucosa of the distal antrum and proximal duodenum, and gradually decrease in frequency throughout the remainder of the duodenum. These are mucus-secreting glands which presumably function to protect the mucosa of the duodenum from the acid outflow of the stomach. Thus, the absence of hyperacidity contradicts the diagnosis of hyperplasia of Brunner's glands (Weinberg, 1965).

Lipomas. These arise from the submucosal layers but frequently develop a pedicle and present as an intraluminal mass (Fig. 10–8). They are usually smooth-surfaced lesions and frequently acquire an elliptical appearance because their softness allows them to conform to the lumen of the bowel. Typically,

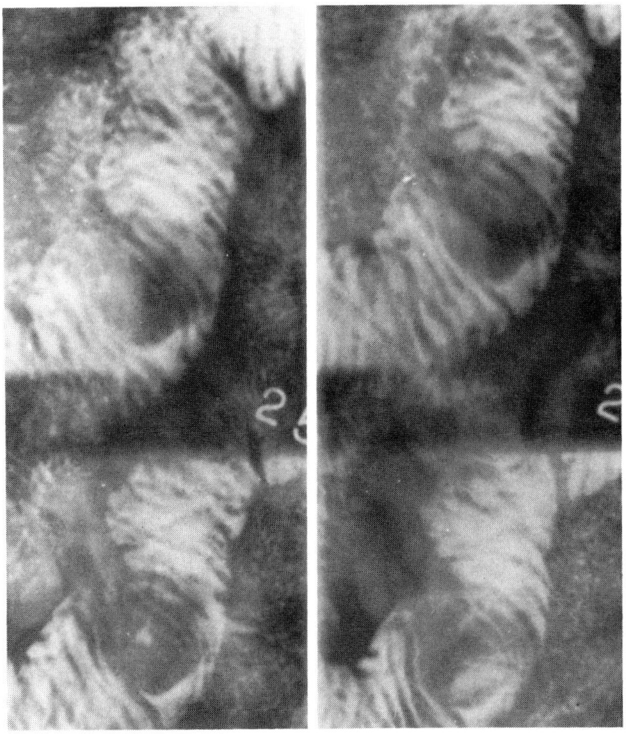

Figure 10–3. Leiomyoma of the fourth portion of the duodenum. Note the typical central ulceration (lower views). (Courtesy of Dr. J. Hanelin, Newton, Mass.)

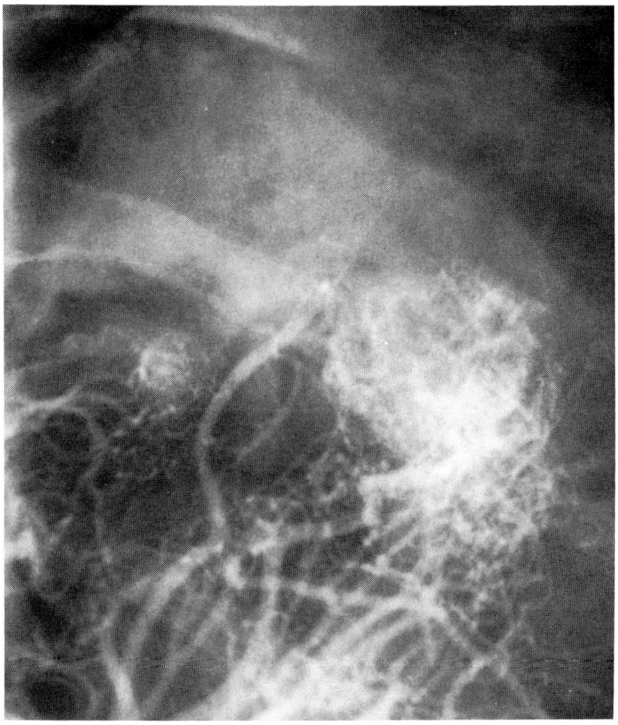

Figure 10–4. Hypervascular leiomyoma of the duodenojejunal flexure demonstrated by angiography. This is often a vascular tumor as seen angiographically, and is associated with a high incidence of gastrointestinal bleeding.

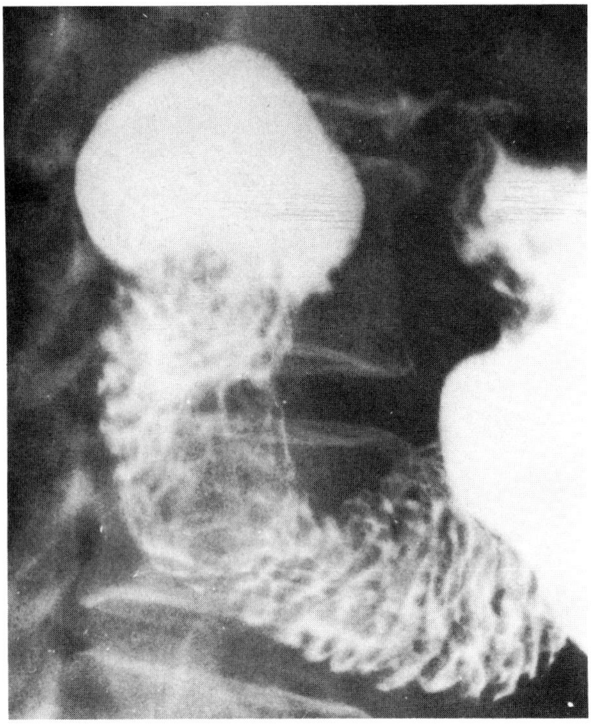

Figure 10–5. Leiomyoma or leiomyosarcoma? This case is analogous to that of an epithelial neoplasm. Despite the grossly benign roentgenographic appearance of spindle-cell tumors, histologically they may be malignant sarcomas. Diagnosis: leiomyosarcoma. (Published by permission of *Radiology.*)

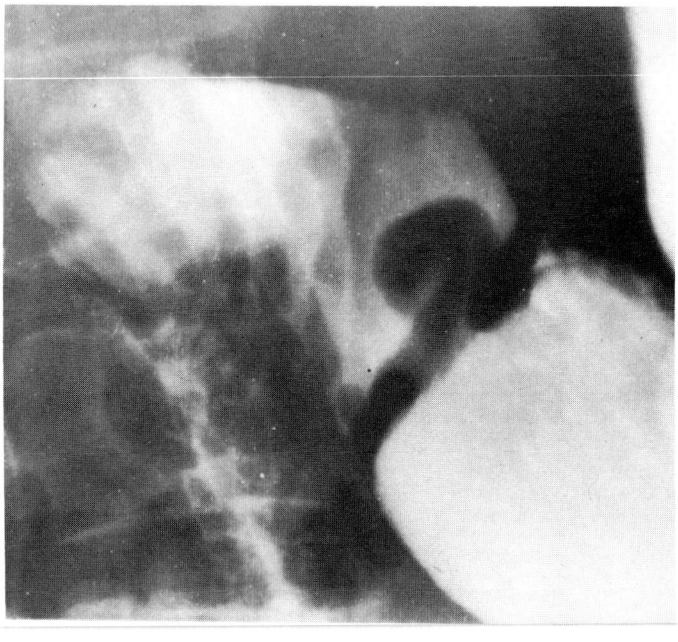

Figure 10–6. Carcinoid-islet cell tumor at the base of the duodenal cap. The smooth intramural appearance is typical though not specific.

lipomas demonstrate a changeable contour on successive films. However, similar variability may occur in duplication cysts and retention cysts (Fig. 10–9).

Ectopic Pancreas and Retention Cysts. These frequently have an intramural appearance and often are indistinguishable from primary tumors (Fig. 10–10). As noted in Chapter 4, p. 133, ectopic pancreas may be recognized by its characteristic central dimple of barium which occasionally shows branch-like extensions over the surface of the mass.

Villous Adenomas. Villous adenomas of the duodenum have a radiographic appearance similar to that of their colonic counterparts. They are usually multinodular, sessile, verrucous filling defects which may extend over a considerable length within the duodenal lumen (Fig. 10–11). A recent report of six duodenal villous adenomas indicated that approximately 50 per cent of them are histologically malignant (Ring, 1972).

Benign Tumors of the Papilla. These are not frequently recorded in the literature (Oh, 1965). They are usually adenomatous polyps but may be associated with considerable inflammatory hyperplasia. Microscopically, foci of low-grade malignancy may be discovered on careful histologic study, and these are generally considered premalignant lesions. Griffen (1968) recently reported five interesting patients with low-grade ampullary obstruction due to "benign duodenal polyps" which histologically showed only hyperplastic inflammatory tissue and were interpreted to be a variant of papillitis rather than true neoplasms.

MALIGNANT TUMORS. As noted above, adenocarcinomas are the most common duodenal malignancies, 80 to 90 per cent of duodenal cancers belonging to this category (Burgerman, 1956; Bosse, 1969; and Bruno, 1970).

Adenocarcinomas. These most commonly arise at or distal to the ampulla of Vater and are less frequently encountered in the proximal duodenum. Clinical manifestations depend on the tumor's relation to the papilla; suprapapillary lesions cause obstruction and bleeding; peripapillary lesions cause ex-

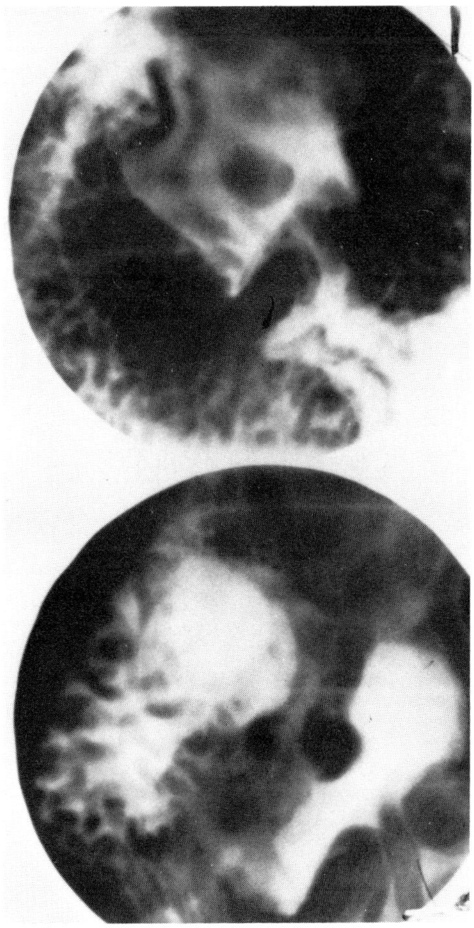

Figure 10–7. Brunner's gland adenoma of the duodenal cap. The smooth-surfaced discrete filling defect is typical but not specific.

trahepatic jaundice; infrapapillary lesions obstruct, ulcerate, and hemorrhage (Ochsner, 1957; Resnick, 1958). Radiographically, carcinoma of the duodenum has the same roentgen characteristics as carcinoma arising at any level in the gastrointestinal tract (Ochsner, 1957). These include polypoid intraluminal masses, annular constricting lesions with overhanging edges, nodular mucosal destruction, and frank ulceration (Figs. 10–13, 10–14, and 10–15).

Carcinoma of the Ampulla. This is difficult to distinguish radiographically as a specific lesion except for its characteristic location on the inner wall of

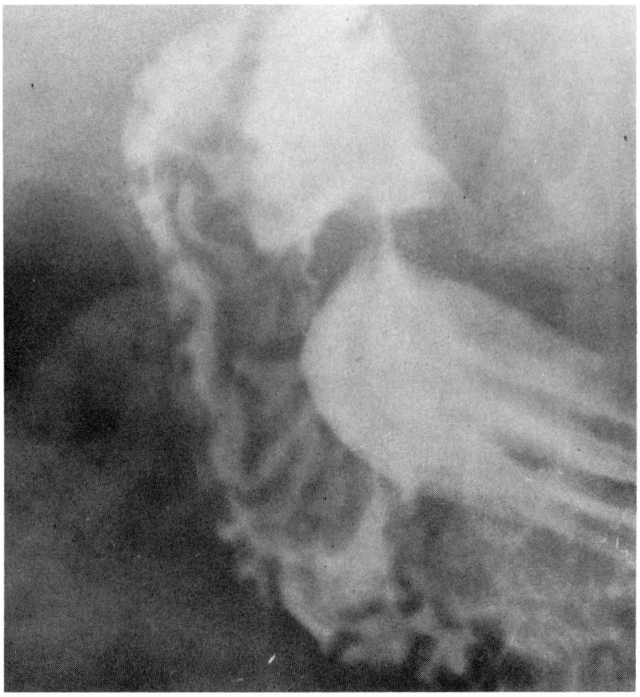

Figure 10–8. Lipoma. Although lipomas arise from submucosal layers, they frequently acquire a pedicle and present as smooth, rounded, or oval intraluminal masses. They may assume an elliptical shape because their softness allows molding by the bowel walls. Typically, there is a changeable contour on serial films.

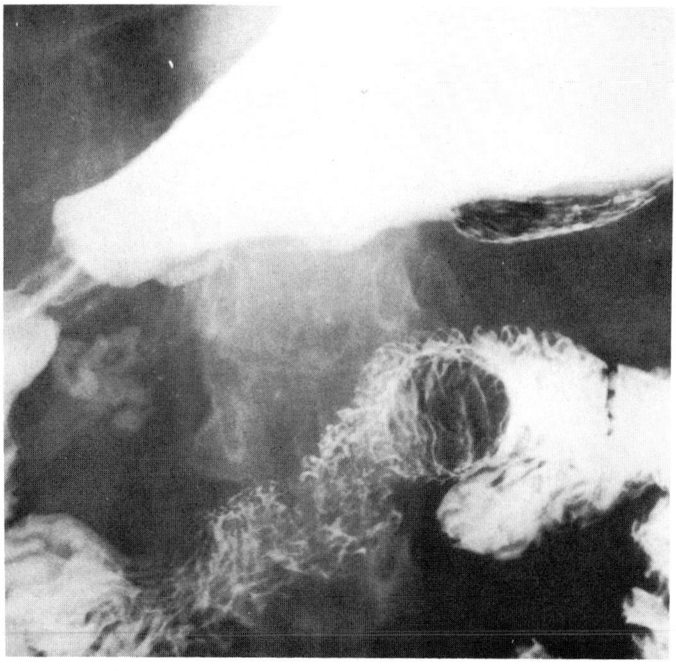

Figure 10–9. Lipoma. This smooth-surfaced lesion could also be an adenomatous polyp, a spindle-cell tumor, or a retention cyst.

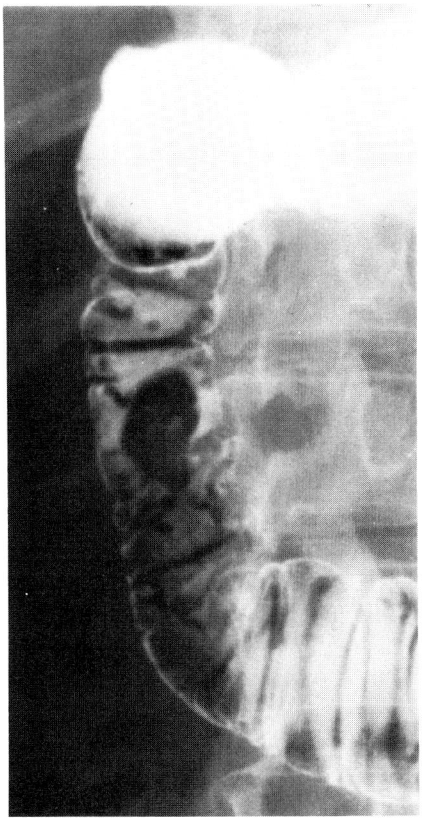

Figure 10–10. Ectopic pancreas. Typically, this is a flat submucosal lesion with slightly undulating margins and a characteristic central dimple of barium, which may show branch-like extensions over the surface of the mass. These are considered to represent the filling of miniature pancreatic ductal structures (see also Fig. 4–60). (Courtesy of Dr. J. Spencer, Providence, R. I.)

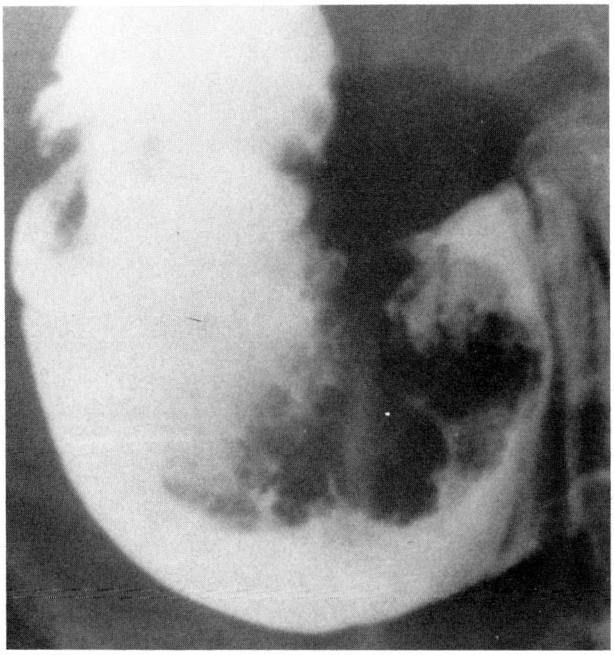

Figure 10–11. Villous adenoma. Note the characteristic multinodular villous excrescences over the surface of this large intraluminal mass. Histologically, this was a benign lesion. (Courtesy of Dr. R. Seidler, Beverly, Mass.)

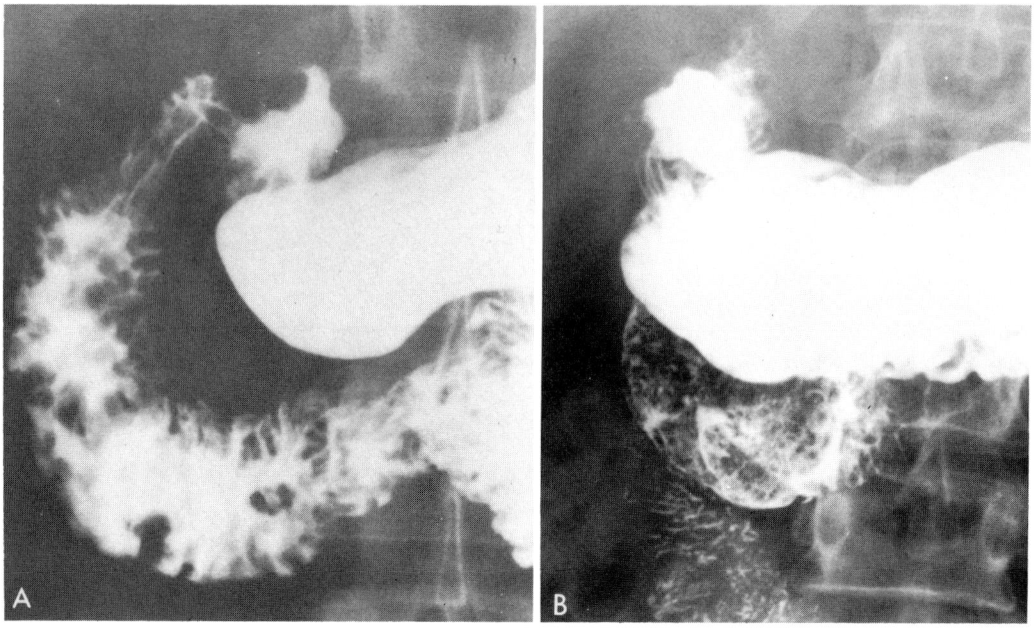

Figure 10–12. Peutz-Jeghers syndrome in two patients. Innumerable tiny hamartomatous nodules are visible.

the duodenal loop. Most of the ampullary lesions actually arise in the biliary or pancreatic ducts rather than from the duodenal mucosa, and produce a clinical picture different from that of duodenal neoplasms—i.e., jaundice is more frequent (Brenner, 1955). These tumors are usually frankly malignant in appearance, presenting as irregular nodular masses often with mucosal destruction or ulceration (Figs. 10–16 and 10–17). Invasion of the duodenal wall and destruction of the muscular fibers of the sphincter of Oddi may permit reflux of barium into the common duct (Fig. 4–65). However, it is frequently difficult for the pathologist to establish the site of origin of an adenocarcinoma involving the Vaterian segment since such a lesion may arise in any one of four different structures within 1 cm. of each other (the duodenum, ampulla of Vater, distal common duct, and pancreas) (Fig. 10–18). Rarely, ampullary carcinoma may present as a deceptively smooth-surfaced enlargement of the papilla, simulating benign inflammatory papillary swelling.

Sarcomas and Lymphomas. These produce little desmoplastic reaction and therefore are not apt to cause luminal constriction. On the other hand, deeply ulcerated lesions may occur and, as in the stomach or small bowel, aneurysmal dilatation of the lumen should lead one to suspect lymphoma or leiomyosarcoma. As noted in Chapter 4, lymphoma may also cause diffuse nodular thickening of the mucosal folds.

Differential diagnosis of malignant duodenal tumors includes carcinoma of the pancreas which usually affects the medial wall of the duodenal lumen. Both annular pancreas and postbulbar ulcer may produce luminal constriction but usually leave the mucosa intact. Secondary neoplastic invasion by contiguous extension to the duodenum from the pancreas, gallbladder, or colon may produce an ul-

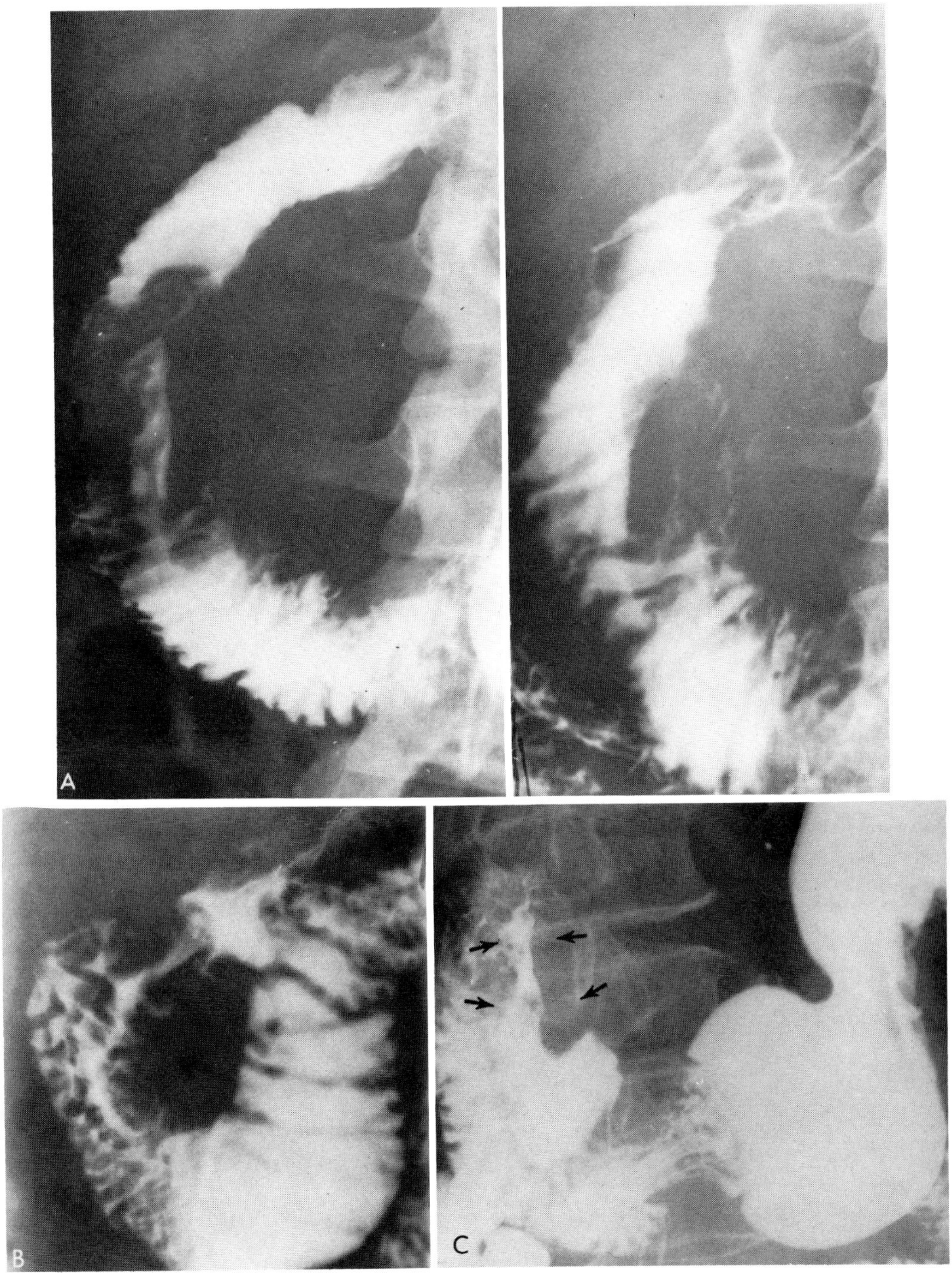

Figure 10–13. Ulcerating carcinoma of the proximal duodenum in three patients. These are typically malignant in appearance, with nodular mucosal destruction, irregular ulceration, and infiltration of the adjacent wall. Because of the location, it is nearly impossible to distinguish it from carcinoma of the ampulla or from carcinoma of the head of the pancreas invading the duodenum.

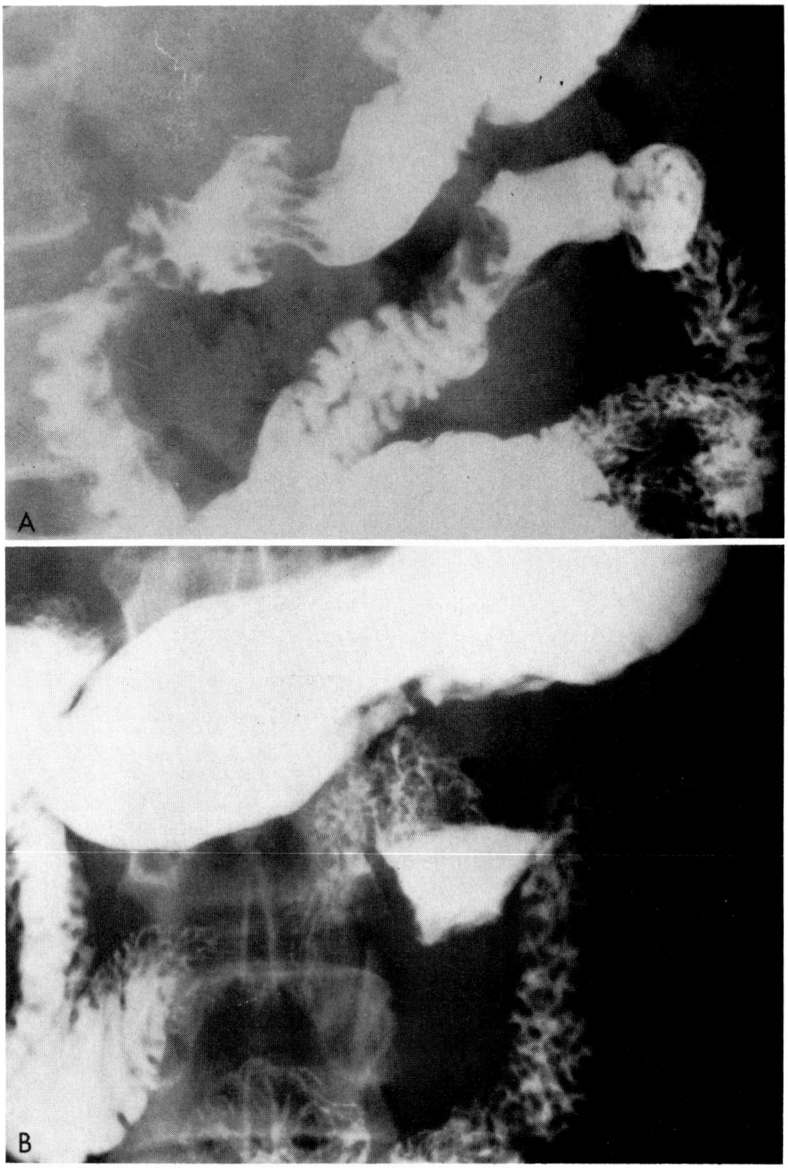

Figure 10–14. Ulcerating carcinoma of the duodenojejunal junction in two patients. This geometric aneurysmal ulceration also occurs in lymphosarcoma.

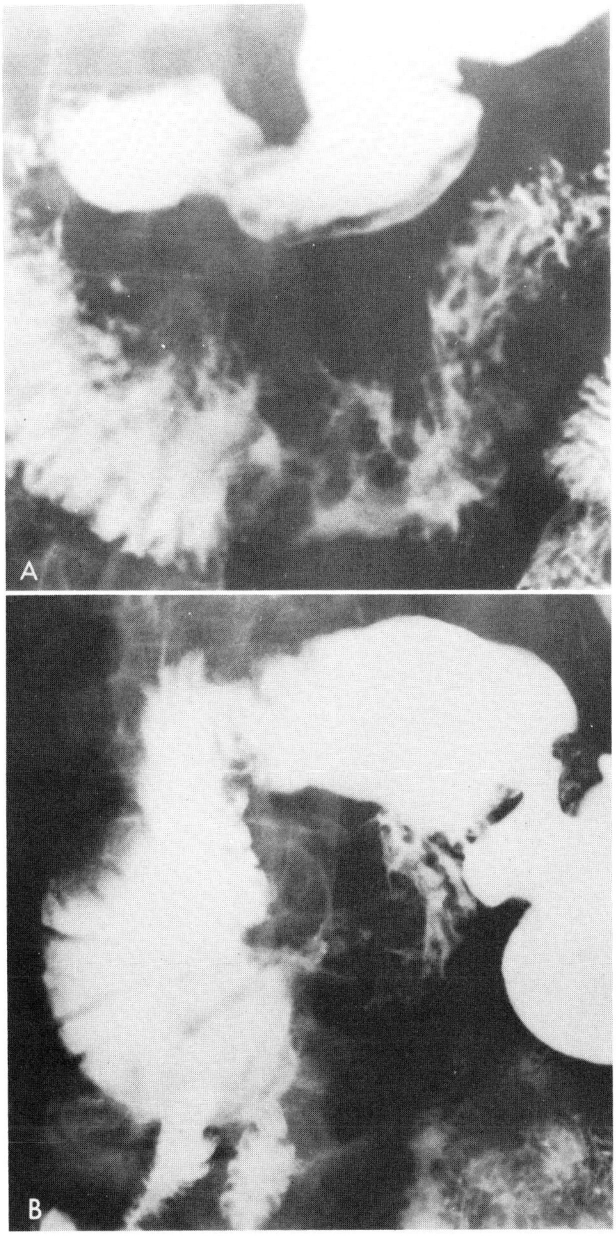

Figure 10–15. Carcinoma of the duodenum in two patients, showing annular constriction with nodular mucosal destruction and overhanging edges.

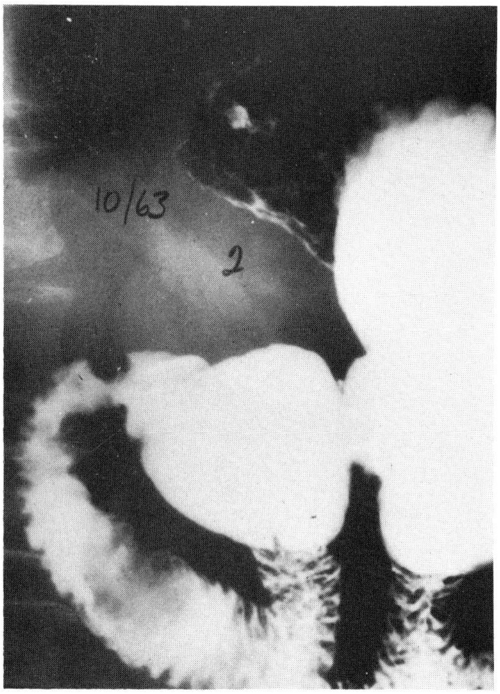

Figure 10–16. Carcinoma of the ampulla of Vater. An irregularly surfaced polypoid filling defect arises from the medial wall of the descending duodenum.

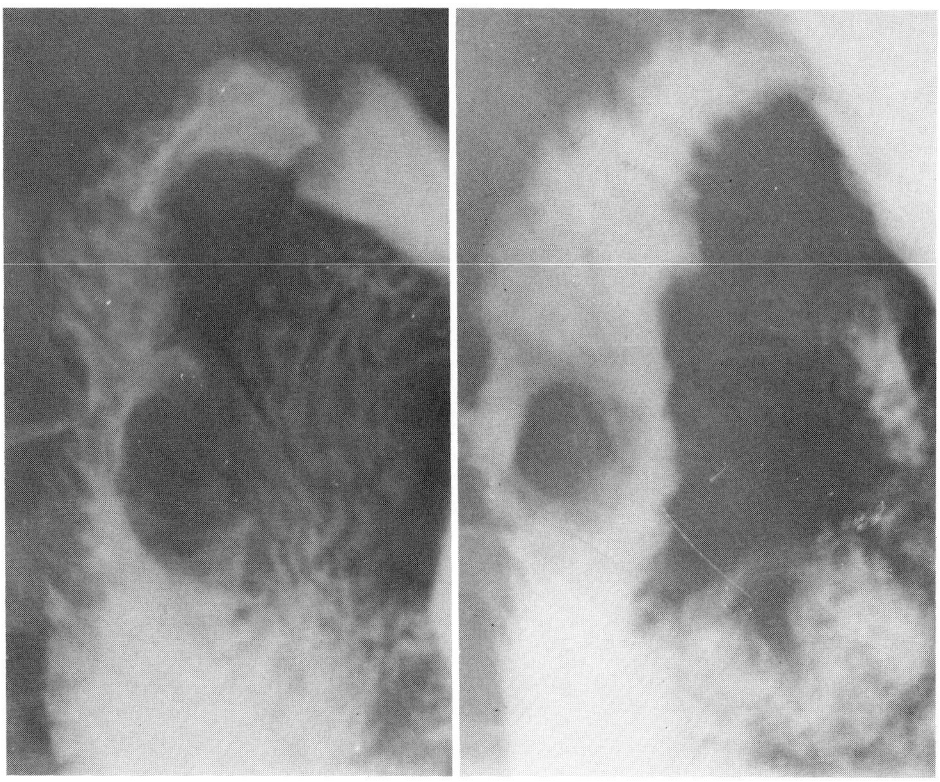

Figure 10–17. Carcinoma of the ampulla. Two views. The slightly irregular surface of this enlarged papilla suggests a malignant lesion.

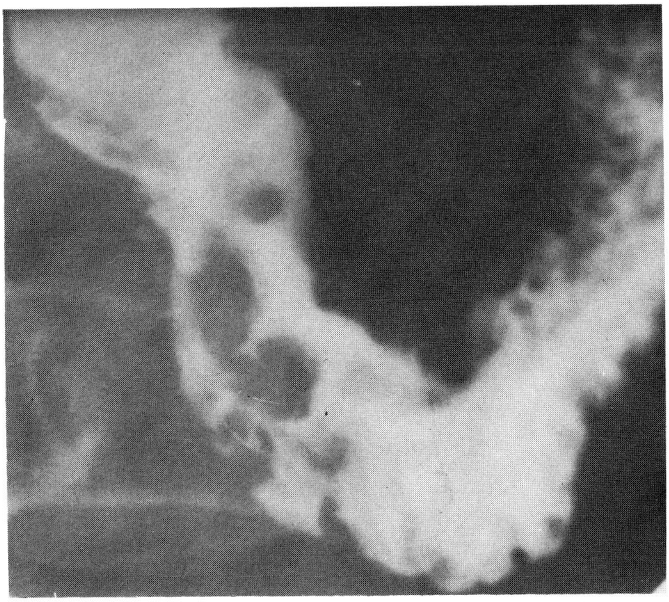

Figure 10–18. Ulcerating carcinoma of the ampulla. Radiographically and pathologically, this lesion is difficult to distinguish from carcinoma of the duodenum or from invading cancer of the pancreas.

cerating constricted lesion indistinguishable from primary duodenal neoplasm.

Management

Management decisions in cases of suspected duodenal tumor are easily made when roentgenographic findings suggest a malignant process. However, when a benign-appearing duodenal tumor is suggested, management must be individualized. A common problem is the apparently incidental discovery of small, smooth-surfaced, intramural types of filling defects in the first or second portion of the duodenum (Fig. 10–19). These are usually ectopic pancreas, Brunner's gland adenoma or carcinoid-islet cell tumors. In the absence of symptoms or objective findings of bleeding or ampullary obstruction, duodenoscopy and careful clinical and radiographic follow-up are minimum measures; surgery should be considered in good-risk patients. Lobulated or ulcerated lesions may be adenomatous polyps or spindle cell tumors but cannot be distinguished from malignancies, and the indications for surgical excision are more clear-cut.

Benign tumors usually can be treated by local excision; a biliary bypass procedure may be required if the excision or subsequent duodenal reconstruction encroaches on the patency of the ampulla. Radical pancreaticoduodenectomy (Whipple procedure) offers the best chance for cure in operable malignancies. Unfortunately, early metastases are frequent; prophylactic palliative bypass procedures will prevent obstruction and offer reasonable palliation (Freedman, 1955).

ACID PEPTIC DISEASE

Although the roentgen manifestations of duodenal ulcer disease and its common complications (perforation and obstruction) are basic knowledge to all radiologists, there are several less widely appreciated variations of duodenal acid peptic disease that have significant clinical implications. These are worthy of further discussion.

Duodenitis

This is considered a legitimate clinical radiologic entity by Fraser and his co-workers (1964) who recognized a syndrome of peptic ulcer symptoms, coarse duodenal mucosal folds, and gastric hypersecretion in 33 patients. These authors confirmed an association of high gastric acid output, low duodenal pH, and in-

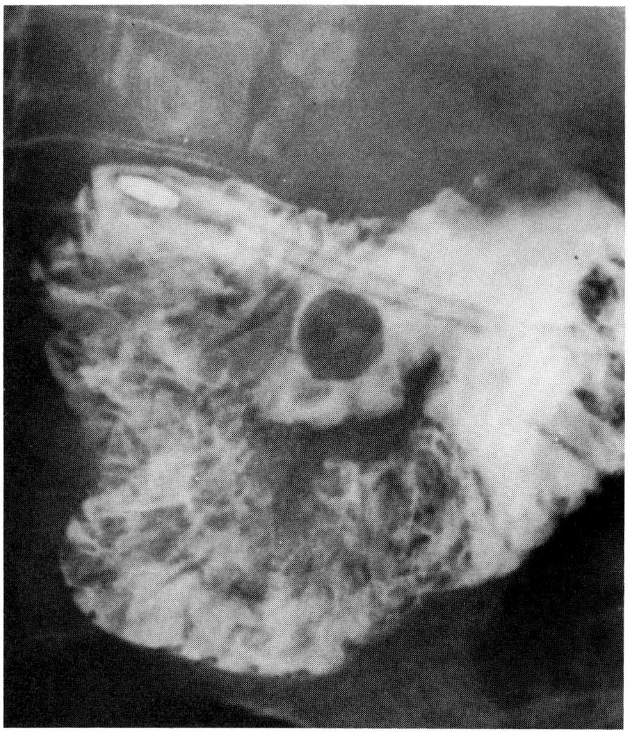

Figure 10–19. How should it be managed? A benign-appearing duodenal filling defect discovered as an "incidental finding." No objective changes (i.e., jaundice, occult blood in the stool).

Follow-up barium study? The minimum.

Duodenoscopy? If available.

Surgical excision? No objection.

Diagnosis: adenomatous polyp of the cap.

(Courtesy of Dr. Roberto Jiminez.)

flammatory histologic mucosal changes in patients with coarsely irregular duodenal folds, but no ulcer crater. They pointed out that ulcer craters may, of course, exist without being demonstrated but that duodenitis without ulcer does exist as a different or perhaps intermediate phase of peptic ulcer disease.

Radiographically, the coarsened folds may involve the cap as well as the descending duodenum, and are associated with irritability and poor barium coating. The coarse folds may be obliterated by compression of the cap, as opposed to thickened-appearing folds in Brunner's gland hyperplasia which are not obliterated by compression and appear constant from film to film. Duodenal varices may also produce lobulated thickening of folds but are seldom visible when the patient is in the erect position (Bateson, 1969).

Giant Duodenal Ulcer

This is a form of ulcer disease with a grave prognosis which frequently is misdiagnosed radiographically. "Giant" duodenal ulcer refers to a crater measuring at least 2 cm. in diameter (Dawson, 1958; Mistilis, 1963; and Kirsh, 1968). Because of its large size and usual round or oval shape, the crater may be misinterpreted as a normal or merely deformed duodenal cap (Fig. 10–20). Pathologically, such craters are walled-off perforations, not uncommonly penetrating into the head of the pancreas.

Radiographically, the crater replaces the bulb but the collection of barium simulating the bulb does not change in size or shape. Mucosal folds are absent and the base of the crater may be nodular where it penetrates into the pancreas. The pylorus is patulous or destroyed, and there is usually a constriction of the duodenal lumen distal to the crater which may be mistaken for the pyloric canal (Fig. 10–21). An important confirmatory finding is the fact that barium is retained in the crater on delayed films taken several hours after the examination (Rosenquist, 1969).

Clinically, there is severe intractable epigastric pain which often radiates to the back and is unrelieved by antacids. Gastrointestinal bleeding is common.

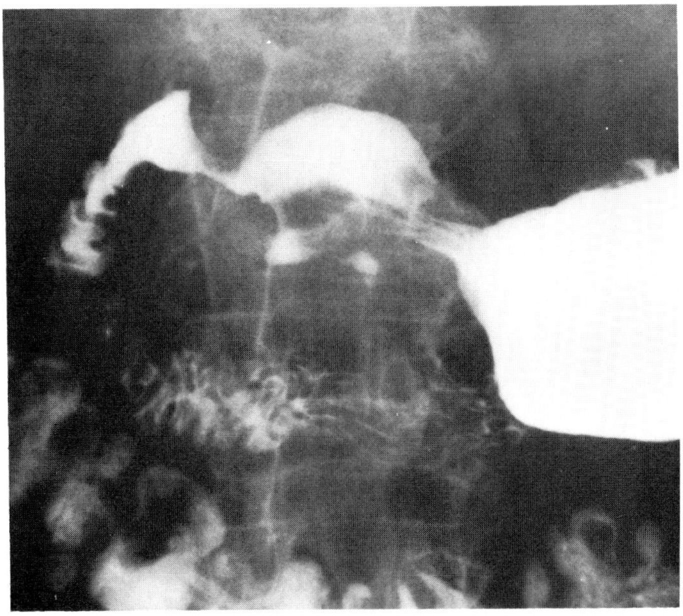

Figure 10–20. Giant duodenal ulcer. The crater replaces almost the entire cap. Mucosal folds are absent, and the base of the crater has a nodular contour.

The prognosis is grave, with a mortality rate ranging from 40 per cent to 67 per cent; the diagnosis of giant duodenal ulcer is considered an indication for surgical intervention (Hirsh, 1968).

In differential diagnosis of giant duodenal ulcer, it is necessary to consider exceptions to the generally accepted dictum that ulcers of the duodenal cap are benign lesions (Mistilis, 1963).

Although rare, primary adenocarcinoma or lymphosarcoma of the first portion of the duodenum may present as a large irregular ulceration (Chassin, 1949; Rider, 1969) (Fig. 10–22). Similarly, carcinoma of the gallbladder, pancreas, or

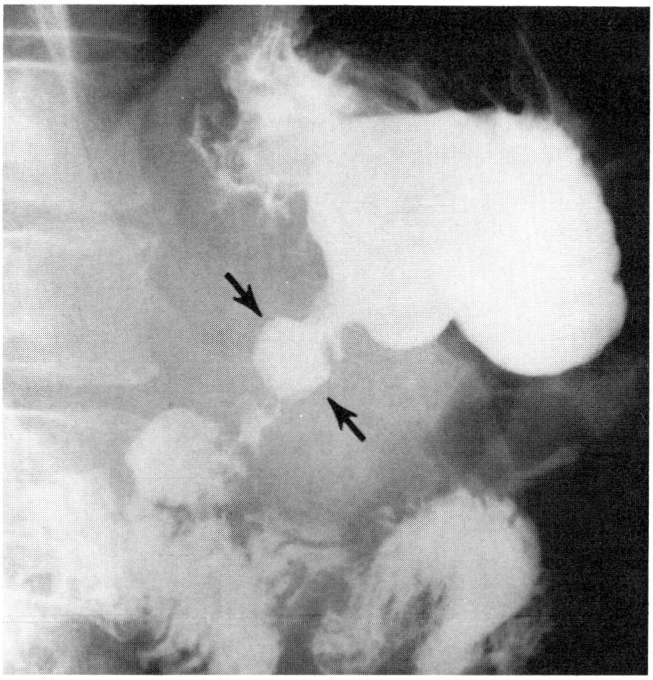

Figure 10–21. Giant duodenal ulcer (*arrows*). Proximally, the pylorus is widened, and the apex of the cap appears constricted. In two previous studies, this appearance was interpreted as a deformed cap.

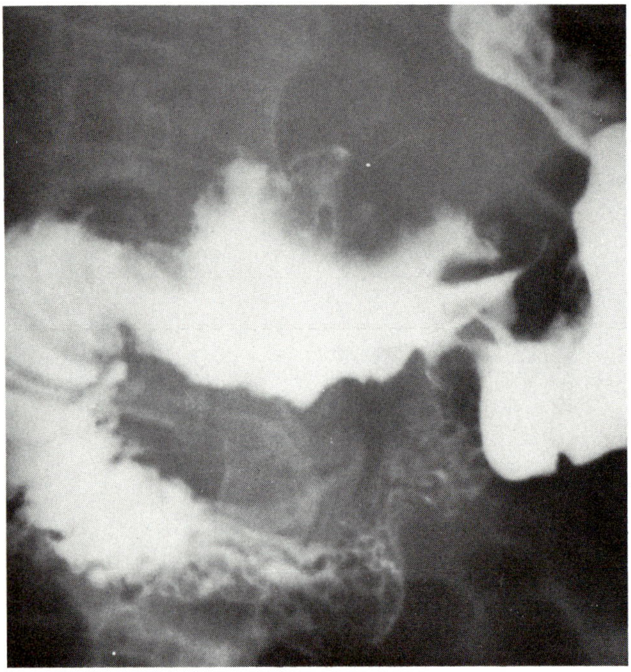

Figure 10–22. Giant duodenal ulcer resulting from primary lymphosarcoma of the duodenal cap. An immense crater with bizarre irregular contours replaces the entire cap. (Rider, R. F.: Giant duodenal ulceration. J.A.M.A., *209*:408, 1969. Copyright 1969, American Medical Association.)

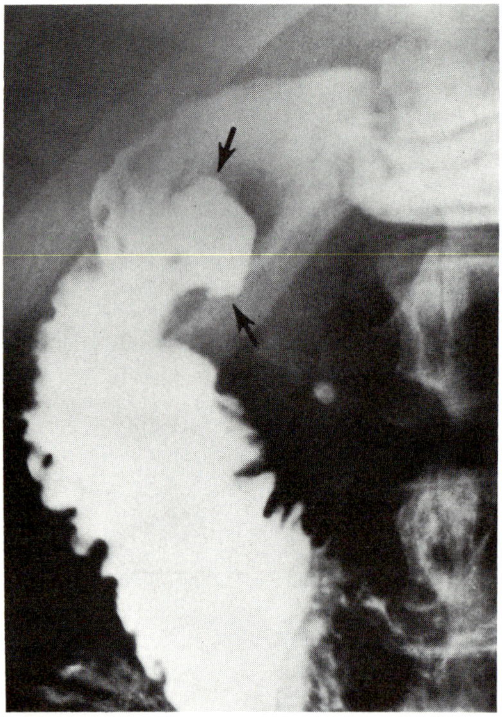

Figure 10–23. Large irregular ulceration at the apex of the cap resulting from recurrent carcinoma of the right colon invading the duodenum.

right colon occasionally invades the duodenal cap and presents as a bizarre or nonhealing ulcer crater (Gottlieb, 1951) (Fig. 10–23).

Postbulbar Ulcer

This is another severe form of ulcer disease with characteristic roentgen findings. Postbulbar ulcerations are reported to occur in approximately 5 per cent of the surgical and necropsy cases, but authorities in the literature agree that the frequency of roentgen recognition is less (Borman, 1943; Ball, 1948; Paterson, 1958; and Bilbao, 1971). Difficulties in roentgen diagnosis are attributable to the presence of peristaltic hyperactivity, mucosal edema, and poor barium coating which may obscure the crater itself. When these secondary signs are noted in patients with a strong ulcer history or upper gastrointestinal bleeding, hypotonic duodenography may be essential for accurate diagnosis (Bilbao, 1971) (Fig. 10–24).

As indicated in Chapter 4, postbulbar ulcers most frequently occur on the inner

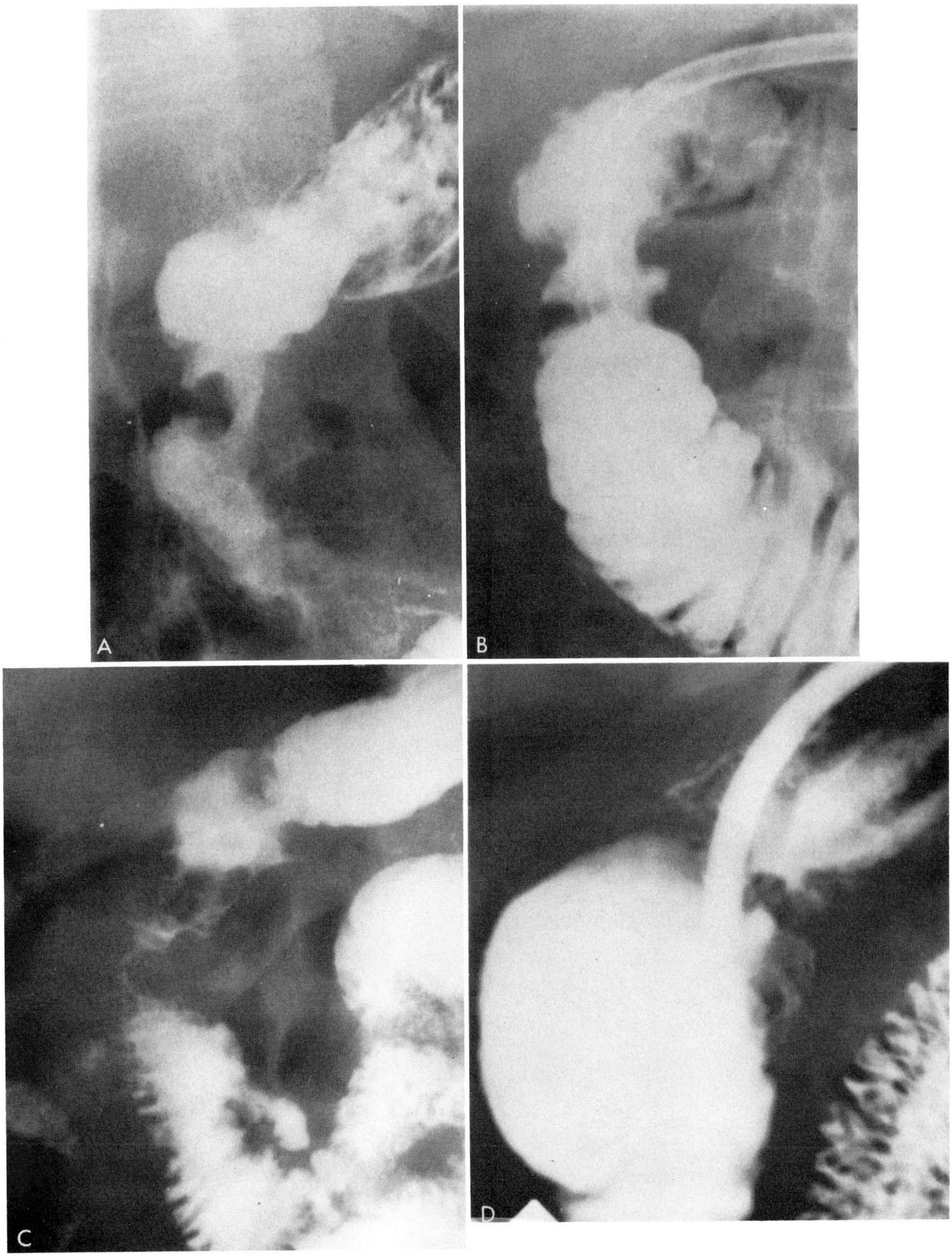

Figure 10–24. Postbulbar ulcer demonstrated by hypotonic duodenography. Two cases. Case 1: *A*, Standard barium meal showing effaced folds medially, and a polypoid defect laterally. The initial diagnosis was duodenal tumor. *B*, Duodenogram demonstrating typical postbulbar ulcer projecting from the medial aspect of the proximal descending duodenum.

Case 2: *C*, Standard barium study showing irregular postbulbar narrowing and edematous folds but no ulcer crater. *D*, Duodenogram one day later showing a small apical ulcer crater with radiating folds. The stenotic area was entirely due to spasm.

duodenal border at the junction of the first and second portions of the duodenum. However, it is occasionally difficult to determine whether a crater involves the apex of the cap or the upper descending duodenum, particularly in instances in which the cap is directed caudally (Borman, 1943). An important roentgenographic sign of the true postbulbar ulcer is a notch-like indentation defect (incisura) on the lateral wall of the duodenum at the level of the crater (Fig. 10–25). This is a manifestation of inflammatory spasm but may persist during and after healing as cicatricial scarring develops. Occasionally, this laterally placed indentation defect appears smooth and rounded, resembling a polypoid mass. Usually the duodenal lumen is retracted medially and eccentrically narrowed as the crater burrows medially into the head of the pancreas. Hence, a subacute pancreatitis frequently coexists. Signs of an associated inflammatory mass in the pancreas include effacement of plical folds on the inner aspect of the loop, a stiff rigid narrowing of the lumen, and an extrinsic pressure defect on the medial duodenal border (Teplick, 1956). The crater itself is usually smooth in outline, and adjacent mucosal folds appear edematous. As noted above, the actual crater may be difficult to visualize, duodenography notwithstanding, and in such cases differential diagnosis from annular pancreas may be difficult. In the presence of an irregular crater or nodular mucosal folds, a malignancy must be considered (Fig. 10–26).

Other considerations in the differential diagnosis include a partially filled or distorted diverticulum. Usually, however, mucosal folds can be seen passing into the neck of the diverticulum; this appearance contrasts with a clear zone of edema around the base of an ulcer crater. In addition, an ulcer niche usually retains a fixed configuration while diverticula vary in shape on serial films. Traction diverticula, showing a typical conical or pyramidal appearance without associated inflammatory changes, have also been recorded (Wilson, 1956).

Occasionally, the niche may present on the lateral convexity of the loop (Pater-

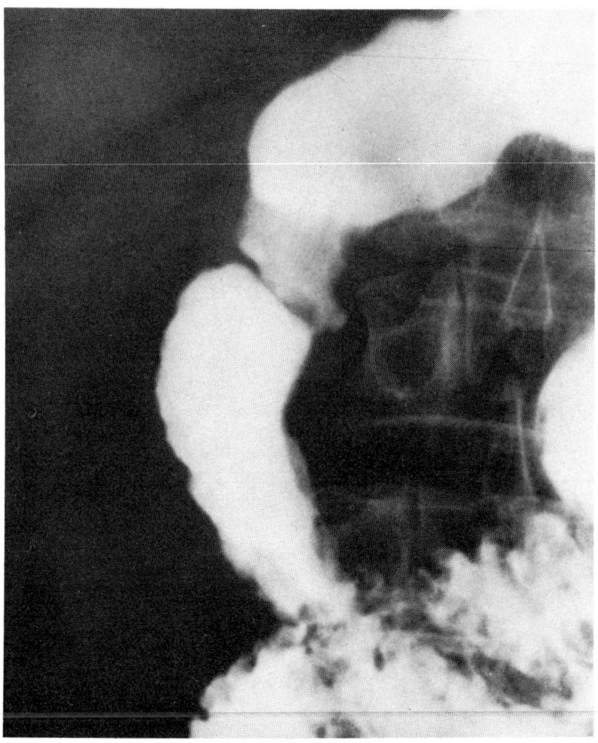

Figure 10–25. Prominent lateral incisura associated with a small postbulbar ulcer. As healing progresses, a ring stricture can be expected.

son, 1958) (Fig. 10–27). Rarely, a crater in the vicinity of the papilla may cause inflammatory changes which destroy the competency of the ampullary sphincter and allow barium to reflux into the common duct (Poppel, 1953).

Clinically, as in the case of giant ulcers of the cap, there is often intractability and a long history before diagnosis (Bilbao, 1971). Pain is characteristically severe, and may be felt primarily in the back. Gross and recurrent hemorrhage occurs twice as often as in bulbar ulcers, ranging from 37 to 86 per cent in reported series, whereas the frequency of hemorrhage in bulbar ulcers ranges from 12 to 44 per cent (Kaufman, 1957; Paterson, 1958). Superficial stress ulcers of the second portion of the duodenum may cause severe bleeding. They are rarely demonstrated on barium study, but the site of bleeding may be shown angiographically (Baum, 1970). See also Chapter 7.

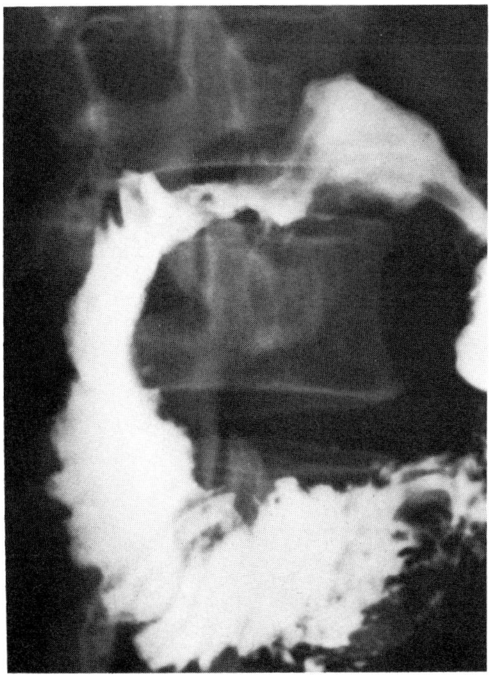

Figure 10–26. Postbulbar ulcer with a mass in the head of the pancreas resulting from invasion of the duodenum by a pancreatic cancer. In this case, the radiographic appearance is indistinguishable from that of a benign peptic ulcer with associated pancreatitis.

Ring Stricture of the Duodenum

This is another manifestation of postbulbar ulceration recently emphasized

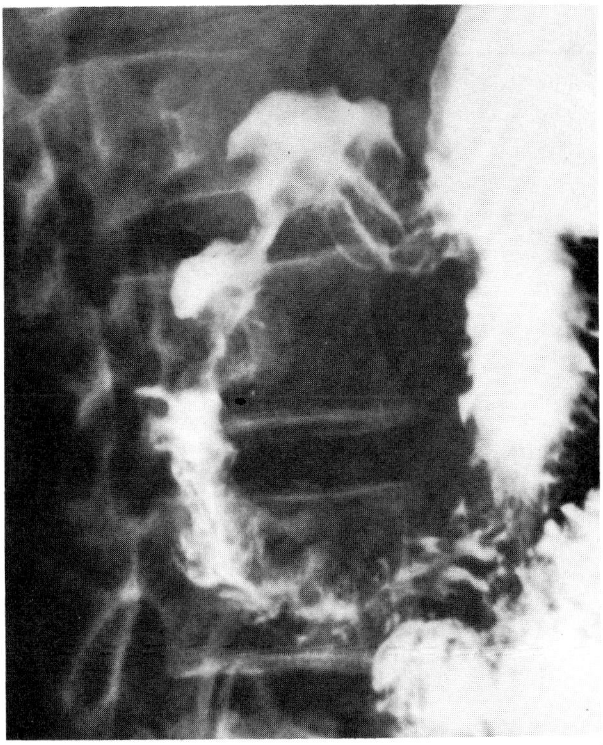

Figure 10–27. Laterally projecting benign postbulbar ulcer. The majority of postbulbar ulcers project from the medial duodenal margin into the head of the pancreas. (Courtesy of Dr. S. M. Wyman, Cambridge, Mass.)

by Bilbao and her co-workers (1971). A discrete circumferential narrowing of the upper descending duodenum to a diameter of 0.5 to 1.0 cm. may be associated with shallow indolent postbulbar ulceration (Fig. 10–28). The actual ulcer is seldom visible radiographically and is usually found only on internal inspection of the duodenum at surgery. These strictures are progressive, strongly symptomatic, and may be missed on conventional barium meal study. Hypotonic duodenography readily demonstrates the lesion by producing full duodenal distention above and below the narrowing.

Zollinger-Ellison Syndrome

This is characterized by a fulminating ulcer diathesis with a characteristic constellation of roentgen findings which may permit the alert radiologist to make a specific diagnosis. This disorder has been exhaustively detailed in the literature and well summarized in reviews by Christoforidis and Nelson (1966), Zollinger and Moore (1968), and Zboralske (1968). Nonbeta islet cell tumors of the pancreas secrete a gastrin-like hormone which stimulates marked gastric hypersecretion, leading to severe peptic ulcer disease with a tendency toward multiple ulcers in unusual locations (the distal duodenum and jejunum) and profound diarrhea due to an acid-related chemical enteritis. The tumors are often multiple, histologically carcinomatous in 60 per cent, adenomatous in 30 per cent, and hyperplastic in 10 per cent. They occur in ectopic locations in 10 per cent of the cases (the stomach, duodenum, and spleen). The frequent association of carcinoid-islet cell tumors of the duodenum and Zollinger-Ellison physiology was noted earlier in this chapter (p. 292). In one-fourth of the cases, the Zollinger-Ellison syndrome coexists with adenomas or hyperplasia in other endocrine glands (multiple endocrine adenomatosis syndrome).

Roentgenographic evidence of peptic ulceration in the second or third portion should lead one to suspect an ulcerogenic tumor of the pancreas (Fig. 10–29). However, in two-thirds of the cases, the duodenal ulcer appears as an ordinary peptic ulcer of the duodenal cap. Secondary signs of hyperacidity are marked. The duodenum is atonic and dilated, with thickened edematous-appearing mucosal folds (Fig. 10–30). Associated

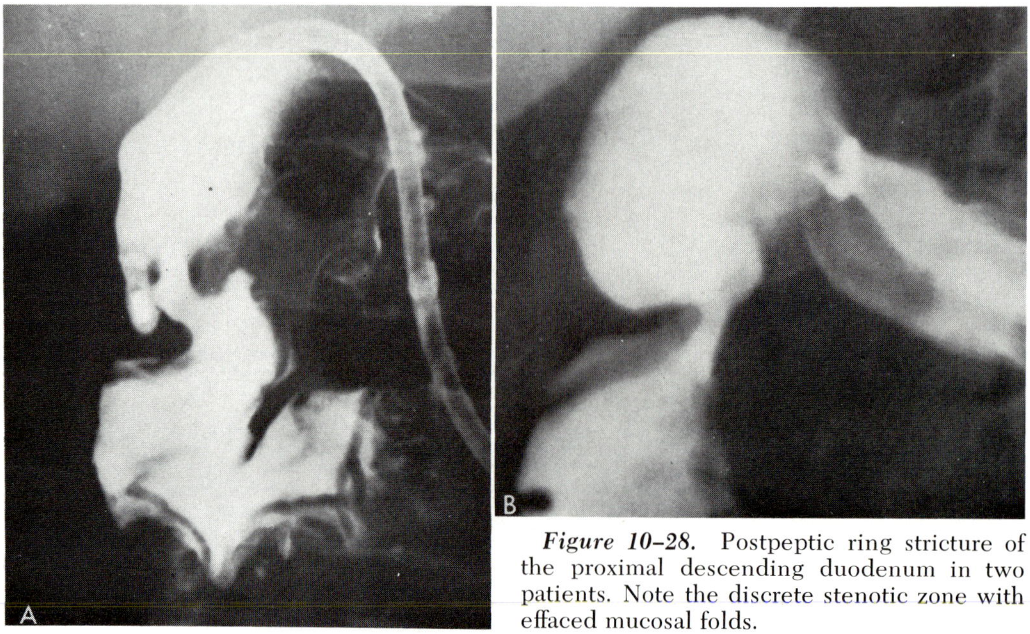

Figure 10–28. Postpeptic ring stricture of the proximal descending duodenum in two patients. Note the discrete stenotic zone with effaced mucosal folds.

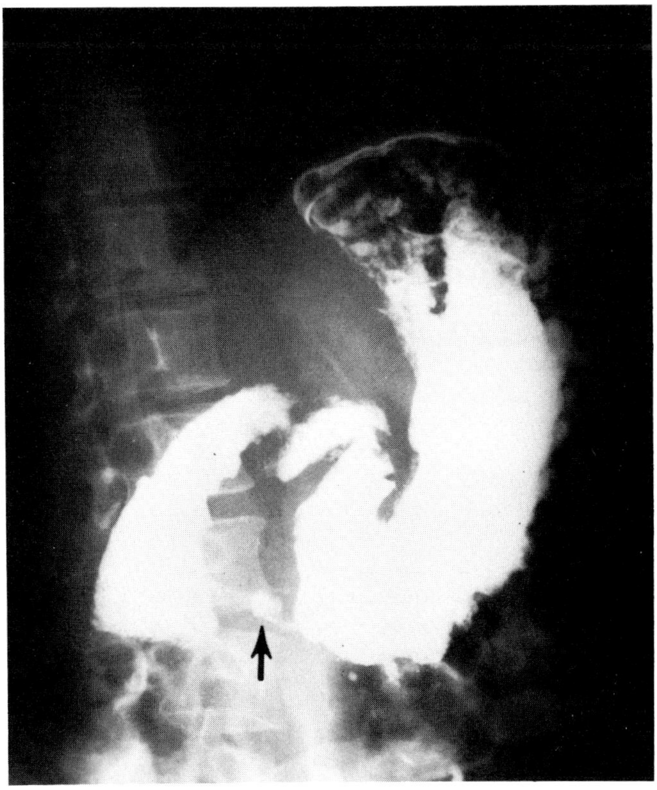

Figure 10–29. Zollinger-Ellison syndrome. An ulcer in the horizontal duodenum is visible (*arrow*). Note the marked hyperrugosity of the gastric folds.

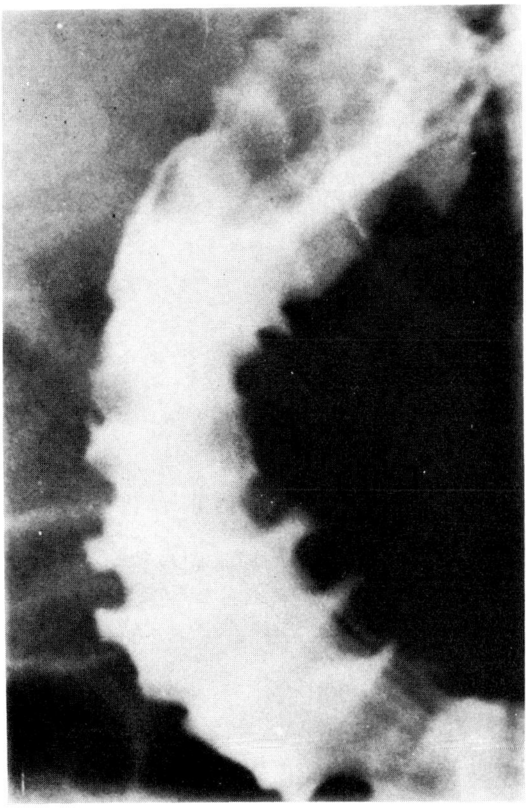

Figure 10–30. Severe thickening of the duodenal fold in the Zollinger-Ellison syndrome. An ulcer crater is not visible.

confirmatory findings include marked gastric hyper-rugosity, excessive gastric secretions, and jejunal ulcerations with mucosal thickening and hypermotility of the upper small bowel.

Clinically, the diagnosis is suspected by the finding of a 12-hour overnight concentration of free hydrochloric acid in the stomach exceeding 100 mEq. per liter (the normal volume is approximately 18 mEq. per liter) and volumes of gastric secretion greater than 2000 cc. (the normal volume is 350 cc.) (Ellison, 1964). This examination should be followed by the augmented histamine test. This ordinarily shows that histamine fails to increase gastric secretion more than 25 per cent over the basal values since the parietal cells are already being maximally stimulated by the ulcerogenic gastrin-like hormone. The diagnosis is further substantiated by the detection of elevated serum gastrin levels, using radioiodine immunoassay techniques (McGuigan, 1968).

Both benign and malignant tumors are frequently vascular, and arteriography is recommended for preoperative localization (Zboralske, 1968).

Since the tumors are often multiple and frequently metastasize to the liver, the treatment of choice is the removal of the target organ (i.e., the stomach) by total gastrectomy. If resection of the tumor short of total pancreatectomy is feasible, then this should be combined with gastrectomy (Ellison, 1964). Even in patients with hepatic metastases, the tumor may have an indolent growth potential. Zboralske (1968) reports two patients with liver metastases who survived more than ten years, and emphasizes the possibility of prolonged survival if the end organ (e.g., the stomach) can be removed.

SPECIFIC INFLAMMATORY DISEASES

Regional Enteritis

This involves the duodenum and usually occurs as a late complication in Crohn's disease after the process is well established elsewhere in the gastrointestinal tract. However, isolated duodenal involvement has been reported (Law, 1964). Although approximately 60 cases of regional enteritis of the duodenum have been recorded in the literature (Law, 1964; Nelson, 1969; and Legge, 1970), the experience of the authors of this monograph indicates that the condition is undoubtedly much more common. In a recent long-term study of 300 patients with Crohn's disease, duodenal involvement occurred in 4 per cent of the cases (Fielding, 1970).

Radiographic findings resemble changes of regional enteritis elsewhere in the alimentary tract, and are usually recognizable as an inflammatory process. Early findings include blunted, thickened, edematous mucosal folds which, on occasion, may assume a polypoid appearance due to the presence of islands of hyperplastic mucosa (Keats, 1957) (Figs. 10–31 and 10–32).

As the disease progresses, the plical fold pattern becomes obliterated, and the duodenum becomes rigid and stiff, finally progressing to an elongated, smooth, tapered stenosis (e.g., "string sign"). Consequently, obstructive dilatation of the proximal duodenum and/or stomach may occur. Skip areas are often visible in the upper jejunal loops (Fig. 10–33), and fistulae into the stomach or colon may occur. An interesting finding recently reported by Legge (1970) is that of barium reflux into the biliary and pancreatic ducts. This occurred in three patients with duodenal involvement presumably due to disruption of the papillary sphincter mechanism by inflammatory cicatrix. In some instances, pancreatitis resulted. Gastric involvement occurs only in the presence of duodenal disease and usually affects the distal antrum in contiguous retrograde fashion. Extension to the stomach occurs in approximately one-half of the cases of duodenal disease and accounts for another characteristic sign coined by Nelson (1969). He applies the term "pseudo-post Bilroth I" appearance to describe a tubular or funnel-shaped narrowing of the antrum, pylorus, and duo-

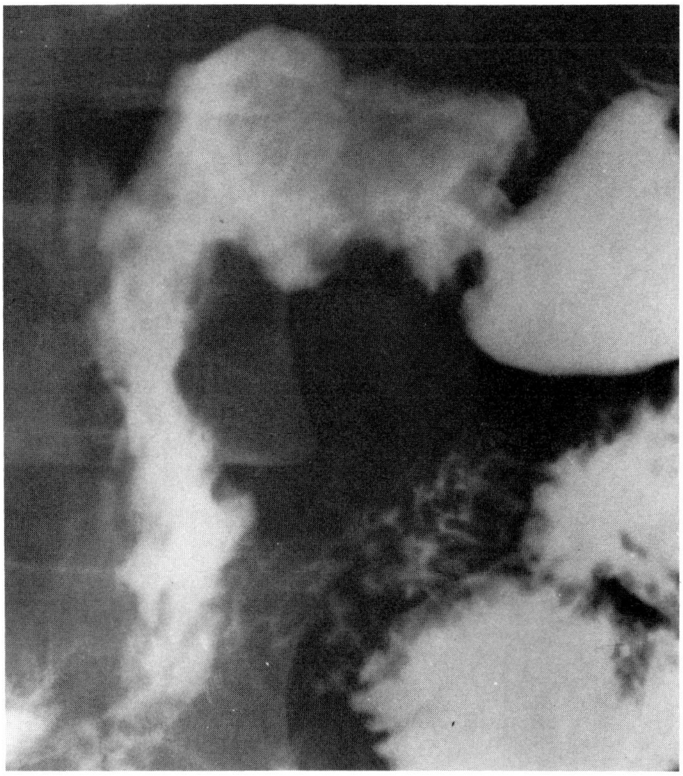

Figure 10–31. Granular, shaggy-appearing thickening of the mucosal folds in regional enteritis of the duodenum. The appearance resembles the changes caused by ulcer disease or pancreatitis.

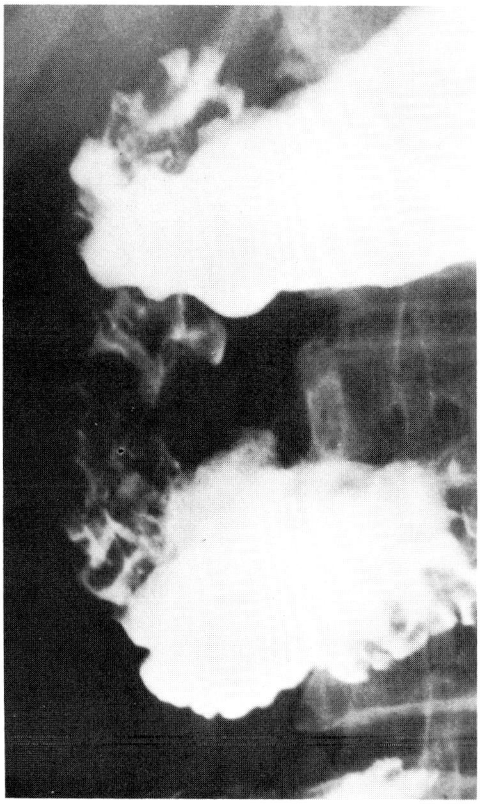

Figure 10–32. Nodular polypoid fold thickening in regional enteritis of the duodenum.

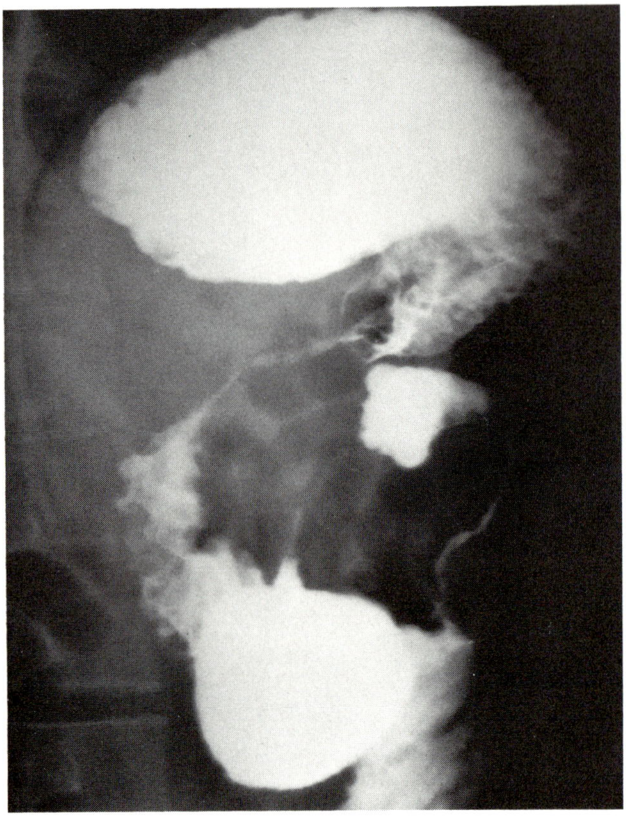

Figure 10–33. Regional enteritis, showing a stenotic segment involving the duodenal cap, pylorus, and gastric antrum, as well as a skip area in the upper jejunum. (From Ferrucci, J. T., and Jonower, M. L.: Localized infiltrating lesions of the stomach. Seminars Roentgen., 6:168, 1971. By permission of Grune & Stratton, Inc.)

denal cap in which all the commonly recognized anatomic landmarks are obliterated (Fig. 10–34). He considers this deformity quite suggestive of Crohn's disease in contradistinction to peptic ulcer disease or neoplasms of the stomach or duodenum which rarely cross the pylorus in either direction. When regional enteritis affects the duodenum as an isolated event, as it rarely may, the differential diagnosis includes peptic ulcer disease, pancreatitis, intramural bleeding, and lymphosarcoma.

Clinically, patients with duodenal involvement usually have crampy epigastric pain, nausea, and vomiting, reflecting high intestinal obstruction (Fig. 10–35). Should medical management fail, a surgical bypass in the form of a gastrojejunostomy may be required.

Tuberculosis

Tuberculosis of the duodenum is extremely rare even in patients with pulmonary or intestinal tuberculosis. Feldman (1957) found duodenal involvement in only 0.5 per cent of autopsied patients with tuberculosis. The distal antrum and pylorus are almost invariably involved in contiguity with the duodenum (Ostrum, 1948; Balikian, 1967), although there have been case reports of isolated duodenal involvement (Ferreira, 1972). The radiographic appearance is variable and is usually interpreted as a carcinoma of the stomach or peptic ulcer disease. The findings include nodular hyperplastic thickening of folds, often with frank ulceration (Fig. 10–36). Luminal narrowing by an inflammatory constrict-

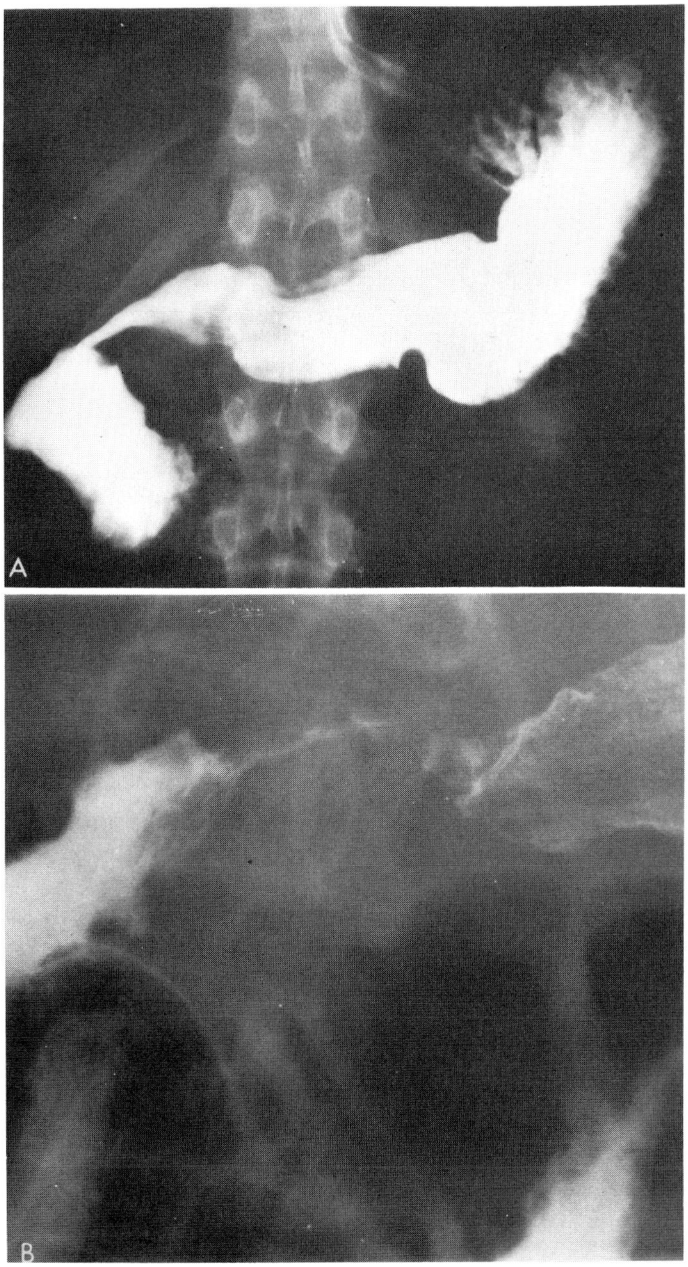

Figure 10–34. Regional enteritis of the proximal descending duodenum, producing a smooth funnel-like narrowing which has been designated the pseudopost Bilroth I appearance in two patients. See also Figure 4–89.

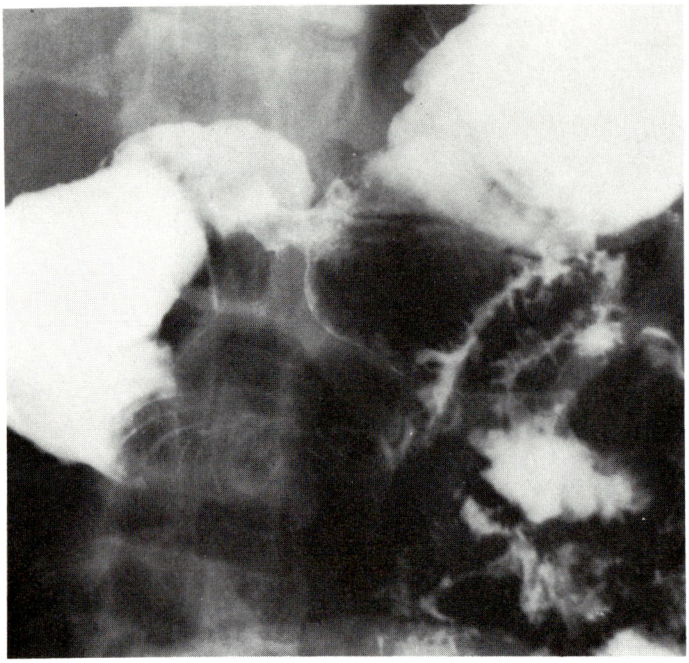

Figure 10–35. Duodenal obstruction secondary to regional enteritis involving the distal duodenum and proximal jejunum.

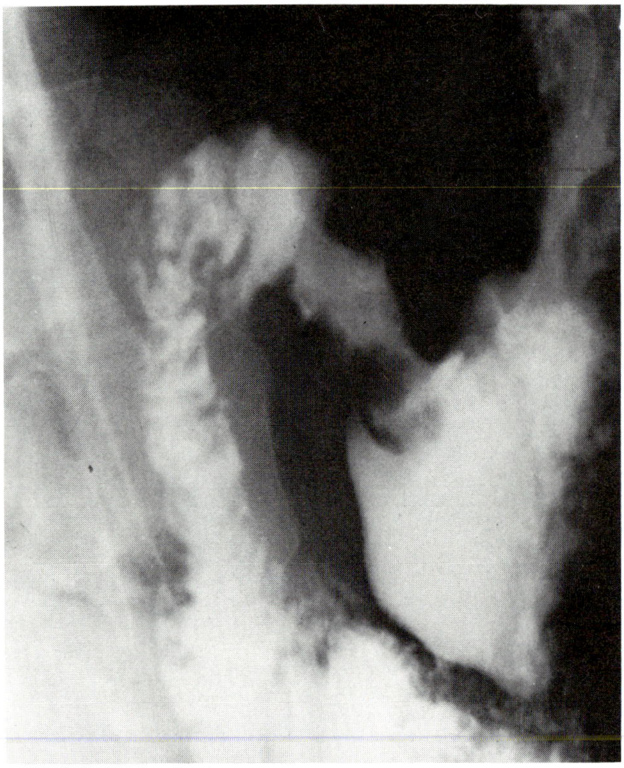

Figure 10–36. Pyloroduodenal tuberculosis. An irregular diamond-shaped ulceration involves the distal antrum, pylorus, and duodenal cap. Films of the chest were normal. (Courtesy of Dr. N. Joffee, Boston, Mass.)

ing mass usually involves the antrum, pylorus, and duodenum. As in regional enteritis, this distribution should distinguish the process from gastric malignancy which rarely crosses the pylorus. Sinus tracts, fistulae, and abscess formation may also occur. In late cases, significant pyloroduodenal obstruction may occur.

Strongyloidiasis

This produces severe duodenitis as part of a more generalized enteritis (Louisy, 1971; Berkmen, 1972). The roentgen findings may simulate regional enteritis and may include mucosal edema and alterations in peristaltic activity, including severe atony. Significant stasis and duodenal dilatation may occur. This has been attributed to periduodenal edema and compression by the superior mesenteric artery (Louisy, 1971).

As in regional enteritis, advanced cases may show ulcerations, stenotic narrowing of the duodenum, and reflux of barium into the biliary ducts. An enteritis pattern is usually visible in the upper small bowel but there is no ileal involvement or fistulae. Other major differential diagnoses include lymphosarcoma and intramural bleeding.

Giardiasis

This is another recently publicized parasitic infestation which causes changes in the duodenum and jejunum resembling mild cases of strongyloidiasis (Marshak, 1968; Babb, 1971). The organism, *Giardia lamblia*, may be a harmless commensal within the intestinal lumen, but in patients with a heavy infestation (often acquired during foreign travel) or predisposing factors, a significant diarrheal disease and malabsorption may occur. Important predisposing conditions are malnutrition, the presence of enteric bacterial infection, and altered immune mechanisms. In the latter case, dysgammaglobulinemia may be associated with lymphoid nodular hyperplasia of the small bowel which is manifested radiographically by numerous tiny mucosal filling defects in the distal ileum.

Roentgen findings in giardiasis are usually confined to the duodenum and jejunum. There is marked hyperperistalsis and increased secretions which produce blurred, thickened, edematous-appearing mucosal folds (Fig. 10–37).

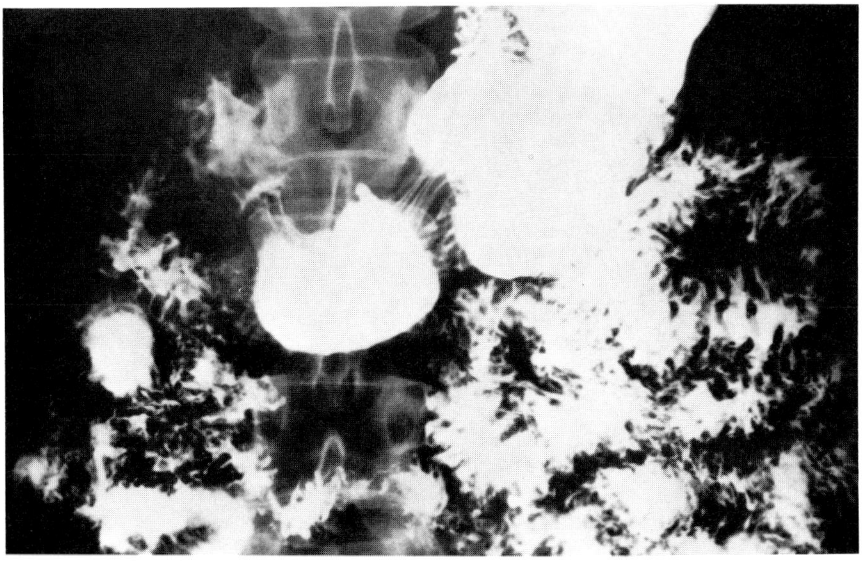

Figure 10–37. Giardiasis. Nodular thickening of folds is visible in the duodenum and jejunum.

The distal ileum appears normal except in patients with associated lymphoid hyperplasia in whom the numerous tiny filling defects may be visible. The organism is found in the stool, and the disorder is reversible following treatment with quinacrine (Atabrine).

SUPERIOR MESENTERIC ARTERY SYNDROME

Forty years of discussion in the literature has failed to dull interest in the superior mesenteric artery syndrome. For the most part, the discussion has centered on the validity of chronic vascular compression of the duodenum (arteriomesenteric occlusion) as a definite and definable entity.

Von Rokitansky is generally credited with first recognizing duodenal vascular compression in 1861. Not until some 60 years later was the syndrome given a legitimate status and name—Wilkie's syndrome—in a careful description of clinical findings and treatment (Wilkie, 1921). Enthusiastic surgeons immediately diagnosed and treated the condition, reporting nearly 100 patients who had undergone surgery in one series but, after the 1930's, interest waned until the late 1950's when a more critical medical community reassessed the entity (Goin, 1956; Bitner, 1958; and Jones, 1960). Several authors expressed "uneasiness" about the validity of the syndrome and proposed that "possibly a disservice has been done" (Fischer, 1960), and that "the role of the superior mesenteric artery is in fact circumstantial" (Cimmino, 1961). It seems likely that many of the cases described prior to 1940 were due to such factors as inflammatory or neoplastic obstruction, electrolyte imbalance, and perhaps scleroderma. Again, within very recent years, a series of articles on an acute form of duodenal vascular compression has appeared, resulting in a new legitimacy for the relations of the artery and the duodenum.

Anatomy and Pathogenesis

Anatomically, the transverse portion of the duodenum is the most fixed portion of the entire alimentary canal. It is situated retroperitoneally, in contact with the aorta and lumbar spine posteriorly at the L3 level where the lumbar lordosis is most pronounced. Anteriorly, the duodenum lies subjacent to the root of the mesentery carrying the superior mesenteric artery and is thus contained in a closed compartment (Fig. 10–38).

In quadrupeds, the mesentery hangs downward and there is no tendency for the mesenteric vessels to compress the duodenum. In the erect posture of humans, the mesenteric vessels drape more tightly over the anterior duodenal wall. Thus, wedged within this aortomesenteric angle, the normal duodenum is precariously situated, and mild duodenal compression could be construed as a normal variant. Not uncommonly, in normal patients, barium is transiently delayed at the midline where the duodenum crosses the spine, and mild inconstant dilatation proximal to this point may occur (Nugent, 1966). Casts of cadaver duodenums may show grooves on the anterior and posterior duodenal walls attributed to impression by the superior mesenteric artery and aorta, respectively. Such grooves occasionally are encountered as incidental findings during barium study of normal patients (Fig. 10–39). Similar groove-like impressions on the pancreas noted at radionuclide scanning have been attributed to impression by midline structures. See Chap. 6.

Any alteration of these anatomic relationships, which tends to close the nutcracker-like jaws of the aortomesenteric angle, will cause some degree of duodenal compression (Jones, 1960). Thus, debilitating illness accompanied by loss of weight and retroperitoneal fat or by conditions leading to relaxation of abdominal wall musculature (such as multiple pregnancies) tends to increase the dragging effect of the mesenteric root and consequently narrow the space anteriorly (Goin, 1956). Prolonged bed

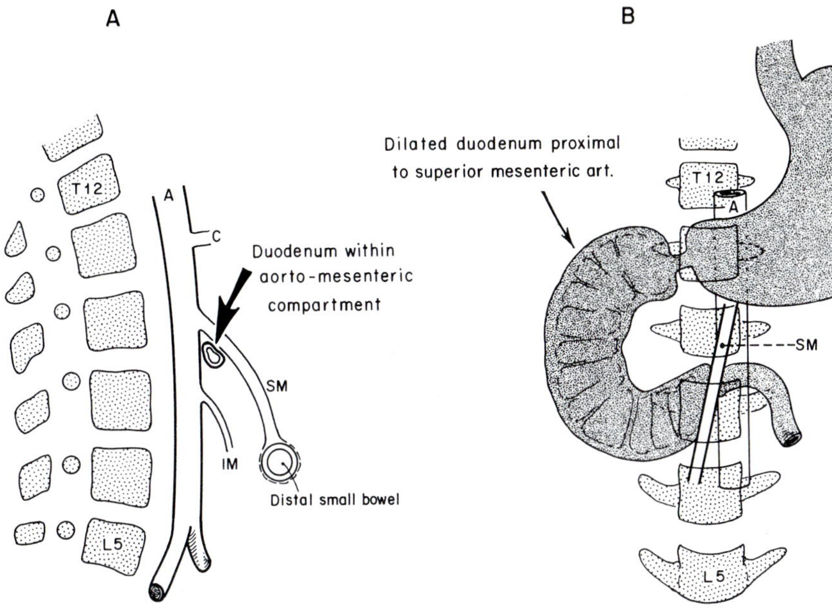

Figure 10–38. Schematic representation of the relationships between the superior mesenteric artery, the aorta, and the duodenum. *A*, Lateral projection; *B*, frontal projection, showing the proximal dilatation characteristic of the superior mesenteric artery syndrome.

rest or immobilization in the supine position allows the mesenteric artery to fall back upon the duodenal wall, compromising the lumen anteriorly. The midline elevation of the spine in this position constitutes another mechanical barrier to the duodenal contents which must flow over it and, together, these two factors may produce considerable duodenal stasis.

This phenomenon has been reported as an acute complication in patients immobilized in a hyperextension body cast (body cast syndrome) (Berk, 1970) and in patients subjected to acute lumbar hyperextension following surgical correction of scoliosis by braces, or skeletal traction (Evarts, 1971). A similar mechanism has also been suggested in two different groups of patients who developed an acute superior mesenteric artery syndrome because of profoundly immobilizing whole-body burns (Wallace, 1970; Ogbuokiri, 1972) (Fig. 10–40). In addition, there can be little doubt that in some instances primary neuromuscular dysfunction contributes to duodenal stasis. In disorders with reduced peristaltic activity—e.g., trauma, acute pancreatitis, and scleroderma—the midline complex of spine, aorta, and superior mesenteric artery may constitute a sufficient barrier to cause significant obstruction at the third portion of the duodenum. Thus, any patient with duodenal hypomotility, when placed supine, may develop the superior mesenteric artery syndrome.

Inflammatory thickening of the bowel wall and of the mesenteric root without frank narrowing of the aortomesenteric angle is a second mechanism whereby duodenal compression may occur. Phlegmonous swelling of soft-tissue structures within the aortomesenteric space has resulted in vascular compression of the duodenum in pancreatitis, regional enteritis, and duodenal ulcer (Simon, 1962) (Fig. 10–41).

Of interest are the various measurements of the aortomesenteric compartment that have been made in vivo, although the clinical significance of these observations remains doubtful. Lateral

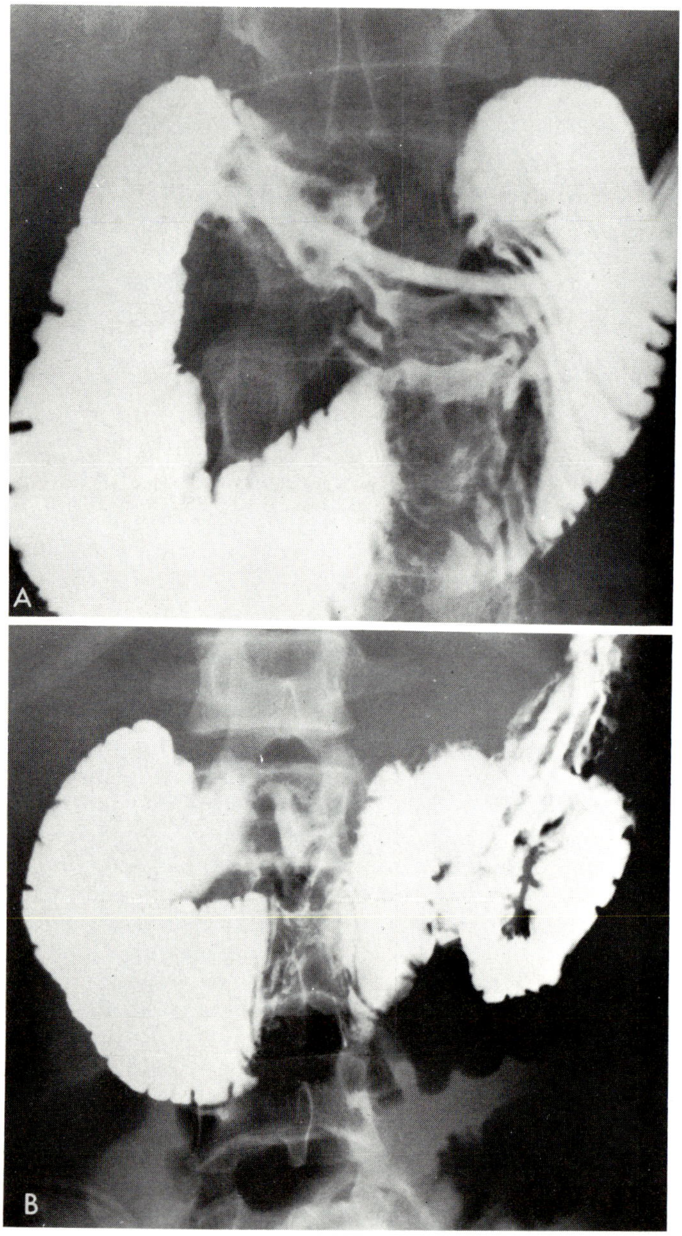

Figure 10–39. Aorto-mesenteric duodenal compression as a normal variant may be seen when duodenal dilatation occurs. The typical midline vascular impression is visible in two patients with duodenal dilatation due to hypotonic duodenography (*A*), and post-traumatic ileus (*B*).

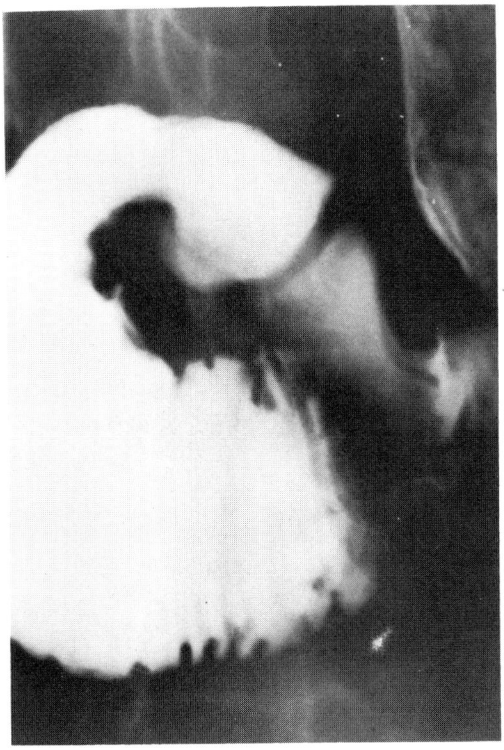

Figure 10–40. Acute superior mesenteric artery syndrome complicating severe burns. Note the typical vertical linear compression defect on the horizontal duodenum, producing complete obstruction. (Courtesy of Dr. W. B. Howard.)

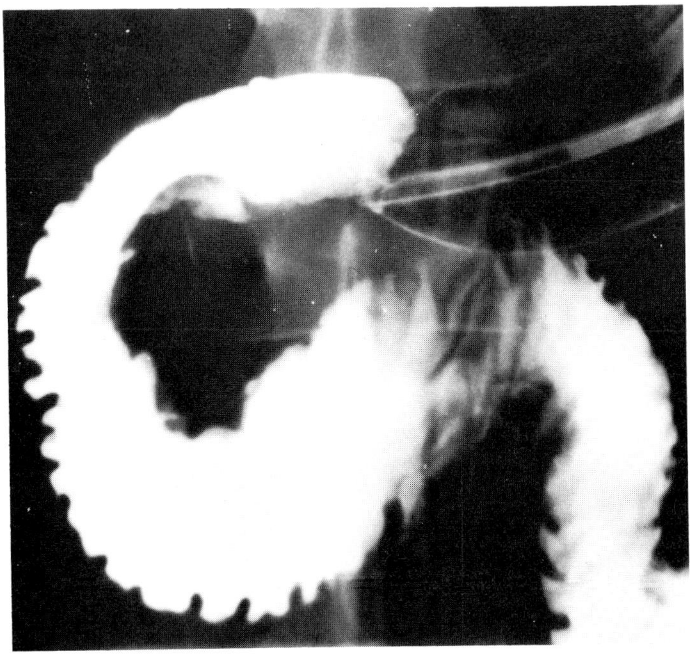

Figure 10–41. Superior mesenteric artery compression complicating acute pancreatitis. Note the mass in the head of the pancreas, and the vertical linear impression on the horizontal duodenum. Mild duodenal dilatation is apparent. These changes are attributed to phlegmonous periduodenal swelling which compresses the duodenum between the aorta and the superior mesenteric artery.

abdominal aortograms have demonstrated an aortomesenteric angle of less than 12° in two symptomatic patients with duodenal ileus; in five normal controls, this angle varied from 45° to 65° (Hearn, 1966).

Roentgen Findings

Radiographically, the findings in the superior mesenteric artery syndrome are quite characteristic and vary little regardless of the underlying process. Dilatation of the first and second portion of the duodenum associated with a vertical linear extrinsic pressure defect in the third portion are the hallmarks of this syndrome (Bitner, 1958) (Figs. 10–42, 10–43, and 10–44). Spot films of the site of obstruction show a narrow compressed lumen with intact mucosal folds. Retention of barium in the duodenal loop, with dilatation and to-and-fro peristaltic activity, may occur; these are nonspecific signs simply reflecting the severity of the condition. Gastric dilatation may also be present. Differential diagnosis from an organic constriction is made by placing the patient in the left decubitus, prone, or knee-chest position, thus decreasing traction drag by the mesentery on the duodenum (Fig. 10–45). In this position, the duodenal contents will be seen to empty promptly, confirming the diagnosis. Resumption of the supine position reproduces the findings. We think that angiographic documentation of the course of the superior mesenteric artery is rarely indicated.

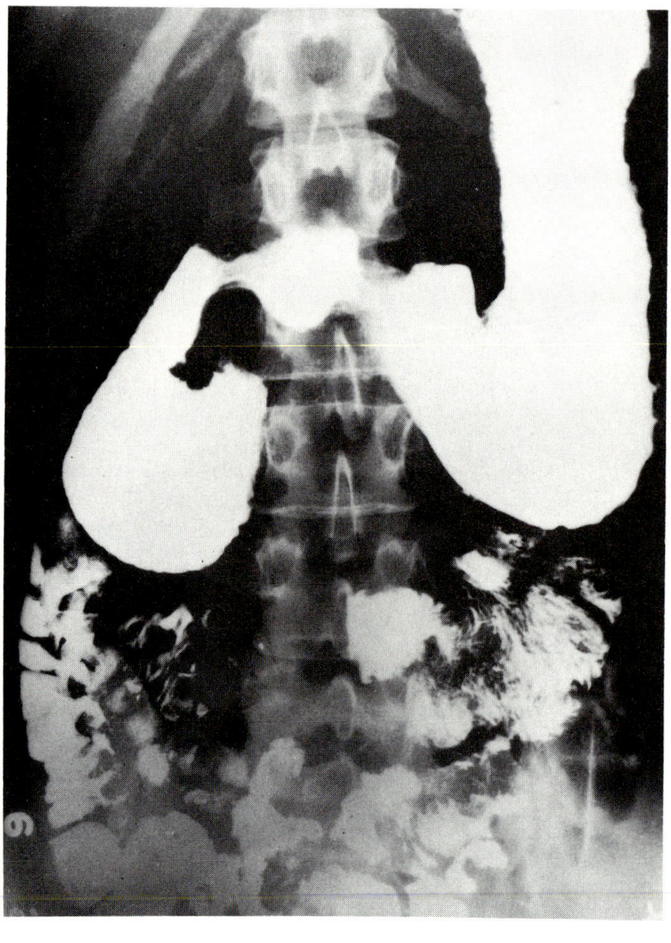

Figure 10–42. Superior mesenteric artery syndrome complicating scleroderma. Note the typical vertical midline compression. The distal small bowel shows characteristic dilatation.

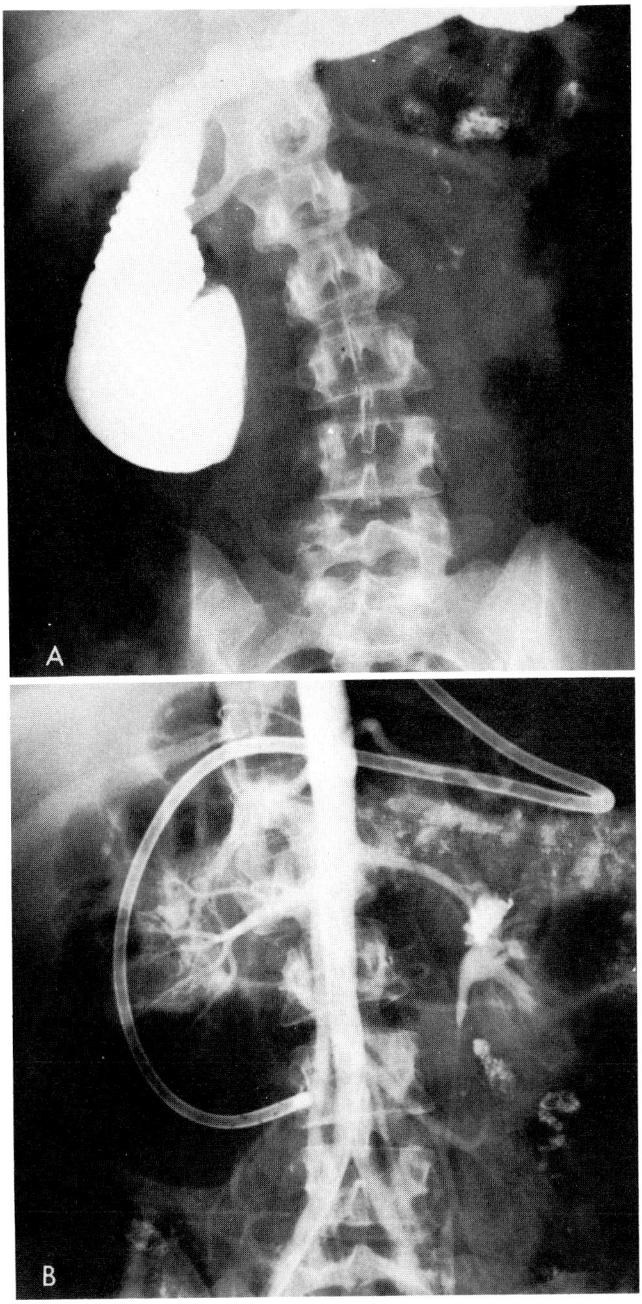

Figure 10–43. Superior mesenteric artery syndrome.
A, Barium study showing typical vertical linear termination of the barium column.
B, Aortogram showing the relationship of the superior mesenteric artery to a duodenography tube passed to the point of obstruction.

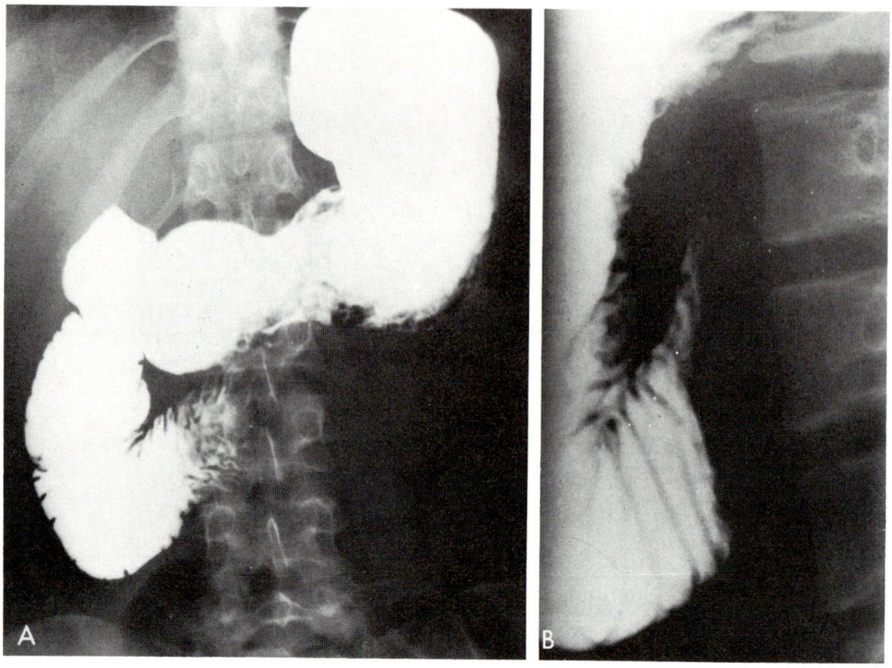

Figure 10–44. Superior mesenteric artery syndrome.

A, Frontal projection showing duodenal dilatation and complete obstruction of further passage of barium.

B, High oblique projection demonstrating the typical vertical linear extrinsic compression defect. The patient was chronically ill as a result of septic complications of lower alimentary tract surgery.

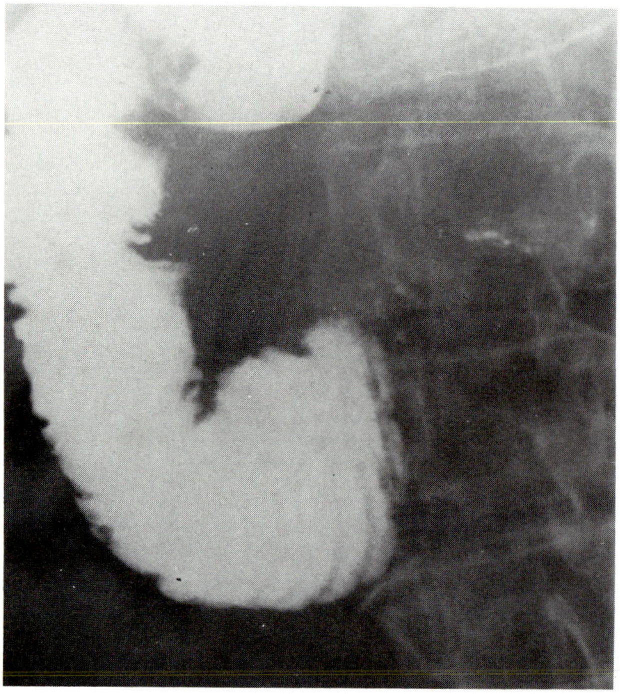

Figure 10–45. Organic duodenal obstruction, simulating the superior mesenteric artery syndrome, resulting from carcinoma of the body of the pancreas. The termination of the barium column reveals only nonspecific external compression resembling compression by the superior mesenteric artery. No emptying occurred in the prone or left decubitus position.

Clinical Considerations

In the authors' opinion, the clinical features of the chronic superior mesenteric artery syndrome as reported in the literature do not coalesce into a discrete entity.

In our experience, an underlying medical disease, often of a debilitating nature (e.g., malignancy, scleroderma, sprue), has been the predominant clinical feature outweighing the significance of duodenal stasis as an isolated problem. It is our belief that the chronic superior mesenteric artery syndrome is rarely, if ever, an independent entity but more often represents a complication of a chronic disease. Hence, surgical bypass is only rarely indicated.

A similar situation exists in the case of the acute superior mesenteric artery syndrome. Here, the severity of the precipitating illness usually causes the phenomenon of duodenal compression to be clearly recognized as a complication of the primary disease—e.g., acute pancreatitis (Brust, 1962; Simon, 1962), burns (Wallace, 1970), severe trauma (Mindell, 1970), and hyperextension traction treatment of scoliosis (Evarts, 1971). Unfortunately, failure to recognize acute duodenal stasis has resulted in a number of fatalities as a result of aspiration.

Accurate radiographic diagnosis followed by adequate nasogastric decompression are important in the management. Fluoroscopic positioning to reduce duodenal obstruction may permit optimal positioning of the patient in bed during the acute phase. If these measures fail, timely surgical intervention in the form of duodenojejunostomy is indicated.

TRAUMATIC LESIONS OF THE DUODENUM

The importance of roentgenologic findings in the diagnosis and management of duodenal injuries has been appreciated only within the last decade. Prior to 1955, only 12 cases of duodenal hematoma were recorded in the literature (Freeark, 1966); the first correct preoperative roentgen diagnosis of duodenal hematoma was reported in 1954 (Felson, 1954).

Two main types of duodenal injuries occur: penetrating injuries and blunt trauma. The former, the result of missiles or stab wounds, is usually managed surgically and does not present a radiologic diagnostic problem. In cases of blunt trauma to the abdomen, however, symptoms and signs of visceral injury may be obscure. In such instances, radiologic examination may provide crucial diagnostic information (Hill, 1965).

Anatomy, Mechanism of Injury, and Pathophysiology

Because the duodenum is fixed retroperitoneally and overlies the vertebral column, it is particularly susceptible to compression or shearing injuries from blunt abdominal trauma. It has been postulated that, when distended with fluid, the duodenum is potentially a closed loop occluded at its upper end by the pyloric sphincter and narrowed distally by the overlying mesenteric root carrying the superior mesenteric vessels. It is therefore easily injured by relatively mild direct blows.

Severe striking forces may cause total disruption of the duodenal wall. Frank rupture of the duodenum usually involves the posterior duodenal wall so that the site of injury is retroperitoneal. Occasionally, complete transection, involving the anterior wall as well, occurs and produces intraperitoneal signs. In such cases, the escape of highly irritating digestive juices will prove rapidly fatal unless recognized and treated promptly. With severe trauma, associated injury to the pancreas is common and varies from contusion with fat necrosis to massive disruption of pancreatic parenchyma. Clinically, combined injury of the pancreas and duodenum carries a grave prognosis and, in a recent surgical series of 13 such patients, the mortality rate was approximately 50 per cent (Roman, 1971).

Blows of lesser severity may effect a partial disruption of the duodenal wall, with a less predictable outcome. Shearing forces which tear the intramural vasculature without disrupting the mucosal or serosal layers permit escaping blood to accumulate within the duodenal wall, producing an intramural duodenal hematoma. Such hematomas may grow to appreciable size since intramural hemorrhage in this area is less likely to tamponade itself than in areas where the entire circumference of the bowel is enclosed in a serosal layer. Thus, obstruction of the duodenal lumen by the mass of the hematoma is a common clinical feature of such injuries.

The most common sites of involvement by the intramural hematoma are the second and third portions of the duodenum, but the hematoma may extend distally into the jejunum or proximally into the descending duodenum, obstructing the biliary and pancreatic ducts and producing jaundice or pancreatitis (Freeark, 1966).

The course of duodenal hematomas is variable. They may increase in size because of persistent bleeding or breakdown of hemoglobin, drawing in fluid in a manner similar to the osmotic swelling of a subdural hematoma. Eventually they may rupture into the free peritoneal cavity or retroperitoneal space. In most instances, the mucosal layer of the bowel remains intact, so that secondary infection or rupture into the intestinal lumen is rare. Commonly, however, when a duodenal hematoma occurs as an isolated injury, spontaneous resolution occurs. The hematoma undergoes gradual liquefaction, and broken-down blood products are reabsorbed over a period of one to two weeks. Careful clinical and roentgenographic monitoring of the evolution of the hematoma is imperative for successful management.

Clinical Features

Three groups of individuals appear particularly susceptible to blunt trauma to the duodenum. These include (1) persons involved in automobile accidents who have sustained steering-wheel injuries; (2) persons under the influence of alcohol who are prone to a variety of bodily injuries; (3) children who may be injured at play, particularly in bicycle accidents. In all of these groups, sudden blows to the abdomen may occur at times when the anterior abdominal muscles are relaxed, so that the usual protection afforded by these structures is absent.

In the case of massive trauma with frank duodenal rupture or major associated injury to the pancreas and other viscera, symptoms and signs usually indicate significant visceral injury, and the need for immediate surgical intervention is apparent. In less severe injury to the duodenum, there is typically a delay in the onset of symptoms, often as long as one week. Characteristically, clinical findings are deceptively benign. Symptoms develop gradually and are often quite nonspecific. Such patients may complain of epigastric pain followed by gradually increasing nausea and bilious vomiting for several days after the traumatic event. Frequently, especially in children and alcoholics, a blow to the abdomen is forgotten or denied, and is not recollected until after surgical or radiologic findings establish the diagnosis. Physical findings include epigastric tenderness or a mass; laboratory studies are of little specific value except for hyperamylasemia as an indication of concomitant pancreatic injury (Freeark, 1966).

Radiographic Findings

Plain film study of the abdomen performed immediately after injury may reveal evidence of retroperitoneal air in cases of duodenal rupture (Gould, 1963; Toxopeus, 1972). This may appear as streaks or bubbles of gas along the psoas margins, kidneys, and transverse mesocolon, and is often located on the right side of the abdomen (Fig. 10–46). Rarely, pneumoperitoneum may occur, with disruption of the anterior duodenal wall and escape of gas into the peritoneal cavity. In cases of suspected duodenal rupture, administration of a water-soluble contrast agent is preferred since extravasation of contrast may be the major

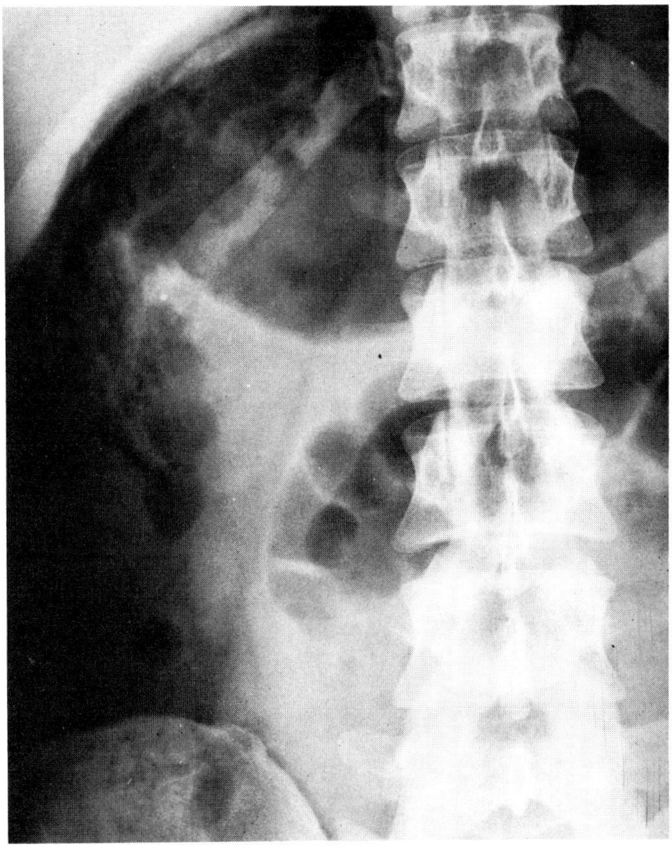

Figure 10–46. Perirenal and retroperitoneal air accumulation associated with acute duodenal rupture.

indication of the site of injury (Fig. 10–47).

Plain film findings in duodenal hematoma include a soft-tissue mass as well as evidence of duodenal obstruction, with dilatation and air fluid levels in the stomach and duodenum. The so-called double-bubble sign of duodenal obstruction may be observed (Fig. 10–48).

On barium meal examination, a variety of findings may be encountered. There may be partial or complete obstruction at any level of the duodenum, with an abrupt or irregular tapered narrowing at the termination of the barium column (Figs. 10–49 and 10–50). Partial duodenal obstruction may be present with a picket-fence configuration and numerous nodular filling defects producing eccentric narrowing of the lumen to the duodenojejunal flexure and beyond (Fig. 10–51). A coiled-spring appearance resembling an intussusception has been described by Felson and Levin (1954) who considered this sign pathognomonic of an intramural duodenal hematoma (Fig. 10–52). The cause of this sign is not entirely clear and, in the experience of the authors of this monograph, it has not been particularly common. Occasionally, the hematoma presents as a large intramural mass simulating a tumor (Fig. 10–53). In one instance, the coiled-spring appearance developed on follow-up barium meal study, after initial examination had disclosed only a nonspecific obstructive configuration (Fig. 10–54). Associated pancreatic injury (e.g., traumatic abscess or pseudocyst) may be manifested by extrinsic mass impression on the gastric or duodenal contour out of proportion to the duodenal abnormalities. This configuration is also suggested in Figure 10–54.

(Text continued on page 331)

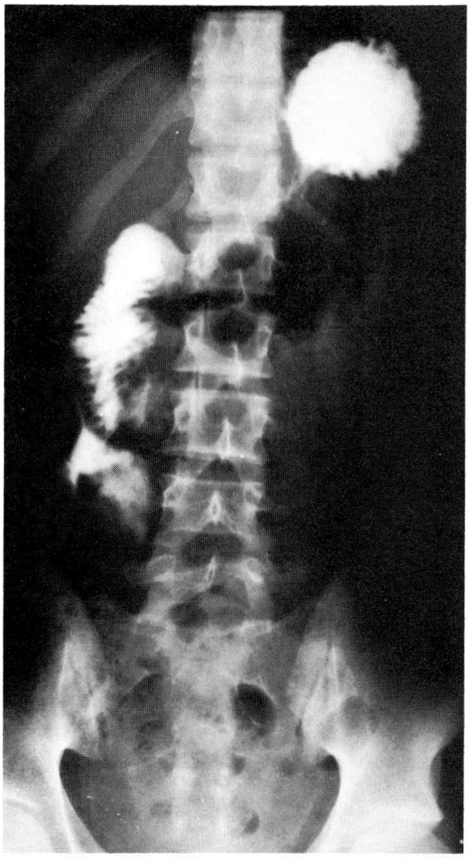

Figure 10–47. Acute rupture of the duodenum following blunt abdominal injury. Contrast extravasation into the right retroperitoneal space.

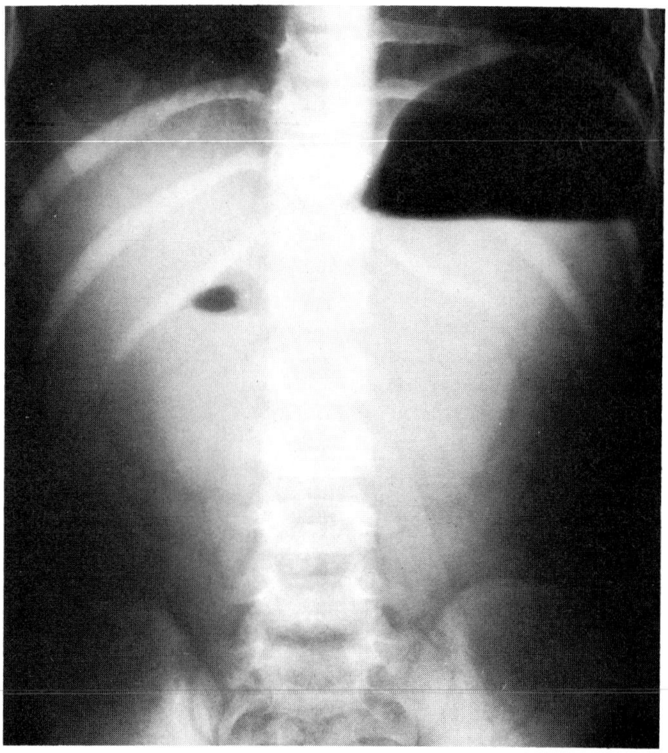

Figure 10–48. Duodenal obstruction associated with intramural hematoma. Note the "double bubble" sign.

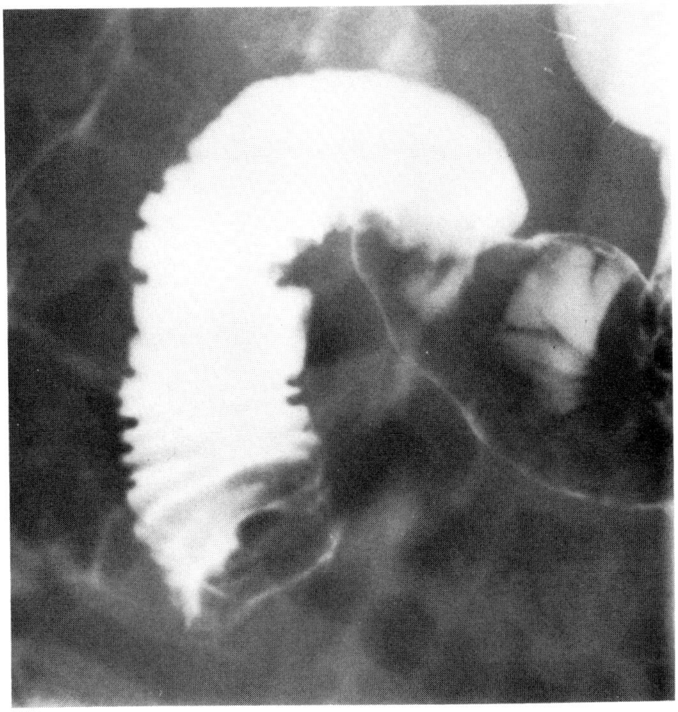

Figure 10–49. Obstructing hematoma of the duodenum. This configuration is unusually abrupt but strongly suggests duodenal injury in a patient examined shortly after abdominal trauma.

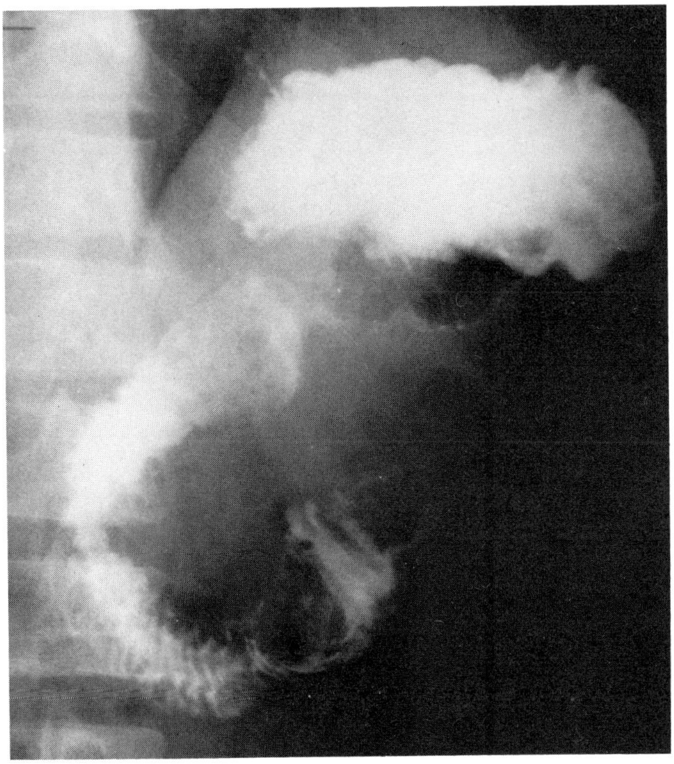

Figure 10–50. Obstructing intramural hematoma of the horizontal portion of the duodenum. Multiple nodular areas of hematoma formation are apparent.

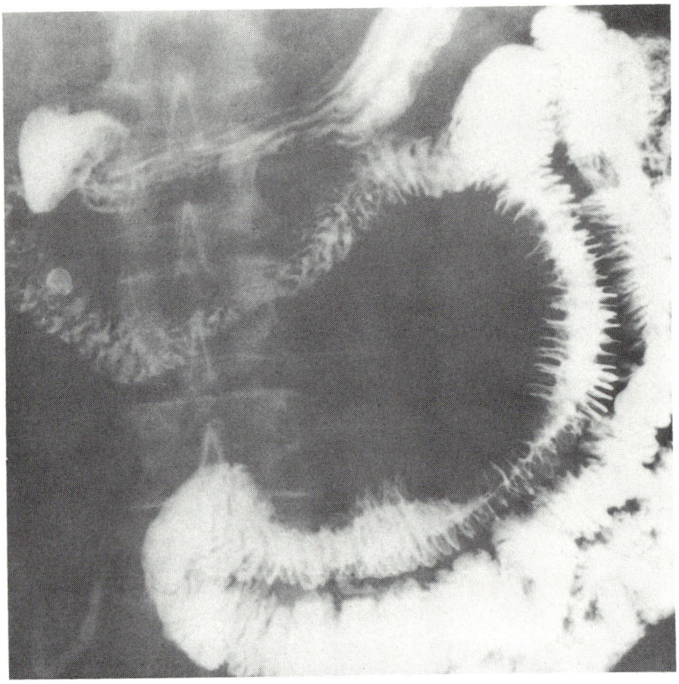

Figure 10–51. "Picket fence" appearance due to traumatic submucosal hemorrhage at the duodenojejunal flexure.

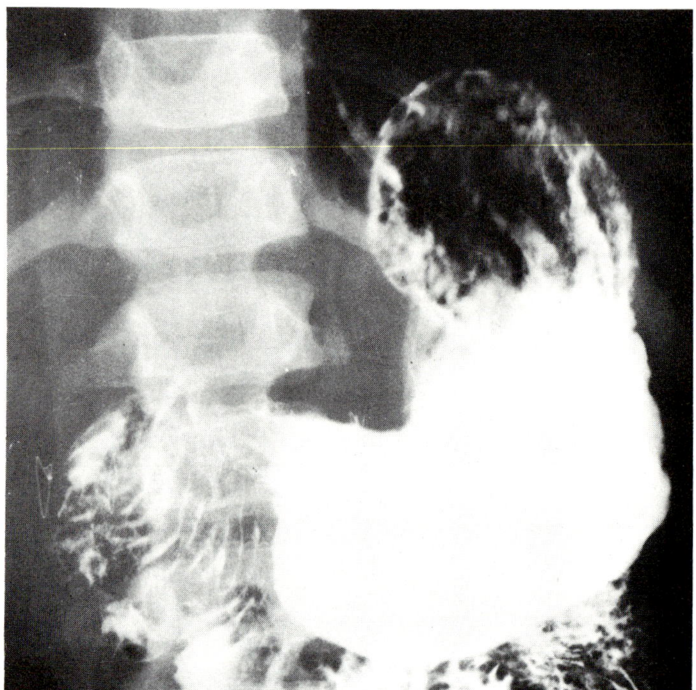

Figure 10–52. "Coiled spring" appearance due to a traumatic intramural hematoma of the descending duodenum. Associated gastric stasis is evident. This sign has been considered pathognomonic of an intramural duodenal hematoma.

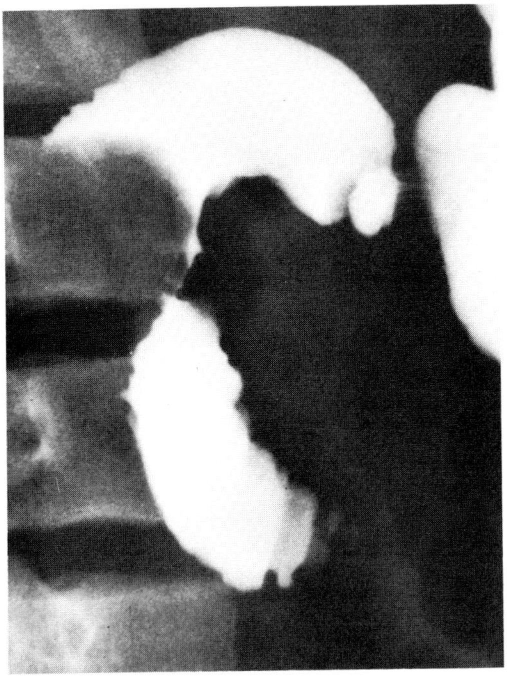

Figure 10–53. Duodenal hematoma simulating intramural tumor. The characteristic "coiled spring" appearance is not present. However, in such cases this sign may appear on follow-up examinations.

Management

When injury to the pancreas or other solid viscera accompanies blunt duodenal trauma, or when frank duodenal rupture is evident, early surgical intervention is mandatory. When repair of duodenal perforation is delayed for more than 24 hours, mortality rates approach 65 per cent, compared with a 50 per cent mortality rate in those patients operated upon within 24 hours. Operative management includes drainage of the hematoma with or without a gastroenterostomy (Roman, 1971).

When the duodenal hematoma is determined to be an isolated injury, nonoperative treatment is often preferred. Conservative management includes nasogastric suction and parenteral alimentation. Serial barium meal studies over a period of one to two weeks will show resolution of the obstructing hematoma in approximately 50 per cent of the cases (Fig. 10–54). If obstruction persists, the hematoma is usually sufficiently liquefied so that surgical evacuation is readily accomplished (Kakos, 1971). Bypass procedures usually are unnecessary.

MISCELLANEOUS

Duodenum Inversum

This is a rare developmental variation of little clinical significance in which abnormal peritoneal fixation permits the descending duodenum to loop laterally and toward the right; this causes the distal duodenum to lie to the right of the descending portion so that the duodenojejunal flexure assumes a high medial location in the left retroperitoneum (Fig. 10–55). The jejunum is in its normal location and the rest of the small bowel is in its normal situs.

Paraduodenal Hernia

Paraduodenal hernias are the result of congenital variations in peritoneal fixation and are the commonest form of internal hernia (Meyers, 1970). Two forms occur, either left or right, depending on the position of the duodenum and the orientation of the opening of the paraduodenal fossa. In left hernias, which are the more common variety, small-bowel loops pass into the paraduodenal fossa posteriorly and into the left mesocolon, producing a collection of small-bowel loops lateral to the ascending duodenum in the left upper quadrant of the abdomen (Fig. 10–56). Right-sided paraduodenal hernias occur less commonly (25 per cent) and are associated with incomplete intestinal rotation (Bartlett, 1971). Radiographically, the duodenojejunal flexure has a faulty, low, right paramedian position, the duodenum is dilated, and the jejunal loops are situated in the right side of the abdomen, extending into the right transverse mesocolon. In both instances, the transverse colon may appear depressed.

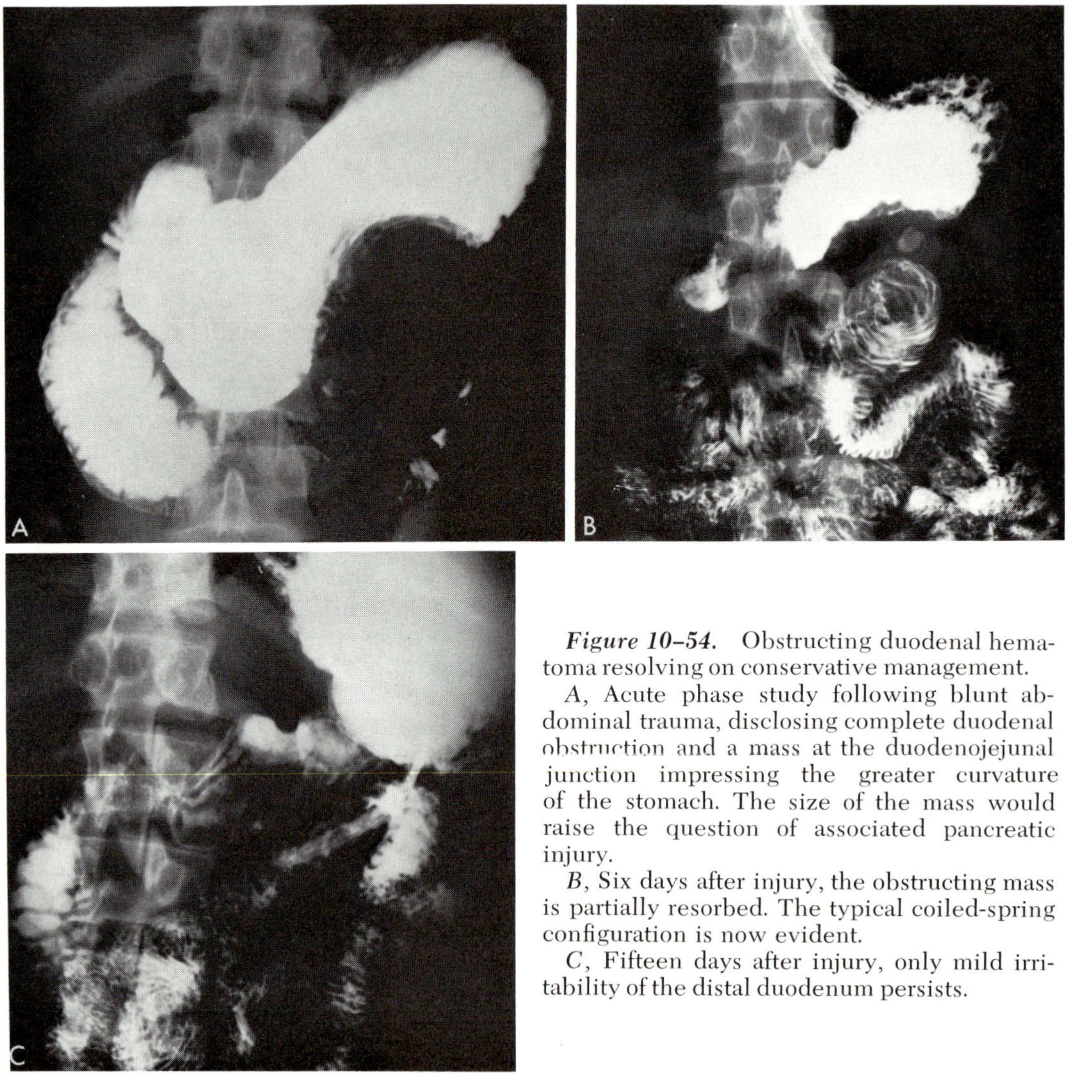

Figure 10–54. Obstructing duodenal hematoma resolving on conservative management.

A, Acute phase study following blunt abdominal trauma, disclosing complete duodenal obstruction and a mass at the duodenojejunal junction impressing the greater curvature of the stomach. The size of the mass would raise the question of associated pancreatic injury.

B, Six days after injury, the obstructing mass is partially resorbed. The typical coiled-spring configuration is now evident.

C, Fifteen days after injury, only mild irritability of the distal duodenum persists.

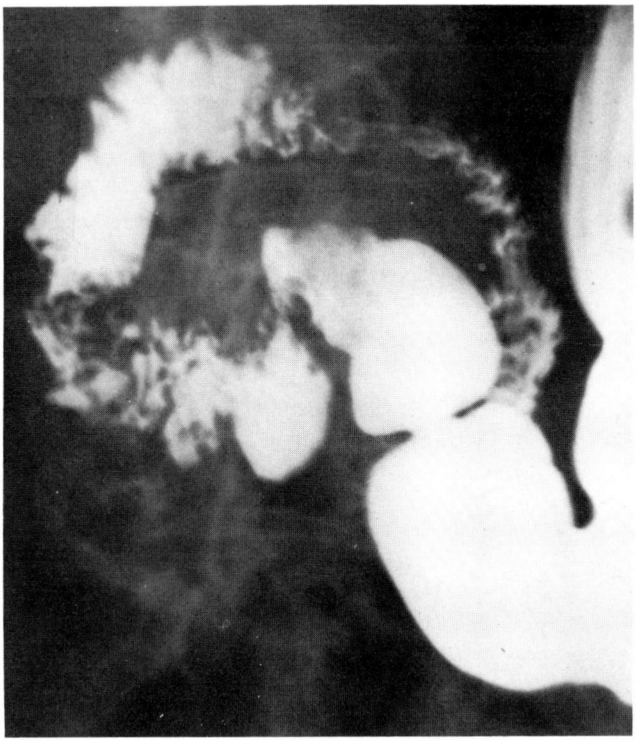

Figure 10–55. Duodenum inversum. Faulty peritoneal fixation causes the second and third portions of the duodenum to appear inverted superiorly.

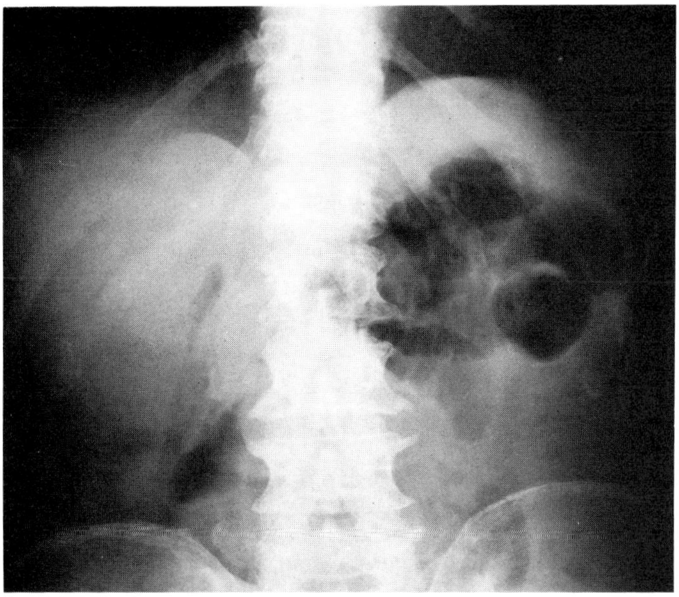

Figure 10–56. Left-sided paraduodenal hernia. Note the dilated loops of small bowel clustered in the left upper abdominal quadrant.

The clinical features vary from mild intermittent digestive complaints to acute intestinal obstruction with volvulus and infarction. A history of previous surgery is frequent since these hernias may be overlooked or inadvertently reduced during surgical exploration. Barium studies are most productive during a symptomatic period. Angiographic features may be striking, consisting of a reversed course of proximal jejunal arteries (Meyers, 1970).

Duodenal Diverticula

Duodenal diverticula are commonly encountered radiographically (1 to 5 per cent of the cases), but infrequently cause symptoms. However, serious complications such as biliary obstruction, perforation, and bleeding may occur and are occasionally life-threatening. The operative mortality in complicated duodenal diverticula approaches 10 per cent (Neill, 1965; Miller, 1970).

Duodenal diverticula are most commonly found along the medial border of the descending duodenum in the periampullary region. They are often multiple, and a significant number occur in the third and fourth portions (30 to 40 per cent); rarely (4 per cent), they occur laterally (Castleman, 1960) (Fig. 10–57). They are acquired lesions consisting of a sac of mucosal and submucosal layers herniated through a muscular defect. They fill and empty by gravity as a result of pressures generated by duodenal peristalsis and are usually identified late during the course of a barium study. The typical smooth rounded shape, frequent changeability, and lack of inflammatory reaction differentiate them from postbulbar ulcers.

Complications are related to pressure on contiguous structures (jaundice, cholangitis, acute and chronic pancreatitis) and inflammation (hemorrhage, perforation, abscess, fistulae) but are infrequently diagnosed radiographically (Neill, 1965; Wolfe, 1972).

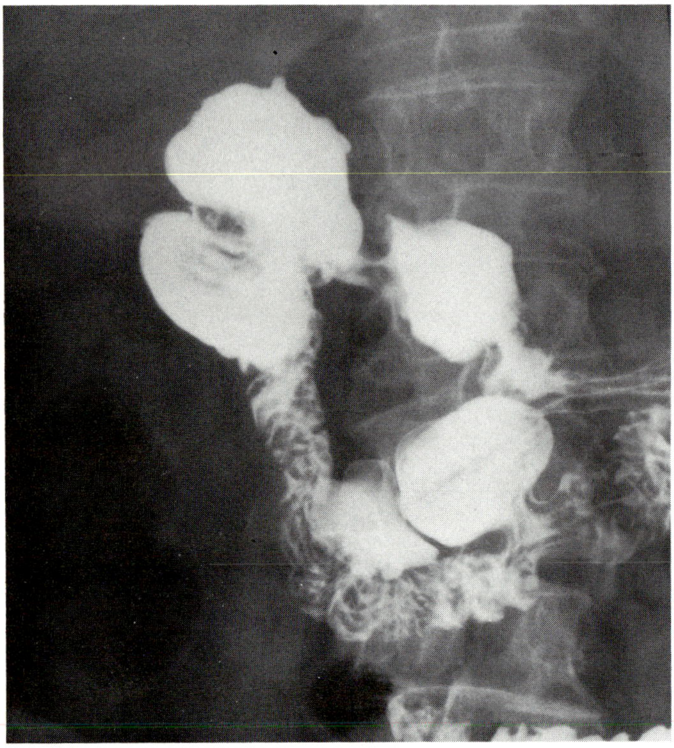

Figure 10–57. Multiple duodenal diverticula creating a bizarre appearance and confusion as to the location of the duodenal cap.

Duodenal diverticula may contain inspissated food particles (enteroliths) (Fig. 10–58) leading to mechanical obstruction of the biliary and pancreatic ducts or to diverticulitis with perforation and bleeding (Curtis, 1966). Diverticular hemorrhage has been demonstrated angiographically (Miller, 1970).

Recently, Costopoulous (1967) has drawn attention to the termination of the common bile and pancreatic ducts into peri-Vaterian diverticula as a cause of cholangitis and pancreatitis. Presumably, this anatomic arrangement interferes with the emptying mechanism of these ductal systems predisposing to stasis and inflammatory sequelae. Disturbance of the ampullary sphincter mechanism probably accounts for the occurrence of spontaneous reflux of barium from the diverticulum into the common bile duct as noted in a case report by Eaton (1969). Usually, the ductal structures enter the neck of the diverticulum but occasionally terminate at the fundus (Culver, 1966) (Fig. 10–59).

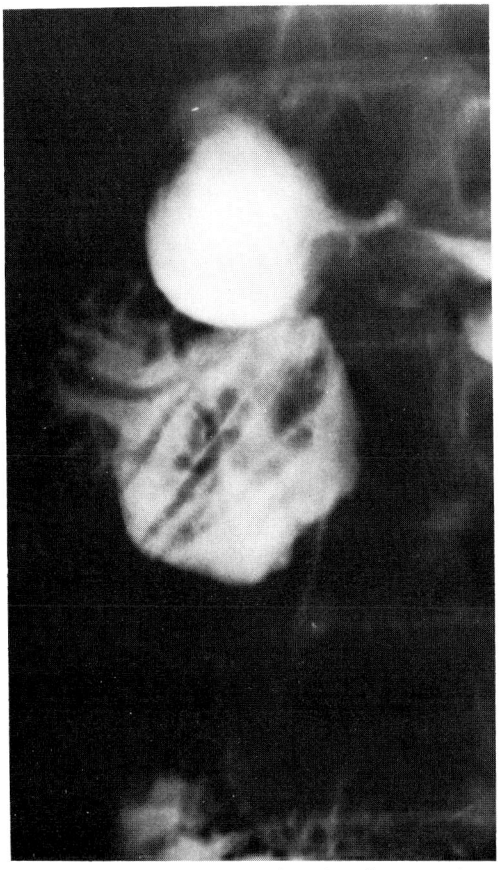

Figure 10–58. Duodenal diverticulum with inspissated material.

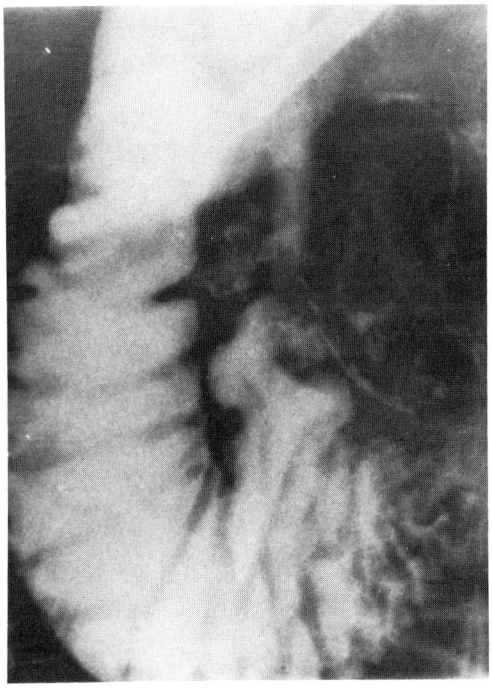

Figure 10–59. Termination of the common bile duct in a periampullary diverticulum. Spontaneous reflux of barium is apparent. This presumably occurs because of the disturbance of the ampullary sphincter mechanism produced by this anatomic configuration. (Reproduced by permission of the *American Journal of Roentgenology and Radium Therapy.*)

REFERENCES

Babb, R. R., Peck, O. C., and Vescia, F. G.: Giardiasis: a cause of traveler's diarrhea. J.A.M.A., *217*:1359–1361, 1971.

Balikian, J. P., Yenikomashian, S. M., and Jidejian, Y. D.: Tuberculosis of the pyloro-duodenal area. A report of four cases. Amer. J. Roentgen., *101*:414–420, 1967.

Ball, R. P., Segal, A. L., and Golden, R.: Postbulbar ulcer of the duodenum. Amer. J. Roentgen., *59*:90–99, 1948.

Bartlett, J. D., Martel, W., and Lindenauer, S. M.:

Right paraduodenal internal hernia. Surg. Gynec. Obstet., *132*:443–449, 1971.

Bateson, E. M.: Duodenal and antral varices. Brit. J. Radiol., *42*:744–747, 1969.

Bayless, T. M., Kapelowitz, R. F., Shelley, W. M., Ballinger, W. F., and Hendrix, T. R.: Intestinal ulceration: a complication of celiac disease. New Eng. J. Med., *276*:996–1002, 1967.

Baum, S., Ward, S., and Nusbaum, M.: Stress bleeding from the mid duodenum. Radiology, *95*:595–602, 1970.

Berk, R. N., and Coulson, D. B.: The body cast syndrome. Radiology, *94*:303–305, 1970.

Berkmen, Y. M., and Rabinowitz, J.: Gastrointestinal manifestations of strongyloidiasis. Amer. J. Roentgen., *115*:306–311, 1972.

Bilbao, M. K., Frische, L. H., Rosch, J., Benson, J. A., and Dotter, C. T.: Post-bulbar duodenal ulcer and ring stricture. Radiology, *100*:27–35, 1971.

Bitner, W. P.: Arteriomesenteric occlusion of duodenum. Amer. J. Roentgen., *79*:807–814, 1958.

Borman, C. N.: Ulcer in the descending duodenum. Amer. J. Roentgen., *50*:752–764, 1943.

Bosse, G., and Neely, J. A.: Roentgenologic findings in primary malignant tumors of the duodenum. Amer. J. Roentgen., *107*:111–118, 1969.

Brenner, R. L., and Brown, C. H.: Primary carcinoma of the duodenum. Gastroenterology, *29*:189–198, 1955.

Bruno, M. S., and Fein, H. D.: Primary malignant and benign tumors of the duodenum. Arch. Intern. Med., *125*:670–679, 1970.

Brust, R., and Chen, K. C.: Acute hemorrhagic pancreatitis complicated by duodenal obstruction. Report of a case. Amer. J. Roentgen., *87*:732–735, 1962.

Burgerman, A., Baggenstoss, A., and Cain, J. C.: Primary malignant neoplasms of the duodenum, excluding the papilla of Vater. Clinicopathological study of 31 cases. Gastroenterology, *30*:421–431, 1956.

Castleman, B.: Case records of the MGH: case 46091. New Eng. J. Med., *262*:462–473, 1960.

Chassin, J. L., and Hinton, J. W.: Primary carcinoma of the duodenal bulb mimicking duodenal ulcer. Gastroenterology, *12*:312–322, 1949.

Christofordisis, A. J., and Nelson, S. W.: Radiological manifestations of ulcerogenic tumors of the pancreas. J.A.M.A., *198*:511–516, 1966.

Cimmino, C. V.: Arteriomesenteric occlusion of the duodenum: an entity? Editorial. Radiology, *76*:828–829, 1961.

Costopoulos, L. B., and Miller, J. D. R.: Insertion of the common bile duct and pancreatic duct into duodenal diverticula. Radiology, *89*:256–262, 1967.

Culver, G. J., and Pirson, H. S.: The roentgenographic findings in 3 cases of termination of the common bile duct in duodenal diverticula. Amer. J. Roentgen., *96*:370–374, 1966.

Curtis, L. E., and O'Grady, T. J.: Duodenal diverticulitis with spontaneous perforation. J.A.M.A., *195*:582–583, 1966.

Dawson, J.: Giant duodenal ulcer. Brit. J. Radiol., *31*:666, 1958.

Eaton, S. B., Berke, R. A., and White, A. F.: Preoperative diagnosis of common bile duct entering a duodenal diverticulum. Amer. J. Roentgen., *107*:43–46, 1969.

Ellison, E. H., and Wilson, S. D.: The Zollinger-Ellison syndrome: re-appraisal and evaluation of 260 registered cases. Ann. Surg., *170*:152, 1964.

Evarts, C. M., Winters, R. B., and Hall, J. E.: Vascular compression of duodenum associated with treatment of scoliosis. J. Bone Joint Surg., *53-A*:431–444, 1971.

Feldman, M.: Clinical Roentgenology of the Digestive Tract. 4th ed. Baltimore, Williams and Wilkins Company, 1957.

Felson, B., and Levin, E.: Intramural hematoma of the duodenum. Radiology, *63*:823–831, 1954.

Ferreira, L. C., and Filho, A. M. S.: Duodenal tuberculosis. Report of a case. Amer. J. Roentgen., *96*:366–369, 1972.

Ferris, D. O., Molnar, G. D., Schnelle, N., Jones, J. D., and Moffitt, E. A.: Recent advances in management of functioning islet cell tumor. Arch. Surg., *104*:443–446, 1972.

Fielding, J. F., Toye, D. K. M., Beton, D. C., and Cooke, W. T.: Crohn's disease of the stomach and duodenum. Gut, *11*:1001–1006, 1970.

Fischer, H. W.: The big duodenum. Amer. J. Roentgen., *83*:861–875, 1960.

Fraser, B. M., Pitman, R. G., Lawrie, J. H., Smith, G. M. R., Forrest, A. P. M., and Rhodes, J.: The significance of the radiological finding of coarse mucosal folds in the duodenum. Lancet, *2*:979–982, 1964.

Freeark, R. J., Corley, R. D., Norcross, W. J., and Baker, R. J.: Unusual aspects of pancreaticoduodenal trauma. J. Trauma, *6*:482–492, 1966.

Freedman, E., Rabwin, M. H., and Sava, M.: Benign and malignant tumors of the duodenum. Radiology, *65*:557–568, 1955.

Goin, L. S., and Wilk, S. P.: Intermittent arteriomesenteric occlusion of duodenum. Radiology, *67*:729–737, 1956.

Gottlieb, C.: Pancreatitis: its pre-operative diagnosis by gastrointestinal roentgenography. Radiology, *56*:528–534, 1951.

Gould, R. J., and Thorwarth, W. T.: Retroperitoneal rupture of the duodenum due to blunt nonpenetrating abdominal trauma. Radiology, *80*:743–747, 1963.

Griffen, W. O., Jr., Schaefer, J. W., Schindler, S., Hyde, G., and Bryant, L. R.: Ampullary obstruction by benign duodenal polyps. Arch. Surg., *97*:444–449, 1968.

Hearn, J. B.: Duodenal ileus with special reference to superior mesenteric artery compression. Radiology, *86*:305–310, 1966.

Hill, M. C.: Roentgen diagnosis of duodenal injuries. Amer. J. Roentgen., *94*:356–361, 1965.

Jones, S. A., Carter, R., Smith, L. L., and Joergenson, E. J.: Arteriomesenteric duodenal compression. Amer. J. Surg., *100*:262–277, 1960.

Kakos, G. S., Grosfeld, J. L., and Morse, T. S.: Small bowel injuries in children after blunt abdominal trauma. Ann. Surg., *174*:238–241, 1971.

Kaufman, S. A., and Levene, G.: Post-bulbar duodenal ulcer. Radiology, *69*:848–852, 1957.

Keats, T. E., and Brady, R. M.: Duodenal involvement in regional enteritis. Amer. J. Roentgen., *77*:639–643, 1957.

Kirsh, I. E., and Brendel, T.: The importance of giant duodenal ulcer. Radiology, *91*:14–19, 1968.

Law, S. W., Searle, N. B., Barton, H. L., and Erickson, E. E.: Regional enteritis of the duodenum. Arch. Surg., *89*:562–569, 1964.

Legge, D. A., Carlson, H. C., and Judd, E. S.: Roentgenologic features of regional enteritis of the upper gastro-intestinal tract. Amer. J. Roentgen., *110*:355–360, 1970.

Louisy, C. L., and Barton, C. J.: The radiological diagnosis of Strongyloides stercoralis enteritis. Radiology, *98*:535–541, 1971.

Marshak, R. H., Ruoff, M., and Lindner, A. E.: Roentgen manifestations of giardiasis. Amer. J. Roentgen., *104*:557–560, 1968.

McGuigan, J. E., and Trudeau, W. L.: Immunochemical measurement of elevated levels of gastrin in the serum of patients with pancreatic tumors of the Zollinger-Ellison variety. New Eng. J. Med., *278*:1308–1313, 1968.

Meyers, M. A.: Paraduodenal hernias: radiologic-arteriographic diagnosis. Radiology, *95*:29–37, 1970.

Meyers, M. A., and King, M. C.: Leiomyosarcoma of duodenum: angiographic findings and report case. Radiology, *91*:788–790, 1968.

Miller, R. E., McCabe, R. E., Salomon, P. F., and Knox, W. G.: Surgical complications of small bowel diverticula exclusive of Meckels. Ann. Surg., *171*:202–210, 1970.

Mindell, H. J., and Holm, J. L.: Acute superior mesenteric artery syndrome. Radiology, *94*: 299–302, 1970.

Mistilis, S. P., Wiot, J. F., and Nedelman, S. M.: Giant duodenal ulcers. Ann. Intern. Med., *59*:155–164, 1963.

Neill, S. A., and Thompson, N. W.: The complications of duodenal diverticula and their management. Surg. Gynec. Obstet., *120*:1251–1258, 1965.

Nelson, S. W.: Some interesting and unusual manifestations of Crohn's disease ("regional enteritis") of the stomach, duodenum, and small intestine. Amer. J. Roentgen., *107*:86–101, 1969.

Nugent, F. W., Braasch, J. W., and Epstein, H.: Diagnosis and surgical treatment of arteriomesenteric obstruction of the duodenum. J.A.M.A., *196*:1091–1093, 1966.

Oberhelman, H. A.: Excisional therapy for ulcerogenic tumors of duodenum. Arch. Surg., *104*: 447–453, 1972.

Ochsner, S., and Kleckner, M. S., Jr.: Primary malignant neoplasms of the duodenum. J.A.M.A., *163*:413–417, 1957.

Oh, C., and Jemerin, E. E.: Benign adenomatous polyps of the papilla of Vater. Surgery, *57*: 495–503, 1965.

Ogbuokiri, C. G., Law, E. J., and MacMillian, B. G.: Superior mesenteric artery syndrome in burned children. Amer. J. Surg., *124*:75–79, 1972.

Ostrum, H. W., and Serber, W.: Tuberculosis of the stomach and duodenum. Amer. J. Roentgen., *60*:315–322, 1948.

Paterson, D. E., and Hancock, D. M.: Duodenal stenosis due to postbulbar ulcer. Brit. J. Radiol., *31*:660–665, 1958.

Poppel, M. H., Jacobson, H. G., and Smith, R. W.: The Roentgen Aspects of the Papilla and Ampulla of Vater. Springfield, Ill., Charles C Thomas, Publisher, 1953.

Resnick, H. P., and Cooper, P. R.: Carcinoma of the duodenum: Review of the literature from 1948 to 1956. Amer. J. Surg., *95*:946–952, 1958.

Rider, R. F.: Giant duodenal ulceration. J.A.M.A., *209*:408–409, 1969.

Ring, E. J., Ferrucci, J. T., Eaton, S. B., and Clements, J. L.: Villous adenomas of the duodenum. Radiology, *104*:45–48, 1972.

Roman, E., Silva, Y. J., and Lucas, C.: Management of blunt duodenal injury. Surg. Gynec. Obstet., *132*:7–14, 1971.

Rosenquist, C. J.: Clinical and radiographic features of giant duodenal ulcer. Clin. Radiol., *20*:324–328, 1969.

Simon, M., and Lerner, M. A.: Duodenal compression by the mesenteric root in acute pancreatitis and in inflammatory conditions of the bowel. Radiology, *79*:75–81, 1962.

Stassa, G., and Klingensmith, W. C.: Primary tumor of the duodenal bulb. Amer. J. Roentgen., *107*:105–110, 1969.

Teplick, J. G.: Duodenal loop changes in posterior penetration of duodenal ulcer. Ann. Intern. Med., *44*:958–974, 1956.

Toxopeus, M. D., Lucas, C. E., and Krabbenhoft, K. L.: Roentgenographic diagnosis in blunt retroperitoneal duodenal rupture. Amer. J. Roentgen., *115*:281–288, 1972.

Wallace, R. G., and Howard, W. B.: Acute superior mesenteric artery syndrome in the severely burned patient. Radiology, *94*:307–310, 1970.

Weichart, R. F., Roth, L. M., Krementz, E. T., Hewitt, R. L., and Drapanas, J.: Carcinoid islet cell tumors of duodenum. Amer. J. Surg., *121*:195–205, 1971.

Weinberg, P. E., and Levin, B.: Hyperplasia of Brunner's glands. Radiology, *84*:259–262, 1965.

Wilkie, D. P. D.: Chronic duodenal ileus. Brit. J. Surg., *9*:204, 1921.

Wilson, J. W., and Wilson, B. J.: Pseudo-ulceration of the stomach and duodenum produced by traction diverticulum. Amer. J. Roentgen., *75*:297–307, 1956.

Wolfe, R. D., and Pearl, M. J.: Acute perforation of duodenal diverticulum with roentgenographic demonstration of localized retroperitoneal emphysema. Radiology, *104*:301–302, 1972.

Zboralske, F. F., and Amberg, J. R.: Detection of the Zollinger-Ellison syndrome: the radiologist's responsibility. Amer. J. Roentgen., *104*: 529–543, 1968.

Zollinger, R. M., and Moore, F. T.: Zollinger-Ellison comes of age. J.A.M.A., *204*:361–365, 1968.

Chapter 11

THE RADIOLOGY OF SELECTED PANCREATIC DISORDERS

The clinical data in any given case affect radiologic evaluation of the patient in at least three major ways. First, the *choice* of examination to be performed must be determined by the type of pathologic condition clinically suspected. Secondly, the technical *performance* of any given examination is influenced significantly by the historic, physical and laboratory data available. Finally, the authors believe that optimal *interpretation* of radiologic examinations requires careful correlation of the radiographic findings with pertinent clinical information.

This chapter attempts to provide a scaffolding of clinical material appropriate for radiologic evaluation of the most important pancreatic disorders. While it is outside the scope of this book to attempt a comprehensive, in-depth clinical analysis of pancreatic disease, it is hoped that these brief accounts, together with the references provided, will serve as a starting point for more clinically oriented pancreatic radiology.

The strictly radiologic material in this chapter has been covered in a brief manner since individual signs have already been discussed at greater length in earlier chapters. Here, however, the radiographic manifestations of more important pancreatic disease conditions are grouped together and treated as components of a specific clinicoradiologic whole. In other words, coverage is "disease-oriented" rather than "sign-oriented" as it has been in previous chapters.

PANCREATIC CANCER

Introduction

While radiologic diagnosis of pancreatic cancer has for many years been a topic of considerable interest to radiologists and clinicians interested in gastrointestinal tract disease, the condition itself has popularly been considered uncommon or even rare. Recently, however, the increasing frequency of this deadly malignancy has become recognized (Stephenson, 1972). Over the past 50 years, the mortality rate due to pancreatic carcinoma has risen at a pace exceeded only by bronchogenic carcinoma (Beall, 1970). Between 1920 and 1965, there was a 383 per cent increment in the age-adjusted mortality rate for pancreatic cancer (Krain, 1970). American Cancer Society statistics indicate that cancer of the pancreas is currently the fourth leading cause of cancer death in men and the sixth leading cause of cancer death in women (Silverberg, 1972). In 1972, 19,100 Americans were estimated to have pancreatic cancer—a value distinctly above that for gastric cancer (16,800) and reasonably close to that for malignancies of the rectum (21,000). Present trends indicate a steady further increase over the coming decade (Silverberg, 1972).

The presentation, course, and prognosis of patients with pancreatic carcinoma depend to a considerable degree on the location of the tumor. Neoplasms arising in the head differ significantly in clinical and radiologic characteristics from those which develop in the remainder of the organ. About 70 per cent of all pancreatic tumors involve the head of the gland; approximately 25 per cent are confined to the body and/or tail while in the remainder the entire gland is involved. Tumors of the head of the pancreas are often included in the "pancreaticoduodenal" category. This grouping includes other neoplasms (such as cancer of the duodenum, ampulla of Vater, and distal common bile duct) which occur within the confines of the duodenal loop. These lesions can produce fairly similar clinical manifestations and may have such similar histologic features that pathologic distinction between them becomes difficult or impossible (Frantz, 1959).

Pancreaticoduodenal Cancer

Clinical Features (Table 11–1)

Most pancreaticoduodenal carcinomas occur in patients within the 50 to 70 age range, but numerous patients under 30 and others over 90 have been reported. Males are somewhat more commonly affected than females (in approximately a 2:1 ratio) (Braganza, 1972). *Jaundice* is the dominant symptom or finding in most cases and occurs in from 60 to 95 per cent of patients in this category depending upon the series analyzed (Eaton, 1970*a*; Bowden, 1972). Such jaundice is usually relentlessly progressive although, in occasional patients with periampullary neoplasms, fluctuations in serum bilirubin may be noted (Warren, 1968). Painless jaundice has long been considered the hallmark of cancer arising in the head of the pancreas, but actually most patients (60 to 75 per cent) suffer

TABLE 11–1. Pancreaticoduodenal Cancer

Symptom	*Incidence (%)*
Jaundice	60–90
Epigastric pain	60–75
Back pain	20
Weight loss	75–80
Anorexia	Usually present
Pruritus	20–40
Physical Finding	
Hepatomegaly	50–70
Palpable gallbladder	5–30
Laboratory Value	
Abnormal glucose tolerance	Up to 90
Amylase	Normal, elevated, or low
Elevated bilirubin	60–90
Elevated alkaline phosphatase	75 or more
Serum albumin, SGOT, LDH, cephalin flocculation	Usually near normal except late in course
Anemia	About 33
Occult stool blood	About 25

from dull, steady, and often intense epigastric *pain.* Radiation to the back is less frequent than in patients with carcinoma of the body or tail, but occurs in about 20 per cent of cases. *Weight loss* (usually associated with *anorexia* and often marked in degree) has been noted by the majority of patients (75 to 80 per cent), and *pruritus* occurs in a significant minority (20 to 40 per cent). *Hepatomegaly* is present in most patients (50 to 70 per cent), but a *palpable gallbladder* can be detected in less than a third (5 to 30 per cent). Over the years, Courvoisier's observation that a palpable gallbladder in the presence of painless jaundice should suggest a malignant periampullary pathologic condition has been well substantiated, but such disease certainly cannot be excluded merely because the gallbladder is not palpable.

Laboratory findings in pancreaticoduodenal cancer are generally nonspecific. An abnormal *glucose tolerance* test is very common in patients with carcinoma of the head of the pancreas (88 per cent in the Cleveland Clinic series) (Rastogi, 1967), but serum *amylase* can be elevated, normal, or low (Klintrup, 1966). If jaundice is present, *hyperbilirubinemia* is frequently intense, but whether "liver chemistries" can reliably detect extrahepatic biliary obstruction is a matter of debate. Classically, in such cases, tests of hepatic excretory function (e.g., direct bilirubin and serum *alkaline phosphatase* levels) will be found to be abnormal, whereas tests reflecting hepatic synthetic function (e.g., serum *proteins, SGOT,* etc.) will remain within normal limits. Warren and his colleagues (1968) feel that this pattern is accurate in the majority of instances, but Rastogi and Brown (1967) have held that arbitrary levels for serum alkaline phosphatase fail to distinguish medical from surgical jaundice. Most authors agree that if jaundice has been present for a lengthy period, laboratory studies are of considerably less value in indicating the nature of the icterus than if jaundice is of recent onset. *Anemia* is present in about a third of all patients with pancreaticoduodenal malignancy and occult *stool blood* can be found in nearly a quarter. Tumors of the duodenum, the ampulla of Vater and also the head of the pancreas can all produce gastrointestinal bleeding which, therefore, has little value in differentiating between them.

Radiologic Features

BARIUM EXAMINATION OF THE UPPER GASTROINTESTINAL TRACT. For the most part, the different types of tumor included in the pancreaticoduodenal category produce indistinguishable findings on barium upper gastrointestinal examination (Hodes, 1954). Lesions arising in this area cause changes involving the distal gastric antrum and the inner aspect of the duodenal loop. The basic roentgen abnormalities include *mass indentation, mucosal fold distortion* and, in some instances, *ulceration, stricture formation,* and even *obstruction.* The prominence of abnormalities demonstrated on barium study bears little relation to the size of the lesion present. Small, strategically placed tumors (i.e., close to the duodenum or stomach) can be shown at a much earlier stage than larger lesions which arise at a point relatively removed from viscera which can be opacified by barium (Russell, 1965).

A detailed description of individual findings, together with a discussion of pertinent differential features, can be found in Chapters 3 and 4. In the stomach, the most typical alteration is an *"antral pad sign"*—an indentation defect on the greater curvature of the gastric antrum (Case, 1940). Extrinsic pressure along the concavity of the duodenal loop is the commonest duodenal finding in patients with pancreaticoduodenal malignancy. Such pressure may take the form of localized *nodular indentation* (Fig. 11–1) or of a larger *mass impression* involving much of the inner duodenal margin. In its subtlest form, only a *"double contour"* effect may be present. This sign results from differential filling of the duodenum: the interfold spaces along the inner aspect of the loop contain less barium than the corresponding spaces along the outer aspect (Eyler, 1962). The *"inverted '3' sign"* of Frostberg (1938) (Fig. 11–2) and generalized widening of the loop are other frequently described abnormalities produced by extrinsic pressure resulting from pancreaticoduodenal malignancy. When the latter is present, the condition is usually far advanced. Other signs usually indicating relatively advanced disease are *postbulbar ulceration* and *obstruction* of the duodenum which are uncommon but occasionally encountered manifestations of tumors in this area.

Salik (1961) emphasized the importance of mucosal fold alterations in the early recognition of pancreatic carcinoma. A brush- or spike-like configuration is one common pattern; this is sometimes referred to as *spiculation* (Eaton, 1970*b*). Orientation of the folds in divergent di-

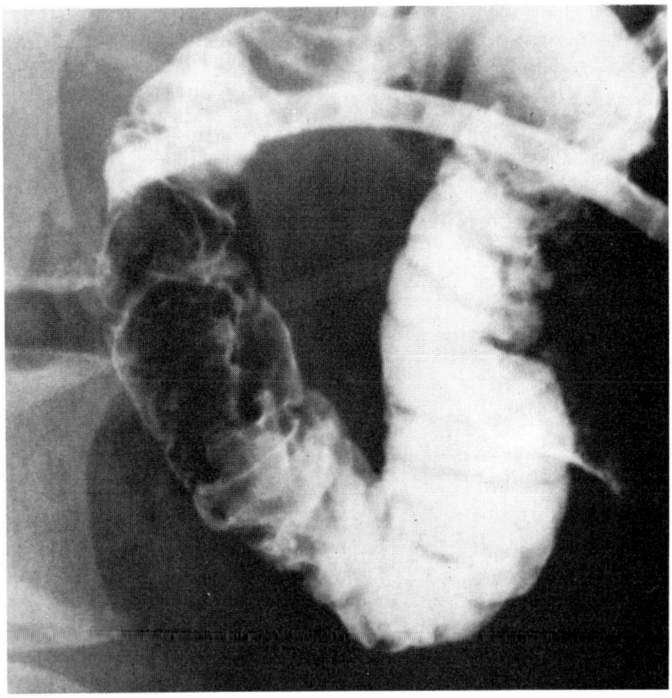

Figure 11–1. Irregularly nodular indentation in area of duodenal papilla produced by periampullary pancreatic carcinoma. Hypotonic duodenogram (conventional upper gastrointestinal barium examination two weeks earlier had been considered "negative"). (Reproduced by permission of *New England Journal of Medicine.* From Current concepts: radiology of the pancreas. New Eng. J. Med., 288:506–510, 1973.)

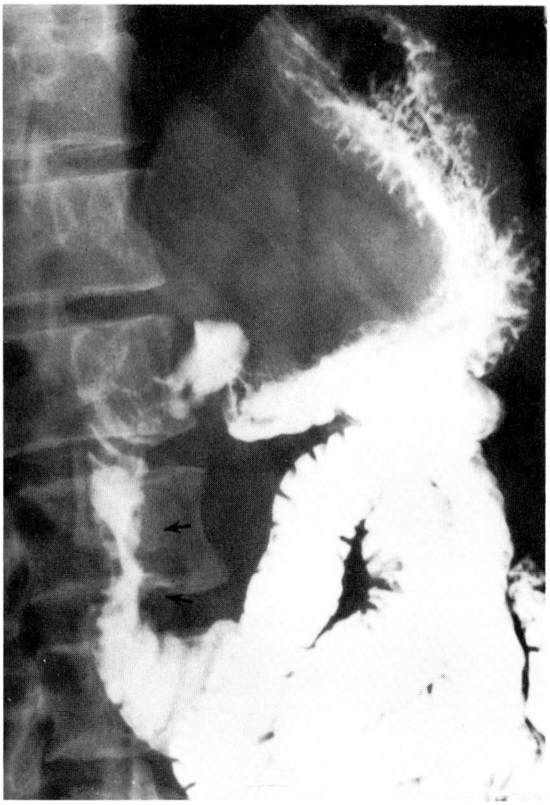

Figure 11–2. Inverted "3" indentation (Frostberg's sign) along inner border of descending duodenum, produced by carcinoma arising in head of pancreas. Conventional upper gastrointestinal barium examination.

rections and elongation of individual folds are other, somewhat less frequent, abnormalities of this nature.

When pancreaticoduodenal malignancies produce extrahepatic biliary obstruction, the resulting enlargement of the common bile duct and gallbladder may produce *indentation deformities* of the duodenum (see Chapter 5). Hodes and his colleagues (1954) described the defect produced by common-duct dilatation as a "pencil-like" extrinsic compression on the immediate postbulbar portion of the duodenum while an enlarged gallbladder usually produces a smooth curved indentation on the outer border of the upper descending duodenum.

Dynamic features (i.e., abnormalities of duodenal motility) have been considered to be valuable signs by some authors (e.g., Salik, 1961; Beranbaum, 1966), but others (e.g., Adler, 1967), including ourselves, have little faith in disordered duodenal peristalsis as an indicator of pancreaticoduodenal cancer.

Prior to 1965, an accurate preoperative diagnosis of pancreaticoduodenal malignancy was made by barium examination in approximately 30 to 50 per cent of the cases (Perez, 1965). As early as 1961, however, Salik (1961) predicted that a correct prospective diagnosis might be made in as many as 75 to 85 per cent of such patients. Eyler and his co-workers (1962) and Perez and his associates (1965) concurred that increased diagnostic accuracy should be possible; they emphasized the importance of satisfactory duodenal delineation and of attention to subtle radiographic abnormalities.

In 1965, a French monograph on hypotonic duodenography appeared (Jacquemet, 1965). The authors analyzed results of their experience with over 500 patients who had been studied by means of this technique. Of their patients with carcinoma of the head of the pancreas, this technique allowed a correct diagnosis in 76 per cent while in their patients with tumors of the ampulla of Vater, accuracy was 92 per cent. American experience with this procedure promptly verified French results. Bilbao and her colleagues (1968) reported 84 per cent and Eaton and his co-workers (1968), 78 per cent correct diagnoses in pancreaticoduodenal malignancy. Subsequently, various other reports (e.g., Martel, 1969; Bourke, 1972) have presented results indicating similar success with hypotonic duodenography. Since the radiographic abnormalities demonstrated by hypotonic duodenography are no different from those shown by conventional upper gastrointestinal barium examinations, the authors feel that these improved results have fully justified the earlier predictions of Salik, Eyler, and Perez.

ANGIOGRAPHY. Angiographic criteria employed for diagnosis of tumors arising in the pancreaticoduodenal area are similar to those used to show lesions in the body or tail of the pancreas and include *arterial stenosis* (encasement or "tumor cuffing"), *arterial occlusion, vascular displacement* (either arterial or venous), tumor *neovascularity,* and *venous compression* or *occlusion.* Since pancreatic adenocarcinoma and the other tumors in the pancreaticoduodenal group are relatively avascular, direct angiographic evidence of malignancy (i.e., neovascularity-tumor vessels or "stain") is uncommon (Nebesar, 1967). The arterial change most characteristic of the disease is an area of serrated, irregular stenosis. Arterial occlusion is another finding relatively specific for carcinoma, but smooth arterial narrowing is nonspecific (being found in some cases of chronic pancreatitis as well as in pancreatic neoplasms). Vascular displacement is seldom pronounced because of the infiltrative (rather than expansile) nature of tumors in this area. The importance of venous stenosis or occlusion for the diagnosis of pancreatic malignancy was first demonstrated by splenoportography (Rosch, 1964). Nebesar and Pollard (1967) felt that the most reliable angiographic evidence of pancreatic malignancy was a combination of arterial and venous abnormalities located in the same vicinity. More recently, Buranasiri and Baum (1972) showed that venous stenosis or occlusion was evident in fully 98 per cent of their documented cases of pancreatic cancer.

Pancreaticoduodenal neoplasms generally produce angiographic abnormalities in the hepatic, gastroduodenal, and pancreaticoduodenal arteries (Fig. 11–3) and in the superior mesenteric and portal veins (Fig. 11–4). When gallbladder enlargement results from pancreaticoduodenal disease, the distended gallbladder can usually be shown during angiographic study either by the configuration of the cystic artery or by demonstration of the gallbladder wall itself during the parenchymal phase of the examination. The accuracy of angiographic diagnosis is slightly lower for pancreaticoduodenal tumors than for carcinoma of the body or tail of the pancreas, because very small tumors located near the common bile duct can produce clinical manifestations while they are still undetectable by angiography. In contrast, tumors of the body or tail of the pancreas usually become quite bulky before producing symptoms which might lead to angiographic study. Such tumors are generally amenable to angiographic demonstration. The angiography of pancreatic disease is discussed in detail in Chapter 7.

The diagnostic accuracy of angiography in patients with pancreatic cancers of all sorts has improved dramatically over the past few years. In 1967, Nebesar and Pollard reported 29 per cent correct prospective diagnoses. In 1969, Bookstein and his co-authors reported preoperative accuracy of 76 per cent. More recently, in 1972, Buranasiri and Baum were able to record a prospective diagnostic accuracy of greater than 90 per cent. As previously noted, angiographic accuracy is slightly lower for pancreaticoduodenal tumors than for lesions of the body or tail of the pancreas, presumably because some of the former are very small lesions whereas nearly all the latter are relatively large by the time patients are referred for angiographic examination.

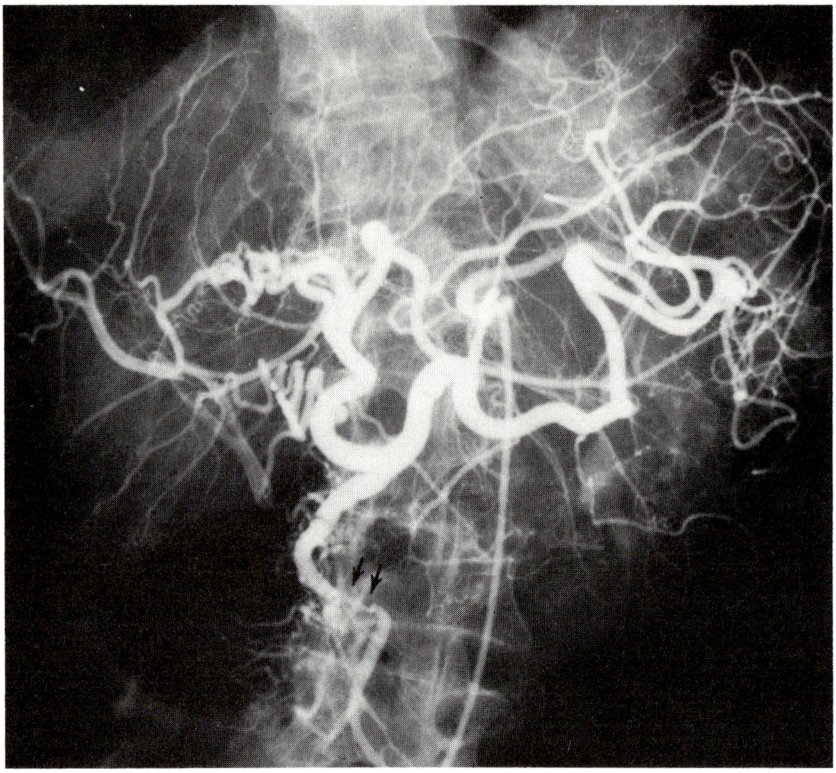

Figure 11–3. Celiac arteriogram. "Encasement" of gastroduodenal artery produced by carcinoma arising in head of pancreas.

Hepatobiliary examinations. In most instances where pancreaticoduodenal malignancies produce jaundice, the degree of hyperbilirubinemia present precludes oral or intravenous cholangiography. In such circumstances, radioisotopic studies may provide useful information and transhepatic cholangiography may allow specific diagnosis. Many patients who present with symptoms suggesting carcinoma of the head of the pancreas undergo radioisotopic *liver imaging* with ^{99m}*Tc sulfur colloid* more as part of their general diagnostic evaluation than in a specific attempt to identify extrahepatic biliary obstruction. Clinicians in such cases are usually looking for evidence of hepatic metastasis or of intrinsic hepatocellular disease. Such evidence—especially the former—is, of course, of great diagnostic significance. There is, however, one scintigraphic finding directly applicable to the diagnosis of extrahepatic biliary obstruction—demonstration of dilated biliary radicals at the porta hepatis (Heck, 1971). Typically, the porta hepatis appears enlarged and differentiation of biliary ductal dilatation from metastatic lymphadenopathy at the porta is impossible under these circumstances. In some instances, however, a characteristic branching pattern is present (Chapter 5) and this finding is essentially pathognomonic for extrahepatic biliary obstruction.

Evaluation of the liver by *radioiodinated rose bengal examination* can provide information regarding the integrity of the extrahepatic biliary ducts when serum bilirubin elevation is far above levels where study by intravenous cholangiography might be considered. Free passage of radioactivity from the liver into the intestinal tract excludes malig-

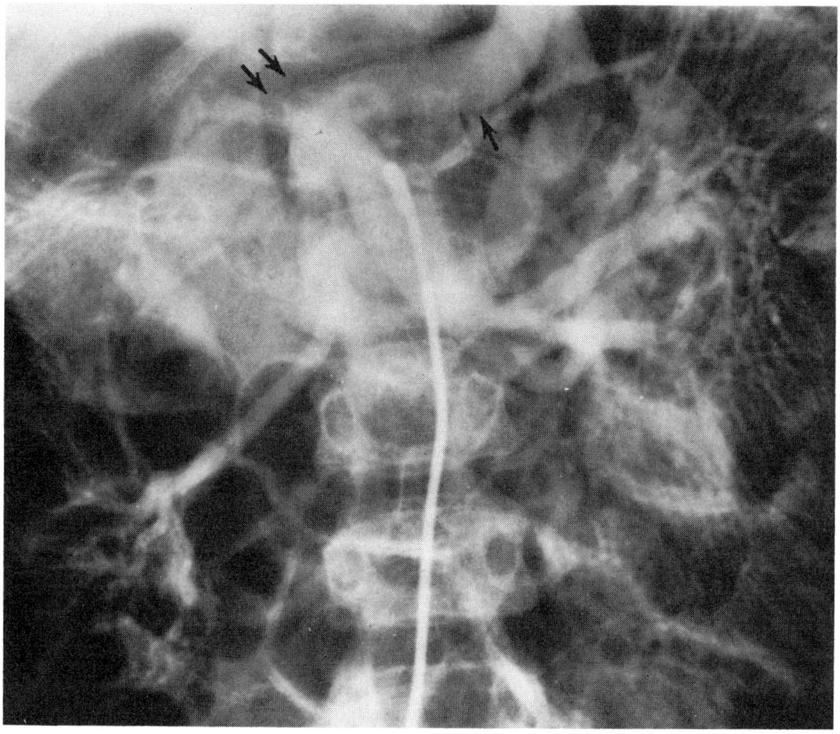

Figure 11–4. Portal vein occlusion (*double arrows*) resulting from carcinoma arising in head of pancreas. Venous phase roentgenogram made after superior mesenteric artery injection. Note hepatofugal flow of contrast into splenic vein (*single arrow*).

nant biliary obstruction with high reliability (Greene, 1972). Failure of radioactivity to appear in the gut, however, can result from either severe hepatocellular disease or from obstruction of the bile ducts. To allow distinction between these alternatives in at least some cases, a hepatic rose bengal clearance determination is carried out shortly after administration of radioiodinated rose bengal. Normally, no more than 55 per cent of the baseline value should remain in the blood 20 minutes after administration. If 90 per cent (or more) of the baseline value remains in a patient who has no passage of radioactivity into the gut, hepatocellular disease is considered the cause. If, in a patient with similar failure of radioactivity to enter the gut, the 20-minute value is 70 per cent (or less) of the baseline, extrahepatic obstruction is diagnosed. In patients whose blood retention falls between 70 and 90 per cent, the results are considered inconclusive and distinction between intra- and extrahepatic obstruction cannot be justified (see Chapter 5).

To an increasing extent, patients with jaundice and in whom a specific diagnosis cannot be established by other diagnostic maneuvers (e.g., barium studies, angiography, etc.) are being studied by *transhepatic cholangiography.* The technique for and possible complications of this procedure are detailed elsewhere (Chapter 5). Pancreaticoduodenal lesions which produce jaundice usually have pronounced dilatation of the intrahepatic biliary radicals and are thus ideal candidates for successful duct opacification. In recent series, the incidence of successful studies under these circumstances has varied from 84 to 92 per cent (Mujahed, 1966; Ritchie, 1969).

The sine qua non for cholangiographic

diagnosis of obstructive jaundice is demonstration of biliary ductal dilatation down to a point of occlusion, marked narrowing, or other distortion with little or no passage of contrast into the duodenum. In most cases of pancreaticoduodenal malignancy, the point of occlusion occurs in the distal common bile duct but, when there has been metastatic spread to the porta hepatis, the obstruction is higher—often at the junction of the right and left hepatic ducts. The configuration of the most distal portion of the opacified duct may be raggedly irregular, asymmetrically tapered, or have a "rat-tail" appearance (see Chapter 5). These patterns are all considered indicative of neoplastic obstruction. In other instances, the end of the common duct may appear smoothly blunted (Fig. 11–5). This pattern is nonspecific but it does provide confirmation of extrahepatic biliary obstruction and this, taken together with other clinical and radiologic features, usually allows a confident diagnosis.

Several recent reports (e.g., Rossi, 1970) have suggested that colloidal hepatic radiopharmaceuticals are capable of demonstrating liver metastasis by hepatic scintigraphy in approximately 80 to 85 per cent of patients in whom such involvement is present. The reliability of this technique for detection of extrahepatic biliary obstruction (as evidenced by ductal dilatation at the porta hepatis) has been well-documented. In a retrospective study, Heck and Gottschalk (1971) derived data suggesting that such diagnosis is possible in approximately 80 per cent of patients with this condition.

Several recent clinical investigations (e.g., Freeman, 1966; Greene, 1972) have suggested that, when serial abdominal images made after administration of radioiodinated rose bengal are analyzed together with blood clearance data from the same patient, extrahepatic biliary obstruction can be identified with greater than 90 per cent accuracy. The combined study is more reliable than either component taken alone (Nordyke, 1965; Eyler, 1965).

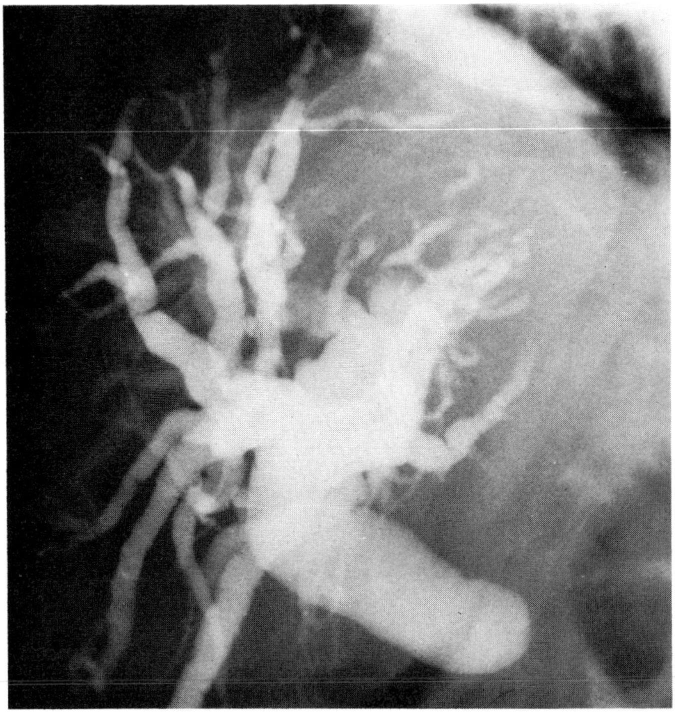

Figure 11–5. Percutaneous transhepatic cholangiogram. Complete obstruction of common bile duct produced by carcinoma arising in head of pancreas. Smoothly blunted ending is nonspecific but is commonly seen in patients with this condition.

Transhepatic cholangiography is "successful" (i.e., achieves satisfactory ductal opacification) in 85 to 90 per cent of patients who have extrahepatic biliary obstruction due to pancreaticoduodenal carcinoma (Ritchie, 1969; Mujahed, 1966). In nearly all of these patients, accurate distinction between obstruction and nonobstructive jaundice is possible as is demonstration of the site of obstruction. Identification of the nature of the underlying pathologic process is more difficult and figures relating to this point are infrequently reported. Seldinger's (1966) data suggest that an exact etiologic diagnosis can be made about 80 per cent of the time.

^{75}Se SELENOMETHIONINE PANCREATIC IMAGING. Normal pancreatic acinar cells have an extremely high rate of amino-acid utilization since their protein synthetic activity (for manufacture of digestive enzyme proteins) is higher than that of any other body tissue. In consequence, ^{75}Se selenomethionine (an effective amino-acid analogue) is rapidly accumulated by normal pancreas. Pancreatic adenocarcinomas are "dedifferentiated" and their protein synthetic activity is much less than that of normal pancreatic acinar tissue. In consequence, pancreatic carcinomas appear as areas of decreased radioactivity on pancreatic scintigrams (in comparison with adjacent normal pancreatic tissue).

Carcinomas of the head of the pancreas tend to decrease pancreatic ^{75}Se selenomethionine accumulation by a second mechanism as well. Most of these tumors produce blockage of the main pancreatic duct (of Wirsung). Such obstruction results in a secondary inhibition of exocrine pancreatic synthetic activity "up stream" from the site of blockage. In consequence, amino-acid incorporation in the body and tail of the pancreas is markedly diminished. Accordingly, abdominal images made after administration of ^{75}Se selenomethionine to patients with pancreaticoduodenal carcinoma often fail to reveal any accumulation of radioactivity in the pancreas. This pattern is observed in approximately 60 per cent of patients with pancreaticoduodenal cancer (McCarthy, 1972). Presumably, in the remainder the main pancreatic duct is not occluded by the tumor mass and, therefore, amino-acid metabolism (and, hence, ^{75}Se selenomethionine uptake) in the majority of the pancreas is unimpaired. In these instances (approximately 40 per cent of all pancreaticoduodenal tumor cases [McCarthy, 1972]), localized "cold areas" in the head of the gland are commonly demonstrated.

Generally speaking, normal pancreatic images are fairly reliable evidence against the presence of pancreatic cancer, but abnormal images are often falsely positive (Bouchier, 1972). In Chapter 6, results of over 2000 pancreatic imaging studies are discussed. An analysis of these data indicates that in about 10 per cent of these examinations, false-negative diagnoses were made while in approximately 30 per cent, false-positive diagnoses were given. Typical recent investigations (e.g., Landman, 1971; McCarthy, 1969) suggest very low false-negative rates (5 to 7 per cent) with regard to the diagnosis of pancreatic cancer, but the incidence of false-positive scintigrams remains high. Abnormal pancreatic images in patients with no pancreatic disease (except for diabetes in some cases) were obtained in 15 to 40 per cent of the examinations. Relative accuracy of pancreatic radionuclide imaging in patients with pancreaticoduodenal neoplasms in comparison with patients whose lesions are in the body or tail of the pancreas has been detailed in only a few articles. If data from four studies (Eaton, 1968; Heslip, 1971; Miale, 1972; and McCarthy, 1972) are pooled, pancreatic scintigraphy was abnormal in 87 of 93 patients with pancreaticoduodenal cancer (94 per cent). It should be noted that tumors of the common bile duct or ampulla of Vater as well as small tumors arising in the head of the pancreas may produce jaundice at a time when ^{75}Se selenomethionine pancreatic images appear normal. The only patients with pancreatic cancer who had false-negative pancreatic scintigrams in the series cited had lesions of this type.

ULTRASONIC EXAMINATIONS OF THE PANCREAS. In Chapter 9, the application of ultrasonic abdominal imaging to the detection of pancreatic disease is discussed in detail. Briefly, most authors (e.g., Filly, 1970; Russell, 1972) feel that the normal pancreas cannot be outlined as a distinct organ. Pancreatic carcinomas greater than 3 cm. in diameter can often be demonstrated as irregular masses in the pancreatic area (Engelhart, 1970). At relatively low ultrasonic intensity, such lesions appear transonic but, when the intensity is increased, ultrasonic inhomogeneity is produced. This helps to distinguish solid from cystic masses since the latter remain transonic (i.e., sonically "hollow") even on high-intensity scans.

Lesions in the head, body and tail of the pancreas seem equally demonstrable by echography (Filly, 1970) but, in pancreaticoduodenal tumors associated with jaundice, gallbladder distention can be readily shown and, in some instances, even dilated intrahepatic biliary radicals are apparent (see Chapter 9). These secondary findings may help point to the correct diagnosis and make abdominal echography especially valuable for evaluation of suspected pancreaticoduodenal malignancy.

Since abdominal echography is truly in its infancy, extensive reliability statistics relevant to detection of pancreatic malignancy are unavailable. In one series (Filly, 1970), four of five pancreatic carcinomas were demonstrated preoperatively. The authors estimate that 3-cm. lesions are the smallest that can currently be detected. In the same investigation, there were 11 other patients in whom pancreatic tumor was clinically suspected. Of these, six had peripancreatic mass lesions. Three of these were ultrasonically indistinguishable from pancreatic carcinoma, two could be identified as masses separate from the pancreas and, in one (a common-duct carcinoma), the echogram was considered normal. In the remaining five patients, none of whom actually had mass lesions, a pancreatic tumor was ultrasonically suspected in one instance. These figures, while limited, may be considered representative of current echographic accuracy in detecting pancreatic cancer.

Carcinoma of the Body and Tail of the Pancreas

Clinical Features (Table 11–2)

Cancer of the body or tail of the pancreas, like pancreaticoduodenal cancer, develops most commonly in patients 50 to 70 years old, but numerous individual patients under 30 and over 90 have been recorded. In most reports (e.g., Mani, 1966), the sex ratio is similar to that for pancreaticoduodenal cancer (approximately a 2:1 male preponder-

TABLE 11–2. Cancer of the Body or Tail of the Pancreas

Symptom	*Incidence (%)*
Abdominal pain	75–95
Back pain	About 40
Weight loss	65–100
Anorexia, weakness	Common
Depression, anxiety	Up to 20
Peripheral venous thrombosis	2–4
Physical Finding	
Jaundice	20
Hepatomegaly	30–60
Upper abdominal mass	20–50
Ascites	10
Laboratory Value	
Abnormal glucose tolerance	Up to 60
Anemia	Up to 60
Occult stool blood	Infrequent
Elevated alkaline phosphatase	Nearly 50
Elevated bilirubin	About 20
Amylase	Normal, elevated, or low

ance). This disease is probably the most insidious of all forms of cancer in onset and early symptomatology (Bowden, 1972). *Abdominal pain* occurs in 75 to 95 per cent of these patients and is usually the presenting complaint (Eaton, 1970*a*; Braganza, 1972). *Radiation of pain to the back* occurs in about 40 per cent of cases. *Weight loss* is another extremely common symptom and is noted in 65 to 100 per cent of patients with cancer of the body or tail of the pancreas, depending on the series analyzed. The amount of weight lost is frequently impressive. *Anorexia, weakness* and other nonspecific symptoms are common.

Many patients with cancer of the body or tail of the pancreas are initially believed to have psychiatric disorders (Bowden, 1972). Depression and anxiety are common in these individuals (Fras, 1968) and their vague abdominal pain is frequently misinterpreted as a psychoneurotic manifestation. In one series (Rastogi, 1967), definite *psychiatric symptoms* were considered to be present in 19 per cent of their patients with pancreatic cancer.

The frequency of *peripheral venous thrombosis* (Trousseau's phenomenon) in carcinoma of the body and tail of the pancreas has been debated since Sproul (1938) called attention to this relationship 35 years ago. In most recent reports (e.g., Ansari, 1968; Rastogi, 1967), the incidence of this phenomenon has been low (e.g., 2 to 4 per cent), yet, as stressed by Warren (1968), patients who present with migratory thrombophlebitis merit pancreatic investigation.

Jaundice develops in approximately 20 per cent of patients with carcinoma of the body or tail of the pancreas, but it differs in important respects from that which can be observed in patients with pancreaticoduodenal cancer. It is rarely the presenting symptom and is almost never painless. Jaundice is usually the presenting complaint in patients with pancreaticoduodenal malignancy and, in 25 to 40 per cent of these cases, there is no associated pain. These differences result from the fact that jaundice in patients with carcinoma of the body or tail of the pancreas nearly always results from metastasis to the porta hepatis and/or liver parenchyma, whereas in pancreaticoduodenal lesions, the primary tumor itself produces mechanical biliary obstruction. For the same reason, the gallbladder is almost never palpable in patients with cancer of the body or tail, although it can be palpated in 5 to 30 per cent of patients with lesions in the head of the pancreas. *Hepatomegaly* occurs in 30 to 60 per cent of patients with tumors of the pancreatic body or tail, and a *palpable upper abdominal mass* separate from the liver is present in approximately 20 to 50 per cent of the patients (Eaton, 1970*a*; Bowden, 1972). *Ascites* can be detected in nearly 10 per cent (Braganza, 1972).

Laboratory studies in carcinoma of the body or tail of the pancreas are seldom of decisive importance. *Glucose tolerance tests* are abnormal in as many as 60 per cent of the patients (Rastogi, 1967). *Anemia* is also common, being present in up to 60 per cent, but is generally mild (Braganza, 1972); positive *stool quaiac tests* are infrequent. Hepatic metastasis produces elevation of *serum alkaline phosphatase* in almost half of the patients, but *hyperbilirubinemia* occurs in only about 20 per cent. *Hyperamylasemia* is occasionally encountered, but serum levels are normal much more often and are sometimes depressed (Klintrup, 1966).

Radiologic Features

BARIUM EXAMINATIONS. Tumors located in the body or tail of the pancreas are almost invariably far advanced before the patient develops symptoms which lead to barium meal examination (Mani, 1966). For this reason, there is a fairly high incidence of positive findings on barium upper gastrointestinal studies performed in such patients. The fundus and body of the stomach, the distal portions of the duodenum, and the duodenojejunal junction are most frequently involved.

The basic changes consist of mass indentation defects, mucosal distortion (including ulceration) and, in some instances, obstruction. Lesions of the pancreatic body usually involve the body of the stomach (sometimes the body and antrum together). Indentation occurs most commonly on the posterior surface of the stomach and often involves the greater curvature as well (Fig. 11–6). An actual contour defect is typical, although in some instances only rugal splaying is evident. Mucosal distortion (other than mere splaying) indicates tumor invasion and may closely simulate primary gastric cancer (see Chapter 3). Tumors of the tail of the pancreas often indent the gastric fundus, frequently near the cardia. Invasion here may produce low-grade esophageal obstruction with dysphagia—a symptom which has occasionally been the presenting complaint of patients with tumors of the tail of the pancreas (Strang, 1953).

Cancers of the body and tail of the pancreas fairly often produce an indentation defect involving the distal duodenum or the duodenojejunal junction (at the ligament of Treitz). Such indentation usually involves the posterosuperior aspect of the duodenum, although sometimes the duodenojejunal junction is indented on its left side. Distortion of mucosal folds (Fig. 11–7), often with associated ulceration, tends to involve the same duodenal margins and, more often than is commonly recognized, proceeds to frank ulceration.

Barium examination of the colon in patients with carcinoma of the body or tail of the pancreas occasionally reveals significant abnormalities. The transverse colon and, especially, the splenic flexure are most often involved. The changes range from simple extrinsic indentation (superiorly and posteriorly), through mucosal irregularity, to actual stricture (see Chapter 3). Since the symptoms of cancer arising in the body and tail of the pancreas are so nonspecific, abnormali-

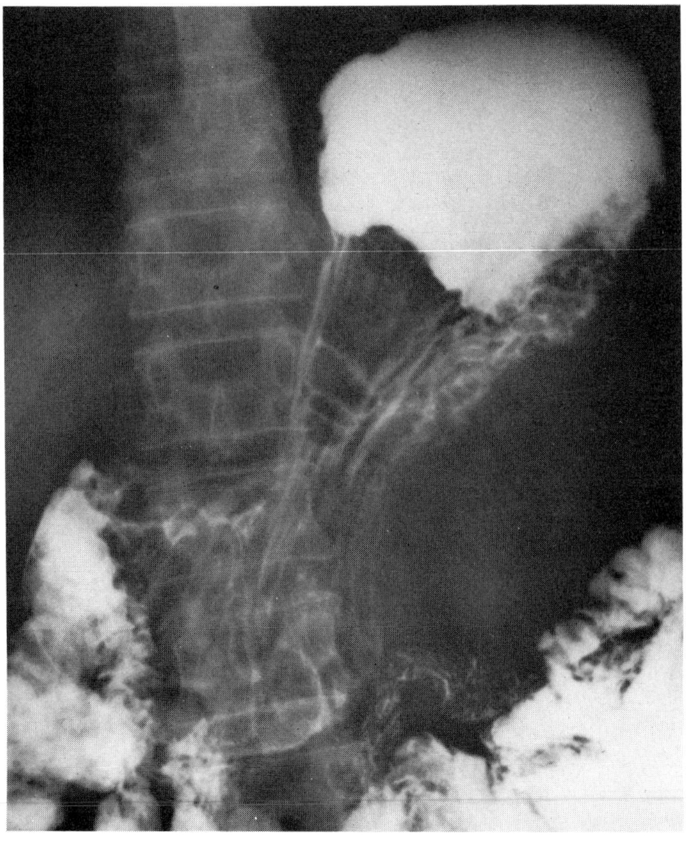

Figure 11–6. Extrinsic indentation on greater curvature of stomach produced by cancer arising in body of pancreas. Conventional upper gastrointestinal barium examination.

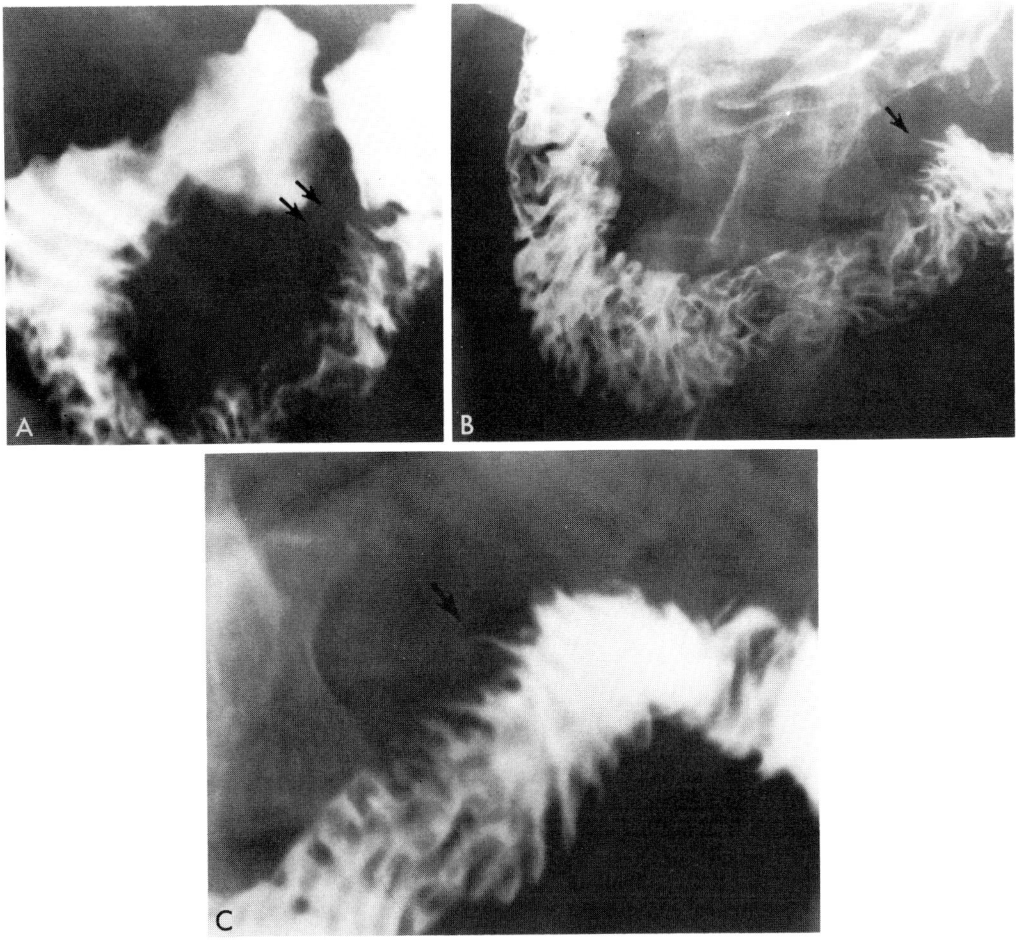

Figure 11–7. Spiculation involving superior border of distal duodenum. This abnormality was suspected on basis of conventional barium upper gastrointestinal examination (*A*) and confirmed by multiple films made during hypotonic duodenography (*B* and *C*). Preoperative diagnosis of carcinoma arising in body of pancreas was based on these subtle findings and confirmed at surgery.

ties demonstrated by barium enema examination may, in some cases, be the first (or only) objective sign of a pathologic condition.

Mani and his co-authors (1966) retrospectively analyzed barium upper gastrointestinal examinations performed in 46 patients with cancer of the body or tail of the pancreas. They identified an extrinsic mass indenting the stomach (with or without splaying of rugal folds) in two-thirds of the patients. Gastric invasion (e.g., mural fixation with edematous, distorted, or frankly ulcerated mucosa) was found in 41 per cent. Evidence of an extrinsic mass adjacent to the distal duodenum (as shown by marginal indentation and/or splaying of the mucosal folds) was found in exactly half of the patients while invasion (as indicated by mucosal distortion, ulceration, or obstruction) was present in 61 per cent. Barium enemas had been performed in 24 of the 46 patients in this series. In nine (38 per cent), there were abnormalities consistent with a pancreatic neoplasm. Extrinsic indentation was most common, but there was frank invasion in two cases, one of which produced colonic obstruction.

Because of its retrospective nature, Mani's series must be considered as a source of data on the *potential* accuracy of barium examination in detecting cancers of the body or tail of the pancreas. No extensive prospective series has been reported, but among the 45 patients studied by Eaton and his co-authors (1968) were five with cancer of the body or tail of the pancreas. Of these, two were correctly identified by conventional barium meal examination, while in the other three cases barium upper gastrointestinal studies were considered normal. One additional patient was incorrectly thought to have carcinoma of the body or tail and thus represented a falsely positive diagnosis. All of these diagnoses were recorded prospectively for purposes of statistical analysis.

It appears that, in everyday practice, preoperative identification of cancer in the body or tail of the pancreas by barium examination remains quite difficult. The findings of Mani and his associates (1966) should thus be viewed as an incentive to improved performance in this area.

Angiography. As previously described (see p. 343; also Chapter 7), the same basic angiographic abnormalities are used to diagnose carcinoma in any part of the pancreas. These consist of *arterial stenosis* (encasement or "tumor cuffing"), *venous compression, arterial* or *venous occlusion, neovascularity* and, occasionally, *displacement* of either arteries or veins. If arterial changes of this sort are demonstrated in the celiac axis, splenic artery, dorsal pancreatic artery, pancreatica magna, or distal transverse pancreatic artery, then a tumor of the body or tail is indicated (Fig. 11–8). Involvement of the splenic or inferior mesenteric vein has similar significance (Fig. 11–9).

Atherosclerosis commonly involves the splenic artery and may produce localized narrowing. In most instances, this narrowing is smooth, but occasionally it is irregular and thus simulates the changes

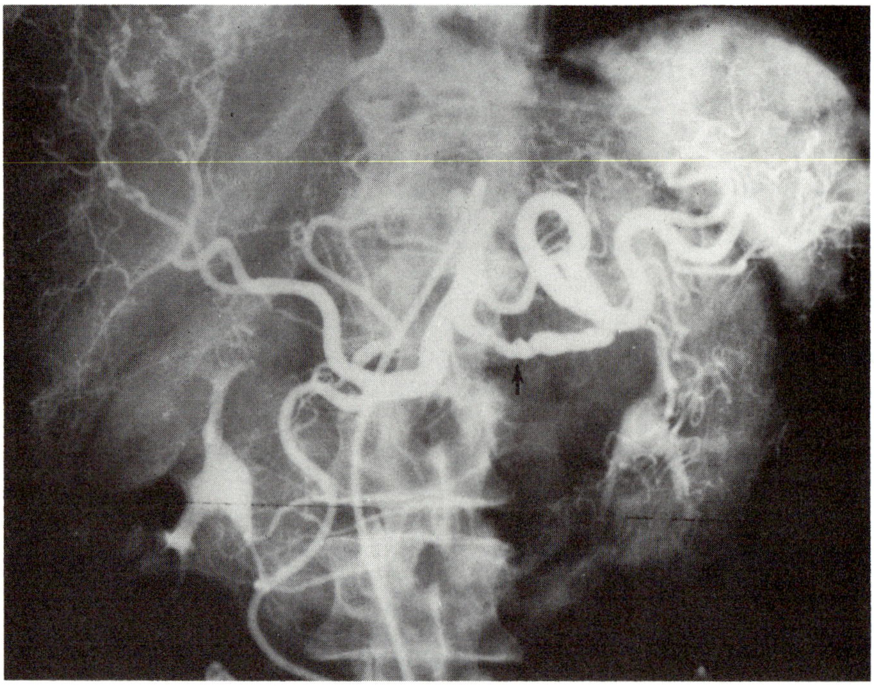

Figure 11–8. Celiac arteriogram, arterial phase. Irregular proximal splenic artery narrowing ("encasement") produced by carcinoma arising in body of pancreas.

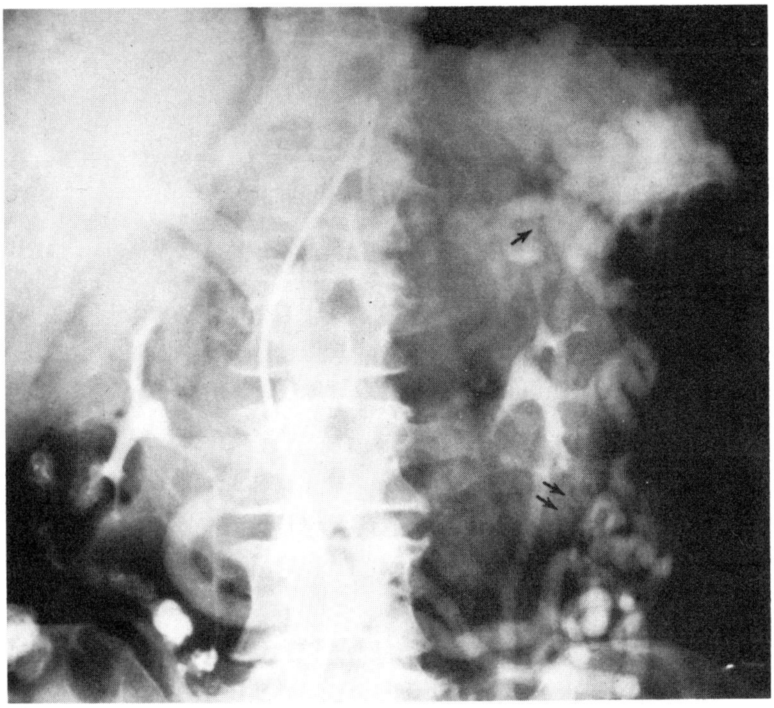

Figure 11-9. Celiac arteriogram, venous phase. Splenic venous occlusion (*single arrow*) produced by cancer arising in tail of pancreas. Prominent venous collateral channels (*double arrows*) have developed. These bridge the obstructed segment and allow opacification of the portal vein.

seen in pancreatic carcinoma (Reuter, 1970). In such patients, splenic venous abnormalities are uncommon, whereas they are the rule in pancreatic cancer (Buranasiri, 1972). Chronic pancreatitis is another condition which can produce encasement similar to that seen in pancreatic cancer (Moskowitz, 1968) and, in contrast to atherosclerosis, venous changes are common in pancreatic inflammatory disease. Often, pancreatitis produces arterial abnormalities over a large segment of the pancreas, whereas those due to carcinoma are generally localized to a relatively small area. Nevertheless, in some cases, angiographic distinction between neoplastic and inflammatory pancreatic disease may be impossible (Reuter, 1972).

If results from two recent reports (Eaton, 1968; Buranasiri, 1972) are pooled, prospective angiographic findings were diagnostic in 16 of 19 patients (84 per cent) with cancer confined to the body and tail of the pancreas. In two additional patients, there were suggestive findings and in only one patient was the angiographic examination considered normal. Venous changes are especially prominent in tumors involving the body and tail. All but one of the patients with such disease in Buranasiri's series had either stenosis or occlusion of the splenic vein, and many had abnormalities of the superior mesenteric vein as well. The single patient without splenic vein involvement had distinctive changes in the portal vein.

^{75}SE SELENOMETHIONINE PANCREATIC IMAGING. In many cases, carcinomas arising in the body or tail of the pancreas are associated with complete failure of pancreatic visualization on ^{75}Se selenomethionine scanning. In other instances, there is a generalized diffuse decrease in uptake of radioactivity resulting in an abnormally faint and poorly defined image. Why tumors located in the body or tail affect protein metabolism in the head of the pancreas is not understood. In practice, however, total failure of or diffuse decrease in pancreatic accumulation of radioactivity has no value in differentiating between malignancy of the body or tail and that occurring in the pancreaticoduodenal region.

In occasional instances, there is normal radioactivity in the pancreatic head and complete or almost complete failure of uptake in the body and tail (Fig. 11–10). Positive scintigrams of this nature are more reliable than those in which there is generalized abnormality. In the latter instance, there is a high incidence of false positives, but the former pattern almost always indicates disease (usually neoplasm, sometimes pseudocyst and, rarely, localized pancreatitis) confined to the body and tail. Pancreaticoduodenal cancer is not associated with scintigraphic findings of this sort.

One pattern which has confused interpretation of ^{75}Se selenomethionine pancreatic images since the examination was introduced is the occurrence of a midline defect near the "neck" of an

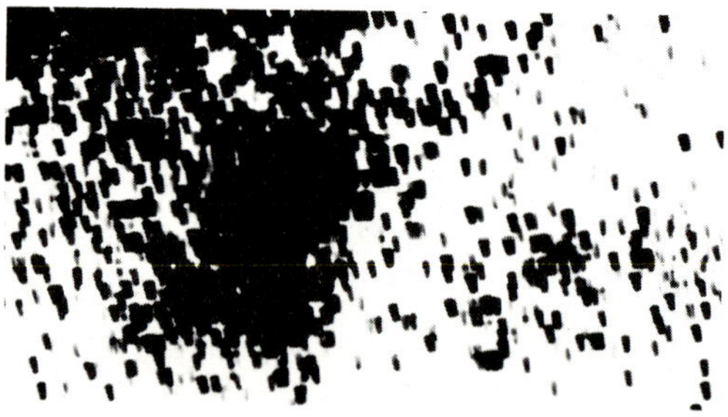

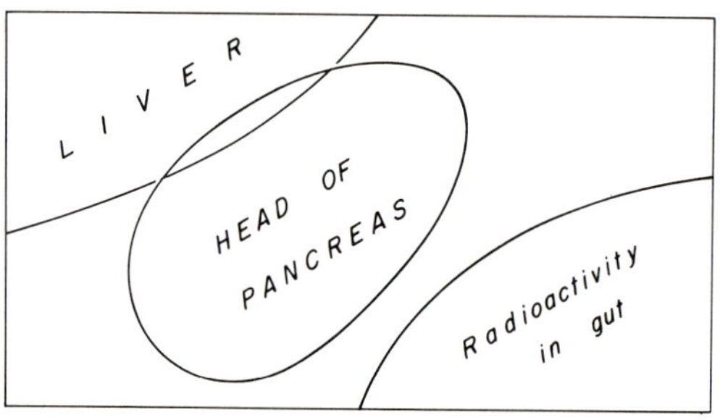

Figure 11–10. ^{75}Se selenomethionine pancreatic scan reveals normal accumulation of radioactivity in head of pancreas, but no radioactivity in body or tail of gland. Abnormal pattern resulted from carcinoma arising in body of pancreas.

otherwise normal pancreatic image (e.g., Eaton, 1967; Riccobono, 1968). In most instances, this pattern results from thinning of pancreatic tissue at the junction of the head and body (see Chapter 1) where the pancreas overlies the aorta and spine. In these cases, Landman and his associates (1971) suggest a bolus injection of ^{99m}Tc pertechnetate given without changing the patient's position to obtain a radionuclide abdominal aortogram. If the localized diminution in pancreatic ^{75}Se radioactivity corresponds to the position of the aorta and the ^{75}Se selenomethionine images are otherwise unremarkable, then the pancreas should be considered normal. If the pancreatic defect is in a portion of the organ away from the aorta, then the examination should be considered abnormal.

Few articles dealing with the accuracy of ^{75}Se selenomethionine pancreatic imaging have divided their cases of pancreatic cancer into those of the head versus those of the body or tail. However, if patients from three studies (Eaton, 1968; Heslip, 1971 and McCarthy, 1972) are pooled, pancreatic scintigraphy was abnormal in 23 of 25 cases (92 per cent) in which malignancy was confined to the body or tail of the gland. Although this figure represents only a limited number of cases, its similarity to figures for scintigraphic detection of pancreatic cancer in general suggests that the ability of this technique to detect pancreatic malignancy does not vary significantly with the portion of the organ involved.

CHRONIC PANCREATITIS

Introduction

The international symposium on pancreatitis held at Marseilles in 1963 defined chronic pancreatitis as a process characterized by permanent pancreatic damage—either functional or anatomic—which persists even when the inciting cause or causes are eliminated. While there has been some tendency toward general adoption of this definition, articles continue to appear in which any patient with recurrent pancreatitis is considered to have chronic pancreatitis regardless of whether or not permanent pancreatic damage has been incurred.

In the United States, the two most important forms of pancreatitis are those associated with alcoholism and biliary tract disease. The former falls into the category of chronic pancreatitis by all definitions because irreversible anatomic and functional changes tend to persist in the pancreas once the disease process becomes established. According to the Marseilles classification, however, pancreatitis related to biliary tract disease would ordinarily be considered "relapsing acute pancreatitis," since the pancreas is usually restored to normal between acute episodes.

Since both of these types of pancreatitis can produce recurrent attacks of abdominal discomfort resulting from pancreatic inflammation, and since their distinction is of considerable importance for planning appropriate therapy, they will be considered together in this section.

Clinical Features (Table 11–3)

According to Howard (1960), just over half of all American patients with chronic pancreatitis are *chronic alcoholics.* Slightly more than a third have *biliary tract disease* (usually with gallstones) and the remainder (about 10 per cent of the total) have one of the rare "causes" of pancreatitis (e.g., hyperparathyroidism, hereditary pancreatitis, or localized ampullary disease) or have no known predisposing condition.

Patients with alcoholic pancreatitis are relatively young. Attacks of abdominal pain begin in the fourth decade of life and complications such as diabetes, steatorrhea, and pancreatic calcification develop around age 40 to 45. In this group, males outnumber females approximately 3:1 (Howard, 1960) to 12:1 (Sarles, 1965). Gallstone pancreatitis affects an older age group, the mean age being about 55 years when acute attacks of pain begin. About 60 per cent of these patients are women.

Over 90 per cent of patients with chronic (or recurrent) pancreatitis have had one or more episodes of *abdominal pain* (Sarles, 1972). The pain can be mild or excruciating; it is usually (about 75 per cent) epigastric, and frequently (50 to 60 per cent) radiates through to the back (Eaton, 1970*a*). About three-fourths of the patients have had more than one painful episode and often there is a history of repeated hospitalization for these attacks. In gallstone pancreatitis, the recurrences generally remain isolated but, in alcoholic patients, a fairly constant low-grade abdominal pain ultimately develops (usually about 5 to 10 years after the first acute attack). A small but definite proportion of patients with chronic pancreatitis may never have suffered pain that is suggestive of pancreatic disease (Fitzgerald, 1972).

Almost all patients with well-established chronic pancreatitis report *weight loss.* In many cases, a significant amount (e.g., 25 to 30 pounds) has been lost over a period of a few months to a year. When painful attacks are intermittent, the patient's weight tends to fluctuate but, once persistent pain develops, significant weight gains are uncommon.

TABLE 11–3. Chronic Pancreatitis

Symptom	*Incidence* (%)
History of alcoholism	Over 50
History consistent with cholelithiasis	About 33
Abdominal pain	90
Back pain	50–60
Weight loss	Nearly 100
Physical Finding	
Jaundice	Rare except during acute exacerbation
Laboratory Value	
Elevated fecal fat	15–20 } "Alcoholic pancreatitis" only
Elevated fasting blood sugar	25–30 } "Alcoholic pancreatitis" only

Transient, low-grade *jaundice* often complicates acute attacks of pancreatitis (Sarles, 1965). A persistent form resulting from inflammatory stricture of the distal common bile duct also occurs (Weinstein, 1963). Howard and Jordan (1960) were able to collect seven cases of painless jaundice due to chronic pancreatitis.

Complications such as *malabsorption* and *diabetes* occur much more commonly in alcoholic pancreatitis than in pancreatitis associated with biliary tract disease. Of patients with alcoholic pancreatitis who develop persistent abdominal pain, about 25 to 30 per cent have overt diabetes and 15 to 20 per cent have steatorrhea. Only about 2 per cent of patients with gallstone pancreatitis develop such symptoms. Over 40 per cent of American patients with alcoholic pancreatitis also have *cirrhosis* (Howard, 1960).

Radiologic Features

PLAIN FILM FINDINGS. When several different reports (Howard, 1960; Warren, 1962) are analyzed, it appears that between 20 and 30 per cent of patients with chronic pancreatitis have *pancreatic calcification* (Fig. 11–11). The radiologic appearance of such calcification is discussed in detail in Chapter 2. In the United States, pancreatic calculi are usually a sign of alcoholic pancreatitis since "gallstone pancreatitis" only rarely gives rise to pancreatic lithiasis, and the other "causes" of pancreatitis which can produce calcification (e.g., hyperparathyroidism and hereditary pancreatitis) are rare in themselves.

Some authorities feel that calcific pancreatitis predisposes to development of pancreatic cancer (e.g., Paulino-Netto, 1960; Ansari, 1968) while others (e.g., Bowden, 1972) disagree. In most comprehensive series, the incidence of cancer developing in calcific pancreatitis varies from 2 to 4 per cent (e.g., Johnson, 1963; Guien, 1972). This value is significantly above that in the general population, of course, but is still sufficiently low that roentgen demonstration of pancreatic lithiasis should be considered an indicator of benign disease.

If data from two pertinent series are

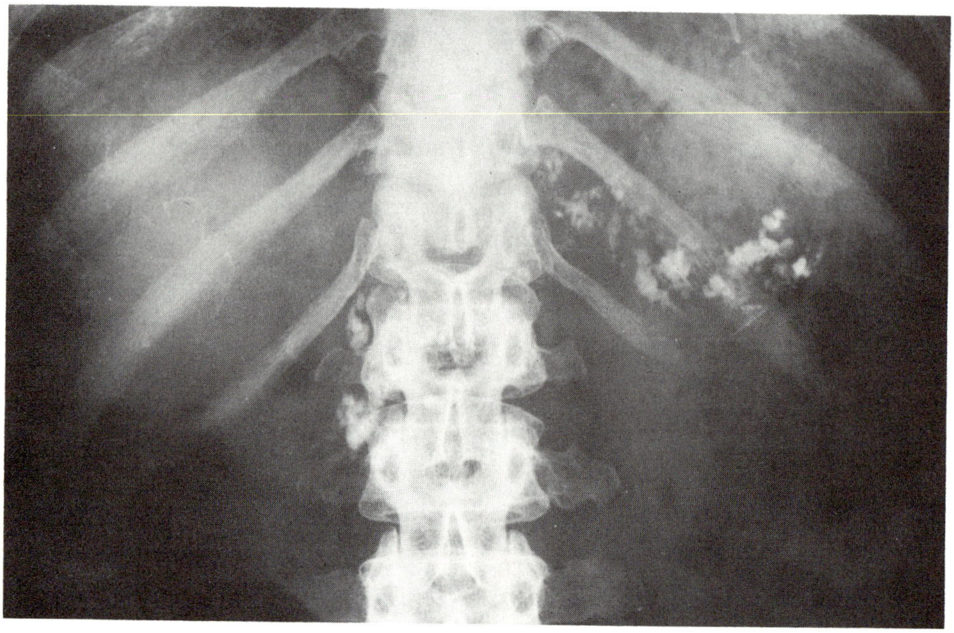

Figure 11–11. Plain abdominal roentgenogram reveals typical pancreatic lithiasis resulting from chronic alcoholic pancreatitis.

combined, approximately 5 per cent of all patients with established chronic pancreatitis will have osseous abnormalities such as *medullary infarcts* and *aseptic necrosis* of the femoral or humeral heads (Gerle, 1965; Bank, 1966). Demonstration of such changes in a patient whose clinical manifestations are inconclusive may help to strengthen a provisional diagnosis of chronic pancreatitis.

BARIUM UPPER GASTROINTESTINAL EXAMINATION. Conventional barium meal examination in patients with chronic pancreatitis is usually unrevealing. In Guien's series (1972), only 16 per cent of the patients had gastric abnormalities (and an unspecified number of these patients also had pancreatic pseudocyst). Indentation along the greater curvature of the antrum was the commonest individual sign. Duodenal changes were demonstrated by conventional barium studies in only 10 per cent of patients reported by Rubinstein and his associates (1971); again the most common sign was an extrinsic indentation defect, in this case, along the inner border of the descending duodenum.

Hypotonic duodenography can demonstrate evidence of chronic pancreatitis in 64 to 80 per cent of the patients in whom it is employed (Eaton, 1968; Rubinstein, 1971). The most specific abnormality is a smooth effacement of the duodenal fold pattern along the upper inner margin of the descending duodenum (Fig. 11–12). Similar changes also occur along the lower inner margin of the descending duodenum but, if restricted to this area, are difficult to distinguish from the normal "straight segment" (Ferrucci, 1970; see Chapter 4). Other findings include a serrated, spiculated appearance of the folds along the inner duodenal margin and enlargement of the duodenal papilla; both of these are nonspecific and can also occur in pancreaticoduodenal carcinoma while impacted ampullary calculi can produce edema of the duodenal papilla. Other abnormalities occasionally encountered include "thumbprint-like" indentation on the duodenal bulb itself and, in some cases, a nodular filling defect in the bulb which may be associated with central ulceration (Guien, 1972).

^{75}SE SELENOMETHIONINE PANCREATIC IMAGING. The pattern of pancreatic amino acid (and hence selenomethionine) uptake in patients with chronic

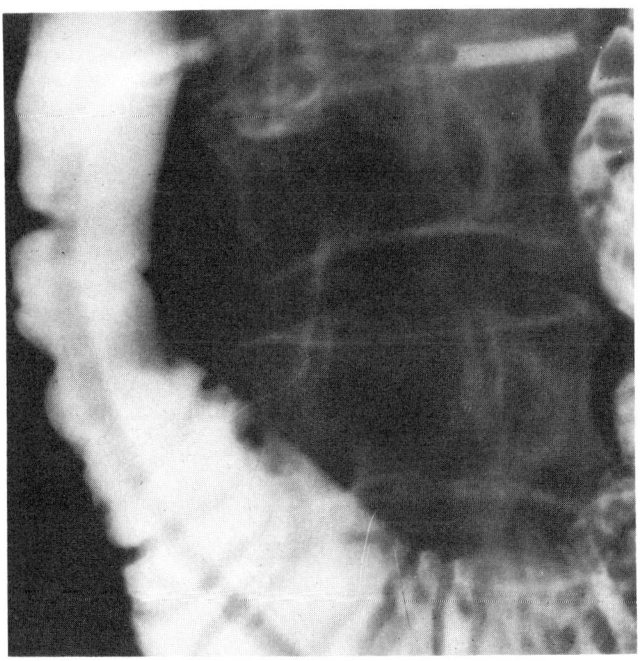

Figure 11–12. Hypotonic duodenogram. Flattening and fold effacement along inner margin of descending duodenum resulting from chronic pancreatitis.

pancreatitis is dependent upon the extent and activity of the disease process. In endstage disease with almost total destruction of the organ and manifest clinical pancreatic insufficiency, there will be no apparent concentration of selenomethionine in the pancreas. In less severe disease, an irregular but generally decreased uptake pattern may be expected. In cases in which there has been a recent episode of acute pancreatitis, there may be complete failure of amino-acid uptake even when relatively little irreversible damage to the gland has occurred (McCarthy, 1969; Eaton, 1971). These scintigraphic patterns are nonspecific and can also be seen in patients with pancreatic carcinoma and with pancreatic pseudocysts.

The value of ^{75}Se selenomethionine pancreatic imaging in patients with chronic pancreatitis lies in its sensitivity; false-negative results (i.e., normal scans) are uncommon and have been found in only 10 to 16 per cent of patients in several series (Eaton, 1968; Riccobono, 1968; Bouchier, 1972; and McCarthy, 1972). As is the case with pancreatic cancer, however, false-positive results are common. Accordingly, a convincingly normal pancreatic scintigram constitutes fairly good evidence against chronic pancreatitis while an abnormal scan merely indicates that the possibility of chronic pancreatic inflammation deserves further diagnostic investigation.

ULTRASONOGRAPHY. In chronic pancreatitis, ultrasonic abdominal scanning is usually unremarkable (Russell, 1972). If echographic examination is conducted during an acute episode, however, it will often reveal an elongated transonic area anterior to the aorta and vena cava. The image conforms to the normal shape of the pancreas and its borders are usually smooth and distinct (Stuber, 1972). The thickness of the pancreatic image in such instances is apparently related to the amount of edema present (Filly, 1970).

PANCREATIC ANGIOGRAPHY. Angiographic abnormalities in patients with chronic pancreatitis are directly related to the duration and severity of disease. In the early stages, no changes are observed (Reuter, 1972; Boijsen, 1972) but, in the majority of patients with longstanding disease, vascular abnormalities are seen (Hernandez, 1967; Reuter, 1969). A beaded appearance of the intrapancreatic arteries where short dilated segments alternate with normal or narrowed segments is considered specific for pancreatitis (Reuter, 1972), although some authorities (e.g., Kyaw, 1970) have noted a similar appearance in pancreatic carcinoma. Other changes include smooth arterial stenoses, arterial tortuosity, aneurysms arising from the intra- and peripancreatic arteries, and venous narrowing and/or occlusion.

The demonstration of aneurysms (which presumably develop as a consequence of enzymatic activity on the arterial wall) is of considerable significance since there are now several reports of gastrointestinal or intraabdominal hemorrhage secondary to rupture of such lesions (e.g., Baum, 1965; Boijsen, 1969). Obstruction of the splenic vein with development of varices is another particularly important finding since it also constitutes a potential source of gastrointestinal bleeding (e.g., Longstreth, 1971). In either event, prophylactic surgery may be contemplated in a patient for whom operative management was not previously considered to be desirable.

TRANSHEPATIC AND INTRAOPERATIVE CHOLANGIOGRAPHY. In those patients in whom chronic pancreatitis has produced extrahepatic obstructive jaundice and in cases in which an intraoperative cholangiogram has been obtained to aid in distinction between pancreatic carcinoma and chronic pancreatitis (a differentiation which may remain unclear after thorough palpation at celiotomy and even after frozen-section histologic analysis [Bowden, 1954]), an appreciation of the cholangiographic appearance of chronic pancreatitis is important. The most characteristic findings include compression and lateral displacement of the distal common bile duct. This usually produces angulation at the junction of the middle and distal thirds of the common duct so that a smooth, undulating, tapered narrowing is created (Fig. 11–13). There is usually some proximal dilatation of the

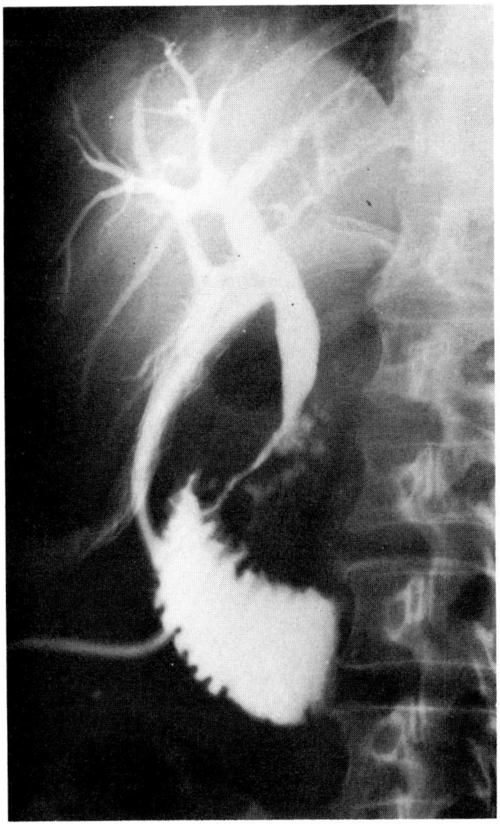

Figure 11–13. Long, tapered, undulating stenosis of distal common bile duct resulting from chronic pancreatitis (see calcifications). Pattern is typical of chronic pancreatitis. Postoperative "T-tube" cholangiogram; percutaneous transhepatic cholangiography can demonstrate similar pattern (see Fig. 5–39, Chapter 5).

biliary radicals and common hepatic duct, but complete common duct obstruction is rare (Sachs, 1956).

ORAL CHOLECYSTOGRAPHY. The natural history of pancreatitis is largely dependent on the etiologic factors which are operating. As long as these persist, further attacks may be expected. Accordingly, recurrent episodes of acute pancreatitis are likely in patients with gallstones until the biliary tract disease has been fully eradicated (Trapnell, 1972) (Fig. 11–14). Radiologic evaluation of the gallbladder in patients with recurrent or chronic pancreatitis requires careful timing. The gallbladders of patients examined during or shortly after an acute episode often fail to opacify even though they are later found to be normal (see Chapter 3). Accordingly, Stein and his co-workers (1959) have recommended that oral cholecystography be carried out in such patients only after bromsulphalein (BSP) retention has become normal and after the gallbladder has been stimulated to empty by giving one or more fatty meals.

As noted earlier in this chapter, about one-third of American patients have chronic pancreatitis associated with biliary tract disease. In England, the percentage is even higher—over 50 per cent in some series (e.g., Trapnell, 1972). Since most of these patients can be cured by cholecystectomy (Anderson, 1969), the importance of oral cholecystography is clearly apparent.

ACUTE PANCREATITIS

Introduction

Acute pancreatitis is a great mimic and can be confused with a number of other acute abdominal conditions (Anderson, 1969; Trapnell, 1972). Acute cholecystitis, perforated peptic ulcer, acute appendicitis, mesenteric vascular accident, dissection or ruptured aortic aneurysm, intestinal obstruction (with or without strangulation), and myocardial infarction are entities not infrequently mistaken for acute pancreatitis (and vice versa). Most of these can produce moderate elevation of serum amylase and, in occasional instances, marked hyperamylasemia develops.

While there are some advocates of early operative intervention in acute pancreatitis, either for diagnosis alone (Trapnell, 1967) or for aggressive treatment (e.g., Waterman, 1968; Lawson, 1970), there is general agreement that nonoperative management is indicated for the patient with acute pancreatitis, and in a high proportion of cases the response is prompt" (Anderson, 1969). Because of the difficulty of establishing a clinical or laboratory diagnosis and because an

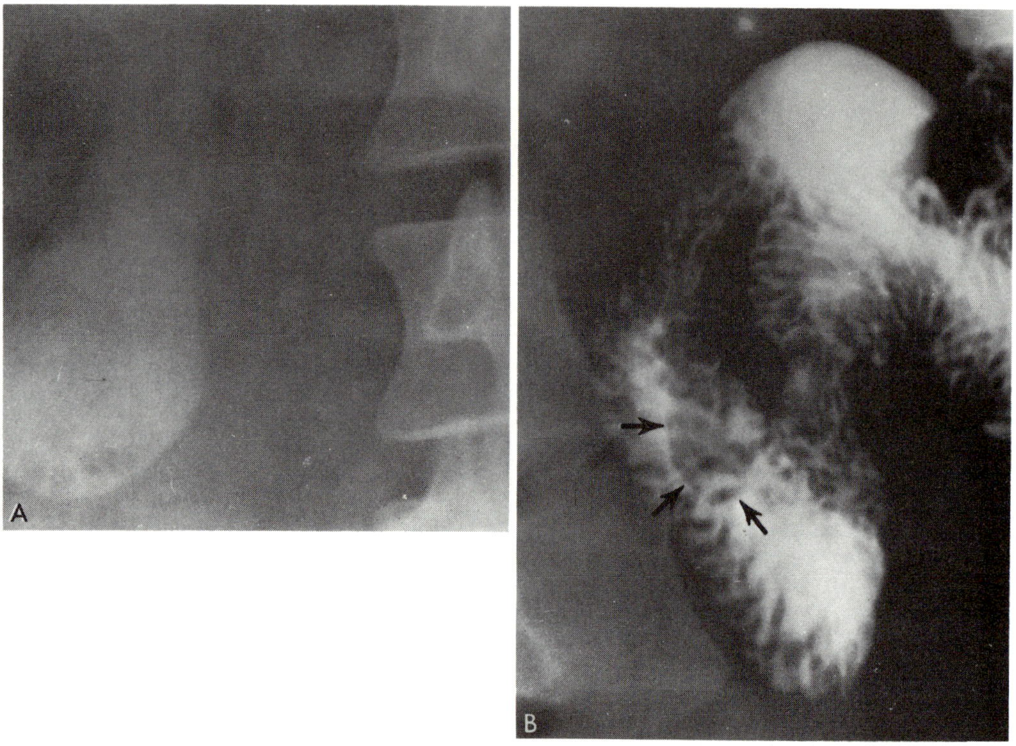

Figure 11–14. Multiple nonopaque calculi demonstrated by oral cholecystography in patient with recurrent "gallstone" pancreatitis (*A*). Conventional barium meal examination demonstrated papillary edema (Poppel's sign) in the same patient during episode of acute pancreatic inflammation (*B*).

accurate diagnosis is necessary for the choice between operative and nonoperative care, any aid available from radiologic techniques is of significant value in patients presenting with clinical features suggestive of acute pancreatitis.

Clinical Features (Table 11–4)

Patients who present with acute pancreatitis average between 40 and 50 years of age, but individuals under 20 and others nearly 90 have been listed

TABLE 11–4. Acute Pancreatitis

Symptom	*Incidence* (%)
Abdominal pain	95
Back pain	Nearly 50
Nausea, vomiting, prostration	Very common
Physical Finding	
Temperature elevation	80
Epigastric tenderness	85
Abdominal guarding and rigidity	About 33
Abdominal distention	20
Decreased or absent peristalsis	20
Shock	5–10
Jaundice	About 10
Laboratory Value	
Leukocytosis	About 50
Elevated bilirubin	25
Elevated alkaline phosphatase, positive cephalin flocculation, prolonged prothrombin time	5–20
Elevated amylase	80–90 (especially first day)
Elevated lipase	About 90
Hypocalcemia	About 25

in series of patients studied for this condition. Acute pancreatitis occurs more often in males than in females, and a history of alcoholic excess can be elicited in men more often than in women. No racial predisposition has been identified. In about 20 per cent of these patients, there is a history of previous episodes consistent with acute pancreatitis (Bockus, 1955).

Upper abdominal pain is present in 95 to 98 per cent of all cases. It is usually sudden in onset and more often constant than intermittent. In nearly half of the patients, there is *radiation of pain to the back. Nausea, vomiting,* and a feeling of *prostration* are other common symptoms. Low-grade *temperature elevation* is usually present and, in the great majority, there is *epigastric tenderness.* In severe cases, there is abdominal guarding and rigidity. *Abdominal distention* is present in about 20 per cent of cases and peristalsis is usually decreased or absent in such patients. In 5 to 10 per cent, *shock* develops.

Leukocytosis is present in approximately half of the patients. About 25 per cent have transient *hyperbilirubinemia* (> 1.5 mg. per 100 ml.) while between 5 and 20 per cent have one or more abnormal *hepatic function tests* (e.g., elevated serum alkaline phosphatase, depressed serum prothrombin concentration, or positive cephalin flocculation) (Bockus, 1955). If a blood sample can be obtained early in the attack, *hyperamylasemia* is present in over 90 per cent of all acute pancreatitis patients. Serum amylase values that are five times the upper limit of normal are usually reliable indicators of pancreatitis, but often the degree of elevation is considerably lower. In these cases, conditions such as acute cholecystitis, perforated duodenal ulcer, mesenteric vascular occlusion and strangulated intestinal obstruction cannot be excluded since they can cause similar rises in the levels of serum amylase. *Serum lipase* elevations are more specific for pancreatitis (Anderson, 1969) but require 24 hours to complete. *Hypocalcemia* may develop during acute pancreatitis, but this finding is more helpful as a guide to prognosis in the severe case than as a generally applicable diagnostic aid (Trapnell, 1972).

Radiologic Features

PLAIN FILM FINDINGS. In many patients with acute pancreatitis, plain roentgenograms of the chest and abdomen are the only radiologic studies obtained. The signs which can be detected on such films are described in detail in Chapter 2. The commonest are abnormalities of the abdominal gas pattern. Felson (1968) first linked a *"gasless abdomen"* to the presence of acute pancreatitis. Like nearly all the plain film findings in acute pancreatitis, this sign is nonspecific and can also be seen in patients with mesenteric vascular accident and in cases of high intestinal obstruction.

Adynamic ileus is more common than the gasless abdomen as a sign of acute pancreatic inflammation. Such ileus can be generalized or localized. The latter form creates a *"sentinel loop"*—a localized segment of gas-filled, dilated small bowel. This finding can occur in any number of acute abdominal disorders but, when ileus is confined to the duodenal loop, much more diagnostic specificity is warranted (Fig. 11–15). *Duodenal ileus* can occur in acute cholecystitis (Weens, 1964) but, in the authors' experience, has almost always indicated adjacent pancreatic inflammation. The *"colon cut-off sign,"* in contrast, has been much less helpful. In our experience, it has only infrequently been seen in patients with acute pancreatitis and has been observed fairly often in patients with mesenteric infarction (and in a fair number of patients without identifiable acute abdominal disease).

One very important, albeit infrequent, sign of acute pancreatic inflammation is the *gas abscess.* In such patients, numerous small air bubbles develop in the area of the pancreas (in extreme cases, an actual pancreatic air fluid level may be present on upright films). Mortality in cases of pancreatic abscess is high (25

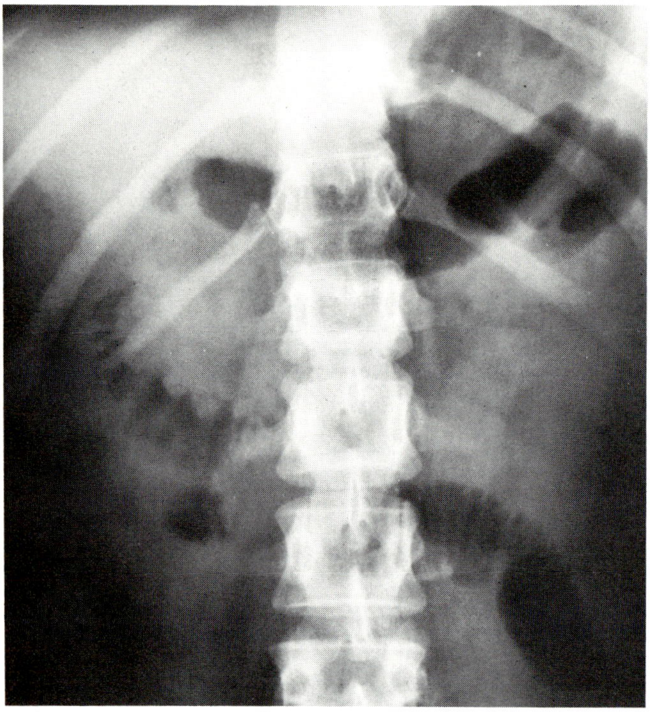

Figure 11–15. Plain abdominal roentgenogram. Duodenal ileus in patient with acute pancreatitis. Note edematous duodenal folds. There is also a jejunal "sentinel loop" phenomenon.

to 50 per cent; see Chapter 2) and early diagnosis is of prime importance. Accordingly, identification of gas in the pancreas is of great value. The most common differential problem is to exclude gas in the stomach or transverse colon as a cause of the findings observed.

Chest findings (e.g., pleural effusion, hemidiaphragmatic elevation, basilar atelectasis, etc.) are common in acute pancreatitis as well as in other acute subdiaphragmatic inflammatory disorders (Fig. 11–16). The most helpful is demonstration of a left pleural effusion, not because of radiologic specificity, but rather because aspiration and determination of amylase content may allow a prompt and accurate diagnosis (Hammansten, 1959; see Chapter 2).

BARIUM UPPER GASTROINTESTINAL EXAMINATION. Barium meal examination may reveal findings which allow a diagnosis of acute pancreatitis in patients whose clinical manifestations are inconclusive and in whom plain abdominal roentgenograms have been unavailing (Fig. 11–17). The commonest individual sign is duodenal paresis (Bergkvist, 1959). By itself, this abnormality is relatively nonspecific, but it is usually associated with edema of the duodenal folds (Schultz, 1963). Other common findings are signs of pancreatic enlargement (e.g., a mass indentation defect on the inner duodenal border) and edema of the duodenal papilla (Poppel's sign). When two or more of these abnormalities occur together, a confident radiologic diagnosis is usually possible. While these signs are most often noted in the descending duodenum, other segments of the upper gastrointestinal tract may be involved. An extrinsic indentation defect on the posterior surface or greater curve of the stomach can be created by marked pancreatic swelling (in acute pancreatitis, the pancreas may enlarge to three times its normal size [Blumenthal, 1959]). Gastric atony is also fairly common while dilatation and fold edema may also be seen in the proximal jejunum.

A negative upper gastrointestinal barium examination cannot exclude acute pancreatitis, but the abnormalities described in the preceding paragraph occur very commonly in patients with this

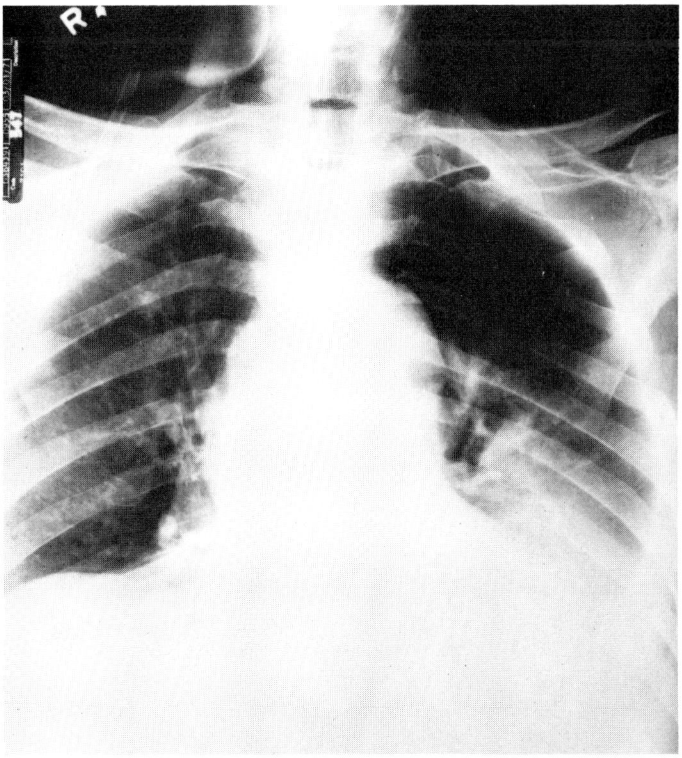

Figure 11–16. Plain chest roentgenogram. Left-sided pleural effusion in patient with acute pancreatitis.

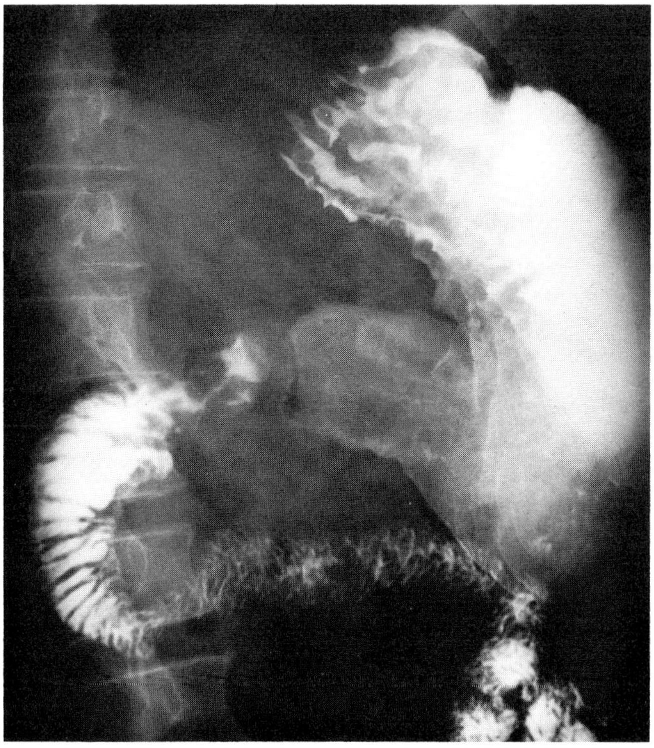

Figure 11–17. Upper gastrointestinal barium examination demonstrates retrogastric mass effect, antral "pad" sign, rugal edema, paresis in descending duodenum and mild edema of folds in distal duodenum. Abnormalities resulted from acute pancreatitis.

condition. In a prospective study, Schultz (1963) found one or more of these signs in 15 of 21 patients (71 per cent). On retrospective review, abnormalities were found in two additional cases so that over 80 per cent of these patients actually had radiographic evidence of pancreatic inflammation at the time of barium examination. This study was not designed to evaluate the incidence of false-positive diagnoses, but Schultz (1963) felt these to be rare and this has been true in the authors' experience as well. We feel an accurate diagnosis by barium meal examination should be made in the majority of patients and that, while a normal study cannot exclude acute pancreatitis, it should prompt a careful re-evaluation of the clinical data to make sure another acute abdominal condition is not, in fact, the cause of the patient's distress. Patients with high serum amylase resulting from any number of nonpancreatic causes have died while being treated conservatively for acute pancreatitis (e.g., Schultz, 1963; Trapnell, 1972).

ORAL CHOLECYSTOGRAPHY. As has been previously discussed identification of gallbladder and biliary tract disease is of great significance for the management of patients with acute pancreatitis. Definitive surgery in such circumstances eliminates further episodes of pancreatic inflammation in the great majority of instances. It is important to remember that biliary tract evaluation should be performed only after acute symptoms have subsided. In patients whose gallbladders are actually normal, oral cholecystography fails to opacify the gallbladder in about 50 per cent during the actual episode of acute pancreatitis. Even with intravenous cholecystography the gallbladder cannot be demonstrated in about a third of such patients (Weens, 1964). Stein (1959) recommends that cholecystography be performed only after BSP retention has become normal and the gallbladder has been stimulated to empty by giving one or more fatty meals.

RADIOISOTOPIC PANCREATIC IMAGING. Scintigraphic examination made after administration of ^{75}Se selenomethionine is nearly always positive in patients with acute pancreatitis (Bouchier, 1972). Because of the relatively high incidence of false-positive results, however, the study is seldom performed in patients in whom the diagnosis is clinically suspected. The technique can be used to follow return to normal function in patients recovering from acute pancreatitis; in some patients, normal uptake can be demonstrated within two weeks of an attack. Persistently positive scans often indicate the presence of chronic pancreatitis (i.e., where irreversible glandular damage is present) or the development of a complicating pancreatic pseudocyst (Bouchier, 1972).

ULTRASONOGRAPHY. The efficacy of echography in detecting acute pancreatitis is directly related to the amount of pancreatic edema present (Filly, 1970) and inversely related to any adynamic ileus which may accompany the process (Leopold, 1972*a*; see Chapter 9). The normal pancreas is not transonic and, therefore, cannot be distinguished from adjacent retroperitoneal structures. In pancreatitis with significant edema, the gland becomes more permeable to sound. In such cases, it often appears as an arc-shaped sonolucent zone anterior to the aorta and vena cava (Fig. 11–18). Unfortunately, air collections present an almost absolute impediment to ultrasonic transmission. Since many patients with acute pancreatitis have associated localized or generalized ileus, adequate demonstration of the pancreatic region is sometimes impossible.

These factors interact in the ultrasonic detection of acute pancreatitis. Filly and Freimanis (1970) detected evidence of pancreatitis in nine of 11 patients with acute disease, and numerous reports (e.g., Stuber, 1972; Russell, 1972) have supported the initial observation that a transonic area conforming to the shape of the pancreas can usually be found in such patients. Leopold and his associates (1972*a*) are less optimistic and feel that ileus often renders ultrasonic examination inconclusive in such cases (see Chapter 9). All authorities concur that echography cannot, at present, distinguish between acute pancreatitis and chronic pancreatitis with acute exacerbation.

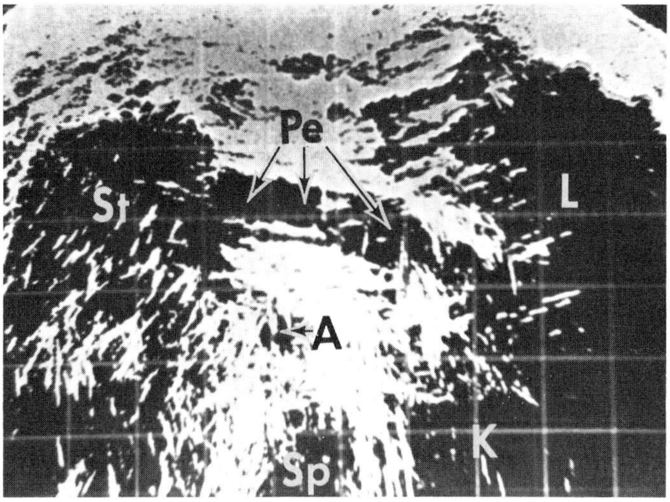

Figure 11–18. Cross-sectional abdominal echogram demonstrates arc-shaped transonic zone (Pe) due to pancreatic edema in acute pancreatitis. The stomach (st), liver (L), aorta (A), right kidney (K) and spine (sp) are also visible. (Reproduced by permission of Filly, R. A., and Freimanis, A. K.: Echographic diagnosis of pancreatic lesions. Radiology, 96:575–582, 1970.)

PANCREATIC ANGIOGRAPHY. In acute pancreatitis, intrapancreatic edema produces subtle displacement of vessels surrounding the gland. There is also inflammatory hypervascularization. The latter findings were unequivocally demonstrated by Aakhus and his associates (1969) who performed paired angiographic studies in 13 patients with acute pancreatitis. Small intrapancreatic vessels were greater in size and number during the acute phase (as opposed to follow-up studies obtained after clinical symptoms subsided) in 11 of the 13 patients. Unfortunately, the absolute number and size of pancreatic vessels is so variable in different individuals that hypervascularity cannot be definitively diagnosed without follow-up studies obtained during a quiescent period (Aakhus, 1969; Boijsen, 1972). For these reasons, angiographic study is infrequently requested for evaluation of patients suspected of having acute pancreatitis.

PANCREATIC PSEUDOCYST

Introduction

Pancreatic pseudocysts, so named because they do not possess an epithelial lining and therefore differ from true cysts, are much more common than any other form of cystic pancreatic lesion. They are usually unilocular and tend to be fairly large; the average cyst found at operation contains several liters of fluid (Howard, 1960). The exact origin of pseudocysts is often impossible to determine at surgery but, in cases where the origin can be identified, about two-thirds to three-fourths arise from the body and tail while the remainder arise from the head of the organ. Pancreatic pseudocysts can "migrate" and have been reported in a number of bizarre locations such as the pelvis and mediastinum; nevertheless, the great majority develop between the pancreas and the stomach.

While 10 to 20 per cent of all pancreatic pseudocysts develop in the absence of any known predisposing pancreatic disorder, most occur in patients who have previously had acute pancreatitis; alcoholic pancreatitis is more commonly complicated by development of pseudocyst than is gallstone pancreatitis. As many as 20 per cent of patients with pseudocysts have had previous pancreatic injury. Blunt abdominal trauma is the commonest contributor to this category but, in a significant number, iatrogenic pancreatic damage has been incurred during previous abdominal surgery.

Clinical Features (Table 11–5)

Pancreatic pseudocysts occur in both pediatric (Kilman, 1964) and geriatric

TABLE 11–5. Pancreatic Pseudocyst

Symptom	*Incidence (%)*
Abdominal pain	90
Radiation to back	Common
Nausea and vomiting	Occasional
Weight loss	30–50
Physical Finding	
Upper abdominal mass	50–70
Epigastric tenderness	60–80
Fever	25–50
Jaundice	10–15
Laboratory Value	
Abnormal glucose tolerance	Over 50
Elevated amylase	40–50
Anemia	15–20
Elevated bilirubin	20–30

patients (Caravati, 1966), but the age incidence parallels that for acute pancreatitis: the condition is most common in patients between 40 and 50 years old (Walker, 1967). Because alcoholism is the commonest single predisposing factor, males usually outnumber females in reported series by 2 or 3 to 1 (e.g., Walker, 1967; Thomford, 1969).

About 90 per cent of patients with pancreatic pseudocysts complain of *abdominal pain.* The pain is usually located in the epigastrium, frequently radiates to the back, and is typically constant rather than colicky. *Nausea and vomiting* are common symptoms and *weight loss* occurs in a third to a half of all patients with pseudocysts. In many instances, the degree of weight loss is pronounced—often 20 pounds or more. An *upper abdominal mass* can be palpated in from one-half to two-thirds of all patients with pseudocysts. Such masses are nearly always tender; even in patients without a palpable mass, *epigastric tenderness* is common. *Fever,* usually low-grade in nature, is suprisingly common, occurring in 25 to 50 per cent of all cases. *Jaundice* develops in from 10 to 15 per cent and, when present, usually indicates compression of the common bile duct by a pseudocyst in the head of the pancreas. In other patients, usually alcoholics, cirrhosis and pancreatic pseudocyst coexist; in these cases, jaundice may be due to hepatocellular disease rather than to extrahepatic biliary obstruction.

Laboratory findings often implicate the pancreas. Indicators of abnormal carbohydrate metabolism (e.g., elevated two-hour postprandial *blood sugar* or abnormal *glucose tolerance test*) are present in over half of the patients (Caravati, 1966), and an elevated *serum amylase* can be detected in 40 to 50 per cent. *Anemia* occurs in 15 to 20 per cent and *hyperbilirubinemia* can be demonstrated in as many as a third of the patients (i.e., in many cases when jaundice is not apparent on physical examination).

Radiologic Features

PLAIN FILM FINDINGS. Pancreatic calcification can be identified in 10 to 20 per cent of all patients with pancreatic pseudocysts. Lithiasis, typical of that encountered in patients with alcoholic pancreatitis, is nearly always the form observed but, in rare cases, actual cyst wall calcification can be detected (see Chapter 2). An epigastric soft-tissue mass density can occasionally be demonstrated on plain abdominal roentgenograms when the pseudocyst is large enough to displace adjacent air-containing viscera (Fig. 11–19). Smaller pseudocysts are harder to detect on plain films; they tend to be poorly defined since they are usually not outlined by extraperitoneal fat (Whalen, 1971). Pulmonary abnormalities are present in about a third of all patients with pancreatic pseudocysts. The most common finding is a left pleural effusion. The amylase content of such effusions is usually markedly elevated (Caravati, 1966), and aspiration can therefore provide prompt and specific diagnosis. Other pulmonary abnormalities are of less help. Hemidiaphragmatic elevation and basilar subsegmental atelectasis are common, albeit nonspecific. They occur more often on the left than on the right.

BARIUM EXAMINATIONS. Barium meal examination can demonstrate 80 to 85 per cent of pancreatic pseudocysts which usually produce extrinsic mass indentation on the stomach or on the inner border of the descending duodenum (Caravati, 1966; Thomford, 1969) (Fig. 11–20). The site of mass effect is determined by the location of the pseudocyst:

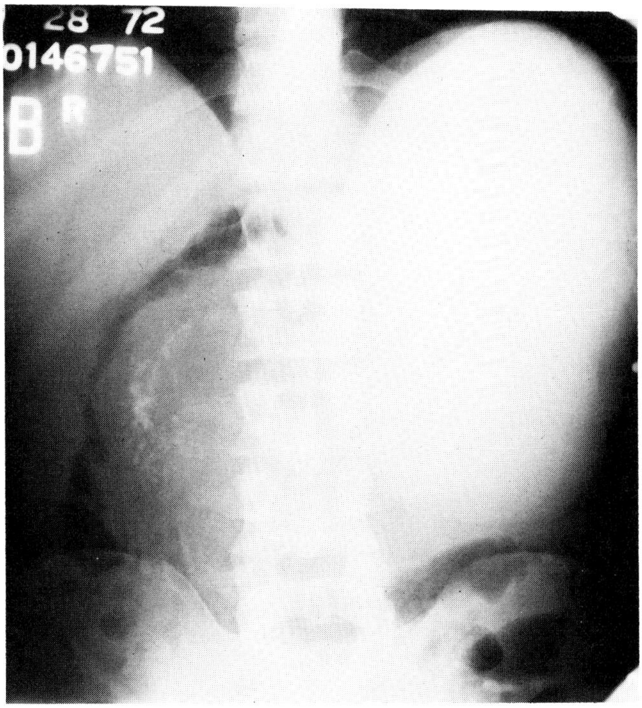

Figure 11–19. Plain abdominal roentgenogram. Pancreatic calcification together with large epigastric and left upper abdominal quadrant soft-tissue mass in patient with chronic alcoholic pancreatitis complicated by development of pseudocyst.

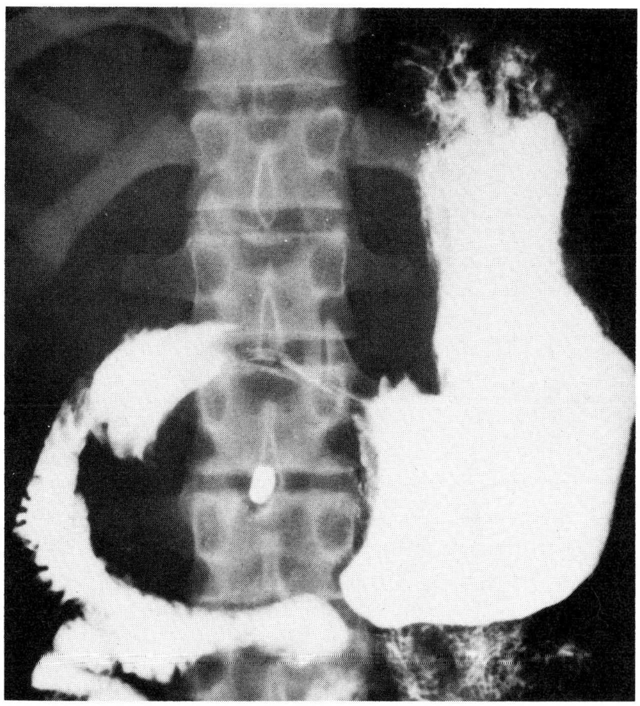

Figure 11–20. Upper gastrointestinal barium examination demonstrates mass in head of pancreas resulting from pseudocyst produced by bullet injury.

those arising from the tail tend to involve the gastric fundus, lesions arising from the body usually indent the body of the stomach, and those developing in the head of the pancreas produce duodenal abnormalities. The most typical form of gastric involvement is an extrinsic mass impression on the posterior surface of the stomach. In general, pancreatic pseudocysts produce smooth-contoured indentations. Such findings indicate mass impression without actual invasion and, as such, are common in patients with pseudocysts. It is well to remember, however, that pancreatic cancers can also indent without invading. Furthermore, pseudocysts can invade adjacent viscera by enzymatic action, pressure necrosis, and intense inflammation (Shockman, 1967). In such cases, the gastric or duodenal wall may appear irregular and ragged. Accordingly, distinction between pseudocysts and tumors on the basis of whether the indentation produced is smooth or irregular is unreliable.

Pseudocysts indent and/or displace the splenic flexure or transverse colon with appreciable frequency—in as many as 40 per cent of instances in some series (e.g., Thomford, 1969). The most frequent abnormality is an inferior displacement of the splenic flexure. In occasional cases, stenosis and even obstruction may be produced (see Chapter 3).

Ultrasonic examination. Echographic examination of the pancreas has proved highly accurate in establishing the diagnosis of pancreatic pseudocyst. Filly and Freimanis (1970) detected six of seven cases prospectively, and subsequent reports have supported the reliability of this technique in identifying all but the smallest of such lesions (e.g., Russell, 1972; Nardi, 1972). Leopold (1972*a*) has reported experience with 13 such cases, all of which were correctly identified. Pancreatic pseudocysts appear as sharply marginated transonic masses on echograms (Fig. 11–21). Because of their homogenous fluid-filled nature, they retain their echo-free appearance even when the transducer sensitivity is increased. It is this feature which allows ultrasonic differentiation from solid pancreatic tumors. These characteristically appear as relatively echo-free areas on scans made at low sensitivity, but "fill in" with small echoes at higher sensitivity settings (Ostrum, 1967).

Because ultrasonic scanning is easily performed and wholly noninvasive, it lends itself to the serial study of patients with pancreatic pseudocyst, and already a body of new information about this

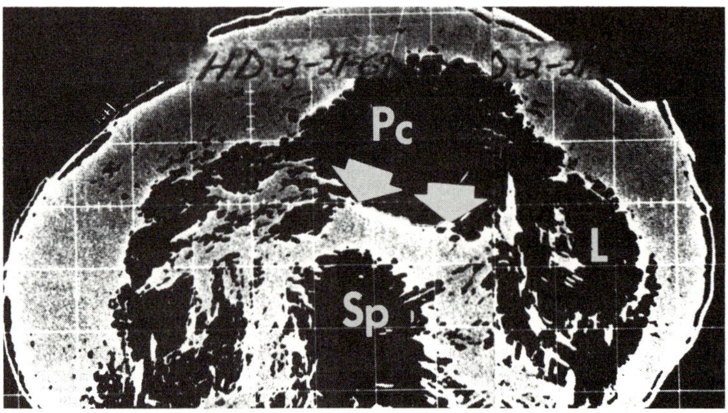

Figure 11–21. Cross-sectional abdominal echogram demonstrates transonic pancreatic mass (Pc) in patient with pancreatic pseudocyst. Liver (L) and spine (sp) are also visible. Arrows indicate increased echo return from behind mass due to compressed tissue effect. (Reproduced by permission of Filly, R. A., and Freimanis, A. K.: Echographic diagnosis of pancreatic lesions. Radiology, 96:575–582, 1970.)

disorder has been accumulated. Evolution of acute pancreatitis into pseudocyst formation has been documented (Leopold, 1972*a*) as has spontaneous resolution by rupture into an adjacent hollow viscus (Leopold, 1972*b*). Furthermore, the lobular or loculated nature of many pseudocysts has been demonstrated (Leopold, 1972*a*); this gross pathologic characteristic was not previously appreciated.

While ultrasonography represents a considerable advance in the diagnostic evaluation of patients with suspected pancreatic pseudocysts, it naturally has limitations. A dilated fluid-filled stomach may lead to misinterpretation. Gastric aspiration can easily settle problems of this nature, but differentiation of pancreatic pseudocysts from other upper abdominal cystic masses presents a more difficult problem. Renal, splenic, and especially adrenal cysts may appear echographically indistinguishable from pseudocysts. Despite these drawbacks, the contribution of ultrasonography to the detection of pancreatic pseudocysts is already unquestioned. Since the technique is still only in its infancy, improvements in instrumentation and further experience in interpretation should increase its value in the future.

Angiography. Since pseudocysts have expansile (rather than infiltrative) growth characteristics, the adjacent arteries become stretched and displaced around them as they enlarge (Fig. 11–22). Smooth stretching of intrapancreatic arteries is fairly specific for pseudocyst and is rarely seen in carcinoma or uncomplicated pancreatitis (Reuter, 1972). The vessels affected depend upon the size and location of the cyst. Very small cysts may displace only the intrapancreatic arteries. Most clinically encountered pseudocysts, however, produce smooth bowing and displacement of major vessels such as the splenic, hepatic, gastroduodenal and/or superior mesenteric branches. Venous compression and occlusion are also common; most frequently the splenic vein is involved (Fu, 1969). In addition, angiographic manifestations of chronic pancreatitis are often present as well.

Angiographic studies appear to detect pancreatic pseudocysts more reliably than any other form of pancreatic pathology. By pooling data from five reports (Nebesar, 1967; Eaton, 1968; Fredens, 1969; Reuter, 1969; and Fu, 1969), 16 of 19 pseudocysts were correctly identified preoperatively (there were also two false-positive diagnoses). In addition to establishing the diagnosis of pancreatic pseudocyst, arteriographic study may demonstrate erosion into major arteries adjacent to the cyst with formation of pseudoaneurysms from which massive gastrointestinal or intraperitoneal hemorrhage may result (e.g., Kadell, 1967). This important information cannot be provided by other roentgen techniques.

FUNCTIONING ISLET CELL TUMOR

Introduction

Neoplastic (or hyperplastic) conditions involving the islets of Langerhans can give rise to a number of intriguing clinical syndromes depending on the humoral substance secreted. The association between islet cell tumors and hyperinsulinism has been known for nearly 50 years (Wilder, 1927), while Zollinger and Ellison (1955) emphasized the link between islet cell tumors and refractory peptic ulcer diathesis almost 20 years ago. At least ten glucagon-secreting islet cell tumors associated with diabetes have been described (Yoshinaga, 1966) and, more recently, a diarrheal syndrome (pancreatic cholera) occurring in patients with islet cell tumors has been identified (Kraft, 1970).

Hyperinsulinism

Pathology

About 70 per cent of islet cell neoplasms associated with excessive secretion of insulin are benign adenomas; about 10 per cent are carcinomas with metastases; and the remainder ap-

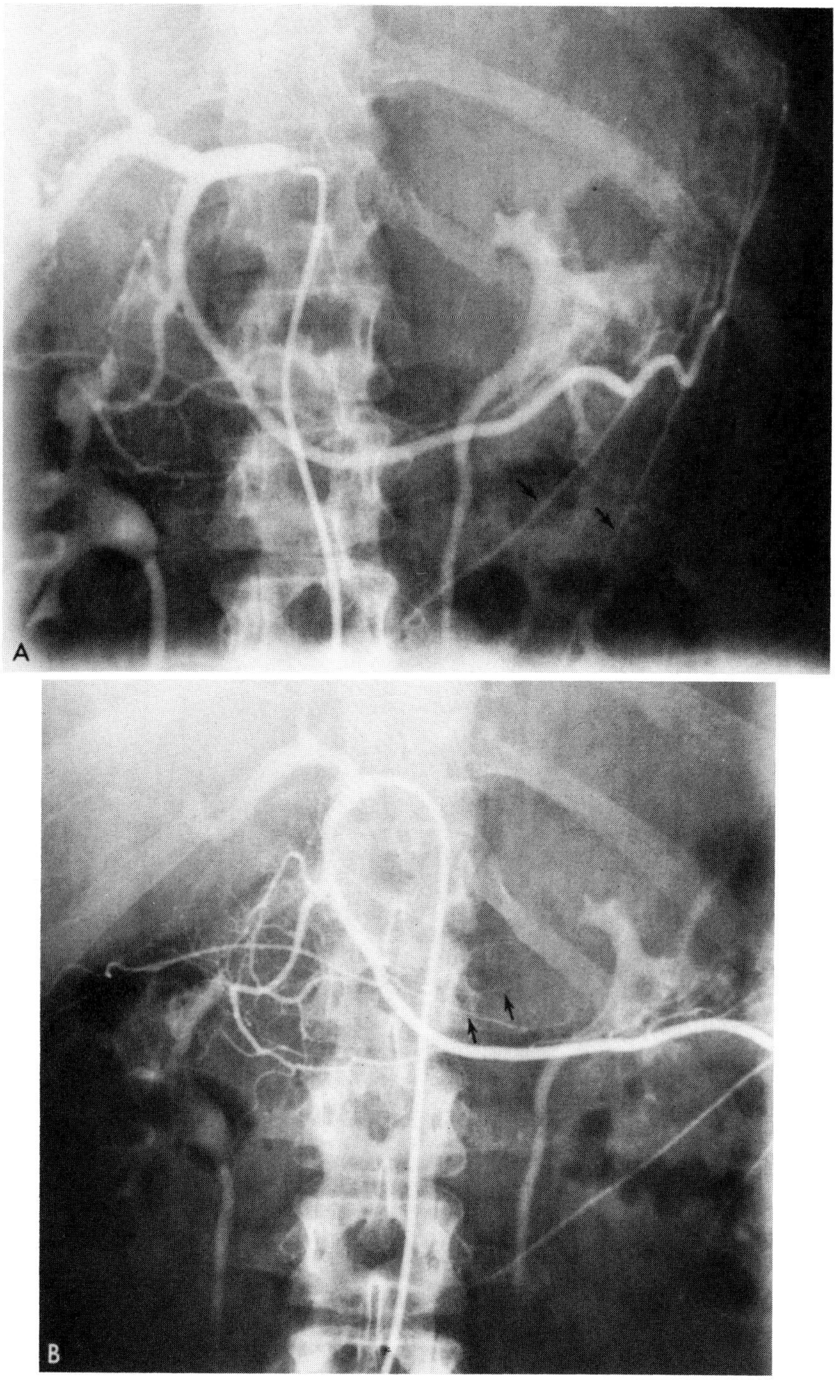

Figure 11–22. Selective hepatic arteriogram (*A*) shows stretching of omental branches of right gastroepiploic artery (*arrows*), while selective gastroduodenal arteriogram (*B*) reveals stretching of intrapancreatic vessels (*arrows*). Changes resulted from large pancreatic pseudocyst.

pear histologically malignant, but grossly and clinically benign (Frantz, 1959). These lesions have a definite predisposition to occur in the body and tail of the pancreas and are usually single (multiple lesions are found in only about 12 per cent of cases). The predominant cellular constituent is the beta-cell which has been shown to represent the site of insulin secretion. In some cases, adenomas of other endocrine glands (e.g., pituitary, parathyroid, etc.) are also present. In these instances, the condition is termed multiple endocrine adenomatosis.

Clinical Features

Insulinomas have been reported in children (e.g., Tuttle, 1972) and in patients over 80 years of age (Hess, 1965), but the majority occur in individuals between 30 and 50. In the typical case, hypoglycemic attacks occur after *exercise* or during a prolonged period of *fasting;* early morning symptoms are especially common. Individual episodes of *fatigue, anxiety, nausea,* and *sweating* may gradually become increasingly frequent and severe or the syndrome may begin with the sudden development of *convulsive seizures* associated with *loss of consciousness.* Between attacks, there are usually no symptoms or signs.

The cardinal clinical feature is the presence of *hypoglycemia* during symptomatic episodes. Symptoms rarely develop unless the blood sugar level is below 50 mg. per 100 ml. and symptomatic remission occurs when carbohydrate (especially intravenous glucose) is administered. When the diagnosis of hyperinsulinism is suspected clinically, a *72-hour fast* is often employed as a diagnostic maneuver. In most instances, this will evoke the patient's symptoms, at which time a blood sugar determination can be made and the effects of intravenous glucose administration observed. The intravenous *tolbutamide test* is another helpful diagnostic maneuver. Tolbutamide is an insulin secretagogue which, in patients with insulinomas, produces a 36 per cent (or more) reduction in the fasting blood sugar level which is prolonged for at least three hours (Fajans, 1961). This test helps differentiate insulinoma from functional hypoglycemia in which blood sugar levels return to baseline values in 90 minutes or less. *Bioassay* and *immunoassay* techniques for evaluating plasma insulin levels are also available (Anderson, 1969).

Radiologic Features

Insulinomas produce no radiographic findings other than those which can be demonstrated by pancreatic angiography. An increasing number of such cases are being subjected to angiographic study because many of these tumors are small and are buried in the substance of the gland. Therefore, angiographic localization of the tumor may be of valuable assistance to the surgeon even in patients in whom the diagnosis has already been established by medical means (e.g., the tolbutamide test).

The characteristic angiographic finding in patients with an islet cell tumor of any type is a rounded, well-circumscribed area of dense staining during the capillary and venous phases of the injection (Fig. 11–23). In certain larger lesions, actual tumor vessels can be identified, but the presence of such vessels has no particular significance. Unless vascular liver metastases can be shown, there are no angiographic criteria which can distinguish between benign and malignant islet cell tumors (Reuter, 1972).

The accuracy of angiography in detecting islet cell tumors has ranged from 38 (Robins, 1973) to 88 per cent (Boijsen, 1970). Based on a review of reported cases, Gray and his co-workers (1970) estimated that angiographic studies are capable of demonstrating just over 60 per cent of all islet cell tumors. In general, large (greater than 2 cm.) lesions with prominent sinusoids and a rich capillary network are most amenable to detection while small (under 1.0 cm.) or hypovascular tumors usually escape

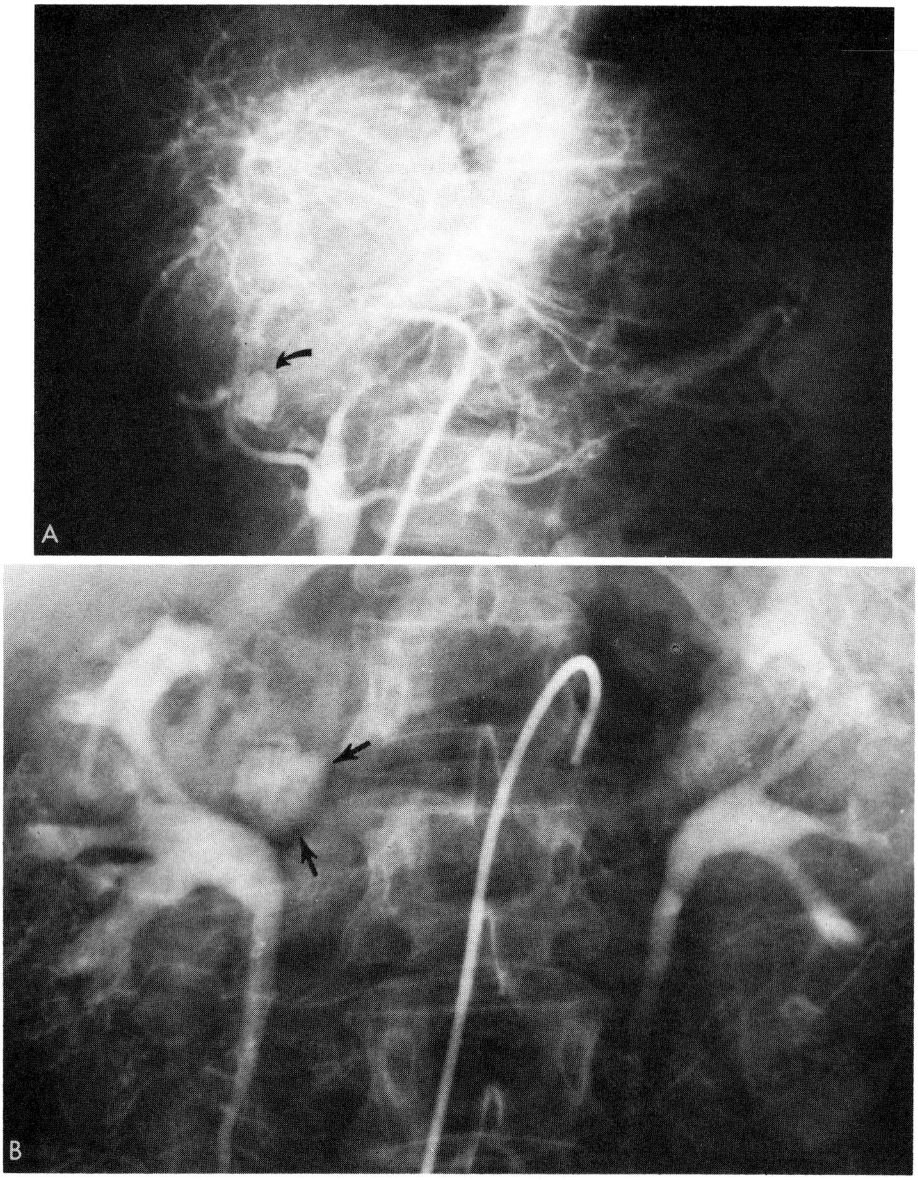

Figure 11–23. Small vascular insulinomas in two different patients. Both were removed from the head of the pancreas at surgery. Selective hepatic (*A*) and superior mesenteric (*B*) arteriograms.

detection. Korobkin and his associates (1971) have emphasized the fact that false-positive diagnoses are possible. In some normal patients, there is an area of hypervascularity in the tail of the pancreas. Accessory splenic tissue and hypervascular metastases to peripancreatic lymph nodes (e.g., from carcinoid tumors) are other potential causes for false-positive diagnosis.

Zollinger-Ellison Syndrome

Pathology

In contrast to insulinomas, over half of all ulcerogenic islet cell tumors are malignant and, of these, two-thirds have metastasized by the time a diagnosis is established (Ellison, 1964). In approximately a third of these patients, multiple tumors are present and in about 10 per cent, the tumors are ectopic in location (e.g., in the stomach, the splenic hilum, and especially the duodenum). The majority of the intrapancreatic lesions occur in the body and/or tail of the gland. The islet cell tumors of Zollinger-Ellison syndrome originate from nonbeta-cell components of the islets (probably from the alpha-cells). The hormonal substance elaborated by these tumors is almost certainly gastrin (Gregory, 1967). This hormone normally occurs in the gastric antral mucosa where it is released in response to local stimulation by food. Its effect is to stimulate secretion of hydrochloric acid by the parietal cells of the stomach. About 20 per cent of all "gastrinomas" are associated with tumors of other endocrine glands (Anderson, 1969).

Clinical Features

Two-thirds of patients with Zollinger-Ellison syndrome are under 50 years old and numerous cases in children under 15 have been reported (Hess, 1965; Zboralske, 1968). More than half of the patients are women. The clinical picture is dominated by *severe ulcer disease.* Over 80 per cent of the ulcers noted in this condition occur in "normal" locations (i.e., the stomach and duodenal bulb), but the relatively high incidence of "ectopic" ulceration has always been considered a hallmark of the syndrome. Multiple ulcers that are active simultaneously is another well known feature. Despite appropriate medical management, the ulcers and their symptoms are remarkably *persistent* and *recurrences* are frequent. Ulcer complications such as perforation and bleeding are also common. Response to conventional surgical therapy is equally poor; *stomal ulceration* developing shortly after gastroenterostomy is a typical feature. *Diarrhea* occurs in about a third of all patients with Zollinger-Ellison syndrome (Zollinger, 1968) and, in as many as 20 per cent, it constitutes the presenting complaint.

When Zollinger-Ellison syndrome is suspected clinically, *12-hour overnight gastric analysis* usually reveals a high volume (as much as 2 to 3 liters) and excessive acid secretion (from three to five times normal). In most instances, *histamine stimulation* produces little or no change in the level of secretion since the stomach is already under maximal hormonal stimulation. *Bioassay* and *immunoassay* techniques (Moore, 1967; McGuigan, 1968) for determination of serum gastrin levels are now available.

Radiologic Features

In most cases, the diagnosis of Zollinger-Ellison syndrome can be strongly suspected on the basis of findings demonstrated by barium examination of the upper gastrointestinal tract (Nelson, 1968; Zboralske, 1968). Peptic *ulceration* is the cardinal feature. Most of such ulcers are in the duodenal bulb or stomach (Fig. 11–24), but craters occur in the esophagus, postbulbar duodenum, and proximal jejunum fairly commonly. Any benign-appearing ulcer detected distal to the duodenal bulb should raise suspicion of the Zollinger-Ellison syndrome. Multiple ulcers occur in about 10 per cent of cases. If the patient has had a previous gastroenterostomy, ulceration often develops at the anastomotic site

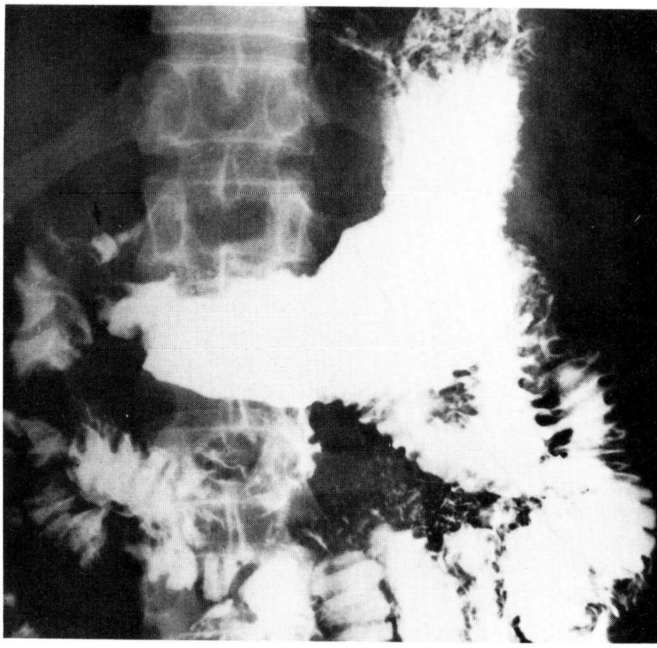

Figure 11–24. Zollinger-Ellison syndrome. Note ulcer crater in apex of duodenal bulb (*arrow*), generalized small-bowel fold thickening and fine granularity of barium in small bowel.

(Fig. 11–25). Such craters are often very large and may resemble large sac-like diverticula. Sometimes multiple ulcers in the region of the stoma can be shown.

The gastric hypersecretion characteristic of this condition produces several radiographic findings. Typically, the stomach contains a good deal of *fluid* despite overnight fasting or even gastric aspiration shortly prior to barium examination. Excessive fluid content in the proximal small bowel is also common. In both locations, *barium appears diluted* and *finely granular* while *mucosal coating is poor.* Excessive gastric acid secretion present in these patients usually produces a reduction in the pH of the duodenal and jejunal contents. As a consequence, a chemical enteritis results with *fold edema* and generalized *dilatation* of the proximal small bowel. *Megaduodenum* is an especially common feature. Another fairly typical result of increased intraluminal acidity is *disordered motility.* The stomach may be atonic and dilated, and hypomotility in the small intestine is also common.

Gastrinomas, like insulinomas, can be demonstrated angiographically as well-circumscribed foci of dense staining visible during the parenchymal and venous phases of celiac or superior mesenteric arterial injection (e.g., Clemett, 1967). Some authorities feel that Zollinger-Ellison tumors are generally less vascular and hence more difficult to demonstrate than insulinomas (Reuter, 1972), but there is currently insufficient data to resolve the issue. Since so many ulcerogenic islet cell tumors are malignant, an especially careful search for vascular hepatic metastases must be made in these patients.

Pancreatic Cholera

This condition, so named by Matsumoto and his colleagues (1966), is characterized by overwhelming diarrhea, marked hypokalemia, and other metabolic derangements associated with severe water and electrolyte depletion. All reported patients have had achlorhydria or hypochlorhydria. Since excessive acid cannot be implicated as a factor in this syndrome, a diarrheogenic hormone has been postulated. Like pa-

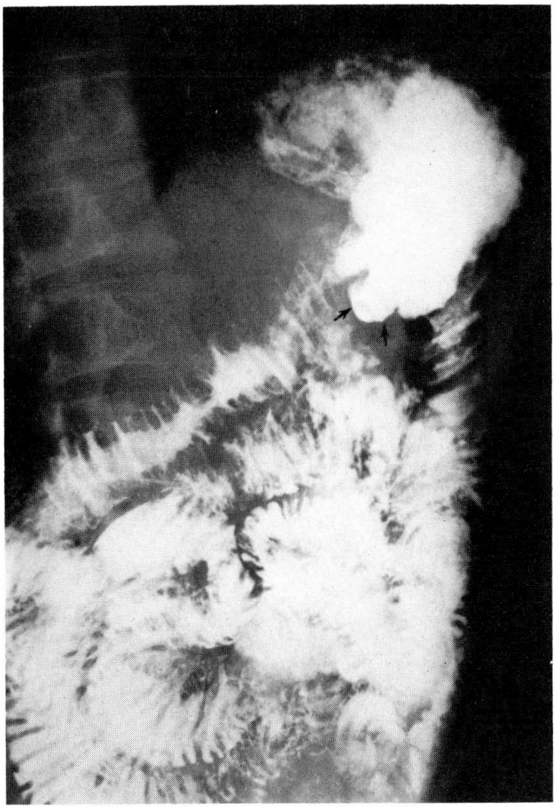

Figure 11–25. Stomal ulceration (*arrows*) in Zollinger-Ellison syndrome. Note associated small-bowel fold thickening and modest small-bowel dilatation.

tients with Zollinger-Ellison syndrome, these individuals (of whom more than 20 have been reported [Kraft, 1970]) have nonbeta-cell tumors of the pancreatic islets. In no instance has gastrin activity been detected when specimens of resected tumor tissue have been assayed. Recently (Zollinger, 1968), it has been suggested that these tumors elaborate secretin; this hormone suppresses gastric acid production and may well represent the diarrheogenic factor.

Review of reported cases (Short, 1973) reveals that dilatation of the small bowel and colon is frequent in these patients. In at least one instance, colonic dilatation was sufficient to simulate megacolon. In most patients, excessive fluid has been present in the small bowel and colon; as in Zollinger-Ellison syndrome, barium dilution and poor mucosal coating result. Gallbladder enlargement has also been present in some instances.

Glucagon-Producing Islet Cell Tumors

At least ten cases of this sort have been reported (Yoshinaga, 1966). The tumors appear to be derived from alpha-cell islet components (McGavran, 1966) and can produce blood glucagon levels 15 to 25 times normal. Glucagon acts by mobilizing hepatic glycogen stores to produce hyperglycemia and diabetes. At least two tumors of this sort have been demonstrated preoperatively by angiographic examination (Anderson, 1969).

REFERENCES

Aakhus, T., Hofsli, M., and Vestad, E.: Angiography in acute pancreatitis. Acta Radiol., 8:119–128, 1969.

Adler, D. C., and Meyers, H. I.: Cineradiographic examination of the upper gastrointestinal tract in obstructive jaundice. J.A.M.A., *199*: 709–713, 1967.

Anderson, M. C.: Review of pancreatic disease. Surgery, *66*:434–449, 1969.

Ansari, A., and Burch, G. E.: A correlative study of proven carcinoma of the pancreas in 83 patients. Amer. J. Gastroent., *50*:456–475, 1968.

Baker, R. J.: Acute surgical diseases of the pancreas. Surg. Clin. N. Amer., *52*:239–256, 1972.

Bank, S., Marks, I. N., Farman, J., and Immelman, E. J.: Further observations on calcified medullary bone lesions in chronic pancreatitis. Gastroenterology, *51*:224–230, 1966.

Baum, S., Greenstein, R. H., Nusbaum, M., and Blakemore, W. S.: Diagnosis of ruptured noncalcific splenic artery aneurysm by selective celiac arteriography. Arch. Surg., *92*:1026–1028, 1965.

Beall, M. S., Dyer, G. A., and Stephenson, H. E.: Disappointments in the management of patients with malignancy of the pancreas, duodenum and common bile ducts. Arch. Surg., *101*:461–465, 1970.

Beranbaum, S. L.: Carcinoma of the pancreas: a bidirectional roentgen approach. Amer. J. Roentgen., *96*:447–467, 1966.

Bergkvist, A., and Seldinger, S. I.: Contrast roentgenography in differential diagnosis between perforated ulcer and acute pancreatitis. Acta Chir. Scand., *118*:137–145, 1959.

Bilbao, M. E., Rosch, J., Frische, L. H., and Dotter, C. T.: Hypotonic duodenography in the diagnosis of pancreatic disease. Seminars Roentgen., *3*:280–287, 1968.

Blumenthal, H. T., and Probstein, R. M.: Pancreatitis. Springfield, Ill., Charles C Thomas, 1959.

Bockus, H. L., Kalser, M. H., Roth, J. L. A., Bogoch, A. L., and Stein, G.: Clinical features of acute inflammation of the pancreas. Arch. Intern. Med., *96*:308–321, 1955.

Boijsen, E., and Samuelsson, L.: Angiographic diagnosis of tumors arising from the pancreatic islets. Acta Radiol. (Diagn.), *10*:161–176, 1970.

Boijsen, E., and Tylen, U.: Angiography in diagnosis. Clinics in Gastroenterology, *1*:85–102, 1972.

Boijsen, E., Gothlin, J., Hallbook, T., and Sandblom, P.: Preoperative angiographic diagnosis of bleeding aneurysms of abdominal visceral arteries. Radiology, *93*:781–791, 1969.

Bookstein, J. J., and Oberman, H. A.: Appraisal of selective angiography in localizing islet-cell tumors of the pancreas. Radiology, *86*:682–685, 1966.

Bookstein, J. J., Reuter, S. R., and Martel, W.: Angiographic evaluation of pancreatic carcinoma. Radiology, *93*:757–764, 1969.

Bouchier, I. A., Youngs, G. R., and Agnew, J. E.: Pancreatic scanning. Clinics in Gastroenterology, *1*:105–118, 1972.

Bourke, J. B., Brown, C. L., Swann, J. C., and Ritchie, H. D.: Exocrine pancreatic function studies, duodenal cytology and hypotonic duodenography in the diagnosis of surgical jaundice. Lancet, *1*:605–608, 1972.

Bowden, L.: Cancer of the pancreas. C. A., *22*: 275–283, 1972.

Bowden, L.: Fallibility of pancreatic biopsy. Ann. Surg., *139*:403–408, 1954.

Braganza, J. M., and Howat, H. T.: Cancer of the pancreas. Clinics in Gastroenterology, *1*:219–237, 1972.

Buranasiri, S., and Baum, S.: The significance of the venous phase of celiac and superior mesenteric arteriography in evaluating pancreatic carcinoma. Radiology, *102*:11–20, 1972.

Caravati, C. M., Ashworth, J. S., and Frederick, P.: Pancreatic pseudocysts. A medical evaluation. J.A.M.A., *194*:572–576, 1966.

Case, J. T.: Roentgenology of pancreatic disease. Caldwell Lecture, 1939. Amer. J. Roentgen., *44*:485–518, 1940.

Clemett, A. R., and Park, W. M.: Arteriographic demonstrations of pancreatic tumor in Zollinger-Ellison syndrome. Radiology, *88*:32–34, 1967.

Eaton, S. B., Benedict, K. T., Ferrucci, J. T., and Fleischli, D. J.: Hypotonic duodenography. Radiol. Clin. N. Amer., *8*:125–137, 1970*b*.

Eaton, S. B., Ferrucci, J. T., and Benedict, K. T.: A comprehensive evaluation of radiologic exploration of the pancreas. C.R.C. Critical Reviews in Radiologic Sciences, *1*:165–205, 1970*a*.

Eaton, S. B., Fleischli, D. J., Pollard, J. J., Nebesar, R. A., and Potsaid, M. S.: Comparison of current radiologic approaches to the diagnosis of pancreatic disease. New Eng. J. Med., *273*: 289–396, 1968.

Eaton, S. B., James, A. E., Potsaid, M. S., and Nardi, G. L.: Evaluation of corrective surgery for pancreatitis by Se^{75} selenomethionine pancreatic imaging. Amer. J. Roentgen., *112*: 678–681, 1971.

Eaton, S. B., Potsaid, M. S., Lo, H. H., and Beaulieu, E.: Radioisotopic "subtraction" scanning for pancreatic lesions. Radiology, *89*:1033–1039, 1967.

Ellison, E. H., and Wilson, S. D.: The Zollinger-Ellison syndrome: reappraisal and evaluation of 260 registered cases. Ann. Surg., *160*:512–528, 1964.

Engelhart, G., and Blauenstein, V. W.: Ultrasound in the diagnosis of pancreatic tumors. Gut, *11*:443–449, 1970.

Eyler, W. R., Clark, M. D., and Rian, R. L.: An evaluation of roentgen signs of pancreatic enlargement. J.A.M.A., *181*:967–971, 1962.

Eyler, W. R., Schuman, B. A., DuSault, L. A., and Hinson, R. E.: The radioiodinated rose bengal liver scan as an aid in the differential diagnosis of jaundice. Amer. J. Roentgen., *94*:469–476, 1965.

Fajans, S. S., Schnieder, J. M., Schtiengart, D. E., and Conn, J. W.: The diagnostic value of sodium tolbutamide in hypoglycemic states. J. Clin. Endocr., *21*:371–386, 1961.

Felson, B.: Letter from the editor. Seminars Roentgen, *3*:215–216, 1968.

Ferrucci, J. T., Benedict, K. T., Page, D. L., Fleischli, D. J., and Eaton, S. B.: Radiographic features of the normal hypotonic duodeno-

gram. Radiology, *96*:401–408, 1970.
Filly, R. A., and Freimanis, A. K.: Echographic diagnosis of pancreatic lesions. Radiology, *96*:575–582, 1970.
Fitzgerald, O.: Painless pancreatitis and other painless pancreatic disorders. Clinics in Gastroenterology, *1*:195–218, 1972.
Frantz, V. K.: Tumors of the pancreas. *In* Atlas of Tumor Pathology, Section VII, Fascicles 27 and 28, Armed Forces Institute of Pathology, Washington, D.C., 1959.
Fras, I., Litin, E. M., and Bartholomew, L. G.: Mental symptoms as an aid in the early diagnosis of carcinoma of the pancreas. Gastroenterology, *55*:191–198, 1968.
Fredens, M., Egeblad, M., and Holst-Nielsen, F.: The value of selective angiography in the diagnosis of tumors of the pancreas and liver. Radiology, *93*:765–769, 1969.
Freeman, L. M., and Kay, C. J.: Radioactive rose bengal abdominal scanning in jaundiced patients. New York J. Med., *66*:1778–1781, 1966.
Frostberg, N.: Characteristic duodenal deformity in cases of different kinds of perivaterial enlargement of pancreas. Acta Radiol., *19*: 164–173, 1938.
Fu, W. R., and Stanton, L. W.: Angiographic study of pseudocysts of the pancreas. J. Canad. Ass. Radiol., *20*:176–179, 1969.
Gerle, R. D., Walker, L. A., Achord, J. L., and Weens, H. S.: Osseous changes in chronic pancreatitis. Radiology, *85*:330–337, 1965.
Gray, R. K., Rosch, J., and Grollman, J. H.: Arteriography in the diagnosis of islet cell tumors. Radiology, *97*:39–44, 1970.
Greene, A. G., and Sadowsky, N. L.: A radiologic approach to the differential diagnosis of surgical and non-surgical jaundice. Amer. J. Roentgen., *116*:368–374, 1972.
Gregory, R. A., Grossman, M. I., Tracy, H. J., and Bentley, P. H.: Nature of the gastric secretagogue in Zollinger-Ellison tumors. Lancet, *2*:543–544, 1967.
Guien, C.: General radiology of the pancreas. Clinics in Gastroenterology, *1*:61–83, 1972.
Hammansten, J. F., Honska, W. L., and Limes, J. L.: Pleural fluid amylase in pancreatitis and other diseases. Amer. Rev. Tuberc. Pulmon. Dis., *79*:606–611, 1959.
Heck, L. L., and Gottschalk, A.: The appearance of intrahepatic biliary duct dilatation on the liver scan. Radiology, *99*:135–140, 1971.
Hernandez, G., Escarlat, B., and Bismuth, V.: L'arterioportographie des affections pancreatiques. J. Radiol. Electr., *48*:327–338, 1967.
Heslip, P. G., and Overton, T. R.: The value of radioisotope scanning in the investigation of suspected carcinoma of the pancreas. Amer. J. Roentgen., *112*:667–677, 1971.
Hess, W.: Surgery of the Biliary Passages and the Pancreas. Princeton, N.J., D. Van Nostrand Company, Inc., 1965.
Hodes, P. J., Pendergrass, E. P., and Winston, N. J.: Pancreatic, ductal and vaterian neoplasms: their roentgen manifestations. Radiology, *62*:1–15, 1954.
Howard, J., and Jordan, G. L.: Surgical Diseases of the Pancreas. Philadelphia, J. B. Lippincott Company, 1960.
Jacquemet, P., Liotta, D., and Mallet-Guy, P.: Early Radiologic Diagnosis of Diseases of the Pancreas and Ampulla of Vater: Elective Exploration of the Ampulla of Vater and the Head of the Pancreas by Hypotonic Duodenography. Springfield, Ill., Charles C Thomas, 1965.
Johnson, J. R., and Zintel, H. A.: Pancreatic calcification and cancer of the pancreas. Surg. Gynec. Obstet., *117*:585–588, 1963.
Kadell, B. M., and Riley, J. M.: Major arterial involvement by pancreatic pseudocysts. Amer. J. Roentgen, *99*:632–636, 1967.
Kilman, J. W., Kaiser, G. C., King, R. D., and Shumacker, H. B.: Pancreatic pseudocysts in infancy and childhood. Surgery, *55*:455–461, 1964.
Klintrup, H. E.: Carcinoma of the pancreas: a statistical, clinical and pathological study. Acta Chir. Scand., *362*:Suppl., 1–96, 1966.
Korobkin, M. T., Palubinskas, A. J., and Glickman, M. G.: Pitfalls in arteriography of islet-cell tumors of the pancreas. Radiology, *100*:319–328, 1971.
Kraft, A. R., Tompkins, R. K., and Zollinger, R. M.: Recognition and management of the diarrheal syndrome caused by non-beta islet cell tumors of the pancreas. Amer. J. Surg., *119*:163–170, 1970.
Krain, L. S.: The rising incidence of carcinoma of the pancreas: further epidemiologic studies. J. Chron. Dis., *23*:685–690, 1971.
Kyaw, M. M.: Personal communication, 1970.
Landman, S., Polcyn, R. E., and Gottschalk, A.: Pancreas imaging: is it worth it? Radiology, *100*:631–636, 1971.
Lawson, D. W., Daggett, W. M., Civetta, J. M., Corey, R. J., and Bartlett, M. K.: Surgical treatment of necrotizing pancreatitis. Ann. Surg., *171*:605–617, 1970.
Leopold, G. R.: Pancreatic echography: a new dimension in the diagnosis of pseudocyst. Radiology, *104*:365–369, 1972*a*.
Leopold, G. R., Berk, R. N., and Reinke, R.:Echographic-radiographic documentation of spontaneous rupture of a pancreatic pseudocyst into the duodenum. Radiology, *102*:699–700, 1972*b*.
Longstreth, G. F., Newcomer, A. D., and Green, P. A.: Extrahepatic portal hypertension caused by chronic pancreatitis. Ann. Intern. Med., *75*: 903–908, 1971.
Mani, J. R., Zboralske, F. F., and Margulis, A. R.: Carcinoma of the body and tail of the pancreas. Amer. J. Roentgen., *96*:429–446, 1966.
Martel, W., Scholtens, P. A., and Lim, L. W.: "Tubeless" hypotonic duodenography: technique, value, and limitations. Amer. J. Roentgen., *107*:119–130, 1969.
Matsumoto, K. K., Peter, J. B., Schultze, R. G., Hakim, A. A., and Franck, P. T.: Watery diarrhea and hypokalemia associated with pancreatic islet cell adenoma. Gastroenterology, *50*:231–242, 1966.
McCarthy, D. M., and Brown, P.: Measurement of

duodenal tryptic activity and Se^{75}-selenomethionine pancreatic scanning compared as tests of pancreatic function. Gut, *10*:913–920, 1969.

McCarthy, D. M., Brown, P., Melmed, R. N., Agnew, J. E., and Bouchier, I. A. D.: 75-Se selenomethionine scanning in the diagnosis of tumors of the pancreas and adjacent viscera: the use of the test and its impact on survival. Gut, *13*:75–87, 1972.

McGavran, M. H., Unger, R. H., Recant, L., Polk, H. C., Kilo, C., and Levin, M. E.: Glucagon-secreting alpha-cell carcinoma of the pancreas. New Eng. J. Med., *274*:1408–1413, 1966.

McGuigan, J. E., and Trudeau, W. L.: Immunochemical measurement of elevated levels of gastrin in the serum of patients with pancreatic tumors of the Zollinger-Ellison variety. New Eng. J. Med., *278*:1308–1313, 1968.

Miale, A., Rodriguez-Antunez, A., and Gill, W. M.: Pancreas scanning after ten years. Seminars Nucl. Med., *2*:201–219, 1972.

Moore, F. T., Murat, J. E., Endahl, G. L., Baker, J. L., and Zollinger, R. M.: Diagnosis of ulcerogenic tumor of the pancreas by bioassay. Amer. J. Surg., *113*:735–737, 1967.

Moskowitz, H., Chait, A., and Mellins, H. Z.: "Tumor encasement" of the celiac axis due to chronic pancreatitis. Amer. J. Roentgen., *104*:641–645, 1968.

Mujahed, Z., and Evans, J. W.: Percutaneous transhepatic cholangiography. Radiol. Clin. N. Amer., *4*:535–545, 1966.

Nardi, G. L., Birnholz, J. C., and Eaton, S. B.: Treatment of pancreatic cyst by gastrostomy and internal drainage. Hosp. Pract., 7:108–114, October, 1972.

Nebesar, R. A., and Pollard, J. J.: A critical evaluation of selective celiac and superior mesenteric angiography in the diagnosis of pancreatic diseases, particularly malignant tumor: facts and "artifacts." Radiology, *89*:1017–1027, 1967.

Nelson, S. W., and Christoforidis, A. J.: Roentgenologic features of the Zollinger-Ellison syndrome: ulcerogenic tumor of the pancreas. Seminars Roentgen., *3*:254–266, 1968.

Nordyke, R. A.: Surgical vs. nonsurgical jaundice: differentiation by a combination of rose bengal I^{131} and standard liver-function tests. J.A.M.A., *194*:949–953, 1965.

Ostrum, B., Goldberg, B., and Isard, H.: A-mode ultrasound differentiation of soft tissue masses. Radiology, *88*:745–749, 1967.

Paulino-Netto, A., Dreiling, D. A., and Barnofsky, I. D.: Relationship between pancreatic calcification and cancer of the pancreas. Ann. Surg., *151*:530–537, 1960.

Perez, C. A., Powers, W. E., Holtz, S., and Spjut, H. J.: Roentgenologic-pathologic correlation of resectable carcinoma of the pancreaticoduodenal region. Amer. J. Roentgen., *94*:438–448, 1965.

Rastogi, H., and Brown, C. H.: Carcinoma of the pancreas. A review of one hundred cases. Cleveland Clin. Quart., *34*:243–263, 1967.

Reuter, S. R., and Redman, H. C.: Gastrointestinal Angiography. Philadelphia, W. B. Saunders Company, 1972.

Reuter, S. R., Redman, H. C., and Bookstein, J. J.: Differential problems in the angiographic diagnosis of carcinoma of the pancreas. Radiology, *96*:93–99, 1970.

Reuter, S. R., Redman, H. C., and Joseph, R. R.: Angiographic findings in pancreatitis. Amer. J. Roentgen., *107*:56–64, 1969.

Riccobono, K. J.: Pancreatic scanning. Seminars Roentgen., *3*:310–317, 1968.

Ritchie, G. W., Jackson, D. C., and Eaglesham, H.: Percutaneous transhepatic cholangiography: experience with 54 cases. Canad. Med. Ass. J., *100*:110–116, 1969.

Robins, J. M., Bookstein, J. J., Oberman, H. A., and Fajans, S. S.: Selective angiography in localizing islet-cell tumors of the pancreas. Radiology, *106*:525–528, 1973.

Rosch, J., and Herfort, K.: Splenoportographic diagnosis of pancreatic disease. Geriatrics, *19*:725–734, 1964.

Rossi, P., and Gould, H. R.: Angiography and scanning in liver disease. Radiology, *96*:553–562, 1970.

Rubinstein, Z. J., Bank, S., Marks, I. N., and Psillos, C.: Hypotonic duodenography in chronic pancreatitis. Brit. J. Radiol., *44*:142–149, 1971.

Russell, J. G. B.: Ultrasound and the pancreas. Clinics in Gastroenterology, *1*:119–124, 1972.

Russell, W. M., and Margulis, A. R.: Impression on the duodenal loop resulting from tumor of the pancreas: a roentgenographic evaluation. Amer. J. Roentgen., *94*:449–452, 1965.

Sachs, M. D., and Partington, P. F.: Cholangiographic diagnosis of pancreatitis. Amer. J. Roentgen., *76*:32–38, 1956.

Salik, J. O.: Pancreatic carcinoma and its early roentgenologic recognition. Amer. J. Roentgen., *86*:1–28, 1961.

Sarles, H., and Gerolami-Santandrea, A.: Chronic pancreatitis. Clinics in Gastroenterology, *1*:167–193, 1972.

Sarles, H., Sarles, J. C., Camatte, R., Muratore, R., Gaini, M., Guien, C., Pastor, J., and Le Roy, F.: Observations on 205 confirmed cases of acute pancreatitis, recurring pancreatitis, and chronic pancreatitis. Gut, *6*:545–559, 1965.

Schultz, E. H.: Aids to diagnosis of acute pancreatitis by roentgen study. Amer. J. Roentgen., *89*:825–836, 1963.

Seldinger, S. I.: Percutaneous transhepatic cholangiography. Acta Radiol., *253*:Suppl., 1–133, 1966.

Shockman, A. T., and Marasco, J. A.: Pseudocysts of the pancreas. Amer. J. Roentgen., *101*: 628–638, 1967.

Short, W. F., Bron, K. M., Eaton, S. B., and Leopold, G. R.: Pancreatic evaluation by roentgenography, ultrasound, and radioisotopes. *In* The Pancreas. Edited by L. C. Casey. St. Louis, Mo., C. V. Mosby Company, 1973.

Silverberg, E., and Holleb, A. I.: Cancer statistics 1972. C. A., *22*:2–20, 1972.

Sproul, E. E.: Carcinoma and venous thrombosis: the frequency of association of carcinoma in the body or tail of the pancreas with multiple venous thrombosis. Amer. J. Cancer, *34*: 566–585, 1938.

Staab, E. V., Babb, O. A., Klatte, E. C., and Brill, A. B.: Pancreatic radionuclide imaging using electronic subtraction technique. Radiology, *99*:633–640, 1971.

Stein, G. N., Kalser, M. H., Sarian, N. N., and Finkelstein, A.: An evaluation of the roentgen changes in acute pancreatitis: correlation with clinical findings. Gastroenterology, *36*:354–361, 1959.

Stephenson, H. E., Jr.: Cancer of the pancreas and stomach: a study in contrasts. Surgery, *71*: 307–308, 1972.

Strang, C., and Walton, J. N.: Carcinoma of body and tail of pancreas. Ann. Intern. Med., *39*: 15–37, 1953.

Stuber, J. L., Templeton, A. W., and Bishop, K.: Sonographic diagnosis of pancreatic lesions. Amer. J. Roentgen., *116*:406–412, 1972.

Thomford, N. R., and Jesseph, J. E.: Pseudocyst of the pancreas. A review of fifty cases. Amer. J. Surg., *118*:86–94, 1969.

Trapnell, J. E.: The natural history and management of acute pancreatitis. Clinics in Gastroenterology, *1*:147–166, 1972.

Trapnell, J. E., and Anderson, M. C.: The role of early laparotomy in acute pancreatitis. Ann. Surg., *165*:49–55, 1967.

Tuttle, R. J., Strasberg, Z., and Cole, F. M.: Angiographic diagnosis of insulinoma in a 6-year-old boy. Radiology, *104*:355–356, 1972.

Walker, L. G., Stone, H. H., and Apple, D. G.: Pseudocysts of the pancreas: a review of 59 cases. Southern Med. J., *60*:389–393, 1967.

Warren, K. W., and Veidenheimer, M.: Pathologic considerations in the choice of operation for chronic relapsing pancreatitis. New Eng. J. Med., *266*:323–329, 1962.

Warren, K. W., Braasch, J. W., and Thum, C. W.: Diagnosis and surgical treatment of carcinoma of the pancreas. Curr. Probl. Surg., June, 1968.

Waterman, N. G., Walsky, R. S., Kasdan, M. L., and Abrams, B. L.: Treatment of acute hemorrhagic pancreatitis by sump drainage. Surg. Gynec. Obstet., *126*:963–968, 1968.

Weens, H. S., and Walker, L. A.: The radiologic diagnosis of acute cholecystitis and pancreatitis. Radiol. Clin. N. Amer., *2*:89–106, 1964.

Weinstein, B. R., Korn, R. J., and Zimmerman, H. J.: Obstructive jaundice as a complication of pancreatitis. Ann. Intern. Med., *58*:245–258, 1963.

Whalen, J. P., Evans, J. A., and Shanser, J.: Vector principle in the differential diagnosis of abdominal masses: the left upper quadrant. Amer. J. Roentgen., *113*:104–118, 1971.

Wilder, R. M., Allen, F. N., Power, M. H., and Robertson, H. E.: Carcinoma of the islands of the pancreas: hyperinsulism and hypoglycemia. J.A.M.A., *89*:348–355, 1927.

Yoshinaga, T., Okuno, G., Shinji, Y., Tsujii, T., and Nishikawa, M.: Pancreatic α-cell tumor associated with severe diabetes mellitus. Diabetes, *15*:709–713, 1966.

Zboralske, F. F., and Amberg, J. R.: Detection of the Zollinger-Ellison syndrome: the radiologist's responsibility. Amer. J. Roentgen., *104*: 529–543, 1968.

Zollinger, R. M.: Zollinger-Ellison syndrome comes of age. Recognition of the complete clinical spectrum and its management. J.A.M.A., *204*:361–365, 1968.

Zollinger, R. M., and Ellison, E. H.: Primary peptic ulceration of the jejunum associated with islet cell tumors of the pancreas. Ann. Surg., *142*: 709–728, 1955.

Zollinger, R. M., Tompkins, R. K., Amerson, J. R., Endahl, G. L., Kraft, A. R., and Moore, F. T.: Identification of the diarrheogenic hormone associated with non-beta islet cell tumors of the pancreas. Ann. Surg., *168*:502–521, 1968.

Chapter 12

TAILORED RADIOLOGIC EVALUATION OF SUSPECTED PANCREATICO-DUODENAL DISEASE

THE PATIENT WHOSE DOMINANT CLINICAL FEATURE IS AN EPIGASTRIC MASS RAISING THE POSSIBILITY OF PANCREATIC PSEUDOCYST
- **Abdominal Ultrasonography**
- **Upper Gastrointestinal Barium Examination**
- **Pancreatic Angiography**

THE ANICTERIC PATIENT IN WHOM ABDOMINAL PAIN CONSISTENT WITH PANCREATIC ORIGIN IS A PROMINENT FEATURE
- **^{75}Se Selenomethionine Pancreatic Imaging**
- **Upper Gastrointestinal Barium Examination**
- **Pancreatic Angiography**
- **Peroral Pancreatography**

THE PATIENT IN WHOM JAUNDICE WHICH MAY BE DUE TO EXTRAHEPATIC BILIARY OBSTRUCTION IS THE DOMINANT CLINICAL FEATURE
- **The Radionuclide "Liver Profile"**
- **Hypotonic Duodenography**
- **Pancreatic Angiography**
- **Peroral Cholangiopancreatography**
- **Transhepatic Cholangiography**

THE PATIENT WITH ACUTE ABDOMINAL DISCOMFORT IN WHOM ACUTE PANCREATITIS IS CONSIDERED A POSSIBILITY
- **Plain Roentgenographic Examination**
  - Study of the Chest
  - Abdominal Films
- **Intravenous Cholangiography**
- **Abdominal Ultrasonography**
- **Upper Gastrointestinal Barium Examination**

THE PATIENT WITH SEVERE ACID-PEPTIC DISEASE IN WHOM ZOLLINGER-ELLISON SYNDROME IS CONSIDERED A POSSIBILITY
- **Gastrointestinal Barium Examination**
- **Angiographic Examination of the Pancreas and Liver**

THE PATIENT WITH CLINICAL AND BIOCHEMICAL FINDINGS WHICH SUGGEST HYPERINSULINISM
- **Pancreatic Angiography**

THE PATIENT WHOSE CONVENTIONAL UPPER GASTROINTESTINAL BARIUM EXAMINATION SUGGESTS PRIMARY DUODENAL DISEASE
- **Hypotonic Duodenography**
- **Fiberoptic Duodenoscopy**

Since radiologic procedures appropriate for evaluation of one suspected pancreatic or duodenal disorder may be poorly suited for demonstrating another condition, the most logical approach to diagnosis of diseases arising in this area is to tailor the radiologic "work-up" to fit the disease condition provisionally considered most likely. Patients referred for radiologic investigation of suspected pancreatic or duodenal disease generally fall into reasonably discrete clinical categories. The historic details, physical findings, and laboratory results which lead the astute clinician to consider carcinoma of the body or tail of the pancreas differ significantly from those which raise the question of pancreaticoduodenal cancer. Patients with pancreatic pseudocysts, chronic pancreatitis, endocrinologically active islet cell tumors, and acute pancreatitis usually manifest still other fairly typical patterns as described in Chapter 11. For the most part, primary duodenal disease other than bulbar ulcer becomes suspected only after the possibility is suggested by conventional barium upper gastrointestinal examination so that subsequent roentgen study in these cases is based on combined clinicoradiologic indications.

This monograph has analyzed the contributions of various radiologic procedures to the diagnosis of pancreaticoduodenal disease. The aim of this concluding chapter is to suggest an appropriate format for radiologic evaluation of patients who present with one of the typical patterns which clinically suggest a disorder involving the pancreas or duodenum. For this purpose, we have followed the same guiding principles of safety, accuracy, and economy which are emphasized in Chapter 5—The Radiology of Jaundice. Ideally, the least hazardous procedures should be employed initially. In addition, the protocol should be designed to minimize patient expense and the time required to establish the diagnosis. These principles are in some ways contradictory and, of course, must be made to fit the clinical setting of the individual case. Nevertheless, it is still possible to draw up a reasonable radiologic format applicable to most situations in which pancreaticoduodenal disease is a likely possibility.

In many cases, radiologic evaluation is best begun on an outpatient basis. Except for patients with acute pancreatitis, the clinical situation is seldom so severe as to require immediate hospital admission, and several noninvasive examinations can easily be performed on outpatients. This approach has the major economic advantage of accomplishing a significant portion of the patient's work-up (and, in many cases, establishing the diagnosis) prior to hospitalization. Furthermore, barium studies can be performed without fear of prolonging the patient's hospital stay merely to clear the bowel of barium in preparation for angiographic study. If outpatient examination indicates the need for more complicated procedures (e.g., angiography), these can be scheduled for the first full hospital day. In most instances, all diagnostic information necessary to make pertinent management decisions can thus be available early in the hospitalization, and it is seldom necessary to delay appropriate surgery beyond the second full hospital day.

It should be emphasized that, although recommended examinations should be employed in a specific sequence, it is not intended that each study be slavishly utilized for every patient. Once the desired information has been obtained, the protocol can be interrupted and therapy begun without reference to further superfluous radiologic studies (see Table 12–1).

THE PATIENT WHOSE DOMINANT CLINICAL FEATURE IS AN EPIGASTRIC MASS RAISING THE POSSIBILITY OF PANCREATIC PSEUDOCYST

ABDOMINAL ULTRASONOGRAPHY. Even though this form of examination is still in its developing stages, it seems clear that echography, where available, should be the initial radiologic study employed for patients falling into this category. As described in Chapters 9 and 11, this mode of examination is very accurate in characterizing the location of clinically palpable epigastric masses and has the additional, highly important capability of distinguishing solid from cystic lesions in most cases. As a wholly noninvasive procedure, this mode of examination is well suited to outpatient application. Ultrasonic studies should be performed prior to barium examination since residual barium interferes with the sonic transmission properties of abdominal viscera (see Chapter 9).

UPPER GASTROINTESTINAL BARIUM EXAMINATION. Prior to the development of ultrasonic techniques, barium

TABLE 12–1. Tailored Radiologic Evaluation of Suspected Pancreaticoduodenal Disease

Epigastric Mass: ? Pancreatic Pseudocyst
- Outpatient Examinations
  - Abdominal Ultrasonography
  - Upper Gastrointestinal Barium Examination
- Inpatient Examinations
  - Pancreatic Angiography

Abdominal Pain: ? Chronic Pancreatitis or Carcinoma Involving the Body or Tail of the Pancreas
- Outpatient Examinations
  - ^{75}Se Selenomethionine Pancreatic Imaging
  - Upper Gastrointestinal Barium Examination
- Inpatient Examinations
  - Pancreatic Angiography
  - Peroral Pancreatography

Jaundice: ? Extrahepatic Biliary Obstruction
- Outpatient Examinations
  - Radionuclide "Liver Profile"
    - ^{99m}Tc Sulfur Colloid Hepatic Imaging
    - Radioiodinated Rose Bengal Examination
  - Hypotonic Duodenography
- Inpatient Examinations
  - Pancreatic Angiography
  - Peroral Cholangiopancreatography
  - Transhepatic Cholangiography

Acute Abdomen: ? Acute Pancreatitis
- Inpatient Examinations
  - Plain Film Studies
    - Chest—PA and Lateral (upright if possible)
    - Abdomen—Supine and Upright (if possible)
  - Intravenous Cholangiography
  - Abdominal Ultrasonography (if available)
  - Upper Gastrointestinal Barium Examination

Severe Acid-Peptic Disease: ? Zollinger-Ellison Syndrome
- Outpatient Examination
  - Upper Gastrointestinal Barium Examination
- Inpatient Examination
  - Angiographic Study of Pancreas and Liver

Hyperinsulinism: ? Pancreatic Insulinoma
- Inpatient Examination
  - Pancreatic Angiography

Questionable Duodenal Abnormality on UGIS: ? Primary Duodenal Lesion
- Outpatient Examination
  - Hypotonic Duodenography
- Inpatient Examination
  - Fiberoptic Duodenoscopy

meal examination was considered the single most helpful diagnostic procedure for patients in whom the diagnosis of pancreatic pseudocyst was clinically suspected. Accordingly, barium upper gastrointestinal study should be the second radiologic procedure employed in this category of patients. Barium examination complements the localization established by ultrasonic scanning and, while it cannot distinguish between solid and cystic pancreatic masses, provides more detailed information concerning the degree of adjacent organ involvement than can be demonstrated by echography.

Like ultrasonic scanning, barium meal examination is well suited for use in outpatients and, when a palpable epigastric mass is a prominent clinical feature, the combined use of these two procedures will establish the diagnosis in the great majority of instances. In many cases, therefore, hospitalization for surgery without further diagnostic evaluation will be appropriate. In other circumstances, however, it may be desirable to perform pancreatic angiography on the first hospital day with surgery scheduled for the next morning.

PANCREATIC ANGIOGRAPHY. As discussed in Chapter 11, angiographic evaluation of the pancreas is an effective means of identifying pancreatic pseudocysts. In patients with palpable abdominal masses who have already been studied by echography and barium upper gastrointestinal examination, the diagnosis will usually have been established but, in rare instances, angiographic study will demonstrate that the mass actually arises from the adrenal or spleen rather than from the pancreas. In all cases, angiography will reveal the relationship of the cyst to the peripancreatic blood vessels. Such information is helpful for planning appropriate surgery. Not infrequently, splenic vein obstruction or development of pseudoaneurysms in arteries adjacent to the pancreas can be demonstrated. If either of these conditions is present, the anticipated surgical procedure can be extended to include correction of the associated vascular disorder.

THE ANICTERIC PATIENT IN WHOM ABDOMINAL PAIN CONSISTENT WITH PANCREATIC ORIGIN IS A PROMINENT FEATURE

For patients to be placed in this category, they must have no visible icterus or significant hyperbilirubinemia. If jaundice is present, then the radiologic work-up should proceed according to the protocol established for jaundiced patients. When restricted in this manner, the most likely pancreatic disorders are chronic pancreatitis or carcinoma of the body and tail of the pancreas. Epigastric pain (often with radiation to the back), weight loss, anorexia, and weakness are clinical features commonly present in both conditions. Similarly, malabsorption and/or diabetes can occur in either form of disease. A history of alcoholism and of previous episodic abdominal pain tends to direct attention to the possibility of chronic inflammation, whereas the insidious development of symptoms in a previously healthy individual suggests malignancy, but in neither case can a clinical diagnosis be made with confidence.

^{75}SE SELENOMETHIONINE PANCREATIC IMAGING. For patients who fall into this category, the appropriate initial radiologic investigation is radioisotopic pancreatic imaging with ^{75}Se selenomethionine. If either chronic pancreatitis or cancer involving the body or tail of the pancreas is present, an abnormal pancreatic scintigram should result approximately 90 per cent of the time. Because of the relatively high incidence of false-positive pancreatic scans, an abnormal result should serve as an indication for further diagnostic effort—not for surgical exploration. On the other hand, a convincingly normal pancreatic image tends to exclude both benign and malignant pancreatic disease with reasonable (~ 90 per cent) reliability. While it still seems appropriate to proceed with barium meal investigation under these circumstances, more complicated and expensive techniques such as pancreatic angiography and peroral pancreatography can reasonably be foregone unless there are unusually convincing clinical features implicating the pancreas.

UPPER GASTROINTESTINAL BARIUM EXAMINATION. Patients with abdominal pain suggesting pancreatic disease deserve study by conventional barium meal technique, not only to search for signs of pancreatic disorder, but also to exclude those extrapancreatic disease processes (such as gastric cancer or peptic ulcer) which can simulate the symptomatology of pancreatic disease and which are also amenable to demonstration by barium upper gastrointestinal examination. When pancreatic disease is suspected, however (e.g., in patients with nonspecific abdominal discomfort and a positive pancreatic scan), the emphasis of barium examination should be placed on detecting pancreatic abnormality. The preliminary abdominal roentgenogram should be closely scrutinized for pancreatic calcification and, if necessary, tomographic sections should be obtained where the plain film is inconclusive. Good quality lateral films to check for evidence of indentation on the posterior surface of the barium-filled stomach should be obtained and the duodenum (including its entire postbulbar extent) should be examined with special care. If equivocal duodenal abnormalities are shown—or if it proves impossible to obtain good quality roentgenograms showing the duodenum—hypotonic duodenography is a logical follow-up outpatient examination. In anicteric patients, however, it seems unnecessary to employ this technique as the primary barium study as is recommended for patients with jaundice.

PANCREATIC ANGIOGRAPHY. When either (or both) ^{75}Se selenomethionine pancreatic imaging or upper gastrointestinal barium examination suggests the possibility of pancreatic disorder, pancreatic angiography can be utilized for further information. In most cases, pancreatic malignancy can be detected by this technique and, while angiography is less successful in demonstrating chronic pancreatitis, inflammatory disease can also be shown in many instances. In addition to establishing or confirming the presence of pancreatic disease, angiographic examination is a valuable predictor of operability. Splenic or portal venous involvement by tumor is generally considered to preclude the possibility of operative resection and, of course, demonstration of hepatic metastases indicates the futility of operation for cure. Conversely, in the case of chronic pancreatitis, angiographic findings such as pseudoaneurysm or splenic venous occlusion may indicate the need for operation in patients for whom surgery would not otherwise have been considered.

PERORAL PANCREATOGRAPHY. This technique may reveal evidence of chronic pancreatitis (and rarely of neoplasm) where all other radiographic techniques are unavailing. As the procedure becomes more widely available, its use in patients falling into this diagnostic category (and especially where radioisotopic pancreatic imaging is positive) seems likely to become widespread.

THE PATIENT IN WHOM JAUNDICE WHICH MAY BE DUE TO EXTRAHEPATIC BILIARY OBSTRUCTION IS THE DOMINANT CLINICAL FEATURE

This category excludes patients with obvious acute hepatitis, well-established cirrhosis, and other straightforward cases of hepatocellular disease. There remain a considerable number of icteric patients in whom the mechanism of jaundice is uncertain. In such individuals, pancreaticoduodenal carcinoma, choledocholithiasis, and the various forms of intrahepatic cholestasis (e.g., "cholangiolytic" hepatitis, drug-induced cholestasis [such as that produced by anabolic steroids or phenothiazine derivatives], primary biliary cirrhosis, etc.) are usually the chief diagnostic possibilities. The clinical problem is simple: is the patient likely to benefit from surgery?

The radiologic approach to patients of this sort has been discussed in detail in Chapter 5, The Radiology of Jaundice. Our recommendations will be reiterated here, but more extensive coverage can be found beginning on page 169.

The radionuclide "liver profile." Radioisotopic examinations with both ^{131}I rose bengal and colloidal agents such as ^{99m}Tc sulfur colloid are of value in jaundiced patients. The latter is best suited for detection of hepatic metastasis or of hepatocellular disease. In many instances, dilated biliary radicals at the porta hepatis can also be shown when jaundice results from extrahepatic biliary obstruction. Examination with radioiodinated rose bengal provides data more directly pertinent to distinction between hepatocellular and "surgical" obstructive jaundice. When there is excretion of radioactivity into the gut by the liver, obstructive disease can be excluded with over 90 per cent reliability. If no such excretion occurs, interpretation depends on the results of blood clearance testing. If there is more than 90 per cent retention of radioactivity at 20 minutes, hepatocellular disease can be accurately predicted, while if retention is less than 70 per cent, extrahepatic obstruction is overwhelmingly most likely. However, the authors feel that if blood retention of radioactivity is between 70 and 90 per cent in a patient in whom no intestinal radioactivity can be detected even on delayed (24-hour) abdominal scintigrams, no diagnostic inference is warranted and further diagnostic study is indicated.

Hypotonic duodenography. If desired, hypotonic duodenography can be performed immediately after the 24-hour rose bengal abdominal scintigram has been made. Barium should not be given before the radioisotopic studies are completed, however, because false-positive liver scans can be created by barium in the colon.

As has been exhaustively described in other portions of this monograph, hypotonic duodenography is highly accurate for detection of pancreaticoduodenal malignancy and can frequently demonstrate the effects of biliary calculi when they are impacted in the distal common duct. The authors feel it is much more sensible to employ this procedure rather than a conventional upper gastrointestinal barium examination when jaundice is the chief reason for radiologic study.

Pancreatic angiography. If outpatient radiologic examinations have failed to establish the nature of a patient's jaundice or if pancreaticoduodenal cancer has been demonstrated but further information regarding the extent of disease and the possibility of resection for cure is desired, pancreatic angiography is the next logical examination. The study should be scheduled at a time when barium will have been cleared from the intestine—ideally on the first full hospital day. Angiographic examination can occasionally demonstrate malignancies located in positions where they produce biliary obstruction without affecting the duodenum. More often, however, angiography will make its chief contribution to patients in this category by alerting the surgeon contemplating operation to the degree of major vascular involvement with which he must be prepared to deal. Angiographic demonstration of gallbladder size usually enables the surgeon to judge preoperatively whether or not a simple cholecystojejunostomy by-pass procedure is feasible. In uncommon instances, demonstration of gallbladder enlargement may provide the only preoperative confirmation that extrahepatic biliary obstruction is, in fact, present.

Peroral cholangiopancreatography. If radiologic procedures have so far been unrevealing and a physician skilled in the performance of peroral ampullary cannulation is available, it would be logical to employ this technique at this point in the work-up. When successful opacification of the biliary tree can be achieved, common-duct calculi located high in the common bile duct, small cholangiocarcinomas, biliary strictures, and conditions such as sclerosing cholangitis may be demonstrated. All of these conditions can easily escape detection by the radiologic techniques previously employed (except for the ^{131}I rose bengal examination), but they are readily appreciated on technically adequate cholangiograms.

Transhepatic cholangiography. At this writing, peroral cholangiopancreatography is being attempted at only a few centers in the United States and the percentage of successful studies is still generally low. In most cases, therefore, when preoperative opacification of the biliary tree is required for diagnosis or in order to allow adequate surgical planning, transhepatic cholangiography will be necessary. The incidence of complications resulting from this examination has been reduced to an acceptably low level by recent technical innovations (see Chapter 5) and the study has been endorsed by numerous texts of gastroenterology, hepatology, surgery, and radiology. Nonetheless, transhepatic cholangiography continues to be woefully underutilized in this country. The same forms of extrahepatic biliary obstruction described in relation to peroral cholangiopancreatography can be identified by transhepatic cholangiography and, in addition, normal biliary radicals can sometimes be shown (in up to 50 per cent of the instances where they are present). It therefore seems eminently logical to employ this procedure when the mechanism of jaundice has remained obscure despite careful radiologic evaluation or when further information concerning the exact level of obstruction seems desirable. If angiography has been performed on the first full hospital day, transhepatic cholangiography (or an alternative technique such as transjugular cholangiography or the "minilaparotomy" approach) can be scheduled for the morning of the second hospital day. The authors feel that time in the operating room should be available later the same morning. If obstruction is demonstrated or if no ductal opacification is achieved, surgery can proceed without delay. If normal ducts are shown, then surgery can be deferred.

THE PATIENT WITH ACUTE ABDOMINAL DISCOMFORT IN WHOM ACUTE PANCREATITIS IS CONSIDERED A POSSIBILITY

Along with those patients who actually have acute pancreatitis, this category will include a large number of individuals who suffer from nonpancreatic disease (e.g., acute appendicitis, perforated peptic ulcer, acute cholecystitis, etc.). Even if the group were restricted to those patients with elevated serum amylase levels, a certain number of extrapancreatic problems would still be included (while some cases of pancreatitis would be missed.) For this reason, most of the radiologic studies advocated are generalized and broadly applicable to nearly all patients with acute abdominal disorders.

Most patients in this category are sufficiently ill that outpatient examination is impractical. Accordingly no separation of outpatient and inpatient studies is suggested. Rather, emphasis is placed on a logical progression of examinations which can be performed promptly and with a minimum of patient manipulation.

PLAIN ROENTGENOGRAPHIC EXAMINATION. For patients with acute abdominal discomfort, erect posteroanterior and lateral chest radiographs as well as supine and upright abdominal films are recommended as the initial radiologic examination. *Study of the chest* may reveal pulmonary disease producing symptoms which simulate acute pancreatitis. More often, such films will show nonspecific abnormalities such as subsegmental atelectasis, hemidiaphragmatic elevation, or pleural effusion which can accompany intraabdominal inflammation. Demonstration of pleural effusion is especially important because aspiration of a pleural fluid sample will allow determination of amylase content. This simple test can quickly and reliably establish the diagnosis of acute pancreatitis (see Chapter 2). Finally, upright chest roentgenograms are excellent for demonstrating the presence of subdiaphragmatic free air.

Supine and upright *abdominal films* may reveal any number of abnormalities bearing on the nature of a patient's acute abdominal discomfort. The most specific signs indicting the pancreas are pancreatic calcification, a pancreatic gas collection, and intraabdominal fat necrosis. Duodenal ileus is another very helpful sign, while a nonspecific sentinel loop, the "colon cut-off" sign, and the "gasless abdomen" also tend to focus attention on the pancreas.

INTRAVENOUS CHOLANGIOGRAPHY. The distinction between acute cholecystitis and acute pancreatitis often poses a difficult problem. In situations of this sort, emergency intravenous cholangiography is recommended. As discussed in Chapter 3, the diagnosis of acute cholecystitis can be established or excluded in approximately 60 per cent of cases where the study is employed for this purpose.

ABDOMINAL ULTRASONOGRAPHY. Although it is not yet widely available (especially on an emergency basis), echographic examination offers a potentially quick and reliable means of establishing the diagnosis of acute pancreatitis. The edematous, inflamed organ can be identified as an arc-shaped transonic zone in the location of the pancreas, whereas the normal pancreas cannot be demonstrated (see Chapter 9). The study could be done before, during, after, or in place of intravenous cholangiography. It should precede any barium examination, however, since barium interferes with normal ultrasonic transmission. When echography becomes generally available, it seems likely that its use for this purpose will become widespread.

UPPER GASTROINTESTINAL BARIUM EXAMINATION. As noted in the previous chapter (page 362), barium studies can establish the diagnosis of acute pancreatitis in over 70 per cent of cases in which the technique is employed. In addition, of course, gastric or duodenal ulceration can be demonstrated. In some circumstances (e.g., where "walled-off" perforation has developed), these conditions can mimic the clinical picture of acute pancreatitis even though no free intraperitoneal air is present on plain film examinations. In those uncommon instances where intrapancreatic gas is suspected on the basis of plain abdominal films, barium study can confirm localization of gas within the pancreas.

For most patients suspected of having acute pancreatitis, it is appropriate that upper gastrointestinal barium examination be employed at this point in the work-up protocol, but there may be cases where angiography should be used instead. Patients with mesenteric vascular accidents may have acute abdominal pain, physical findings similar to those of pancreatitis, and massive hyperamylasemia. In cases where both mesenteric infarction and acute pancreatitis are considered likely, aortography should certainly precede barium examination.

THE PATIENT WITH SEVERE ACID-PEPTIC DISEASE IN WHOM ZOLLINGER-ELLISON SYNDROME IS CONSIDERED A POSSIBILITY

GASTROINTESTINAL BARIUM EXAMINATION. In most instances where Zollinger-Ellison syndrome is considered a possibility, the patient will already have had one or more upper gastrointestinal barium examinations. The presence or absence of characteristic radiographic findings can usually be determined from these alone, but occasionally an additional barium study—perhaps including special examination of the small bowel—may be desirable. In either event, this phase of the work-up can be conducted on an outpatient basis.

ANGIOGRAPHIC EXAMINATION OF THE PANCREAS AND LIVER. Arteriographic study can often identify the islet cell tumor(s) of Zollinger-Ellison syndrome (see Chapter 7) and, in those cases where the lesion is malignant, can frequently demonstrate the presence of hepatic metastasis. Where questions remain after clinical investigation and conventional barium meal examination, angiography may "clinch" the diagnosis. Even in those cases where the presence of the syndrome has been established (e.g., by immunoassay or bioassay techniques), it seems reasonable to proceed with arteriography so that a detailed preoperative assessment of the case can be made. In some situations (e.g., when only a single tumor is shown and no evidence of hepatic metastasis is present), it may be desirable to attempt tumor resection in addition to (or even in place of) total gastrectomy.

THE PATIENT WITH CLINICAL AND BIOCHEMICAL FINDINGS WHICH SUGGEST HYPERINSULINISM

Pancreatic angiography. The accuracy of techniques such as the tolbutamide test and the serum insulin assay is now so great that the presence of hyperinsulinism can be established beyond doubt in the overwhelming majority of patients with this condition. Nevertheless, preoperative arteriography is considered mandatory for proper evaluation of these individuals since the underlying pancreatic tumor may easily be missed at surgical exploration. This is due to difficulty in palpating the pancreas, to the small size of most islet cell adenomas, and to the tactile similarity between small adenomas and lobules of normal pancreatic tissue. Extrapancreatic retroperitoneal tumors (e.g., leiomyosarcomata) may also produce hyperinsulinism so that an aortogram (and indicated selective injections) should be obtained in all cases where pancreatic angiography itself is unrevealing. Nonangiographic radiologic studies have not been shown to be of value in patients with pancreatic insulinomas.

THE PATIENT WHOSE CONVENTIONAL UPPER GASTROINTESTINAL BARIUM EXAMINATION SUGGESTS PRIMARY DUODENAL DISEASE

Patients ultimately found to have primary duodenal disorders (other than bulbar ulceration) usually have clinical and laboratory findings of such a nonspecific nature that the possibility is first raised by upper gastrointestinal barium examination requested in anticipation of demonstrating more common forms of abnormality such as acid-peptic disease, gastric neoplasia, or the like. In such circumstances, the initial barium study may or may not adequately demonstrate the radiographic findings. The choice between alternative follow-up procedures depends largely on the quality of the initial barium meal examination.

Hypotonic duodenography. In most instances of this sort, the initial demonstration leaves something to be desired and, in these cases, hypotonic duodenography should be employed next. This technique can eliminate nonlesions produced by the effects of spasm, normal peristaltic activity, incomplete filling, or other circumstances. Multiple views from different projections—with or without air contrast delineation, and without interference by peristaltic activity or barium in overlying stomach or mesenteric intestine—will nearly always confirm or exclude the presence of a lesion. In most instances, a reasonable formulation of differential diagnostic possibilities can also be made.

Fiberoptic duodenoscopy. When the initial barium examination convincingly demonstrates a duodenal lesion or after the presence of a questionable abnormality has been confirmed by hypotonic duodenography, it is often desirable to visualize (and even biopsy) the pathologic process endoscopically. This is especially true when the patient involved is not a good candidate for surgical exploration or when, despite optimal radiographic study, it is still impossible to tell with certainty whether or not a lesion is actually present (e.g., when a possible pathologic mass may represent merely a large, prominent, but otherwise normal duodenal papilla).

In the hands of experienced endoscopists, fiberoptic duodenal visualization can be successfully accomplished in a very high percentage of cases in which it is attempted (see Chapter 8). The authors feel that patients with primary duodenal abnormalities constitute ideal prospective beneficiaries of this new diagnostic modality.

INDEX

Page numbers in *italics* refer to illustrations.